WITHDRAWN

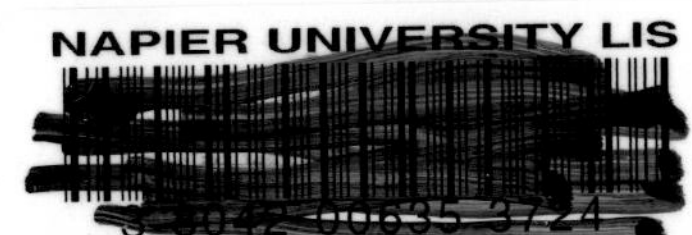
NAPIER UNIVERSITY LIS

Nursing Care of the PEDIATRIC TRAUMA PATIENT

Nursing Care of the PEDIATRIC TRAUMA PATIENT

Patricia A. Moloney-Harmon, RN, MS, CCNS, CCRN, FAAN
Advanced Practice Nurse/Clinical Nurse Specialist
The Children's Hospital at Sinai
Baltimore, Maryland

Sandra J. Czerwinski, RN, MS, CCRN
Nursing Administrative Director
All Children's Hospital
St. Petersburg, Florida

SAUNDERS
An Imprint of Elsevier Science

SAUNDERS
An Imprint of Elsevier Science

11830 Westline Industrial Drive
St. Louis, Missouri 63146

NURSING CARE OF THE PEDIATRIC TRAUMA PATIENT 0-7216-7372-4

NOTICE

Nursing is an ever-changing field. Standard safety precautions must be followed, but as new research and clinical experience broaden our knowledge, changes in treatment and drug therapy may become necessary or appropriate. Readers are advised to check the most current product information provided by the manufacturer of each drug to be administered to verify the recommended dose, the method and duration of administration, and contraindications. It is the responsibility of the licensed health care provider, relying on experience and knowledge of the patient, to determine dosages and the best treatment for each individual patient. Neither the publisher nor the editor assumes any liability for any injury and/or damage to persons or property arising from this publication.

Library of Congress Cataloging in Publication Data

Nursing care of the pediatric trauma patient/[edited by] Patricia A. Moloney-Harmon, Sandra J. Czerwinski.
p.; cm.
Includes bibliographical references and index.
ISBN 0-7216-7372-4
1. Children—Wounds and injuries—Nursing. 2. Pediatric nursing. I. Moloney-Harmon, Pat. II. Czerwinski, Sandra J.
[DNLM: 1. Pediatric Nursing—methods. 2. Wounds and Injuries—nursing—Child. WY 159 N97393 2003]
RD93.5.C4 N876 2003
610.73'62—dc21

2002036461

Vice President and Publishing Director, Nursing: Sally Schrefer
Acquisitions Editor: Susan R. Epstein
Senior Developmental Editor: Maria Broeker
Publishing Services Manager: John Rogers
Designer: Kathi Gosche
Cover Art: Jennifer Brockett

KI / MVY

Printed in the United States of America

Last digit is the print number: 9 8 7 6 5 4 3 2 1

DEDICATION

To my husband, Tom,
who helps make all of these projects happen;
to my dear friend, Karen,
who taught me many lessons, including how to live a life full of joy,
and
to my family and friends,
who are always there for me.
PMH

To my husband, John,
my family and friends,
who encourage and support me
in everything I do.
SJC

Contributors

Teresa Beck, RN, BSN, CRRN, MEd
Clinical Rehabilitation Specialist
Children's Seashore House
of the Children's Hospital of Philadelphia
Philadelphia, Pennsylvania

Debbie Brinker, RN, MS, CCNS, CCRN
Clinical Nurse Specialist, PICU
Deaconess Medical Center
Spokane, Washington

S. Louise Bowen, RNC, ARNP, MSN
Director of Pediatric/Neonatal Transport Team
All Children's Hospital
St. Petersburg, Florida

Franco A. Carnevale, RN, PhD
Head Nurse, Pediatric Intensive Care Unit
Montreal Children's Hospital
Associate Professor, McGill University
Montreal, Quebec, Canada

Michael W. Day, RN, MSN, CCRN
Outreach Educator/Clinical Nurse Specialist
Northwest MedStar
Spokane, Washington

Rosemary Eikov, RN, MSN, CRNP
Care Coordinator
Primary Care Center
The Children's Hospital of Philadelphia
Philadelphia, Pennsylvania

Emily Frosch, MD
Assistant Professor
Johns Hopkins University
School of Medicine
Baltimore, Maryland

Rita Giordano, ARNP, MSN
Clinical Nurse Specialist
Acute Pain Service
Sarasota Memorial Hospital
Sarasota, Florida

Naomi Higuchi, RN, MSN, CRNP, CS
Nurse Practitioner, Department of Radiology
The Children's Hospital of Philadelphia
Philadelphia, Pennsylvania

Mary C. Hoffman, MSN, RN
Administrative Director
All Children's Hospital
St. Petersburg, Florida

Susan Nudelman Kamerling, RN, MSN, CCRN
Trauma Clinical Nurse Specialist
The Children's Hospital of Philadelphia
Philadelphia, Pennsylvania

Ruth M. Lebet, RN, MSN, CRNP, CEN
Education Nurse Specialist
The Children's Hospital of Philadelphia
Philadelphia, Pennsylvania

Linda A. Lewandowski, PhD, RN
Associate Professor
Johns Hopkins University
School of Nursing
Baltimore, Maryland

Monica Artiles Liebman, RN, MSN, PHRN
Clinical Nurse Specialist
Trauma Program
The Children's Hospital of Philadelphia
Philadelphia, Pennsylvania

Denise Poirer Maguire, RN, PhD
Director, Nursing Education and Research
All Children's Hospital
St. Petersburg, Florida

Kimberly J. Mason, RN, MSN
Director, Patient Care Systems and Standards
The Children's Hospital of Philadelphia
Philadelphia, Pennsylvania

Regina Muir, RN, MS, CEN
Nurse Practitioner, Newborn Nursery
Parkland Memorial Hospital
Dallas, Texas

Carolyn M. Perry, RN, CS, MS
Infection Control Clinical Nurse Specialist
All Children's Hospital
St. Petersburg, Florida

Bonnie A. Rice, ARNP, MSN, CCRN, CCNS
Clinical Nurse Specialist, Surgical ICU
All Children's Hospital
St. Petersburg, Florida

Lisa A. Rupp, RN, CCRN, EMT
Pediatric/Perinatal Flight Nurse
Northwest MedStar
Spokane, Washington

Shari Simone, RN, MS, CRNP, FCCM, CCRN
Pediatric Critical Care Nurse Practitioner
Pediatric Intensive Care Unit
University of Maryland Medical System
Baltimore, Maryland

Jennifer Thorpe, MBA, RD, CSP
Clinical Dietitian
The Children's Hospital of Philadelphia
Home Care Department
Philadelphia, Pennsylvania

Paula M. Timoney, RNC, MN, ARNP
Director of Advanced Practice Nursing
All Children's Hospital
St. Petersburg, Florida

Deborah A. Town, RN, ADN, CCRN
Clinical Research Coordinator, Critical Care Services
Children's Medical Center of Dallas
Dallas, Texas

Tara Trimarchi, MSN, RN, CRNP
Nurse Practitioner
Pediatric Intensive Care Unit
The Children's Hospital of Philadelphia
Lecturer
The University of Pennsylvania, School of Nursing
Philadelphia, Pennsylvania

Judy Trivits Verger, RN, MSN, CRNP, CCRN
Pediatric Critical Care Nurse Practitioner
The Children's Hospital of Philadelphia, PICU
Philadelphia, Pennsylvania

Paula Vernon-Levett, RN, MSN, CCRN
Staff Nurse II
University of Iowa Hospitals and Clinics
Iowa City, Iowa

Sally Jo Zuspan, RN, MSN
Trauma Consultant
Salt Lake City, Utah

Reviewers

Cynthia J. Abel, RN, MSN, CEN
Trauma Nurse Specialist
Rush-Copley Medical Center
Aurora, Illinois

Lisa Marie Bernardo, RN, PhD, MPH
Associate Professor
University of Pittsburgh School of Nursing
Pittsburgh, Pennsylvania

Kathleen D. Shinners, BSN, MEd
Nursing Education Associate
Dartmouth-Hitchcock Medical Center
Lebanon, New Hampshire

PREFACE

Pediatric trauma nursing has evolved tremendously over the last several decades. The complexity of caring for this special patient population mandates that nurses have specialized knowledge and skill. *Nursing Care of the Pediatric Trauma Patient* is a state-of-the-art text, written to provide a comprehensive reference for nurses caring for critically injured infants and children. The foundation for this book is the clinical expertise of the contributors. They are able to provide expert knowledge with a strong nursing focus.

Nursing Care of the Pediatric Trauma Patient is divided into four sections that cover all aspects of pediatric trauma nursing.

Section I: The Scope of Pediatric Trauma provides a foundation for the practice of pediatric trauma nursing. There is a discussion of the evolution of pediatric trauma care along with injury prevention, which is essential when examining the entire continuum of care. In addition, ethical concepts surrounding care of the critically injured child are presented.

Section II: Clinical Concepts focuses on issues that are germane to all pediatric trauma victims, regardless of the body system that is affected. Pediatric anatomic and physiologic differences are discussed, along with the effect those differences have on care. Mechanism of injury, initial resuscitation, transport, and rehabilitation ensure that issues across the continuum are addressed. Violence and its effect on the child and family are presented. Discussion of the impact of injury on child development and families guides the nurse in providing interventions that create a humanistic environment. Pain management and nutrition support also ensure that the child's needs are met in the most comprehensive and caring manner.

Section III: System Injuries addresses state-of-the-art nursing care for injuries within each body system. The etiology, pathophysiology, and evidence-based collaborative management are presented in a comprehensive manner. The information provides the nurse with the information to balance the art and science of care.

Section IV: Multisystem Issues addresses the needs of children experiencing multisystem injury. The complexity of these injuries presents special challenges to the trauma team. In addition, the physical and psychologic sequelae of traumatic injury are discussed, providing the nurse with evidence-based interventions.

Caring for the pediatric trauma victim presents challenges, which require evidence-based nursing practice. Our goal in writing this text will be met if readers gain the knowledge that they need to provide excellent care to critically injured children and families.

Patricia A. Moloney-Harmon
Sandra J. Czerwinski

Contents

SECTION I

THE SCOPE OF PEDIATRIC TRAUMA

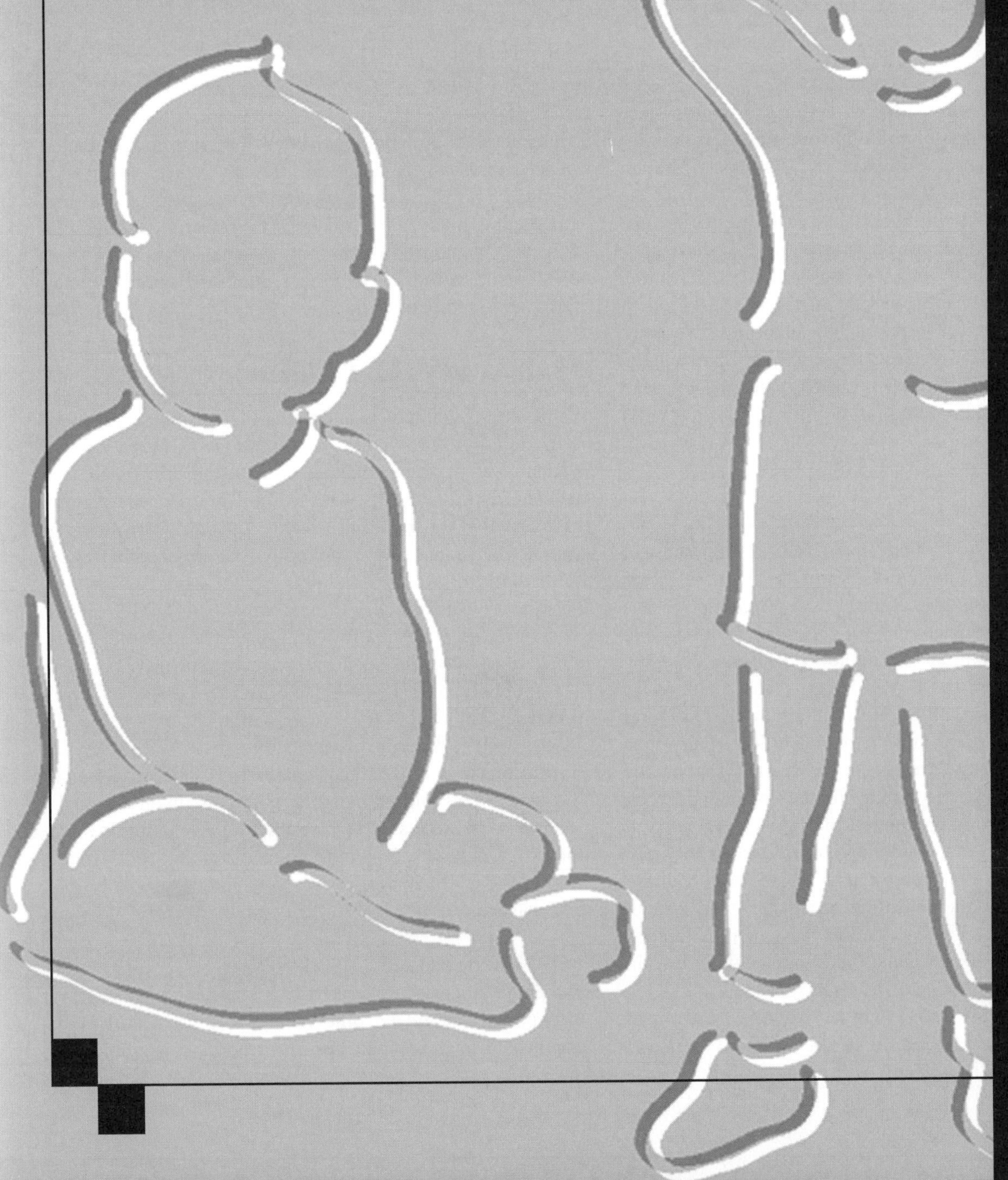

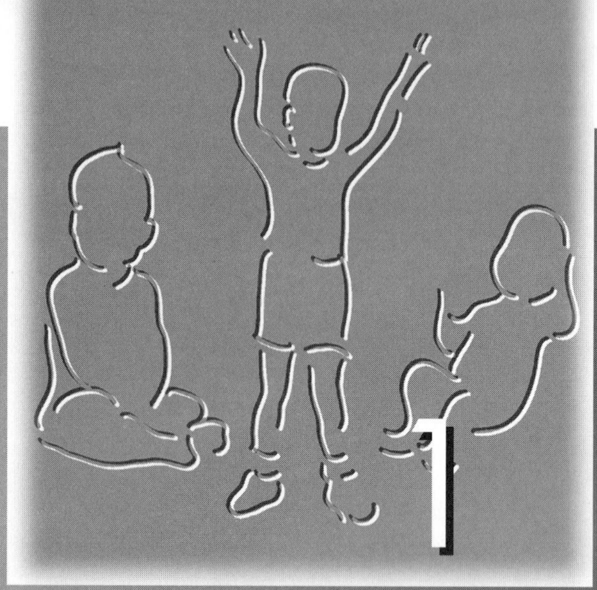

Pediatric Trauma: An Evolving Specialty

Mary C. Hoffman

Nursing leaders in pediatric trauma programs face numerous challenges and opportunities to accommodate change with new processes and systems. Although trauma programs range from pediatric to adult, many of the economic, legal, and political obstacles encountered are similar. Effective cost containment in the managed care environment continues to threaten the viability of trauma programs across the nation, forcing managers and leaders to be on the cutting edge with resourceful and innovative ideas. Changing the delivery of trauma care to a more systematic approach, along with improved triage assessments, can lead to decreased morbidity and mortality for pediatric trauma patients.

HISTORY

Trauma, a Greek word for body injury, is the leading cause of death in children and adults younger than 44 years (Emergency Nurses Association, 1995). According to the American Trauma Society (1999), 100,000 individuals will die and another 8 million to 9 million will sustain disabling injuries each year in the United States. Trauma care as we know it today began with the U.S. military in the 1950s and 1960s during the Korean and Vietnam conflicts. Helicopters were used to expedite treatment for injured soldiers by bringing emergency care rapidly to the soldier and then promptly transporting the injured to Mobile Army Surgery Hospital (MASH) units, bypassing the battlefield front lines. This acceleration of care resulted in fewer casualties. Military physicians brought their wartime experiences and knowledge home to the civilian world after recognizing that accident victims were not receiving the same lifesaving care in the private nonmilitary sector (ACSCOT, 1999).

In a report published in 1966 by the National Academy of Sciences, trauma became known as "the neglected disease of modern society." The account was a cry for help to the American people. The plea was to develop a national committee focused on reducing the devastation from trauma on society. In 1968 the American Trauma Society (ATS) was founded, consisting of physicians, nurses, paramedics, and emergency medical technicians to research, teach, and enhance neighborhood trauma services. With more than 2700 members today, ATS receives funding by grants, donations, and membership dues.

TRAUMA SYSTEMS DEFINED

Until recently, all efforts and energies for trauma care concentrated on improving the care of severely injured trauma patients seeking care at a single institution designated as a *trauma center.* Patients with minor injuries were often discounted. This approach became known as the *exclusive trauma center,* negating trauma care provided at other institutions. In this system only 60% of all trauma victims survived until reaching the trauma center (ACSCOT, 1999). These preclusive trauma programs have recently undergone a metamorphosis from exclusive centers to inclusive systems. They are fully integrated with all health care providers, from prehospital to posthospital rehabilitation centers (ACSCOT, 1999). Today's trauma programs are networks of several institutions with different designated levels of care to match the needs of all injured patients. They contain all the medical resources necessary to care for trauma victims despite the extent of injury or geographic location. Further expansion of today's inclusive system, to include pediatric hospitals, will achieve the highest quality outcomes for children.

Formal Systems

The development of trauma systems is based on the concept that optimal care and outcomes for injured patients, from onset of injury through rehabilitation and return of ideal functioning, can be achieved when essential components of treatment are integrated into an organized system (Mullins & Mann, 1999). The opportunity to improve health care outcomes for the severely injured is greatly enhanced by organizing community health resources into trauma systems, at the local, regional, or state levels. These systems must be designed appropriately and administered within the legal authority to establish and enforce policy. A data system that facilitates the evaluation of system effectiveness is also essential (Bazzoli, 1999).

The American College of Surgeons (ACS) has recommended key criteria for trauma system development. These criteria have been used as the basis of several studies. Briefly, the criteria address issues related to (1) authority, (2) process, (3) ACS standards, (4) use of out of area surveyors, (5) use of preestablished triage protocols, (6) monitoring of performance, and (7) statewide coverage (Bazzoli, Meersman, & Chan, 1996; Bass, Gainer, & Carlini, 1999).

Within a system, the various resources are typically identified by level of intensity of needed resources. Experience has shown that as severity and volume increase, more human and financial resources are required to provide optimal outcomes. Many different guidelines are used for developing trauma programs and identifying the various levels within the program or system. Three are nationally recognized and used throughout the United States by institutions and states for accreditation of trauma programs.

The American College of Surgeons Committee on Trauma (ACSCOT) developed the most widely recognized criteria for trauma center designations. In 1976 they published the first set of criteria necessary for a three-tiered trauma program. Initially, the tiers were identified as optimal, intermediate, and minimal levels. These tiers later matured into what is now known as level I, level II, and level III centers. In 1999 ACSCOT expanded and revised their criteria to include a level IV, promoting a network-linked statewide system that includes rural communities. The U.S. Department of Health and Human Services, Public Health Services also provides a foundation for system evolution that some facilities use when preparing for designation. In 1988 The American College of Emergency Physicians created guidelines for trauma care systems similar to those created by ACSCOT. Many facilities use this set of criteria, which affords more comprehensive guidelines for prehospital elements for their program.

State Systems

Some individual states have developed their own criteria, many of which are more stringent than those set forth by ACSCOT. Maryland, Florida, and Illinois were among the first to develop regionalized emergency services programs that include trauma. These programs were made possible through grants provided by the National Highway Safety Act of 1966. They have expanded to include 24 states with statewide-organized trauma systems and 19 with current funding dedicated to trauma (Bass et al., 1999).

Pediatric Trauma Centers

The Emergency Nurses Association cites trauma as the leading cause of death in children younger than 4 years. According to Hulka (1999), approximately one fourth of all trauma patients are children. Pediatric trauma patients present many unique challenges to emergency physicians, nurses, trauma surgeons, and other health care team members. They have individual needs and specific principles that must be identified early in prehospital care and that must extend to immediate stabilization and beyond.

The special needs of the injured pediatric patient may be ideally met by a children's hospital that has an established commitment to trauma care. Although many outstanding children's hospitals are located throughout the country, many of these do not have the personnel and resources necessary to provide comprehensive care to the pediatric trauma patient. Our current reality is that, because of the limited number and geographic distribution of children's hospitals, all injured pediatric patients cannot be cared for in these specialized hospitals. Other facilities must be available to provide this resource to the community and system of trauma care (ACSCOT, 1999).

Children's hospitals may take a leadership role in the care of the injured child. Children's hospitals that are trauma centers must interact effectively with all hospitals providing care for severely and minimally injured children. These institutions must establish working relationships with other centers that provide pediatric care (ACSCOT, 1999). There is no one "ideal" center for care of the injured child. The most important component of such a facility is a staff of multidisciplinary specialists who are committed to the care of injured children. In addition to providing state-of-the-art care, these specialized pediatric centers must provide leadership and direction for the entire region they serve (Arensman, Statter, Ledbetter, & Vargish, 1995).

Only 20 states have designated pediatric trauma centers (Hulka, 1999). Trauma centers with a pediatric commitment provide superior service to infants and children. Some states, such as Florida, are trying new unique ideas for the delivery of trauma care to children. According to Florida State Approval Standards, a state-approved pediatric trauma referral center (SAPTRC) may be located in a level I center, a level II center, or a pediatric hospital. A joint effort in St. Petersburg, Florida, capitalizes on the unique strengths of two well-established institutions. A joint SAPTRC designation was granted to the tertiary children's hospital and the adjoining level II adult hospital so that they could become one trauma referral center for children. This unique, formal arrangement is being looked to for future trauma development within Florida because it may represent a model that better meets the needs of injured children.

ECONOMICS

From any perspective, trauma is expensive. Unintentional injury is estimated by The National Safety Council to cost $120 billion per year (Harris, Bass, & O'Brien, 1996). Acute medical care for intentional and unintentional traumatic injuries is estimated to cost the United States in excess of $16 billion per year (Elliott & Rodriguez, 1996). According to

Harris et al. (1996), 7% of all U.S. health care expenditures is attributable to trauma. That represents 2.3% of the gross national product. Individual states spent more than $161.6 million on Emergency Medical System (EMS) and trauma in fiscal year 1996 (Goodspeed, 1997).

Death and disability resulting from injuries cost the United States even more than money paid out for patient care. According to Elliott and Rodriguez (1996), annual costs resulting from deaths, disability, lost wages and taxes, and acute medical care secondary to trauma in this country have been estimated to exceed $150 billion. Of the 57 million Americans injured every year, more than 2 million are hospitalized and more than 150,000 die.

Mortality statistics alone do not tell the whole story. Trauma does not always kill. Trauma often disables, disfigures, or otherwise permanently affects victims by the incident (Goodspeed, 1997).

The impact of childhood injury is enormous. Of all pediatric admissions and hospital inpatients, 21% are attributable to injury. This is more than any other condition. The cost for pediatric injury not only includes hospitalization but also the economic loss to society from lost work years and chronic care. In addition, death and disability striking the youngest and most vulnerable of our society carry a significant emotional toll (Harris et al., 1996). The expenses of trauma are multiple: loss of productive lives, permanent disability, pain and suffering, and the consumption of health care resources (Elliott & Rodriguez, 1996).

The financial drain created by trauma care is significant and has raised much concern. A number of urban trauma centers have closed since the late 1980s. Overwhelming financial strain was the primary reason for these closures (Sartorelli, Rogers, Osler, Shackford, Cohen, & Vane, 1999). Currently, three factors are putting financial strain on trauma centers. First is the high cost of trauma care. The cost of care for the average acutely ill patient is more than one third less than the cost of caring for a single trauma patient. The intensity, diversity, and duration of resources needed to provide optimal recovery and a return to normal functioning for the trauma patient all contribute to these costs (Rogers, Osler, Shackford, Cohen, & Camp, 1997).

The second factor is the high percentage of trauma patients who are uninsured. Within the trauma patient population, a disproportionate amount of indigent care exists. This is particularly true in urban settings. It was estimated in 1990 that 30% of trauma patients in the United States were uninsured. This represents $8.3 billion in nonreimbursed care. Because children are one of the largest groups of Americans affected by poverty, they often have inadequate health care coverage (Sartorelli et al., 1999).

The third factor contributing to the financial strain of trauma is the declining levels of reimbursement under Medicaid, Medicare, and other third-party payers. Reimbursement for trauma care has been and continues to be a problem. As injury severity increases, costs and charges increase. Reimbursement, however, has not keep pace with these increased charges. Typically, reimbursement from diagnosis-related groups (DRGs), per diem, capitation, and self-pay arrangements do not cover the true costs of caring for patients (Sartorelli et al., 1999). An estimated loss of $25,000 for each patient with an injury severity score of greater than 15 was the average finding in a Rutledge study done in 1996 (Rutledge, Shaffer, & Ridky, 1996). Not only is reimbursement generally lower for trauma, it is also slower. The resulting costs associated with carrying these debts further decreases reimbursement (Harris et al., 1996).

Declining health care reimbursement in the 1990s, along with erosion in funding from public programs, may forecast a new wave of trauma center closures as hospitals seek to eliminate unprofitable services (Bazzoli et al., 1996; Mullins, 1999). It is imperative that solutions be identified so that the intensive level of care that trauma systems demand can be provided in a manner that is both clinically effective and cost efficient (O'Keefe, Jurkovich, & Maier, 1999).

POLITICAL ISSUES

The development of a trauma system is very complex and fraught with a variety of obstacles. The political issues and intricacies are formidable. There are a diverse groups of stakeholders who are affected by any decision made about the structure and operation of the trauma system (Bazzoli, 1999; Bazzoli et al., 1996).

According to Mullins (1999), "Trauma systems should be perceived as a public health care experiment." The past 30 years of trauma system development has inexorably linked trauma system implementation with public policy. Trauma systems are a prime example of "public assertion of control." Before their evolution, an individual physician had total control of patient placement. Government influence over medical care is epitomized by the designation of trauma centers networked as a trauma system (Mullins, 1999).

In essence, trauma systems are health care policies. They are intended to benefit all citizens residing in the region over which a particular policy has jurisdiction (Mullins & Mann, 1999). Trauma systems demand a level of administrative oversight that is typically provided by a designated state agency. The funding of such agency, by definition, creates a political approval process (Lowe, 1999).

Our trauma systems exist today in great part because of the political process. Congress enacted the National Highway Safety Act in 1966 and gave the Department of Transportation (DOT) the authority, money, and direction to carry out the law. In 1990 Congress specifically allocated federal funding to support publicly administered trauma systems. The Trauma Care Systems and Development Act was intended to provide health care planning support by developing a Model Trauma Systems plan (Mullins, 1999). In 1996 Congress rescinded all funding for trauma as part of the deficit reduction plan (Goodspeed, 1997).

Funding trauma systems is also a politically contentious issue in many states. Most of the states do not address trauma system funding specifically. Trauma system funding is handled by most states within the EMS budget. Typically, the EMS budget fails to fund trauma initiatives. EMS, in turn, usually represents a combination of federal grant monies and state general funds. The federal monies are generally derived from the Department of Transportation, Preventive Health and Human Services Block Grants, the National Highway Traffic Safety Administration, and EMS for Children Grants (Goodspeed, 1997).

As a result of pressure imposed by the establishment of the federal Emergency Medical Services for Children program, in collaboration with the Emergency Medical Services Division of the National Highway Traffic Safety Administration, all but a few states and territories have now embarked upon comprehensive programs of education and training in the early care of injured children (Cooper, 1999).

The future success of trauma care systems depends on the successful collaboration of all relevant stakeholders, medical specialties, and related resources at the local state and national levels. Both public and private partnerships are necessary. The unrestricted access of injured patients to trauma care, without regard to means of payment and the needs of the trauma care system, must be supported by legislation at the national and state levels. This legislation must include ongoing funding for infrastructure, research, and evaluation of outcomes (American College of Emergency Physicians Board of Directors, 1999).

COMPONENTS OF TRAUMA SYSTEMS

A system is composed of a collection of interrelated, interdependent, and corresponding subsystems. The sum total is greater than the individual part. A trauma system is composed of the following key components: prevention, access, hospitals, triage, rehabilitation, and research.

Prevention

The scope and number of injury prevention and wellness programs for children are increasing as health care workers become more proactive in promoting wellness within the community. Prevention is an extremely important part of decreasing mortality, morbidity, and costs associated with the treatment of trauma patients. This is especially meaningful for children when one considers that more than 70% of pediatric trauma deaths occur in the field (Hulka, 1999).

Trauma centers have an obligation to provide both public and professional education regardless of their designation level. Data gathered through the trauma registry should identify deficiencies in community knowledge and provide a basis for neighborhood education. Further discussion on the scope and functions of a trauma registry may be found elsewhere in this chapter. Many programs are available for the public; these programs deal with topics ranging from first aid to cardiopulmonary resuscitation (CPR). Many emergency services personnel are presenting educational programs at schools, sports events, camps, and other community affairs. To maintain market shares in today's evolving trends, trauma centers must review current practices and identify innovative concepts, along with alternative programs for providing community wide education. See Chapter 2 for a more comprehensive discussion of injury prevention strategies.

Access

Access to appropriate trauma care is crucial to the survival of pediatric trauma patients. It begins with a call to 911 for help and a prompt response. Many advanced life caregivers and prehospital providers are insecure about their ability to perform advanced pediatric skills, and many others lack the specialized pediatric equipment and experience. Trauma systems requiring that pediatric hospitals with subspecialty physicians, pediatric equipment, and trained pediatric ancillary resources be bypassed to get the injured pediatric patient to a designated trauma center located in an adult facility have been criticized. Many of these systems are beginning to recognize these problems and have fostered a new collaboration between adult and pediatric facilities to provide the best access for pediatric patients. Many pediatric facilities are working closely with EMS to provide specialized pediatric training, knowledge, and skills necessary to make the critical triage decisions in the field.

Hospitals

It is important to have hospitals within a trauma system that are designated to provide various levels of care. This allows the system to avoid duplication and squandering of valuable medical resources. A level I institution is the primary hospital, that is, a tertiary referral center. It accepts transfers from the lesser acuity regional hospitals. Criteria for level I designation includes 24-hour in-house availability of trauma surgeons, a neurosurgeon, anesthesia, and resources to provide optimal care. This institution must take the key role in education, research, and prevention.

A level II hospital has the expertise of a level I hospital, but it does not require trauma surgeons and other medical resources to be in house 24 hours a day. It allows for resources to be "on call" or available within a short notice. The level I and level II centers must work closely to coordinate care that allows patients to move through the continuum of the two facilities.

Level III trauma centers must have general surgeon coverage and should be capable of providing initial care to the trauma patient. These centers are also expected to actively participate in community prevention programs. Level IV centers are located in rural communities and subsidize the care of the trauma centers. These facilities provide the initial assessment and stabilization, and they transfer most patients to a higher-level facility where more advanced and specialized resources are available.

Pediatric tertiary care facilities are also available in some areas for initial stabilization. These facilities may have transfer agreements with several trauma centers so that they can receive the pediatric patient and provide specialized care after the immediate assessment and evaluation is complete.

Triage

Triage is the method used to sort and classify patients according to the severity and urgency of their injuries as a way of determining who is treated first. The term was derived from the French word *trier.* Triage originated in the battlefields during wars and was first initiated in emergency departments in the 1950s and 1960s, when increased volumes of nonacute patients presented to emergency departments for care. Today's hospitals depend on a reliable triage system both in the field and in the emergency department to distinguish between the emergent, urgent, and nonurgent patients.

Triage for trauma patients should begin in the field with EMS personnel using preestablished protocols. The region should have clear guidelines for determining the destination of trauma patients according to the severity of injuries and resources available in the region. Rapid on-scene triage, assessment, and transportation can mean life or death to a severely injured trauma patient. This requires advanced training and education for EMS personnel so that they can identify patients requiring prompt medical attention and dedicated medical command from physicians at the trauma centers.

Accurate assessment in the emergency department by the triage nurse is equally important in identifying patients with life-threatening conditions. The triage nurse must possess extraordinary assessment skills and the ability to intervene appropriately. It is inappropriate and dangerous to put the least experienced and weakest nurse at triage.

Rehabilitation

With modern technology and expanded knowledge, many more trauma victims are surviving today than in the past. Individuals return to society after horrendous injuries. They are expected to resume activities of daily living and function to the maximum capacity consistent with that which their injuries will allow. If these goals are to be achieved, rehabilitation programs must have a comprehensive, multidisciplinary scope.

Rehabilitation should begin the moment the patient enters the trauma center. Many trauma victims are transferred from the acute care hospital to a rehabilitation center within a few days after the accident. Successful rehabilitation programs make significantly affect trauma care in terms of outcome and cost. There are huge cost savings to be obtained when contrasted with the cost of long-term custodial care. Although surviving the hospital admission has always been the model for measuring outcomes in trauma centers, perhaps measuring function at recovery to preaccident functioning status might be a more valuable outcome for review (ACSCOT, 1999).

Research

Trauma is a domain rich in research opportunities that can enhance knowledge and improve patient outcomes. There are many avenues such as prevention, acute care therapies, clinical nursing practice, and rehabilitation for clinicians to pursue when designing research projects. Research is a requirement for trauma designation at most level I and level II centers. Institutional Review Boards (IRBs) exist in many institutions to protect the patient, to ensure scientific methods are used, and to secure the integrity of the data. Numerous grants are available from federal agencies such as the National Institutes of Health and the National Highway Safety Administration to fund research projects.

SUMMARY

Trauma care for pediatric patients requires prior preparation to ensure that systems are in place throughout the continuum to provide specialized resources and skills necessary for advanced care. Although differing guidelines and criteria exist, an integrated regional or statewide inclusive trauma system is one structure many states use to provide optimal trauma care for pediatric patients. Some states are attempting new innovative approaches for pediatric trauma programs by partnering adult and pediatric facilities in a joint trauma venture. It is evident that there is still much research needed in the pediatric trauma arena to ensure that advanced pediatric comprehensive trauma care is available.

BIBLIOGRAPHY

American College of Emergency Physicians. (1988). *Guidelines for trauma care systems.* Dallas: American College of Emergency Physician.

American College of Emergency Physicians Board of Directors. (1999). American College of Emergency Physicians policy statement: Trauma care systems development, evaluation and funding. *The Journal of Trauma: Injury, Infection and Critical Care, 47*(3), S110.

American College of Surgeons Committee on Trauma (ACSCOT). (1999). *Resources for optimal care of the injured patient.* Chicago: American College of Surgeons.

American Trauma Society. (1999). *History and structure.* Available at: www.amtrauma.org/history.html.

Arensman, R., Statter, M., Ledbetter, D., & Vargish, T. (Eds.). (1995). *Pediatric trauma: Initial care of the injured child.* New York: Raven Press.

Bass, R., Gainer, P., & Carlini, R. (1999). Update on trauma system development in the United States. *The Journal of Trauma: Injury, Infection and Critical Care, 47*(3), 15-20.

Bazzoli, G. (1999). Community-based trauma system development: Key barriers and facilitating factors. *The Journal of Trauma: Injury, Infection and Critical Care, 47*(3 Suppl.), S22-S24.

Bazzoli, G., Meersman, P., & Chan, C. (1996). Factors that enhance trauma center participation in trauma systems. *The Journal of Trauma: Injury, Infection and Critical Care, 41*(5), 876-885.

Committee on Trauma, and Committee on Shock, Division of Medical Sciences, National Academy of Sciences/National Research Council (US). (1966). *Accidental death and disability: The neglected disease of modern society.* Washington, DC: National Academy of Sciences.

Cooper, A. (1999). Toward a new millennium in pediatric trauma care. *The Journal of Trauma: Injury, Infection and Critical Care, 47*(3), S90-S91.

Doolin, E., Browne, A., & DiScala, C. (1999). Pediatric trauma center criteria: An outcomes analysis. *Journal of Pediatric Surgery, 34*(5), 886-890.

Elliott, D., & Rodriguez, A. (1996). Cost effectiveness in trauma care. *Surgical Clinics of North America, 76*(1), 47-62.

Emergency Nurses Association (ENA). (1992). *Triage: Meeting the challenge.* Parkridge, IL: ENA.

Emergency Nurses Association (ENA). (1993). *Emergency nursing pediatric course provider manual.* Parkridge, IL: ENA.

Emergency Nurses Association (ENA). (1994). *Emergency nursing core curriculum* (4th ed.). Philadelphia: WB Saunders.

Emergency Nurses Association (ENA). (1995). *TNCC trauma nursing core course provider manual.* Parkridge, IL: ENA.

Emergency Nurses Association (ENA). (1999). *Trauma coordinators resource manual.* Parkridge, IL: ENA.

Goodspeed, D. (1997). Benchmarking emergency medical services/trauma system funding in the United States. *Best Practices and Benchmarking in Health Care, 2*(2), 45-51.

Harris, B., Bass, K., & O'Brien, M. (1996). Hospital reimbursement for pediatric trauma. *Journal of Pediatric Surgery, 31*(1), 78-81.

Health Care Finance Agency. (1985). *Emergency medical treatment and active labor act.* Section 1867 of the Social Security Act.

Hulka, F. (1999). Pediatric trauma systems: Critical distinctions. *The Journal of Trauma: Injury, Infection and Critical Care, 47*(3), 86-91.

Imami, E., Cleavenger, F., Lampard, S., Kallenborn, C., & Tepas, J. (1997). Throughput analysis of trauma resuscitations with financial impact. *The Journal of Trauma, Injury, Infection and Critical Care, 42*(2), 294-298.

Jurkovich, G., & Mock, C. (1999). Systematic review of trauma system effectiveness based on registry comparisons. *The Journal of Trauma: Injury, Infection and Critical Care, 47*(3), 46-55.

Kissoon, N., Tepas, J., Peterson, R., Pieper, P., & Gayle, M. (1996). The evaluation of pediatric trauma care. *Pediatric Emergency Care, 12,* 272-276.

Lanoix, R., & Golden, J. (1999). The facilitated pediatric resuscitation room. *The Journal of Emergency Medicine, 17*(2), 363-366.

Lowe, D. (1999). Trauma system development: The critical need for regional needs assessments. *The Journal of Trauma: Injury, Infection and Critical Care, 47*(3), S106-S107.

Miller, L., RN Trauma Coordinator, Riverside Regional Medical Center. (1999). Personal Interview.

Mullins, R. (1999). A historical perspective of trauma system development in the United States. *The Journal of Trauma: Injury, Infection and Critical Care, 47*(3), S8-S14.

Mullins, R., & Mann, N. (1999). Introduction to the academic symposium to evaluate evidence regarding the efficacy of trauma systems. *The Journal of Trauma: Injury, Infection and Critical Care, 47*(3), S3-S7.

Mullins, R., Mann, C., Hedges, J., Worrall, W., & Jurkovich, G. (1998). Preferential benefit of implementation of a statewide trauma system in one of two adjacent states. *The Journal of Trauma: Injury, Infection and Critical Care, 44*(4), 609-617.

O'Keefe, G., Jurkovich, G., & Maier, R. (1999). Defining excess resource utilization and identifying associated factors for trauma victims. *The Journal of Trauma: Injury, Infection and Critical Care, 46*(3), 473-478.

Rogers, B., Osler, T., Shackford, S., Cohen, M., & Camp, L. (1997). Financial outcome of treating trauma in a rural environment. *The Journal of Trauma: Injury, Infection and Critical Care, 43*(1), 65-73.

Rutledge, R., Shaffer, V. D., & Ridky J. (1996). Trauma care reimbursement in rural hospitals: implications for triage and trauma system development. *The Journal of Trauma: Injury, Infection and Critical Care, 40*(6), 1002-1008.

Sartorelli, K., Rogers, F., Osler, T., Shackford, S., Cohen, M., & Vane, D. (1999). Financial aspects of providing care at the extremes of life. *The Journal of Trauma: Injury, Infection and Critical Care, 46*(1), 483-487.

Schweer, L., & Ose, B. (1995). Implementation of a regional pediatric trauma center. *AORN Journal, 61*(3), 558-671.

Vernon, D., Furnival, R., Hansen, W., Diller, E., Bolte, R., Johnson, D., & Dean, M. (1999). Effects of a pediatric trauma response team on emergency department treatment time and mortality of pediatric trauma victims. *Pediatrics, 103*(1), 20-24.

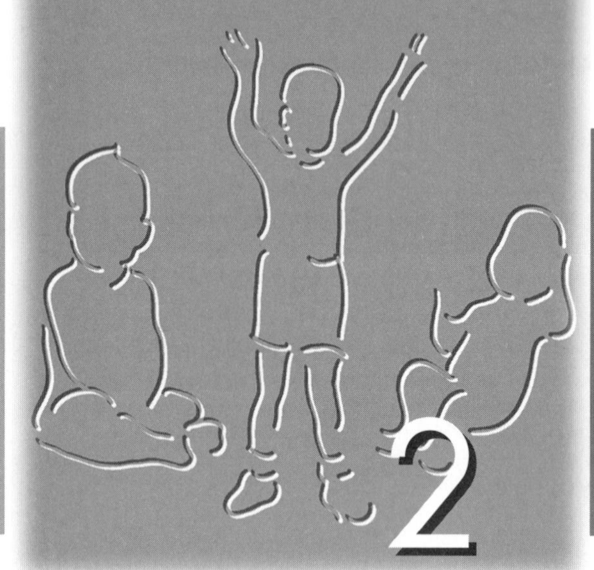

2 Pediatric Injury Prevention

Bonnie A. Rice

Injuries in children occur for a multitude of reasons, and injury prevention is a complex issue with no simple solution. Children have a natural curiosity about the environment in which they live, as well as a phenomenal energy level. Their abilities are developmentally based and individual to each child. A 3-year-old may choose to explore the world with his or her mouth, whereas the precocious 10-month-old may be walking and climbing. Parental vigilance and anticipatory guidance from health care providers play significant roles in injury prevention. They are not the only avenues to greater safety for our children, however. Incorporating safety features into product design and lobbying for legislation aimed at environmental modifications that have been shown to reduce pediatric morbidity and mortality are perhaps the most effective methods of creating a safer world for children (Haddon, 1980).

Each child is a unique individual within the context of a larger family unit. Children vary in disposition, intelligence, impulsiveness, and spatial perception (Fox, 1997). It is conceivable that certain children may be more inclined to take risks that result in injury. Consequently, if guidance offered by health care providers is to be effective, it should be highly individualized and specific.

It is difficult for a health care provider to remain nonjudgmental when treating injuries that were potentially avoidable. Poor parenting skills are often blamed when a child is injured. However, health care providers should recognize that injuries can occur within a few seconds and that most parents feel tremendous guilt regardless of their involvement with the injury.

This chapter addresses the scientific evidence related to genetic makeup and risk-taking, discusses a theoretical framework for injury analysis, and applies that framework to a common subset of pediatric admitting diagnoses. The individual injury categories will specifically direct the trauma nurse in providing appropriate advice for the prevention of injury.

ATTITUDES AND INJURY

An *accident* can be defined as an event that is unplanned or unexpected (Kauffman, 1987). Injury control experts have discouraged the use of this term because it suggests that injuries can not be predicted or prevented (Girasek, 1999). However, it is possible to predict the risk of an injury, and many investigators have looked at this issue scientifically. Coggan, Disley, and Patterson (1998) compared the injury rates of sober teenagers with rates for those who chose to drink alcohol. These researchers found that teenagers who drank alcohol demonstrated a greater risk of injury to themselves and a higher proportion of aggression directed at others than the teens who did not drink. Meropol, Moscati, Lillis, Ballow, and Janicke (1995) found that 22% of adolescents presenting to a trauma center had positive serum ethanol levels. The Centers for Disease Control and Prevention (CDC, 1997a) reports that 50% of all motor vehicle accidents involving teenagers are associated with drivers under the influence of alcohol. Providing teenagers with descriptive statistics concerning injury rates, demographics, and the risks of ethanol ingestion may influence behaviors in the future. It is beneficial to make the public aware that risk factors are being studied and analyzed and will give us more information about the risks that surround us. This information is particularly beneficial for parents raising children.

Behavioral genetics is the science of discovering if certain genes are related to types of human behavior. Gene sequences have been implicated in multiple types of pathologic behaviors, such as compulsive overeating and pathologic pleasure-seeking (Holden, 1998). Studies in animals have shown that certain rodents with a specific genetic sequence mutation are unable to nuture their young (Brown, Ye, Bronson, Dikkes, & Greenberg, 1996). There is some evidence that a particular genetic composition could also result in the development of behaviors that produce greater risk (Blumstein, 1999).

Sensation-seeking in adult men has been associated with a higher percentage of criminality and mortality (El-Sheikh, Ballard, & Cummings, 1994). Bower (1996) cites a study in which researchers hypothesized that many subjects who exhibit novelty-seeking behaviors have altered dopamine receptors. During a study involving juvenile delinquents,

Gabel, Stadler, Bjor, Shindledecker, and Bowden (1995) discovered that youths with antisocial or substance-abusing fathers had altered dopamine metabolism. These studies strongly suggest that a neurotransmitter alteration is closely associated with risk-taking.

Psychologic studies involving risk-taking have primarily centered on drug users who have human immunosuppression virus (HIV). Adolescents who participate in intravenous drug use are more likely to be sexually promiscuous (Turner, Ku, Rogers, Lindberg, Pleck, & Sonenstein, 1998). Durant, Smith, Krieter, and Krowchuk (1999) researched the age when substance abuse began in comparison to other risky behavior. Their research demonstrates that the younger a child is when he or she engages in substance abuse, including tobacco use, the higher the risk will be for the development of other risk-taking behaviors, such as carrying a concealed weapon, abusing other substances, not wearing a helmet when riding a bicycle, or riding with a drunk driver.

Interplay between sibling personalities has been shown to encourage risk-taking behaviors. Morrongiello and Bradley (1997) found that an older sibling can influence the decision making of a younger sibling. They concluded that the influence resulted in children choosing a course of action with heightened risk.

Interpersonal relationships between a child and his or her peers or siblings may play a role in the decision-making process and result in behaviors that are more likely to produce injuries. Placing oneself in harm's way may be a means of establishing a social position within a group. The childhood taunt of "I dare you" is often more a test of bravado than strength. It specifically challenges the child to take a risk to establish a more significant position within the peer or family group. Children believe that they will have a higher social standing if they accept the dare and accomplish it without injury.

Health care providers must remain nonjudgmental and accepting, especially when counseling adolescents about safety and lifestyle choices. Teenagers become alienated easily and often feel isolated and alone. Many teens take risks to test their abilities and values (Lightfoot, 1997). Fear of reprisal or condemnation of behavior can result in a noncompliant teenager who avoids seeking health care. A nonpunitive, straightforward style encourages honest communication regarding recent activities. This relationship may facilitate the diagnosis and improve the outcome.

Accident-Prone Children

The validity of using the term *accident prone* in relation to children has been questioned (Fox, 1997). Many childhood injuries are multifactorial and often associated with specific activities or developmental milestones. Some risk factors for higher injury rates have been more frequently associated with lower socioeconomic status, specific environments, cultural differences, and developmental or perceptual delays. Increased injury rates have been linked to single-parent households, presumably because of the reduced supervision a single parent can provide (Overpeck, Jones, Trumble, Scheidt, & Bijur, 1997). In rural areas there is a greater incidence of injury as a result of ethanol ingestion and identification of thrill-seeking behaviors in adolescents (Riley, Harris, Ensminger, Ryan, Alexander, Green, & Starfield, 1996). Risk factors for injury identified among urban adolescent youths include carrying a weapon for protection and living in an unsafe neighborhood (Svenson, Spurlock, & Nypaver, 1996). Infants and children in urban environments are most likely injured by house fires and gunshot wounds (Weesner, Hargarten, Aprahamian, & Nelson, 1994). Weesner et al. (1994) also report that children raised in rural environments are more commonly injured in motor vehicle accidents. Caucasian children are more prone to injury in an overcrowded environment. Hispanic children are most frequently injured when their primary caregiver does not speak English (Anderson, Agran, Winn, & Tran, 1998). Children with perceptual or developmental delays are unable to recognize environmental clues and are often unaware of impending danger. DiScala, Lescohier, Barthel, and Li (1998) suggest that children with attention-deficit/hyperactivity disorders are at increased risk for pedestrian injury and that a statistically significant number of these injuries are severe. The diversity of injury-associated risk factors in children underscores the need for highly individualized teaching for injury prevention.

Cultural Differences

Cultural beliefs should be explored before teaching injury prevention. Some cultures, including some sects of Islam and Hinduism, have deep-rooted beliefs in fatalism. The concept of fatalism is that each person's life is predetermined and therefore nothing can be done to change the outcome (Maher, 1996). Southeast Asians believe that evil spirits may influence the behavior of their children, which limits their ability to prevent injury (Fox, 1997). Some Cambodians believe that certain behaviors are the result of spells have been placed on their children (Fox, 1997). It is more difficult to stress accountability for personal decision making and injury prevention if one believes there is some greater force guiding one's destiny.

Social Acceptance of Death-Defying Behavior

In American society, children receive conflicting messages about risk-taking. Despite the community's best efforts at safety promotion, children get a clear message from the media that risk-taking is desirable and will be rewarded. Action movies are often filled with death-defying behaviors, and no consequences are shown for risk-taking behaviors (National Television Violence Study, 1995). Superhero cartoons, which target boys 3 to 5 years of age, highlight unrealistic behaviors and outcomes. Children in this age group are unable to synthesize the relationship between cause and effect and often try to mimic superhero maneuvers, only to place themselves at risk for injury (Parker & Zuckerman, 1995). Parents should consider the child's developmental level when choosing appropriate television programs, compact discs, and computer games. Real-life consequences for death-defying behavior should be discussed with the child as the program is viewed to allow for a comparison of reality and fantasy.

Public service announcements promoting firefighters and police as everyday heroes also send a message that risk-taking is rewarded. Sports heroes are often admired for their courage and fearlessness, particularly where injury is involved. These figures are elevated to superhuman status, and playing while injured is portrayed very positively. Many sports, such as wrestling or boxing, are based on the level of injury a person can sustain without becoming incapacitated. Society cannot continue to promote these activities as desirable while at the same time expecting children to avoid activities that place them at risk.

THEORETICAL FRAMEWORKS FOR INJURY PREVENTION

Epidemiology of Childhood Injuries

Epidemiology is the study of the distribution and determinants of health and disease within a population (Swanson & Albrecht, 1993). Epidemiology, as it pertains to injury prevention, tracks and analyzes injury patterns so that preventive safeguards can be developed and recommended. The epidemiology triangle (Figure 2-1) examines injury from the perspective of host, vector/agent, and environment (Gordon, 1949).

The host is the child at risk for injury. Host factors can be considered intrinsic factors to the child that predispose him or her to injury. These factors may influence the child's exposure, susceptibility, or response to harmful agents (Lilienfeld & Lilienfeld, 1980). Some host factors frequently evaluated for the cause of injury are age, sex, genetic makeup, ethnic groups, preexisting disability, and types of human behavior.

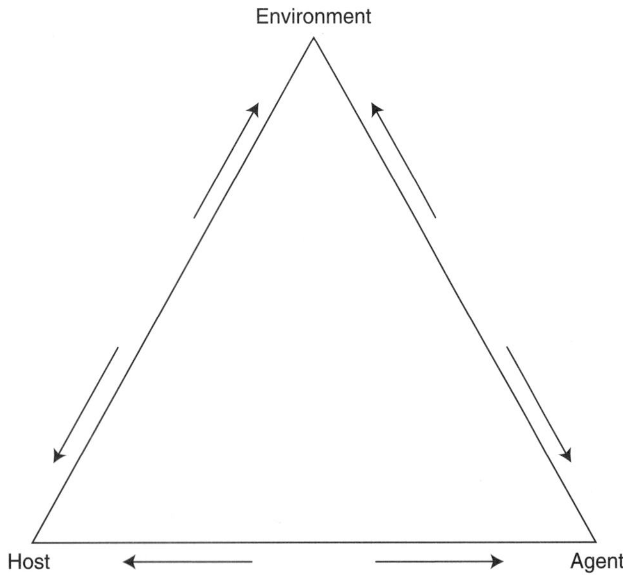

FIGURE 2-1 Epidemiologic triangle.

The agent or vector is the injurious force or object. The agent actually causes the physical trauma and has been described as the etiologic factor necessary to produce the specific damage resulting in injury (Haddon, 1980). Gibson (1961) defines the vector in terms of physical energy release: thermal, kinetic, radiation, or chemical. Vector etiology is also of prime importance because research in this area has yielded many passive environmental safeguards, such as infant car seats and electrical socket guards, which have been shown to be most effective (Haddon, 1980).

Environment also plays an integral role in ascertaining the cause of injury. The area in which the injury occurs plays an important role in the extent of physical damage. A fall from 50 feet can produce no tissue damage to catastrophic tissue damage, depending on the type of surface that breaks the impact. Environment can be examined from a simple physical perspective, such as playgrounds, stairways, or swimming pools. The social environment also has great preventive potential. Legislation relating to automotive safety, building codes, and bike helmets has prevented a huge toll in human disability and death.

The epidemiologic triangle permits a full analysis of injuries and their causative relationships. A multifaceted approach to safety promotion is more likely to result in successful prevention of pediatric injuries.

Haddon Matrix

The Haddon Matrix was first developed to categorize highway safety phenomena (Haddon, 1972). This model facilitates injury analysis from a perspective of multiple causation. It uses the epidemiologic triangle and superimposes primary, secondary, and tertiary prevention levels. This approach surrounds the issue of childhood injuries with a greater number of preventive strategies. The Haddon Matrix also includes a cultural and social perspective in an attempt to promote aggregate activities that have been shown to prevent injuries. These activities include legislative modification of the environment, product design to promote safety, building code changes, and community education campaigns.

Public health nursing has often categorized preventive strategies into primary, secondary, and tertiary levels of prevention. *Primary prevention* activities are those that prevent injury as it occurs. Primary prevention is analogous to a preevent strategy because it prevents contact with the energy, which could cause tissue damage. An example of primary prevention is additional street lighting to reduce pedestrian injury.

Secondary prevention focuses on interventions that occur when the injury is actually taking place. Secondary prevention is considered an event strategy because it lessens the damage associated with the actual energy contact. It encompasses interventions that communities endorse to limit the actual physical harm caused by traumatic energy release. Breakaway guardrails and impact-safe playground surfacing are examples of secondary prevention strategies.

Tertiary prevention refers to limiting the impact of the injury after it has occurred and is considered a postevent strategy. It includes putting mechanisms in place to limit the sequelae of pediatric trauma, such as bystander cardiopulmonary resuscitation and the availability of pediatric emergency medical services.

Public health agencies are collecting the data required to dissect and analyze injury events. The nurse must use a systems thinking approach to injury prevention. This includes participation in data collection; assessment of specific community needs; use of national guidelines for health maintenance guidance; and intervention at the primary, secondary, and tertiary levels of prevention (Eichelberger, 1993).

Finally, outcomes assessment involving the patient, the nurse, and the system should be continually performed to evaluate the effectiveness of particular intervention strategies (Curley, 1998). Injury prevention outcomes could include things such as assessing the percentage of a particular injury rate and tracking morbidity and mortality of a group of children or parents after injury avoidance guidance is provided. Systems outcomes involve the effect of injury-related trauma on the health care system, the community, and the nation. Analysis of system outcomes defines the issues by using epidemiologic data, resource allocation, and public awareness.

Geographic Considerations and Injury Prevention

The geographic characteristics of the United States are diverse. Flora and fauna vary, and these environmental characteristics affect the type and number of injuries. Trauma nurses must be aware of these characteristics and the specific recreational, cultural, or biological hazards within their location of practice. Table 2-1 provides an overview of potential injuries related to geographic factors.

Trauma Nursing and Health Maintenance

Trauma nurses are in an excellent position to act as change agents for individuals at high risk for injury. Trauma nurses need to rely on specific nursing competencies that are driven by the needs and individual situations of each family (Curley, 1998). The characteristics of the pediatric patient, the family dynamics, and the social and physical environments must all be considered as the nurse seeks to facilitate the learning process regarding injury prevention. Parents and children may also benefit from community-funded programs that provide free environmental safeguards. Information from health care providers is often necessary to assist families with accessing these programs. A history of frequent severe injuries that require hospitalization or involve fractures are suspicious and should be followed carefully. A screening of a child's home environment for safety hazards may be helpful; however, any child with severe, frequent injuries should be evaluated for abuse and/or neglect.

Health care guidance can take three forms: anticipatory guidance addressing host factors, preventive guidance addressing agent factors, and community guidance addressing physical and social environmental factors. Counseling should contain pertinent information from each of the three guidance domains.

Anticipatory Guidance

Health care providers often discuss developmental stages and age-specific environmental dangers with parents. They teach parents what to expect and to anticipate certain events. Anticipatory guidance centers around the host or child with the potential for injury. It includes normal developmental milestones and safety implications. This is extremely useful for the first-time parent. It allows the environment to be modified as the child becomes more mobile and demonstrates improved manual dexterity.

Preventive Guidance

Preventive guidance examines agent or vector issues. It usually involves the recommendation of passive environmental safeguards, such as electrical outlet socket caps or window guards. Preventive guidance attempts to alter the agent contacting the host in a continuous fashion. There is almost always some cost associated with preventive guidance, unless funded sources can be identified within the community. The benefit of preventive guidance is that it accounts for the child's size, developmental level, and statistical risk profile. It shifts the focus from strict parental vigilance to the safety needs of that individual child and family. Passive environmental safeguards have been shown to be the most effective injury prevention strategy in children (Eichelberger, 1993; Haddon, 1980).

TABLE 2-1 **Geographic Considerations for Injury Prevention Counseling**

Geographic Location	Recreational and Environmental Factors	Animal-Related Injuries
Northwestern United States	Mountain-climbing, snow skiing, hang gliding	Bear, coyote, and wolf attacks
Southwestern United States	Rodeo activities, horseback riding, surfing, scuba diving, desert hazards (dehydration, sunburn)	Shark attacks Poisonous snake bites Poisonous jellyfish and sea anemones/coral
Northeastern United States	Agricultural injuries, tractor pulls, motor cross biking, alpine skiing and snowboarding, ice skating	Leaches, jellyfish, tick, and poisonous spider bites Mountain lion and bear attacks
Southeastern United States	Sailboarding, jet ski boating, water skiing, snorkeling, and scuba diving Sun and heat exposure hazards	Spider and snake bites Scorpion stings Alligator attacks

Community Guidance

Community guidance consists of providing safety information within the context of a group or class. Community guidance is usually free, concerns physical or social environment issues, and is sponsored through a charitable or civic organization. Group needs are addressed, and prevention advice is presented concerning specific activities or areas. Community guidance may involve dissemination of information through the media or public service announcements. Unfortunately, it is not always applicable to every child. Examples of community guidance include parent instruction on first aid and cardiopulmonary resuscitation and Safe Kids Coalition events.

PREVENTIVE STRATEGIES FOR SPECIFIC INJURY CATEGORIES

In the following section, specific injury types are categorized by examining epidemiology, major risk factor stratifications, and preventive strategies. The Haddon Matrix is presented in table format to review primary, secondary, and tertiary prevention strategies. Suggestions for anticipatory, preventive, and community guidance are reviewed to facilitate prevention education offered by the trauma nurse.

Motor Vehicle Crashes

Epidemiology

Motor vehicle crashes (MVCs) are the leading cause of death in children from birth to 14 years of age (National Center for Health Statistics, 1997b). MVCs caused 18% of all children's deaths in 1996 (National Center for Health Statistics, 1997b).

Risk Factor Stratification

Although MVCs have numerous causes, not wearing a safety restraint and drinking alcohol and driving are the two main factors that contribute to MVCs involving children and teens. Of all motor vehicle fatalities, 67% involve children not wearing the proper restraints (National Highway Traffic Safety Administration, 1996). Children studied were more likely to be unrestrained in cars driven by unrestrained adults. Children were placed in improperly installed car seats 21% of the time (National Highway Traffic and Safety Administration, 1996). Children must be properly seated and restrained to prevent injury during MVCs (Haddon, 1980).

Alcohol ingestion was involved in one fourth of the MVCs that resulted in a child's death between 1985 and 1997 (CDC, 1997a). An intoxicated driver was implicated in 70% of the crashes (CDC, 1997a).

The teenage driver is 18 times more likely to be involved in an MVC than are persons aged 30 to 34 years (CDC, 1997a). This higher incidence has been attributed to a lack of judgment and driving experience and a greater propensity for risk-taking (National Center for Injury Prevention and Control, 1997c). One solution to teenage crash rates is a graduated license; a graduated license initially has certain restrictions that are lifted in a systematic fashion as driving experience is acquired (CDC, 1997a). There would be a complete loss of driving privileges for teenagers driving under the influence of alcohol (Phebo & Dellinger, 1998).

The Haddon Matrix is a useful format for teaching various prevention strategies for MVCs (Table 2-2). Intervention and education when minor crashes occur may help highlight the importance of parental involvement in crash prevention with the current licensing system. The nurse should also review the salient aspects of anticipatory, preventive, and community guidance and individualize the guidance as much as possible for each family's particular situation (Box 2-1).

Pedestrian Injuries

Epidemiology

In 1996, 25% of all pedestrian deaths occurred in children younger than 16 years (CDC, 2000). Pedestrian injuries most frequently occur in boys between the ages of 5 and 7 years (National Highway Traffic Safety Administration, 1997c). Of

TABLE 2-2 Haddon Matrix Applied to Motor Vehicle Crashes

Prevention Type	Host	Agent/Vector	Physical Environment	Social Environment
Primary prevention: preevent strategy	Teach older children basic first aid and crash positioning	Use rear-facing car seats positioned in the center back seat until the child weighs 10 kg or is 1 year of age	Assess intersections and highways for safety records and campaign for improvements	Support zero tolerance laws and encourage traffic safety classes
Secondary prevention: event strategy	Use appropriate child-restraint devices, properly installed	Never place an infant seat in the front passenger side with an air bag	Promote breakaway side rails and highway barriers, and reduce speed limits	Primary child-restraint laws and child-endangerment charges if driving under the influence of alcohol
Tertiary prevention: postevent strategy	Teach child how to call 911	Teach child safe exiting from the vehicle once the crash has occurred	Live in a community with access to pediatric EMS	Parental education in first aid and CPR

Data from American Academy of Pediatrics, Committee on Injury and Poison Prevention (1996); Bauer, Whitfield, & Ferguson (1998); Fox (1997); and NHTSA (1997b).

BOX 2-1 Nursing Recommendations for Parental Education on Motor Vehicle Crashes

Anticipatory Guidance

- Place car seats/restrained child in middle of back seat.
- Car seats should be facing the rear until child weighs 10 kg or is 1 year of age.
- Children should never ride unrestrained in any type of vehicle (including pickup truck beds).
- Children should not ride in the front seat with an air bag until they are 13 years of age.
- Infants should never be nursed or held while riding in a car. It is impossible to hold onto the infant even in low-speed crashes.

Preventive Guidance

- Child restraints should be the appropriate size.
- Children <20 kg should be restrained in a car seat.
- Children who weigh more than 20 kg or are 40 inches tall should use a booster seat.
- Car seats must be installed properly to prevent injury.
- Routine preventive maintenance should be performed on all motor vehicles.

Community Guidance

- Support community education campaigns providing free instruction on proper installation of car seats.
- Support universal car seat legislation.
- Encourage car manufacturers to place air bag disabling devices in cars.
- Participate in teaching parent first aid and CPR.
- Fund free car seat/booster seat programs for disadvantaged families.

Data from American Academy of Pediatrics (1996); CDC (1998); Fox (1997); and NHTSA (1997b).

TABLE 2-3 The Haddon Matrix Applied to Pediatric Pedestrian Injury

Prevention Type	Host	Agent/Vector	Physical Environment	Social Environment
Primary prevention: preevent strategy	Prekindergarten safety classes.	Reflective clothing Driver's education	Pedestrian islands, overpasses and bridges	Increase street lighting Simplify and reduce traffic flow
Secondary prevention: event strategy	Increase length of walk signals at stop lights Walk child to destination	Antilock braking systems Daytime running lights Cellular phone access to 911	Slower speed limits on streets with heavy pedestrian traffic	Stringent DUI laws; legal limit laws for pedestrians
Tertiary prevention: postevent strategy	Parent/bystander first aid and CPR	Track pedestrian injury locations and redesign roadways	Pediatric EMS available	Increased penalties for hit and run or multiple traffic violations

Data from Fox (1997); Lightstone et al. (1997); and NHTSA (1997c).

all pedestrian injuries, 22% involve a child younger than 16. Of these injuries, 13% occur at an intersection. Childhood injuries are most likely to occur in urban areas (Insurance Institute for Highway Safety, 1997).

Risk Factor Stratification

The two most important factors associated with pedestrian injury are low socioeconomic status of the victim and negligent motor vehicle operators. Children from poor, single-parent households with a large number of siblings are the group most likely to be hit by a car (MacPherson, Roberts, & Pless, 1998). Of all pediatric pedestrian injuries, 80% occur close to home, with 25% of those occurring during the walk to or from school (Fox, 1997). When adults walk to school with children, the number of pediatric pedestrian injuries is reduced (Roberts, 1995).

Approximately half of the drivers who hit children are found to be negligent (Fox, 1997). One study demonstrated that 73% of drivers involved in a pedestrian injury had a history of traffic violation (Lightstone, Peek-Asa, & Kraus, 1997). Stiffer penalties associated with multiple traffic infractions and rigorous punishment of hit-and-run drivers may result in a reduction of pedestrian injuries and fatalities.

A child's education about the rules of traffic safety should begin at a young age. Guidance should stress the importance of looking both ways before crossing, waiting for the walk signal, and never playing in the street or a driveway. This education should be started at the preschool level.

The Haddon Matrix (Table 2-3) addresses the issue of pediatric pedestrian injury. The suggested highlights for parental teaching are presented in Box 2-2.

Asphyxiation and Airway Obstruction

Epidemiology

Asphyxiation and foreign body airway obstruction occurs in approximately 5 in every 1 million children (Altmann & Nolan, 1995). The leading causative agents of injury are cords and ropes, entrapment, foreign object aspiration, and facial occlusion resulting in suffocation.

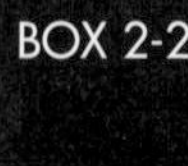

BOX 2-2 Nursing Recommendations for Parental Education on Pedestrian Injury

Anticipatory Guidance

- Accompany child on school journey or provide alternative transportation.
- Avoid highways with high volume of traffic.
- Never allow children to play in the street or driveway.

Preventive Guidance

- Dress children in white or reflective clothing.
- Adopt neighborhood traffic control, such as parental supervision and orange traffic awareness cones.
- Fence yards.

Community Guidance

- Lobby for pedestrian overpasses and walk bridges in areas proven to be unsafe.
- Support zero tolerance laws.
- Support stringent penalties for hit-and-run drivers.
- Teach community education regarding parental first aid and CPR.

Data from NHTSA (1997c) and Roberts (1995).

Risk Factor Stratification

The three main risk factors for asphyxiation in children are sleeping with their parents, being strangled by rope swings, and choking on food pieces. Infants are at particular risk for suffocation, especially during sleep. Infants who sleep in their parents beds or sleep on waterbeds have a higher rate of asphyxiation (American Academy of Pediatrics, 1999). Toddlers and older children often strangle on rope swings or drawstrings on clothes. Another risk factors for suffocation is entrapment in folding cots or hammocks, car trunks, and toy chests (Altmann & Nolan, 1995). Food-related airway obstruction is prevalent from birth to 3 years of age and often involves nuts, carrots, apples, and hard candy (Altmann & Nolan, 1995).

The Haddon Matrix related to asphyxiation and foreign body airway obstruction is presented in Table 2-4. The suggested highlights for parental teaching are presented in Box 2-3.

Fires, Burns, and Scalds

Epidemiology

Burns are the second leading cause of death in children from 1 to 4 years of age and the fifth leading cause of death from birth to 19 years of age (Fox, 1997). Boys between the ages of 5 and 13 years are at highest risk (Fox, 1997). Fifty-six percent of burns are due to scalds, but most fatal burns are the result of house fires (National Institute of Occupational Safety and Health and the University of Missouri–Columbia Extension, 1999). A house burns down every 67 seconds in the United States, and the average person can anticipate enduring two house fires in their lifetime (National Institute of Occupational Safety and Health and the University of Missouri–Columbia Extension, 1999).

TABLE 2-4 The Haddon Matrix Applied to Asphyxiation and Foreign Body Airway Obstruction

Prevention Type	Host	Agent/Vector	Physical Environment	Social Environment
Primary prevention: preevent strategy	Lay infants on their back to sleep Do not allow children to eat nuts, hard candy, etc.	Cut food into small portions Use a firm crib mattress	Lock car trunk at all times Do not use homemade rope swings Cut loops in miniblind and drapery cords	All cribs should be approved by the U.S. Consumer Product Safety Commission
Secondary prevention: event strategy	Observe children younger than 3 years while eating Remove baby's bib before placing in crib	Choose a toy chest without a lid or holes in sides to allow air flow Never prop a baby bottle	Do not use heavy comforters or pillows in crib Never chew gum while swimming	Legislate the avoidance of small toy parts to children younger than 5 years
Tertiary prevention: postevent strategy	Perform Heimlich maneuver or back blows and chest thrusts if the child is choking and unable to vocalize	Do not blind finger sweep an infant or child's airway Attempt to ventilate until EMS arrives	Pediatric emergency medical services available	Recall cribs, clothing, or toys shown to pose a threat to children Report choking on toy parts to the U.S. Consumer Product Safety Commission

Data from Altmann & Nolan (1995); Altmann & Ozanne-Smith (1997); Fox (1997); and Juvenile Products Manufacturer's Association (1997).

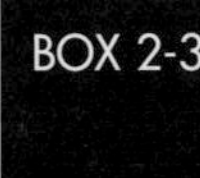

Nursing Recommendations for Parental Education on Asphyxiation and Foreign Body Airway Obstruction

Anticipatory Guidance

- Never use a cord to affix a pacifier to the child's clothes.
- Choking on food is common in children younger than 5 years.
- Do not allow children to put balloons in their mouths.
- Store grocery and garbage bags out of reach.

Preventive Guidance

- Crib gyms should be abandoned once the infant can push up on his or her hands and knees.
- Do not use cribs with cutouts on the end panels or corner posts.
- Do not buy clothing with drawstrings.
- Do not use homemade rope swings.
- Only use cots with safety latches that prevent accidental closure.

Community Guidance

- Mandate appropriate warnings on toys that pose a choking hazard.
- Day-care providers should be certified in pediatric first aid and CPR.
- Assist with parental first aid and CPR classes.
- Teach parents rescue breathing and back blows and chest thrusts.
- Promote safe designs in children's products.

Data from American Public Health Association and the American Academy of Pediatrics (1992).

Risk Factor Stratification

Smoking cigarettes and children obtaining and playing with matches, as well as unsafe use of kitchen appliances and noncentralized space heaters, have all been implicated in burns. Smoking cigarettes is the leading cause of home fires (CDC, 1997c). Parents who drink alcohol and smoke cigarettes are at high risk to cause house fires (CDC, 1997c; Warda, Tenebaein, & Moffatt, 1999). Squires and Buscettil (1996) studied fatalities from fires involving children from birth to 5 years. They discovered that 40% of burns were the direct result of actions such as children playing with ignitable materials. They also found that improper disposal of smoking materials frequently resulted in the death of older children.

Kitchen appliances have also been associated with childhood burns (National Institute of Occupational Safety and Health and the University of Missouri–Columbia Extension, 1999). Children who were permitted to independently prepare food on a stove or in a microwave also were at greater risk for burns. The risk for scald injuries was higher for children who prepared hot drinks or ran their own baths (Harre, Field, & Polzer-Debruyne, 1998).

Electrical burns contribute to 2% to 4% of the overall burn rates in children (Rabban, Blair, Rosen, Adler, & Sheridan, 1997). These burns most often occur in children from birth to 6 years and are usually the result of oral contact with an electrical cord. Despite these statistics, no significant design improvements to electrical cords have occurred in the last 20 years.

Space heaters, wood stoves, and steam radiators also increase the likelihood of childhood burns. In a study by Quinlan (1996), the researchers discovered that 16% of radiator burns occurred because the bed was placed too close to an unprotected radiator.

Table 2-5 provides an overview of prevention strategies for burns, scalds, and fires. Box 2-4 outlines suggested guidance for parents.

Sports Injuries

Epidemiology

Approximately 600,000 annually children are injured during recreational activities and participation in sports (Overbaugh & Allen, 1994). Athletic participation ranks as the fourth leading cause of injury in adolescents (American Medical Association, 1994). Of all head injuries in children, 43% are related to sports and recreational activities (Fox, 1997). The four sports that carry the greatest risk of injury are football, gymnastics, wrestling, and ice hockey (Fox, 1997).

Risk Factor Stratification

Older children who frequently engage in contact sports are most prone to injury. Each sport carries its own patterns of injury type and location. Guidance must be individualized to consider the age and developmental level of the child and the inherent risks of the activity. Physical activity should be encouraged, and children will naturally want to participate to the best of their physical ability; however, the risk of injury from trauma and overuse syndromes must be discussed (Overbaugh & Allen, 1994). This situation makes sports counseling more challenging.

Head injury is a serious consequence of participation in contact sports. Trainers and coaches should have specialized training to recognize subtle signs of concussion and spinal cord injury. Guidelines for managing concussion should follow the recommendations of the American Academy of Neurology (1997). Players should be warned to report any symptoms associated with head injury so that second impact syndrome can be detected. The Haddon Matrix (Table 2-6) provides an overview of sports injury prevention, and guidance areas for injury prevention are presented in Box 2-5.

Animal-Related Injuries

Epidemiology

Many animals can cause injury to humans. Children are at particular risk for predatory attacks. There are more than 50 million domesticated dogs in the United States (Weiss, Friedman, & Coben, 1998), and they are implicated in the majority of animal-related injuries. Every year, close to 5 million people are bitten by dogs, and children and infants are at highest risk for

TABLE 2-5 Haddon Matrix Applied to Burns, Scalds, and Fires

Prevention Type	Host	Agent/Vector	Physical Environment	Social Environment
Primary prevention: preevent strategy	Use summer sun protection Teach children not to play with matches or lighters	Keep hot foods and drinks away from counter edges Do not place beds near space heaters Store flammable items out of reach of children	Install and maintain smoke detectors on each level of the home and outside each bedroom Test smoke detectors every month Teach appliance safety	Use approved electric toys (Underwriter's Laboratory) Enforce safe building codes
Secondary prevention: event strategy	Teach children during a fire to crawl to a window, open it, and signal for help if they cannot escape from a room	Reduce water heater temperature to 120° F Teach children to exit a burning house as soon as possible, without personal items	Buy flame-retardant clothing Practice two different escape routes from your home Teach children to test for heat before opening a door	Support legislation for federal safety mandates for chew-proof electrical cords Develop self-extinguishing cigarettes less likely to ignite upholstery
Tertiary prevention: postevent strategy	Teach children to stop, drop, and roll if their clothes catch on fire Teach children how to call 911	Teach children that if burned, they should remove the causative agent and run cool water on the area; do not apply ice Remove any clothing involved with the fire	Set up a meeting place outside in the event of a fire Phone the fire department from a neighbor's house Live in a community with pediatric EMS and a pediatric burn center	Participate in tobacco cessation programs for parents Legislate child-proof caps on caustic chemicals

Data from CDC (1997c) and National Institute of Occupational Safety and Health (1999).

BOX 2-4 Nursing Recommendations for Parental Education on Burns, Scalds, and Fires

Anticipatory Guidance

- Do not allow children to play in the kitchen during meal preparation.
- Never hold a child and a hot drink at the same time.
- Test all food/bottles heated in the microwave, and stir to avoid "hot spots."
- Do not allow toddlers to turn on the bathtub faucet without supervision.
- Do not leave matches/lighters within reach of children.
- Preplan house fire escape routes and conduct drills.

Preventive Guidance

- Use 15 SPF sunscreen and cover up for prolonged sun exposure.
- Purchase smoke detectors and fire extinguishers for every level of your home.
- Use Underwriter's Laboratory approved appliances, lamps, and toys.
- Purchase irons, coffee pots, and curling irons with automatic shut-off feature.
- Place guards around fireplaces, space heaters, and radiators.
- Place safety caps over electrical outlets.

Community Guidance

- Teach parental first aid and CPR.
- Conduct holiday safety classes, avoid dry Christmas trees, and do not use indoor lights outside.
- Encourage tobacco cessation within the community.
- Promote reducing hot water heater temperatures to 120° F.

Data from CDC (1997c) and Fox (1997).

TABLE 2-6 Haddon Matrix Applied to Sports Injuries

Prevention Type	Host	Agent/Vector	Physical Environment	Social Environment
Primary prevention: preevent strategy	Specialized exercises to strengthen knees and ankles Warm up before exercising	Use padding and protective gear Use trained spotters, coaches, and trainers	Avoid sports on slippery surfaces Avoid running on uneven surfaces Keep bike and running trails well maintained and free of debris	Provide safe areas for skateboarding Encourage the popularity of noncontact sports Strictly enforce playing by the rules
Secondary prevention: event strategy	Teach children how to stop abruptly on skates and skis No activity past the point of pain	Use helmets and mouth guards Coaches should be aware of standards of care for spinal cord injury or concussion	Restrict skiing and snowboarding in poor conditions Use proper floor padding and foam cubes for gymnastics	Mandate helmet use for bicycles, skateboards, and roller blades Ban the sale of home trampolines Encourage parents to avoid reckless motivation of children
Tertiary prevention: postevent strategy	Restrict activity for appropriate length of time Tape involved joint during period of rehabilitation	Provide written instruction on proper sports technique	Pediatric EMS Air ambulance capabilities Advanced registered nurse practitioners and physicians at sporting events	Promote media representation of helmet use Community funding for playground maintenance

Data from CDC (1997e); Fox (1997); and Overbaugh & Allen (1994).

BOX 2-5 Nursing Recommendations for Parental Education on Sports Injuries

Anticipatory Guidance

- Encourage warm ups and cool downs.
- Obtain information on proper sports techniques.
- Provide coaches with training in injury prevention.
- Limit practice times.
- Downplay competitiveness.
- Avoid running on slippery or uneven surfaces.

Preventive Guidance

- Wear appropriate footwear for sport.
- Use protective gear, helmets, and mouth guards.
- Do not purchase snowboards for younger children.
- Use chest guards when playing football.

Community Guidance

- All coaches and trainers should be trained in first aid and CPR.
- Support mandatory helmet use for bicycling, skateboarding, inline skating, and ice hockey.
- Present injury data to local school boards.

Data from Overbaugh & Allen (1994).

mortality related to these bites (Sacks, Kresnow, & Houston, 1996). Children are most likely to be disfigured from dog bites on the face, head, and neck (Weiss et al., 1998).

RISK FACTOR STRATIFICATION

Boys between the ages of 5 and 7 years have the highest incidence of dog bites, and most of the bites occur at the victim's home by a free-roaming dog (Weiss et al., 1998). Dogs that bite are most likely to be male and unneutered (Gershman, Sacks, & Wright, 1994). The three breeds of dog most frequently implicated in biting incidents are pit bulls, rottweilers, and German shepards (CDC, 1997b).

A careful analysis of all animal injuries is presented in Table 2-7. The anticipatory, preventive, and community guidance for education is presented in Box 2-6.

TABLE 2-7 **Haddon Matrix Applied to Animal-Related Injuries**

Prevention Type	Host	Agent/Vector	Physical Environment	Social Environment
Primary prevention: preevent strategy	Use caution when bringing a dog into the house of a toddler Delay acquiring a dog if a child is fearful or apprehensive	Spay and neuter all dogs as they are less aggressive Consider dog obedience training Spend time with a dog before bringing it home	Children should wear long pants, socks, and boots when hiking Keep areas around the house free of debris or wood piles Report dog packs to the ASPCA	Support animal control programs Support specialized restrictions on owners of aggressive breeds
Secondary prevention: event strategy	Supervise children playing with a dog Never run from a dog Teach children to stop, drop, and roll into a ball using arms to cover ears and face	Avoid direct eye contact with a dog Do not play aggressive games with a dog	Keep dogs restrained on a leash or in a fenced yard	Promote public education regarding choosing a dog breed: Consult the ASPCA or a vet Parents should be aware of the wildlife in their community
Tertiary prevention: postevent strategy	Children should be instructed, if bitten by a dog, to immediately seek attention from an adult	All dog bites that pierce the skin should be examined by a health care provider Dogs with a history of aggression are inappropriate in households with children	Report dog bites to the ASPCA for data surveillance Pediatric EMS in area Parental first aid and CPR	Enforce leash laws Provide education in preschool on backing away from aggressive animals and bite prevention Support legislation for irresponsible dog owners

Data from CDC (1997b) and Sacks et al. (1996).

BOX 2-6 **Nursing Recommendations for Parental Education on Animal-Related Injuries**

Anticipatory Guidance

- Most dog bites occur on the victim's property on the weekend.
- Use caution when bringing a dog into a home with an infant or toddler.
- Teach children not to approach an unfamiliar dog.

Preventive Guidance

- When hiking, use insect repellent and wear long pants, socks, and boots.
- Consider dog obedience training.
- Restrain your dog with a leash or a fence.
- Separate dogs and young children with baby gates.
- Spay or neuter your dog.

Community Guidance

- Provide community educational programs on canine behavior/bite prevention in school system.
- Support your local ASPCA.
- Legislate fines for negligent dog owners.
- Support dangerous dog laws.
- Teach parents CPR and first aid.

Data from Sacks et al. (1996) and Weiss et al. (1998).

Falls and Playground Safety

Epidemiology

A child is taken for medical attention for a fall every 2 minutes in the United States, and 35% of these injuries are classified as severe (CDC, 1999). Falls result in 50% of all head injuries in children (Fox, 1997). Each year, approximately 211,000 children in the United States receive emergency care for injuries related to playground equipment (CDC, 1999).

Risk Factor Stratification

Three of the identified risk factors for falls are unsafe playgrounds, unguarded stairways and windows, and the use of infant walkers. Playground overcrowding, mixing of preschool and school-age children, and the lack of adult supervision have been implicated in playground trauma (Fox, 1997). Hard surfacing on playground surfaces has been recognized as a source for serious trauma. The National Program for Playground Safety (Mack, Thompson, & Hudson, 1998) demonstrated that fewer than half of the playgrounds surveyed had padded or soft surfaces to prevent head trauma in the event of a fall (CDC, 1999).

Safety gates to separate toddlers from unsafe areas could prevent falls. All ungated stairways represent a hazard to children younger than 3 years. Children should also be restrained with a waist and crotch strap when riding in strollers or shopping carts or when sitting in high chairs. An infant who falls 2 to 3 feet can receive significant trauma resulting in permanent disability (CDC, 1999).

Infant walkers are extremely dangerous because they permit mobility before children are fully aware of their environmental surroundings. Walkers have been implicated in serious falls down stairways and into swimming pools. Thein, Lee, Tay, and Ling (1997) demonstrated a 12.5% injury rate associated with infants using walkers. The majority of the trauma they sustained was to the face and head.

Education regarding various environmental hazards related to falls should be included when health care providers interact with parents. The Haddon Matrix provides multiple avenues for fall prevention (Table 2-8), and guidance for parents is presented in Box 2-7.

Toy-Related Injuries

Epidemiology

Every year in the United States, more than 100,000 injuries are directly related to playing with toys (CDC, 1997f). In the United States, 13 children died as a result of toy-related injuries in 1996 (CDC, 1997f). Most of these fatalities involved children from birth to 4 years (CDC, 1997f).

Risk Factor Stratification

Toy-related injuries are often the result of children playing with balloons or young children playing with toys intended for an older age group. Projectile toys have also been recognized as

BOX 2-7 Nursing Recommendations for Parental Education on Fall Prevention

Anticipatory Guidance

- Never leave an infant in a swing unattended.
- Be sure tubs are free of soap residue.
- Infants should not be left unattended on changing tables, and a restraining strap should be used.
- Always keep the drop side up when baby is in a crib.
- Keep high chairs away from a table or wall where children can push off.

Preventive Guidance

- Purchase infant swings with strong legs and a wide stance.
- Block doorways/stairs with baby gates.
- Avoid accordion-style baby gates.
- Choose a stroller with a wide wheel base that does not tip.

Community Guidance

- Support maintenance and safety evaluations of city parks and playgrounds.

Data from Juvenile Products Manufacturer's Association (1998).

TABLE 2-8 Haddon Matrix Applied to Fall Prevention

Prevention Type	Host	Agent/Vector	Physical Environment	Social Environment
Primary prevention: preevent strategy	Teach playground safety: taking turns, no pushing, etc. Always secure waist and crotch straps in strollers and shopping carts	Moving parts of teeter totters should be enclosed, and all sharp edges should be covered	Metal slides should always be placed in the shade Swings should have a nine feet clearance in all directions	Regulate playground overcrowding
Secondary prevention: event strategy	Never allow a baby to stand up in a high chair Do not use infant walkers	Swings should have soft, flexible seats	Playground equipment should have regular maintenance Install nonslip floor coverings	Place safety signs and crosswalks around playgrounds
Tertiary prevention: postevent strategy	Teach children to immediately seek attention from an adult for abrasions/injuries obtained on the playground	Surround playgrounds with mulch, sand, or rubber matting	Provide adult playground monitors with first aid training Live in an area with pediatric emergency services	Older playground equipment, if found to cause injury, should be replaced

Data from American Public Health Association and American Academy of Pediatrics (1992) and Juvenile Products Manufacturer's Association (1997).

TABLE 2-9 Haddon Matrix Applied to Toy Safety

Prevention Type	Host	Agent/Vector	Physical Environment	Social Environment
Primary prevention: preevent strategy	Children should be directly supervised during balloon play Young children should not be given toys with projectiles Children should put toys away after play	Do not give young children toys appropriate for older children Parents should avoid buying toys with sharp edges, small parts, or heating elements	Toy purchases for older children should be kept out of reach of younger siblings	Heed choking hazards warning labels Buy products with age-appropriate labeling
Secondary prevention: event strategy	Supervise children while they are playing	Frequently aspirated objects are small balls, marbles, and balloons; these should not be given to children younger than 5 years	Tricycles and riding toys should not be used unsupervised near stairs or swimming pools	Report injuries to the Consumer Product Safety Commission Disseminate information regarding toys known to cause injury
Tertiary prevention: postevent strategy	Discard any toy that causes injury Know first aid	Report injuries to the Consumer Product Safety Commission	Teach parents first aid and CPR Pediatric EMS available	Support legislation to ban infant walkers Ban the sale of BB and pellet guns to minors

Data from CDC (1997f); Fox (1997); and McNeill & Annerst (1995).

BOX 2-8 **Nursing Recommendations for Parental Education on Toy Safety**

Anticipatory Guidance

- Toys should never fit entirely in the child's mouth.
- Monitor toy use by children, and allow use of toy only for intended purpose.

Preventive Guidance

- Buy toys with age-appropriate labels.
- Do not buy BB or pellet guns for minors.

Community Guidance

- Participate in community awareness programs regarding the dangers of balloons and infant walkers.
- Disseminate information regarding recalls of toys.

Data from CDC (1997f).

unsafe for small children (CDC, 1997f). Half of the injuries caused by toys are lacerations (CDC, 1997f).

Children playing with balloons result in 7 to 10 deaths annually in the United States (CDC, 1997f). Parental supervision should be continuous when children play with balloons. It is important to deflate and discard balloons after use. Balloons should be stored out of reach. The Haddon Matrix and parental guidance are presented in Table 2-9 and Box 2-8.

Drowning

Each year in the United States, there are 500 drownings and 3000 near-drownings in swimming pools involving children younger than 5 years (National Center for Health Statistics, 1997a). It is the leading cause for death for children younger than age 5 in Florida, Arizona, and California (Ellis & Trent, 1997). Further information on epidemiology and risk factor stratification can be found in Chapter 20. The Haddon Matrix as applied to drowning is presented in Table 2-10, and parental guidance can be found in Box 2-9.

Ingestion/Poisoning

Most episodes of ingestion of a harmful or poisonous substance involve children in the home environment. Usually, a routine household product is involved (National Center for Health Statistics, 1997a). Ingestion and poisoning in the pediatric population involve such diverse risks as caustic and poisonous chemicals and plants, lead exposure within the environment, and intentional ingestion. The Haddon Matrix and parental guidance are presented in Table 2-11 and Box 2-10.

Firearm Injuries

One child is killed by a gun every 90 minutes. Fifteen children lose their lives every day (Powell, Sheehan, & Christoffel, 1996). A more thorough discussion of gun-related injuries can be found in Chapter 13. The Haddon Matrix and parental guidance are reviewed in Table 2-12 and Box 2-11.

SUMMARY

Childhood morbidity and mortality rates associated with traumatic injury are an indication of society's inability to reduce environmental dangers. Successful injury prevention must encompass behavioral modifications, passive environmental safeguards, and societal modifications. Every

TABLE 2-10 Haddon Matrix Applied to Drowning

Prevention Type	Host	Agent/Vector	Physical Environment	Social Environment
Primary prevention: preevent strategy	Teach children to swim or float Teach basic water safety (no running around pools, using personal flotation devices on boats)	Install an unclimbable fence on all four sides of the pool with a self-latching gate	Check water depth before entering Check weather forecast before boating	Enforce legal drinking age around recreational activities involving water Take a pool safety class when buying a pool
Secondary prevention: event strategy	Never swim alone Never rely on water wings to keep a child from drowning	Install pool alarms and leave them armed	Empty any buckets containing liquid Swim at public beaches with lifeguards	Support pool and hot tub industries to develop more effective prevention technologies
Tertiary prevention: postevent strategy	Begin artificial respiration as soon as possible Be aware of the time period that the child was without respiration	Install telephone near poolside in case of emergency	Parents should know first aid and CPR Pediatric EMS available	Support legislation requiring pool fencing with pool building permit

Data from Ellis & Trent (1997).

BOX 2-9 Nursing Recommendations for Parental Education on Drowning

Anticipatory Guidance

- Children should not be left unattended in the pool or bathtub.
- Empty cleaning buckets immediately after use.
- Even children who know how to swim are not drown-proof.

Preventive Guidance

- Do not use water wings.
- Fence hot tubs as well as pools.
- Pool covers and alarms cannot be depended on to prevent drowning.
- Pool fences should meet standards set by the Uniform Building Code.

Community Guidance

- Promote public service announcements that warn of the dangers of adolescents drinking alcohol and swimming or boating.
- Include pediatric drowning and near drowning education in CPR classes.

Data from National Center for Injury Prevention and Control (1999a) and O'Flaherty & Pirie (1997).

TABLE 2-11 Haddon Matrix Applied to Ingestion

Prevention Type	Host	Agent/Vector	Physical Environment	Social Environment
Primary prevention: preevent strategy	Teach young children about the danger of poisoning and medicine	Product modification and package redesign of caustics and insecticides	Rid your home of all nonessential poisonous substances Discard expired medications Remove poisonous plants from the home	Have houses built before 1978 inspected for lead Begin poison prevention programs in kindergarten
Secondary prevention: event strategy	Have children tested for lead at well-child visits between 12 and 36 months Buy only containers with signal words such as *poison, danger,* or *caution*	Syrup of Ipecac should be available in every home; replace every year Do not keep iron-fortified children's vitamins in the home	Discard dehumidifying packets when products are purchased	Promote awareness classes on substance abuse and suicide Support community teen hotline

Continued

TABLE 2-11 Haddon Matrix Applied to Ingestion—cont'd

Prevention Type	Host	Agent/Vector	Physical Environment	Social Environment
Tertiary prevention: postevent strategy	Keep prescribed tricyclic antidepressants out of children's reach	Poison control center number should be posted by the phone Live in a drug-free safe neighborhood	Environmental clean-up of lead contamination	Increase accessibility of mental health services, community-based family services, and educational outreach programs

Data from AAP (1996) and Liller, Craig, Crane, & McDermott, 1998.

BOX 2-10 Nursing Recommendations for Parental Education on Ingestion

Anticipatory Guidance

- Children are at highest risk for poisoning between the ages of 1 and 6 years.
- Teenage girls are most likely to take an overdose and usually ingest acetaminophen or antidepressants.
- Throw out any nonessential household products such as cleaning products, cosmetics, personal hair care products, plants, and over-the-counter medications.
- Crawl around your home to be sure all poisons are out of children's reach.
- Realize that most cases of lead poisoning occur in the northeast United States.

Preventive Guidance

- Attach safety latches on cabinets.
- Affix warning stickers to poison containers.
- Have your children test for lead exposure at well-child visits.
- Buy only containers with child-proof caps.

Community Guidance

- Encourage poison control classes for kindergartens and the school system.
- Support funding for poison control centers.
- Teach that the ingestion of caustics may have permanent health ramifications within the community setting. Examples are toilet bowl cleaners, metal cleaners, hair dye, drain cleaners, and battery acid.

Data from Liller et al. (1998) and National Center for Injury Prevention and Control (1999b).

TABLE 2-12 Haddon Matrix Applied to Firearm Injuries

Prevention Type	Host	Agent/Vector	Physical Environment	Social Environment
Primary prevention: preevent strategy	Children should never carry a weapon Practice noncorporal punishment within the home, and teach children to solve problems without violence Decrease violence in the media	Use locks on firearms and load indicators that allows easy identification of loaded weapons	Use metal detectors at school entrances	Support firearm control legislation Teach consequences of criminal behavior (cause and effect)
Secondary prevention: event strategy	Teach conflict resolution in the school system Limit violence between siblings	Safely store weapons and ammunition in separate locked areas Teach children that if they find a gun to stop, leave the area, and tell an adult	Increase police surveillance of unsafe neighborhoods	Support gun industry reform Track firearm-related injuries through the National Electronic Injury Surveillance System
Tertiary prevention: postevent strategy	Teach children self-protective behaviors (drop down and lie still)	Bystander and parent first aid and CPR	Penalties for gang behavior Pediatric EMS	Place guns under the jurisdiction of the Consumer Product Safety Commission

Data from CDC (1997d) and Fox (1997).

BOX 2-11 Nursing Recommendations for Parental Education on Firearms

Anticipatory Guidance

- Having a gun in the home makes the home less safe.
- If you must own a gun, always treat the gun as if it is loaded.
- Never put your finger on the trigger until you are ready to shoot.

Preventive Guidance

- Trigger locks and load indicators should be present on all guns purchased.
- Store and lock ammunition and guns separately.
- Buy handguns with high trigger resistance that resist trigger movement by a small child.
- Take a gun safety course.

Community Guidance

- Join Mothers Against Senseless Shooting (MASS).
- Hold gun owners responsible when children access their guns.
- Support legislation that mandates safer gun design.

health care provider is responsible for providing information to parents and other caregivers in an effort to promote a safer environment for children. However, advice may have a marginal effect on the child's safety if the parents have learning or financial barriers. Passive environmental safeguards funded through state and local governments are the fairest and most effective form of injury prevention.

Humans continue to take risks despite centuries of injury prevention education. It may be, however, that risk-taking has improved the condition of humankind through the discovery of new foods, medicinal herbs, and prime agricultural areas. It is also important to understand that survival of humankind depends on the ability to avoid dangers within the environment. This may explain the results of research demonstrating that environmental safeguards are more effective than behavior modification (Haddon, 1980). Pediatric trauma nurses play critical roles in prevention strategies and can use their unique knowledge base and skills to prevent injury, as well as to participate in treatment after the injury has occurred.

BIBLIOGRAPHY

Altmann, A., & Nolan, T. (1995). Non-intentional asphyxiation deaths due to upper airway interference in children 0-14 years. *Injury Prevention, 1*(2), 76-80.

Altmann, A., & Ozanne-Smith, J. (1997). Non-fatal asphyxiation and foreign body airway interference in children 0-14 years. *Injury Prevention, 3*(3), 176-182.

American Academy of Neurology. (1997). Summary of recommendations for the management of concussion in sports. *MMWR Morbidity and Mortality Weekly Report, 46*(10), 3-4.

American Academy of Pediatrics. (1999). Infants at increasing risk of suffocation death. Available at: http://www.aap.org/advocacy/releases/mayinf.htm.

American Academy of Pediatrics, Committee on Injury and Poison Prevention. (1996). Selecting and using the most appropriate car safety seats for growing children: Guidelines for counseling parents. *Pediatrics, 97*(5), 761-762.

American Medical Association. (1994). *Guidelines for adolescent preventative services (GAPS)* (pp. 30-38). Baltimore: Williams & Wilkins.

American Public Health Association and American Academy of Pediatrics. (1992). *Caring for our children: National health and safety performance standards.* Washington, DC: American Public Health Association and American Academy of Pediatrics.

Anderson, C. I., Agran, P. F., Winn, D. G., & Tran, C. (1998). Demographic risk factors for injury among Hispanic and non-Hispanic white children: An ecologic analysis. *Injury Prevention, 4*(1), 33-38.

Blumstein, D. (1999). Enhanced: Selfish sentinels. *Science, 284*(5420), 1640-1644.

Bower, B. (1996). Gene tied to excitable personality. *Science News, 149*(1), 4.

Bauer, E. R., Whitfield, R., & Ferguson, S. A. (1998). Seating positions and children's risk of dying in motor vehicle crashes. *Injury Prevention, 4*(3), 181-187.

Brown, J. R., Ye, H., Bronson, R. T., Dikkes, P., & Greenberg, M. E. (1996). A defect in nurturing in mice lacking the immediate early gene fosB. *Cell, 86*(2), 297-309.

Centers for Disease Control and Prevention. (1997a). Alcohol-related traffic fatalities involving children-United States. *MMWR Morbidity and Mortality Weekly Report, 46*(48), 1130-1133.

Centers for Disease Control and Prevention. (1997b). Dog bite related fatalities—U.S. 1995-1996. *MMWR Morbidity and Mortality Weekly Report, 46*(21), 463-467.

Centers for Disease Control and Prevention. (1997c). National Fire Prevention Week, October 5-11. *MMWR Morbidity and Mortality Weekly Report, 46*(38), 901-902.

Centers for Disease Control and Prevention. (1997d). Rates of homicide, suicide and firearm-related death among children—26 industrialized countries. *MMWR Morbidity and Mortality Weekly Report, 46*(5), 101-105.

Centers for Disease Control and Prevention. (1997e). Sports-related recurrent brain injuries—U.S. *MMWR Morbidity and Mortality Weekly Report, 46*(10), 224-227.

Centers for Disease Control and Prevention. (1997f). Toy-related injuries. *MMWR Morbidity and Mortality Weekly Report, 46*(50), 1185-1189.

Centers for Disease Control and Prevention. (1998). Improper use of child safety seats. *MMWR Morbidity and Mortality Weekly Report, 47*(26), 543-544.

Centers for Disease Control and Prevention. (1999). Playground safety—United States, 1998-1999. *MMWR Morbidity and Mortality Weekly Report, 48*(16), 329-332.

Centers for Disease Control and Prevention. (2000). Fact book for year 2000. Motor vehicle related injuries. Available at http://www.cdc.gov/ncipc/pub-res/FactBook/fkmve.htm.

Coggan, C., Disley, B., & Patterson, P. (1998). Community-based intervention on adolescent risk-taking: Using research for community action. *Injury Prevention, 4*(1), 58-61.

Curley, M. A. (1998). Patient-nurse synergy: Optimizing patient outcomes. *American Journal of Critical Care, 7*(1), 64-71.

DiScala, C., Lescohier, I., Barthel, M., & Li, G. (1998). Injuries to children with attention-deficit hyperactivity disorder. *Pediatrics, 102*(6), 1415-1421.

Durant, R. H., Smith, J. A., Krieter, S. R., & Krowchuk, D. P. (1999). The relationship between early onset of initial substance use and engaging in multiple health risk behaviors among young adolescents. *Archives of Pediatric/Adolescent Medicine, 153*(3), 286-291.

Eichelberger, M. (Ed.). (1993). *Pediatric trauma: Prevention, acute care, and rehabilitation* (pp. 11-16). St. Louis: Mosby.

El-Sheikh, M., Ballard, M., & Cummings, E. M. (1994). Individual differences in preschoolers' physiological and verbal responses to videotaped angry interactions. *Journal of Abnormal Child Psychology, 22*(3), 303-320.

Ellis, A. A., & Trent, R. B. (1997). Swimming pool drownings and near-drownings among California preschoolers. *Public Health Reports, 112,* 73-77.

Fisher, K. J. & Balanda, K. P. (1997). Care giver factors and pool fencing: an exploratory analysis. *Injury Prevention, 3*(4), 257-261.

Fox, J. (1997). *Primary health care of children* (pp. 187-216). St. Louis: Mosby.

Gabel, S., Stadler, J., Bjor, J., Shindledecker, R., & Bowden, C. (1995). Homovanillic acid and dopamine-beta-hydroxylase in male youth: Relationships with paternal substance abuse and antisocial behavior. *American Journal of Drug and Alcohol Abuse, 21*(3), 363-378.

Gershman, K. A., Sacks, J. J., & Wright, J.C. (1994). Which dogs bite? A case control study of risk factors. *Pediatrics, 93*(6), 913-917.

Gibson, J. (1961) The contribution of experimental psychology to the formulation of the problem of safety. In H. Haddon (Ed.), *Behavioral approaches to accident research* (pp. 77-89). New York: Association for the Aid of Crippled Children.

Girasek, D. C. (1999). How members of the public interpret the word accident. *Injury Prevention, 5*(1), 19-25.

Gordon, J.E. (1949). The epidemiology of crashes. *American Journal of Public Health, 39,* 504-515.

Haddon, W. (1972). A logical framework for categorizing highway safety phenomenon and activity. *The Journal of Trauma, 12*(3), 193-207.

Haddon, W. (1980). Advances in the epidemiology of injuries as a basis for public policy. *Public Health Reports, 95*(5), 411-421.

Harre, N., Field, J., & Polzer-Debruyne, A. (1998). New Zealand's children's involvement in home activities that carry a burn or scald risk. *Injury Prevention, 4*(4), 266-271.

Holden, C. (1998). New clues to alcoholism risk. *Science Magazine, 280*(5368), 1348-1349.

Insurance Institute for Highway Safety. (1997). *Facts: 1996 fatalities—Pedestrians.* Arlington: Insurance Institute for Highway Safety.

Juvenile Products Manufacturer's Association (JPMA). (1997). *Safe and sound for baby: A guide for product safety, use and selection.* Juvenile Products Manufacturer's Association. Available at http://www.jpma.org/public/safe-sound.html.

Kauffman, L. (Ed.). (1987). *Webster's dictionary.* Bridgewater: Harbor House Publishers.

Lightfoot, C. (1997). *The culture of adolescent risk-taking* (pp. 161-165). New York: The Guilford Press.

Lightstone, A. S., Peek-Asa, C., & Kraus, J. F. (1997). Relationship between driver's record and automobile versus child pedestrian collisions. *Injury Prevention, 3*(4), 262-266.

Lilienfeld, A. M., & Lilienfeld, D. (1980). *Foundations of epidemiology* (pp. 47-48). New York: Oxford University Press.

Liller, K. D., Craig, J., Crane, N., & McDermott, R. J. (1998). Evaluation of poison prevention lesson for kindergarten and third grade students. *Injury Prevention, 4*(3), 218-221.

Mack, M. G., Thompson, D., & Hudson, S. (1998). Playground injuries in the 90s. *Parks & Recreation, 33,* 88-95.

MacPherson, A., Roberts, I., & Pless, B. (1998). Children's exposure to traffic and pedestrian injuries. *American Journal of Public Health, 88*(12), 1840-1845.

Maher, M. (1996). *Fatalism. The Catholic encyclopedia* (pp. 1-4). New Advent, Inc. Available at: http://www.csn.net/advent/cathen/05791 a.html.

McNeill, A. M., & Annerst, J. L. (1995). The ongoing hazard of BB and pellet gun-related injuries in the U.S. *Annals of Emergency Medicine, 26*(2), 187-194.

Meropol, S., Moscati, R., Lillis, K., Ballow, S., & Janicke, D. (1995). Alcohol-related injuries among adolescents in the emergency department. *Annals of Emergency Medicine, 26*(2), 180-186.

Morrongiello, B. A., & Bradley, M. D. (1997). Sibling power: Influence of older siblings' persuasive appeals on younger siblings judgements about risk-taking behaviors. *Injury Prevention, 3*(1), 23-28.

National Center for Health Statistics. (1997a). *National Center for Health Statistics (1996-97) and injury chartbook.* Hyattsville, MD. Available at http://www.cdc.gov/nchs/data/hus/hus96_97.pdf

National Center for Health Statistics. (1997b). *National mortality data, 1995.* Hyattsville, MD: Centers for Disease Control and Prevention. DHHS Pub No. (PHS)97-1232.

National Center for Injury Prevention and Control. (1997c). *Teenage motor vehicle deaths.* Atlanta: National Center for Injury Prevention and Control.

National Center for Injury Prevention and Control. (1999a). *Drowning fact sheet.* Atlanta: National Center for Injury Prevention and Control.

National Center for Injury Prevention and Control. (1999b). *Facts about poisoning.* Atlanta: National Center for Injury Prevention and Control. Available at: http://www.cdc.gov/ncip/factsheets/poi2.html.

National Highway Traffic Safety Administration. (1996). *Traffic safety facts—Children, 1996.* Washington, DC: National Highway Traffic Safety Administration.

National Highway Traffic Safety Administration. (1997a). *National occupant protection use survey—1996.* Washington, DC: National Highway Traffic Safety Administration.

National Highway Traffic Safety Administration. (1997b). *Observed patterns of misuse of child safety seats. Traffic tech.* Washington, DC: National Highway Traffic Safety Administration.

National Highway Traffic Safety Administration. (1997c). *Traffic safety facts—1996.* Washington, DC: National Highway Traffic Safety Administration.

National Institute of Occupational Safety and Health and the University of Missouri–Columbia Extension. (1999). *Prevention and treatment of burns—Miscellaneous causes.* The National Agricultural Safety database. Available at: http://www.cdc.gov/niosh/nasd/nasd.home.html.

National Rifle Association. (1999). *Information for parents, teachers, and administrators.* Available at: http://www.eddie@nrahq.org.

National Television Violence Study. (1995). Available at: http://www.facts@mediascope.org.

O'Flaherty, J. E., & Pirie, P. L. (1997). Prevention of pediatric drowning and near-drowning: A survey of the members of the American Academy of Pediatrics. *Pediatrics, 99*(2), 169-174.

Overbaugh, K. A., & Allen, J. G. (1994). Adolescent athlete. Part II: Injury patterns and prevention. *Journal of Pediatric Health Care, 8,* 203-211.

Overpeck, M. D., Jones, D. H., Trumble, A. C., Scheidt, P. C., & Bijur, P. E. (1997). Socioeconomic and racial/ethnic factors affecting nonfatally medically attended injury rates in U.S. children. *Injury Prevention, 3*(4), 272-276.

Parker, S., & Zuckerman, B. (1995). *Behavioral and developmental pediatrics* (pp. 6-9). Boston: Little, Brown.

Phebo, L., & Dellinger, A. M. (1998). Young driver involvement in fatal motor vehicle crashes and trends in risk behaviors, United States, 1988-1995. *Injury Prevention, 4*(4), 284-287.

Powell, E. C., Sheehan, K. M., & Christoffel, K. K. (1996). Firearm violence among youth: Public health strategies for prevention. *Annals of Emergency Medicine, 28*(2), 204-212.

Quinlan, K. (1996). Home radiator burns among inner city children—Chicago, Sept. 1991-April 1994. *MMWR Morbidity and Mortality Weekly Report, 45*(38), 814-815.

Rabban, J., Blair, J., Rosen, C., Adler, J., & Sheridan, R. (1997). Mechanisms of pediatric electrical injury. *Archives of Pediatric/Adolescent Medicine, 5,* 696-700.

Riley, A. W., Harris, S. K., Ensminger, M. E., Ryan, S., Alexander, C., Green, B., & Starfield, B. (1996). Behavior and injury in urban and rural adolescents. *Injury Prevention, 2*(4), 266-273.

Roberts, I. (1995). Adult accompaniment and the risk of pedestrian injury on the school-home journey. *Injury Prevention, 1*(4), 242-244.

Routledge, D. A., Repetto-Wright, R., & Howarth, C. I. (1996). The exposure of young children to accident risk as pedestrians. *Injury Prevention, 2*(2), 150-161.

Sacks, J. J., Kresnow, M. I., & Houston, B. (1996). Dog bites: How big a problem? *Injury Prevention, 2*(1), 52-54.

Shepard, G., & Klein-Swartz, W. (1998). Accidental and suicidal adolescent poisoning deaths in U.S., 1979-1994. *Archives of Pediatric/Adolescent Medicine, 152,* 1181-1185.

Squires, T., & Buscettil, A. (1996). Can child fatalities in house fires be prevented? *Injury Prevention, 2*(2), 109-113.

Svenson, J., Spurlock, C., & Nypaver, M. (1996). Factors associated with the higher traumatic death rate among rural children. *Annals of Emergency Medicine, 27*(5), 625-632.

Swanson, J., & Albrecht, M. (1993). *Community health nursing: The health of aggregates* (pp. 80-108). Philadelphia: WB Saunders.

Thein, M. M., Lee, J., Tay, V., & Ling, S. L. (1997). Infant walker use, injuries, and motor development. *Injury Prevention, 3*(1), 63-66.

Turner, C. F., Ku, L., Rogers, S. M., Lindberg, L. D., Pleck, J. H., & Sonenstein, F. L. (1998). Adolescent sexual behavior, drug use and violence: increased reporting with computer survey technology. *Science, 280*, 867-871.

Warda, L., Tenebaein, M., & Moffatt, M. E. (1999). House fire injury prevention update. *Injury Prevention, 5*(2), 145-150.

Weesner, C. L., Hargarten, S., Aprahamian, C., & Nelson, D. R. (1994). Fatal childhood injury patterns in an urban setting. *Annals of Emergency Medicine, 23*(2), 231-236.

Weiss, H. B., Friedman, D. I., & Coben, J. H. (1998). Incidence of dog bite injuries treated in emergency departments. *Journal of the American Medical Association, 279*(1), 51-53.

NATIONALLY RECOGNIZED INJURY PREVENTION RESOURCES

American Academy of Pediatrics
Department of Federal Affairs
601 13th St., NW
Suite 400 North
Washington, DC 20005
http://www.aap.org

Emergency Nurses Association
915 Lee St.
Des Plaines, IL 60016-6569
http://www.ena.org

ENCARE (Emergency Nurses Care)
205 S. Whiting St.
Suite 403
Alexandria, VA 22304
http://www.ena.org/encare

National Highway Traffic Safety Administration
400 7th St., SW
Washington, DC 20590
http://www.nhtsa.dot.gov/

National Institutes of Health
Bethesda, Maryland 20892
http://www.nih.gov

National Safe Kids Campaign
1301 Pennsylvania Ave., NW
Suite 1000
Washington, DC 20004-1707
http://www.safekids.org

U.S. Consumer Product Safety Commission
Washington, DC 20207-0001
http://www.cpsc.gov

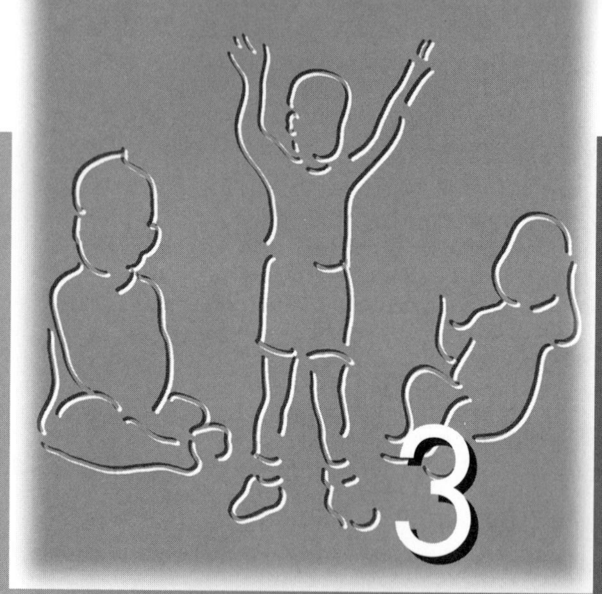

3 Ethical Competencies for Pediatric Trauma Nursing Care

Denise Poirier Maguire

Trauma nurses typically thrive on the excitement of a fast-paced work environment where issues of life and death occur daily. These nurses manage patients who present with grossly abnormal and life-threatening physical and physiologic illnesses with skill and expertise. Although they may be sensitive to the impending death of their patients and the emotional suffering of parents, trauma nurses learn that some children with severe injuries will not survive. Furthermore, pediatric trauma nurses accept that with each situation, parents with difficult questions and extraordinary challenges must be supported, guided, and counseled.

Pediatric trauma nurses face situations unique to their patient population. With increasing frequency, situations occur in which a parent may have purposely inflicted the injury. These situations require nurses to behave professionally at all times and put aside their personal feelings about the individuals suspected of child abuse. Unfortunately, pediatric brain death is routinely encountered by nurses caring for trauma victims and presents extensive ethical issues that challenge both medical and legal professionals (Dorr, 1997). Informed consent is another complicated issue in pediatric settings, largely because of the wide variation of individual levels of patient competency and the obligation to seek consent only when the intent is to weigh the child's decision seriously (American Academy of Pediatrics [AAP], 1995). Other situations that pediatric trauma nurses commonly encounter include organ transplantation, withdrawal of life support, family presence during resuscitation, the child's role in treatment decisions, costs of care in times of limited resources, whistle-blowing, the impact of religious beliefs and cultural practices on the standard of trauma care, and patient advocacy in conflict with hospital loyalty (Claassen, 2000). Each of these situations is likely to pose an ethical dilemma for at least one trauma nurse on the case, and all should be prepared for the possibility. Clearly, clinical skill alone does not describe or encompass the full breadth of an experienced trauma nurse's expertise. Knowledge of self, personal values, and health care ethics are critical to the influence and healthy longevity of pediatric trauma nurses in the emergency department, the critical care unit, and finally the medical/surgical unit.

Just as trauma nurses learn and practice their clinical skills, they must recognize and practice ethical decision making for dilemmas they face, as well as those faced by patients, families, and colleagues. Caring for pediatric trauma victims requires an "ethical commitment to the mastery of relevant knowledge and technical skills, an agreement to safeguard the patient, and a promise to provide highly qualified care" (Wagner & Hendel, 2000). Nursing ethics is an essential component of orientation to pediatric trauma nursing. Orientation provides an excellent opportunity to discuss the relevant decision-making processes unique to each setting and to develop, refine, or review the ethical competency of new staff members.

ETHICAL APPROACHES USED BY PEDIATRIC TRAUMA NURSES

Many approaches or philosophic theories of ethical decision making are used in health care. Decisions may be based on principles, obligations, virtues, rights, consequences, communities, relationships, or cases (Beauchamp & Childress, 2001). The theory, or focus, determines how the dilemma is approached and what is of greatest import. People who espouse different theories come to different conclusions about what is the "right" way to solve an ethical dilemma. Often, their own personal belief system and their religious or cultural background shape how they approach an ethical dilemma. For example, people who are driven by principles are not as concerned about the outcome to the individual as those who live by a relationship-based theory. The former may be guided by "do no harm," whereas the latter may be much more concerned about the effect of any potential decision upon the family, as a unit and for each individual. Recognizing the different theories each of us brings to the clinical setting is the first step toward collaborative decision making. Nurses who are aware of their own culturally grounded behavior are more sensitive to cultural behavior in others (Wong, Hockenberry-Eaton, Wilson, Winkelstein, Ahmann, & DiVito-Thomas, 1999).

Every ethical issue faced by the pediatric trauma team can be characterized as an issue or challenge of an ethical principle. These principles are general guides that provide opportunity for judgment in specific cases (Beauchamp & Childress, 2001). They initially derived from the common morality within the medical tradition. *Morality* refers to the social conventions about right and wrong human conduct. They are widely shared and form a stable consensus. Still, principles are interpreted individually using an ethical theory, usually based on one's value system. Several philosophic theories of ethical decision making are common in health care. The three most commonly known in health care are utilitarianism, deontology, and the ethic of care.

Utilitarianism is an ethical theory also called *situation ethics*. The two major tenets of utilitarianism are the greatest good for the greatest number and the ends justifies the means (Beauchamp & Childress, 2001). Utilitarians believe that the right act is the one that produces the most good. Each act is judged within the context of the situation. Deontology is based on moral rules. Persons must act from obligation rather than fear of consequences to be morally correct (Beauchamp & Childress, 2001). In this system it is not the outcome of the act that makes it right or wrong, it is strict adherence to the principles.

The "ethic of care" theory may be most useful when dealing with pediatric trauma because it is a relationship-based theory. Relationship-based theories place emphasis on the traits valued in relationships, such as sympathy, compassion, and fidelity. It is a theory congruent with the values of family-centered care because the family is supported in the decisions they choose as right for them. The similarities and connections to nursing are obvious. Caring is a concept central to many definitions of nursing (Kikuchi, Simmons, & Romyn, 1996). Nurses take care of others by building trusting relationships with patients and families. Family-centered care is often a stated value of pediatric nurses and facilities. It also is based on relationship building. Pediatric nurses must include the family in the plan of care to achieve the goals of therapy. The ethic of care captures the philosophy of basic nursing practice, especially that of pediatric nursing. The ethic of care is a context in which ethical dilemmas in pediatric trauma can be managed by all members of the health care team. The ethic of care, however, is probably an incomplete model because it lacks a focus on the individual (Omery, 1995). The model presented here incorporates ethical principles to advance the depth of this model and to guide decision making.

ETHICAL PRINCIPLES ENCOUNTERED IN PEDIATRIC TRAUMA NURSING

The major ethical principles encountered in pediatric trauma are autonomy, nonmaleficence, beneficence, and justice. They are helpful when analyzing issues of informed consent, competency, emancipation, limits to the standard of care, withdrawal from life support, futility, and holistic or alternative medicines. A brief review of these principles illustrates the role of ethical principles in the model (Figure 3-1).

AUTONOMY

Autonomy refers to a person's individual freedom to choose his or her own course and make personal decisions (Beauchamp & Childress, 2001). It is a well-respected principle in the adult population, but it is always challenging and problematic in the pediatric population (Wagner & Hendel, 2000). Autonomy has limitations set not only by society (laws) and parents (house rules) but also by health care providers who hold authoritative positions over young patients. Health care providers continually make decisions for their young patients about what treatments they will take and how they will take them. Many health care providers assume that the child does not and perhaps cannot know what is best for him or her. Indeed, children mature in their capacity for self-determination at different times, some later than others. When should the child be included in discussions about how to proceed with treatment options? The Belmont Report (National Commission for the Protection of Human Subjects of Biomedical and Behavioral Research, 1979) provides federal guidelines about "assenting" children who are eligible to participate in investigational research, concurrently with obtaining informed consent from one or both parents. Even so, children have no federal rights in the United States. Instead, the government defines specific requirements to protect human subjects (*Code of Federal Regulations*) regarding ethical conduct and informed consent (U.S. Department of Health and Human Services, 1991).

Applying the concept of autonomy in a pediatric trauma situation requires thoughtful consideration of many

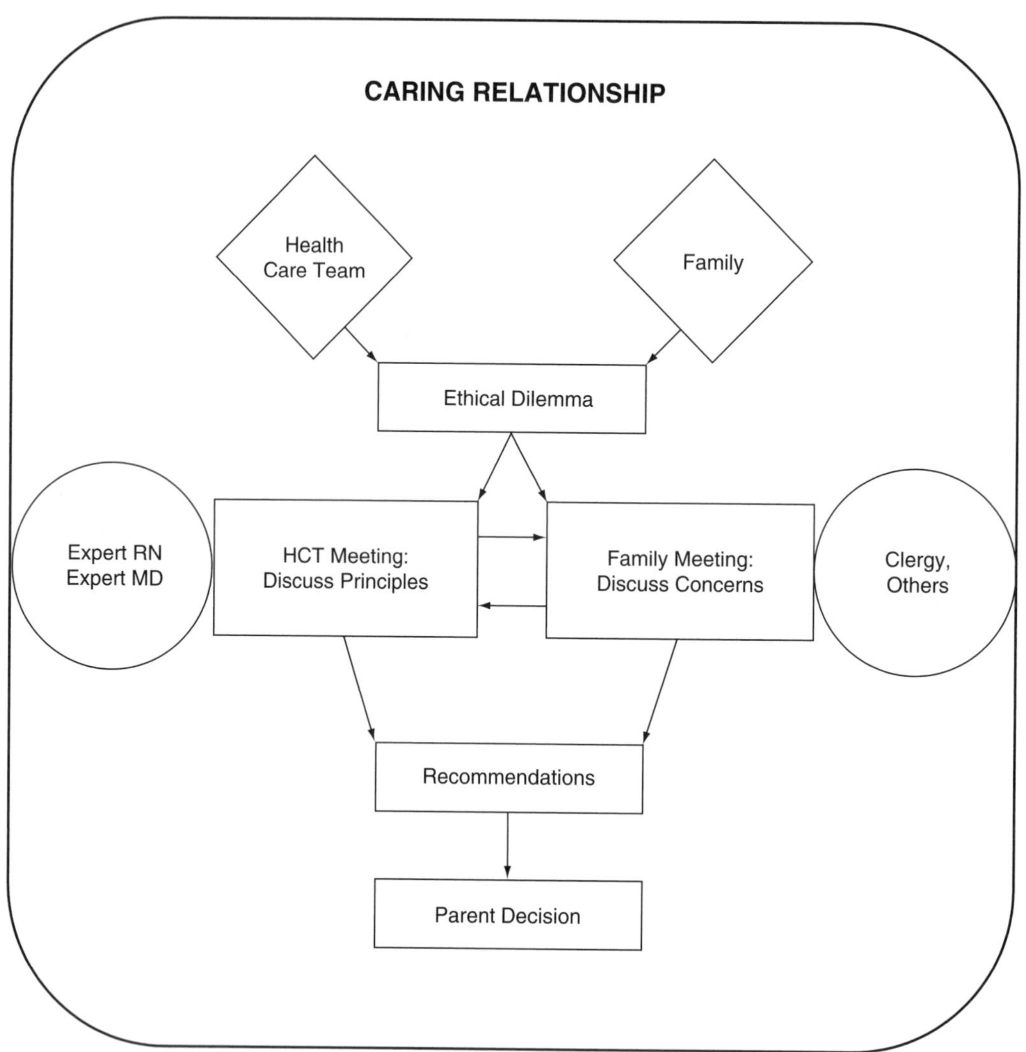

FIGURE 3-1 Model of family-centered care for ethical decision making in pediatric trauma.

variables. First, considering age, cognition, and developmental level, is the child mentally capable of self-determination? Are there some aspects of the decision that are within the child's mental capacity and others that are not? How much should the child's religious beliefs and cultural practices affect the standard of trauma care? How does a trauma nurse weigh hospital loyalty when it appears to be in conflict with the nurse's role as patient advocate? What is the usual pattern of decision making in the family structure? How do family values and beliefs affect the child's autonomy? Finally, does the health care team identify a dilemma, or can they honor any decision made by the family and child? Using the ethic of care as the guiding theory, autonomy of the child is considered in relation to the traditional role the child plays in his or her family structure. Families are encouraged to involve the child in making decisions as much or little as he or she finds comfortable. The pediatric trauma nurse must take time to discover the parents' wishes about the level of involvement their child will have in the decision-making process. They should involve the child in decision making only if they intend to consider and weigh it heavily. No one should make a decision without fully understanding the facts (Graham, 1994).

Another interesting challenge that may be associated with the principle of autonomy is family presence during resuscitation. Many members of the pediatric trauma team may have very strong positive and negative feelings about this request. The Emergency Nurses Association (2001) issued a position statement supporting the option of family presence during resuscitative efforts. They recognize that the family system is the major source of support for their patients and that the presence of family members enables the patient and family to comfort and to be comforted. Little research exists about the effect of family presence during resuscitation, but most families, if well supported, perceive it as a positive experience for which they are grateful (Hanson & Strawser, 1992; Meyers, Eichhorn, Guzzetta, Clark, Klein, Taliaferro, & Calvin, 2000). Health care consumers expect to be treated autonomously, and pediatric trauma nurses should be prepared when families ask for this type of unconventional participation.

Nonmaleficence

The second principle, nonmaleficence, is the obligation not to inflict intentional harm (Beauchamp & Childress, 2001). Health care providers may misinterpret this principle when they subject pediatric trauma patients to treatments that cause pain, such as whirlpool for debridement, physical therapy, and dressing changes. However, this principle would be violated only if they intentionally withhold pain medication so that the patient might suffer. The usual circumstance is that pediatric nurses diligently assess their patients for pain and titrate the opioids to successfully manage pain (Senecal, 1999). Instead, the related issues of nonmaleficence in pediatric trauma may include the withholding and withdrawal of life-sustaining treatments and organ donation.

Withholding care refers to not beginning a treatment because it is considered inappropriate for a person. *Withdrawing treatment* is the removal of a treatment because it is not effective or is worsening the problem. There is no moral difference between starting treatment and stopping it (Caplan, Capron, Murray, & Penticuff, 1987). Rather, it is the consequences of those actions that should be considered. Nonmaleficence, the duty to do no harm, will guide pediatric trauma nurses to thoughtfully examine the consequences of potentially hurtful interventions. When information is limited because of the nature or newness of the trauma, it is morally acceptable to initiate a potentially hurtful intervention, as long as all members of the trauma team believe it is morally acceptable to stop the therapy if it is hurtful or not helpful.

Organ transplantation also raises issues of nonmaleficence. Brain death can be difficult to establish in pediatric trauma victims, even when there is no hope for recovery. The case presentation described later in this chapter illustrates such a dilemma. The family members are devastated by the grim prognosis, but they may be able to find some comfort in organ donation so that another child may live. Criteria of pediatric brain death are based on measurable, physiologic parameters, but who can say with certainty the precise moment that brain death occurs? How much decreased cerebral blood flow can a child sustain and still recover? If a child does not fully meet the criteria but has no hope of recovery, are we doing harm by continuing hurtful treatment until the criteria are met? Do we decide organ transplantation is not an option and steal away what little comfort the family may be able to find? Do we avoid doing harm or invite it by declaring the child a candidate for organ donation? Unfortunately, the legal issues surrounding organ donation will not resolve the dilemma. Occasionally, a concern is raised that may be a matter of law, such as a Jehovah's Witness who refuses a transfusion. Without the transfusion, survival greatly diminishes and risk unnecessarily increases. The law clearly protects autonomous decisions, especially those concerning religious freedom.

Futility

Futility also raises the issues of withholding or withdrawing life-sustaining treatments, as well as extraordinary and ordinary treatments. Futility is often difficult to determine and rarely straightforward. Evidence of brain death provides measurable, objective criteria of futility. In infants younger than 1 week old, however, there is no consensus on brain death criteria (AAP, 1987). The dilemma faced by parents and health care providers is characterized by questioning whether the patient will recover to some level of functioning if life-sustaining treatments are used or whether an inevitable death, and possibly pain, is simply being prolonged. Similarly, there is no consensus on the meaning of extraordinary and ordinary treatments. Technologies such as antibiotics that were once extraordinary have become ordinary. *Extraordinary* usually refers to mechanical systems of life support or that, which if used, would not offer a reasonable hope of benefit (Beauchamp & Childress, 2001). Sometimes these distinctions cause much stress for the trauma nurse in the intensive care unit (ICU). "Extraordinary" care accounts for much of the trauma nurse's practice, and the nurse may feel morally obligated to provide that standard of care to all patients. Using the ethic of care as a framework, the trauma team would first come to a consensus of extraordinary and ordinary, discuss the options with the family, and support their decision.

Beneficence

The third important principle to incorporate into pediatric trauma nursing practice is that of beneficence. Simply stated, beneficence means "do good" (Beauchamp & Childress, 2001). Persons are obligated to take actions that benefit others, which is different than not doing any harm. In health care, beneficence is interpreted as protecting the rights of others, preventing harm, removing harmful conditions, rescuing persons in harm, and helping persons with disabilities (Beauchamp & Childress, 2001). Beneficence guides the pediatric trauma nurse toward actions and interventions that protect. Children usually are protected by their parents, but this is not the case for many pediatric trauma victims. Parents cannot always be presumed to "do good" or to make the appropriate decisions for their children (Dorr, 1997). When practice is guided by the ethic of care, beneficence obligates the pediatric trauma nurse to nurture a relationship with the patient and family. This may be a formidable challenge when the child is a victim of abuse and may lead to moral distress for the trauma nurse.

Justice

The last principle to consider is that of justice. *Distributive justice* refers to fair, equitable, and appropriate distribution of benefits and burdens, such as resources, privileges, and opportunities (Beauchamp & Childress, 2001). As it relates to pediatric trauma, the principle of justice asserts that persons should be treated equally, despite any and all differences to others. Opportunity for expensive, highly technical interventions is the same for the governor's son as it is for the abandoned ward of the state. Dilemmas may arise when resources are limited and cannot be distributed equally. How are intensive care beds allocated and prioritized? Is health care a right or a privilege? What weight do prognosis and quality of life bring to bear? The principle of justice helps clarify the perspective that pediatric trauma nurses should consider when faced with an ethical dilemma. Justice eliminates the tendency to consider value judgments that may unnecessarily complicate the decision. Furthermore, the relationship-based ethic of care focuses the discussion around the family values.

DEVELOPMENT OF ETHICAL SKILLS

Any ethical model that guides pediatric trauma nursing care should be based on ethical principles, be collaborative in nature, and be family focused. The ethic of care forms the basis of the caring relationship between the health care team and the family (see Figure 3-1). Pediatric trauma team nurses and physicians must focus on developing a trusting relationship with the family during every encounter.

Bishop and Scudder (1996) contend that ethics is integral to nursing, a view echoed in the drafted (no. 9) *Code of Ethics for Nurses* (American Nurses Association, 2000). Nursing is a practice with an inherent moral sense. This view of nursing ethics is broad and encompasses being a good nurse, having a caring presence, being "called" to nursing, and therapeutically fostering the well-being of the client. Their work explores how the moral sense of nursing affects patient care and encourages new possibilities and visions of the good that will direct their future caring practices (Bishop & Scudder, 1996). This is not a book about application of nursing ethics; rather, the purpose is to raise consciousness about the value of ethics in nursing practice. Irving and Snider (2002) assert that the values associated with professional practice have never been more crucial to nursing, yet the ability required to deal with the issues of right and wrong is now perceived as less important than the mastery of facts. These authors believe that teaching the value of ethics begins with nurse educators, who are obligated to translate and transfer the standards and principles to their nursing students. One does not think about breathing unless breathing becomes a problem. Likewise, nurses do not think about ethics until an ethical dilemma presents itself. Bishop and Scudder (1996) advance our understanding of the ethical character required of all nurses so that we may participate in the intimate, complex relationships of patient care.

ETHICAL COMPETENCY

Pediatric trauma nurses must help their peers become skilled in ethical decision making. As in clinical practice, there are different levels of ethical competency that develop only with deliberate attention. Rubin (1996) describes experienced critical care nurses who have severely restricted ethical judgments, as evidenced by a lack of awareness of the ethical implications of their nursing interventions. Nurses in this study consistently confused ethical considerations with legal concerns. Rubin contends that they have not accepted responsibility for their nursing practice, as evidenced by consistently attributing responsibility for their decisions to others. For example, the physician who orders a large dose of morphine for a terminally ill patient provides the authorization needed for action. Nurses with limited ethical competency do not acknowledge any ethical dilemma in administering the morphine, only concern that it may be legal or illegal. This lack of responsibility has severely impeded their ability to develop a moral sense of their nursing practice. As a group, these nurses did not appreciate the good they did for their patients or how they influenced patients' desires (Rubin, 1996). Their clinical practice evolved from the task-oriented phase of a beginner nurse, but their lack of ethical competencies severely limited development of expert skills.

In contrast, expert nurses who were knowledgeable about the law and nurse practice act considered only patient and family needs when caring for a patient who was to be removed from life support. Nurses with ethical competence placed the patient and family's comfort above all other concerns, including professional security (Rubin, 1996). They readily distinguished qualitative differences in situations and expressed the salient aspects of an ethical dilemma for themselves, as well as the perspective of the patient and family. Ethically competent nurses know they make a difference in the lives of their patients and families, rather than believing they are unimportant members of the team whose only contributions are following orders. This is obviously an important characteristic of a pediatric trauma nurse, but one that cannot be achieved without deliberate attention.

Penticoff and Walden (2000) described similar results in a study of the influence of the practice environment and nurse characteristics on nurses' responses to perinatal ethical dilemmas. Nurses in this study were more likely to be involved in dilemma resolution when they perceived themselves to have more influence in their practice environments and when they had higher levels of concern about the ethical aspects of the situations. The researchers call for organizational strategies that increase nurses' perceptions about how they might influence practices of the multidisciplinary team. Although the participants in this study were perinatal nurses, the conclusions have relevance for any nurse who works in an environment fraught with ethical dilemmas.

LEARNING ACTIVITIES

Developing the skills necessary to participate in the full experience of pediatric trauma nursing requires acknowledgment of ethical learning needs, planned learning activities, and peer and administrative support. An environment that supports and expects a moral practice of nursing may originate from the manager but must be operationalized by the staff. A moral practice may be described as one in which the nurse is knowledgeable about and is an active participant in ethical decision making. Hiring trauma nurses who demonstrate their moral responsibilities will build and strengthen a supportive environment. Behavioral interview techniques may uncover evidence of ethical competency and moral responsibility. For example, asking an applicant to talk about a previous experience involving caring for a child who was declared brain dead or was a victim of child abuse or dealing parents with cultural beliefs that challenge the standards of trauma practice will provide evidence about the level of ethical competency the applicant will bring to the position. Novice and beginner nurses are expected to have limited ethical competency; experienced trauma nurses should have highly developed ethical competency skills.

Educational activities such as ethics grand rounds, journal clubs, and case presentations focus thinking on nursing ethics and provide nurses opportunities to develop moral competency and eventual expertise. Perhaps the most effective mechanism to support and develop ethical competency is to debrief with those persons involved in an ethical dilemma and to invite those new to the staff to experience the process. Debriefing sessions should always be facilitated by a trusted and respected member of the health care team who is ethically competent. The debriefing itself acknowledges the importance of ethical competency and enables a critique of the process used to manage the dilemma. If they have not realized it already, trauma nurses will begin to appreciate how they influence the decisions made by trauma victims and their families. Furthermore, the debriefing socializes trauma nurses into a supportive milieu where participation and collaboration in ethical dilemmas are expected and supported.

Managing Moral Distress

Pediatric trauma nurses are at high risk to experience moral distress because of the nature of their work. Jameton (1993) defines *moral distress* as a nurse's feeling of constraint that prevents nursing actions that normally should occur. Moral distress was reported in a study of pediatric nurses who described dilemmas in which all possible decisions would lead to equally poor results (Twomey, 2000). Moral distress is a serious concern that should not be ignored. It can be a precursor or symptom of "burnout," especially if trauma nurses believe their practice has little importance.

Staff members who are experiencing moral distress may be helped and supported by debriefing sessions because they provide an opportunity to share uncomfortable feelings and emotions with peers who experienced the same situation. Under the leadership of a trusted, ethically competent colleague, members of the trauma team may be able to talk openly about the stressful issues that haunt pediatric trauma nurses. A more intense intervention, such as professional intervention by a psychologist, may be necessary when members of the peer group are unable to provide support to each other. Most important, interventions specific to the culture and situation may be necessary to manage moral distress, and its presence must be recognized and acknowledged.

A Model of Family-Centered Care for Ethical Decision Making

Models of nursing care serve to illustrate relationships surrounding nursing practice issues. A model that operationalizes the ethic of care within a multidisciplinary team may enhance nurses' ethical competencies and provide a mechanism to prevent or minimize moral distress (see Figure 3-1). The model of family-centered care for ethical decision making in pediatric trauma illustrates the application of this model in an ethical dilemma encountered during the management of a pediatric trauma victim. A collaborative, family-centered care approach is used to establish a trusting relationship with the family, and the ethical principles provide a standard to guide decision making.

Case Presentation

Baby D, age 6 months, was securely fastened in her car seat facing backward in the rear seat of her mother's car when her side of the car was struck by a truck moving at high speed. Cardiopulmonary resuscitation (CPR) was performed at the scene. The infant was airlifted to the nearest trauma center, where the massive, crushing head injury was treated, but her prognosis was grave. Baby D required CPR several times in the ICU during the first 24 hours. Neurologic examination was consistent with brain death. At first, her parents did not accept the possibility of organ donation. On the second day, however, they came to understand the severity of her condition and decided organ donation was what they wanted. Within hours, Baby D met all the criteria for brain death except the brain flow study. Because the guidelines for certain brain death include absence of blood flow to the brain, plans for organ donation were put on hold. Two days after the accident, while the parents gathered family and friends to the hospital, the trauma team held a care conference to discuss the options available to them.

When an ethical dilemma is identified, a care conference or series of conferences should be convened to discuss the issues. First, who identified the dilemma and why? Does the dilemma involve the child, the family, the trauma nurse, the doctor, or a combination? Is the dilemma shared by others? What is the nature of the dilemma? In the case of Baby D, all members of the team shared the dilemma. They could not pursue organ donation without a negative brain flow study, yet it was clear the patient could not recover. The pain of the family permeated the ICU, and the staff wanted to intervene in a caring and meaningful manner.

Once the dilemma is confirmed as legitimate and not a personal issue for a single member of the team, the trauma team should discuss the situation in relation to the ethical principles of autonomy, nonmaleficence, beneficence, and justice. Talking about the dilemma from the perspective of the principles allows clarification of the nature of the dilemma and often eliminates some of the alternative solutions or actions. The goal of the care conference should be to raise concerns and biases, yet come to consensus on the message brought to the parents to preserve the trusting and caring relationship. When the trauma team met to discuss their concerns about Baby D's case, they believed that the evidence supported brain death and that the life support systems maintaining her fragile life were no longer hurtful to her (nonmaleficence). There was consensus on the futility of further medical and surgical interventions. They were concerned, however, with beneficence: They wanted to do good. In their estimation, "doing good" translated to fulfilling the parent's wishes for organ donation to end the nightmare the parents were living in the ICU. They believed, in their experienced medical and nursing judgment, that continuing life support would not be in Baby D's best interest. They also conceded that organ donation may still be an option. Those members of the heath care team who cannot come to consensus because of their religious beliefs or values should be able to remove themselves from the decision. This was not a factor in Baby D's case.

The care conference provides the opportunity for the trauma team to develop consensus and articulate the message that will be brought to the parents. The message may be a nonjudgmental overview of the available options or a recommendation for the family. When the recommendation to withhold or withdraw life-sustaining treatment is considered, a consultation from an attending physician and expert pediatric trauma nurse who are not directly involved in the case will support or suggest that more evidence is needed. Van Marter (1998) describes such a collaborative consultation in her review of neonatal ethical decision making. The sensitive nature of ethical dilemmas in pediatric nursing and the general infrequency of these occurrences may warrant using such an innovative mechanism to exhaust all possibilities before a decision is made.

Baby D's case raised issues that may be common in pediatric trauma nursing. Is there enough physiologic evidence to confirm and satisfy everyone's requirements of futility? Does the hospital policy regarding brain death determination allow room for medical judgment? Requesting a consultation from an expert nurse and physician colleague who have not been directly involved in the case enables a nonbiased viewpoint. They may find in support of the trauma team or request additional examinations to confirm. Two such experts examined Baby D and reviewed her medical record and consultation reports. They also spoke with the parents to assess their understanding of the situation. They suggested repeating the flow study, although the results did not change. They were in full agreement with the trauma team and documented their assessment in the medical record.

At the same time the trauma team is holding the care conference, the family should be encouraged to seek support and guidance from other family members and clergy. A family meeting after the care conference, to discuss the family's concerns, will help maintain an atmosphere of trust and caring. The team from the care conference that meets with the family should be multidisciplinary, but it is suggested that there be no more than three team members to avoid overwhelming the family. An attending physician and the pediatric trauma nurse are imperative to the discussion and be responsible for supporting the decision. Baby D's family began to gather soon after the accident, and their clergy also joined the vigil. The trauma team developed a plan of communication at the conclusion of the care conference. They decided that the attending physician, the primary nurse, and the hospital chaplain would hold the family meeting.

Requirements of the Pediatric Trauma Nurse

Pediatric trauma nurses should be ethically competent. They should have basic knowledge of the ethical principles described earlier and of their own system of values and beliefs. A knowledge of self is critical to the collaborative nature of the model. One must be comfortable with uncertainty and respect the beliefs and traditions from different cultures. The nurse must understand that another person's values cannot be changed to make him or her conform to a common standard. The trauma nurse must accept that it does not matter what he or she would do in the situation, even if the family seeks this information. The ethically competent nurse distances his or her own values and beliefs from the situation and attempts to consider the case without those biases. Furthermore, the nurse requires the same of his or her colleagues, if the discussion warrants. The trauma nurse must have skilled listening techniques to understand the family's concerns and share them with other members of the health care team as they discuss the ethical dilemma.

The pediatric trauma nurse must be familiar with the policies of the facility regarding ethical dilemmas. The policy may specify a chain of command or the patient bill of rights, which may influence how ethical dilemmas are managed. The ethics committee in the facility may be available to review cases, listen to family concerns, or provide education for staff. Pediatric trauma nurses who are able anticipate potential dilemmas through their experiences in continuing education or case presentation will become more familiar with the process. Thinking about potential situations beforehand enables a range of discussion among members of the entire health care team, which may increase comfort in actual situations. Finally, a willingness to "debrief" together as a health care team or among pediatric nurses will identify opportunities for improvement and educational needs. The debriefing also serves to acknowledge the work and outcomes of the team, which may increase team effectiveness in the future.

THE MODEL AS A PROFESSIONAL PRACTICE STANDARD

The first statement in the *Code for Nurses* (American Nurses Association, 1985) states, "The nurse provides services with respect for human dignity and the uniqueness of the client unrestricted by considerations of social or economic status, personal attributes, or the nature of health problems." Pediatric trauma nurses are a critical component of the ethical decision-making process. Their role enables a strong, trusting relationship with families that supports family-centered care. This model illustrates nurses' equal role with physicians and other members of the health care team when they are fully prepared to participate. They must be able to separate from their personal biases, be willing to dissociate from the team if they cannot be open to any decision, and know how to apply ethical principles. The model also acknowledges and enables expert nurses to provide consultation to their colleagues. The eighth statement in the *Code for Nurses* reads, "The nurse participates in the profession's efforts to implement and improve standards of nursing." Using this model, pediatric trauma nurses will apply a professional practice standard for children and families who are faced with an ethical dilemma. Finally, the first line of the most recent draft (no. 9) of the *Code of Ethics for Nurses* is "Ethics is the foundation upon which nursing is built" (American Nurses Association, 2000). Our direction could not be more clearly stated.

BIBLIOGRAPHY

American Academy of Pediatrics. (1987). Guidelines for the determination of brain death in children. American Academy of Pediatrics Task Force on Brain Death in Children. *Pediatrics, 80,* 298-300.

American Academy of Pediatrics, Committee on Bioethics. (1995). Informed consent, parental permission, and assent in pediatric practice. *Pediatrics, 95*(2), 314-317.

American Nurses Association. (1985). *Code for nurses.* Washington, DC: American Nurses Association.

American Nurses Association. (2000). *Code of ethics for nurses, draft no. 9.* Retrieved August 23, 2000, from http://www.ana.org/ethics.code9.pdf.

Beauchamp, T. L., & Childress, J. F. (2001). *Principles of biomedical ethics* (5th ed.). New York: Oxford University Press.

Bishop, A. H., & Scudder, J. R. (1996). *Nursing ethics: Therapeutic caring presence.* Sudbury, MA: Jones and Bartlett.

Burkhardt, M. A., & Nathaniel, A. K. (1998). *Ethics and issues in contemporary nursing.* Albany, NY: Delmar.

Caplan, A., Capron, A. M., Murray, T. H., & Penticuff, J. (1987). Deciding not to employ aggressive measures. *Hastings Center Report, 17*(6), 7-9.

Claassen, M. (2000). A handful of questions: Supporting parental decision making. *Clinical Nurse Specialist, 14*(4), 189-195.

Dorr, P. (1997). Outcomes manager: Brain death criteria in the pediatric patient. *Critical Care Nursing Quarterly, 20*(1), 14-21.

Emergency Nurses Association. (2001). *Position statement: Family presence at the bedside during invasive procedures and/or resuscitation.* Developed April 1994; Revised May 1996, from http://www.eha.org/services/posistate/statements/FamilyPresene.html

Graham, J. P. (1994). Children: Problems in pediatrics. In J. H. Hattah (Ed.), *Ethics and child mental health* (pp. 189-198). Israel: Gefen Publication House.

Hanson, C., & Strawser, D. (1992). Family presence during cardiopulmonary resuscitation: Foote Hospital emergency department's nine-year perspective. *Journal of Emergency Nursing, 18*(2), 104-106.

Irving, J. A., & Snider, J. (2002). Preserving professional values. *Journal of Professional Nursing, 18*(1), 5.

Jameton, A. (1993). Dilemmas of moral distress: Moral responsibility and nursing practice. *AWHONNS Clinical Issues in Perinatal and Women's Health Nursing, 4*(4), 542-551.

Kikuchi, J. F., & Simmons, H. (Eds.). (1992). *Philosophic inquiry in nursing.* Thousand Oaks, CA: Sage Publications.

Kikuchi, J., Simmons, H., & Romyn, D. (1996). *Truth in nursing inquiry.* Thousand Oaks, CA: Sage Publications.

Meyers, T. A., Eichhorn, D. J., Guzzetta, C. E., Clark, A. P., Klein, J. D., Taliaferro, E., & Calvin, A. (2000). Family presence during invasive procedures and resuscitation. *American Journal of Nursing, 100*(2), 32-40.

National Commission for the Protection of Human Subjects of Biomedical and Behavioral Research. (1979). *The Belmont Report: Ethical principles and guidelines for the protection of human subjects of research.* Washington, DC: U.S. Department of Health, Education, and Welfare.

Omery, A. (1995). Care: The basis for a nursing ethic? *Journal of Cardiovascular Nursing, 9*(3), 1-10.

Penticoff, J. H., & Walden, M. (2000). Influence of practice environment and nurse characteristics on perinatal nurses' responses to ethical dilemmas. *Nursing Research, 49*(2), 64-71.

Rubin, J. (1996). Impediments to the development of clinical knowledge and ethical judgment in critical care nursing. In P. Benner, C. A. Tanner, & C. A. Chesla (Eds.), *Expertise in nursing practice: Caring, clinical judgment, and ethics* (pp. 170-192). New York: Springer.

Senecal, S. (1999). Pain management of wound care. *Nursing Clinics of North America, 34*(1), 847-860.

Twomey, J. G. (2000). Ethical voices of pediatric mental health nurses. *Journal of Pediatric Nursing, 15*(1), 36-46.

U.S. Department of Health and Human Services. (1991). Title 46, protection of human subjects. In *Code of federal regulations* (pp. 4-17). Washington, DC: U.S. Department of Health and Human Services, National Institutes of Health, Office for Protection from Research Risks.

Van Marter, L. J. (1998). Decision making and ethical dilemmas. In J. P. Cloherty & A. R. Stark (Eds.), *Manual of neonatal care* (4th ed.). Philadelphia: Lippincott-Raven.

Wagner, N., & Hendel, T. (2000). Ethics in pediatric nursing: An international perspective. *Journal of Pediatric Nursing, 15*(1), 54-59.

Wong, D. L., Hockenberry-Eaton, M., Wilson, D., Winkelstein, M. L., Ahmann, E., & DiVito-Thomas, P. A. (1999). *Whaley & Wong's nursing care of infants and children* (6th ed.). St. Louis: Mosby.

SECTION

CLINICAL CONCEPTS

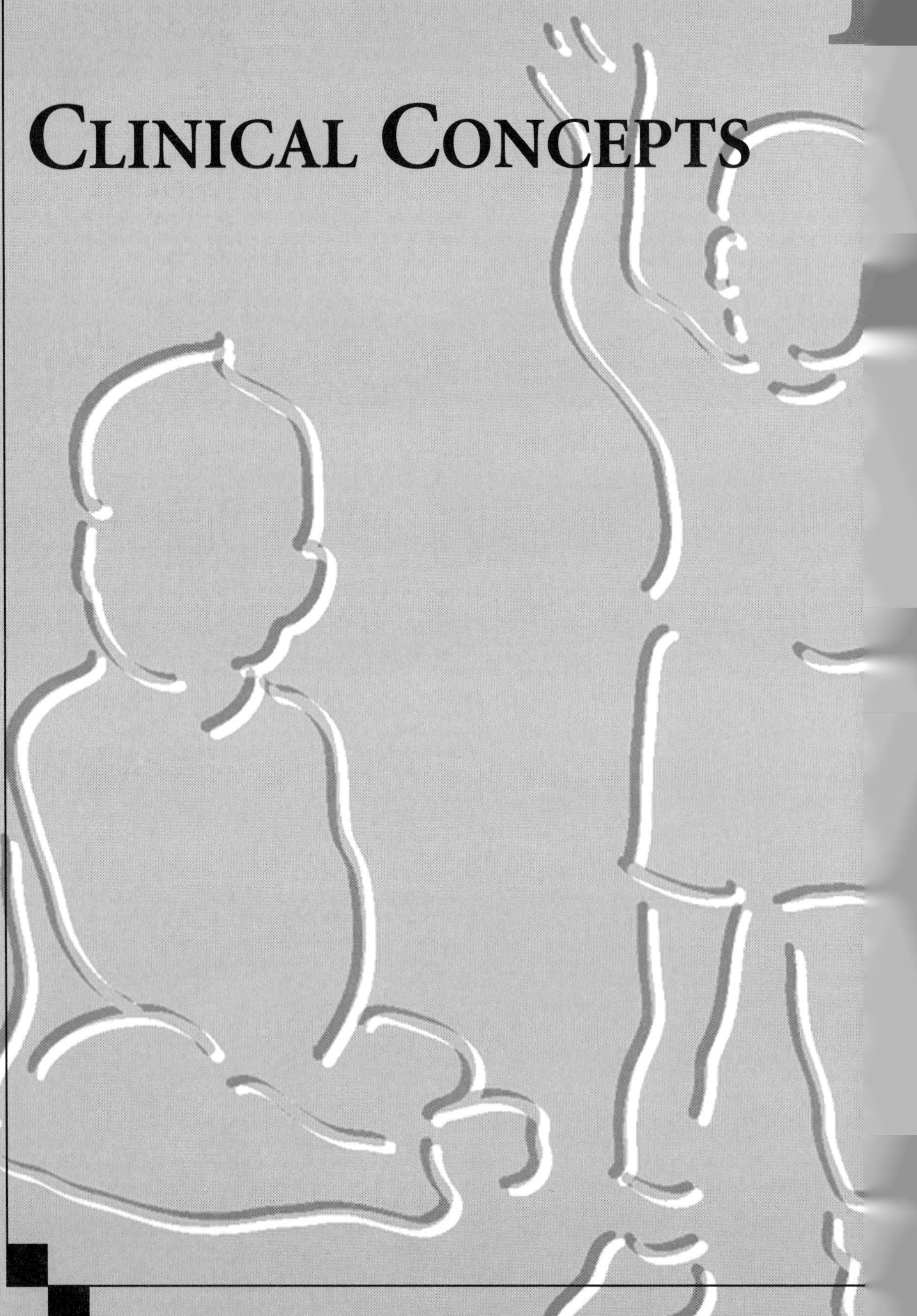

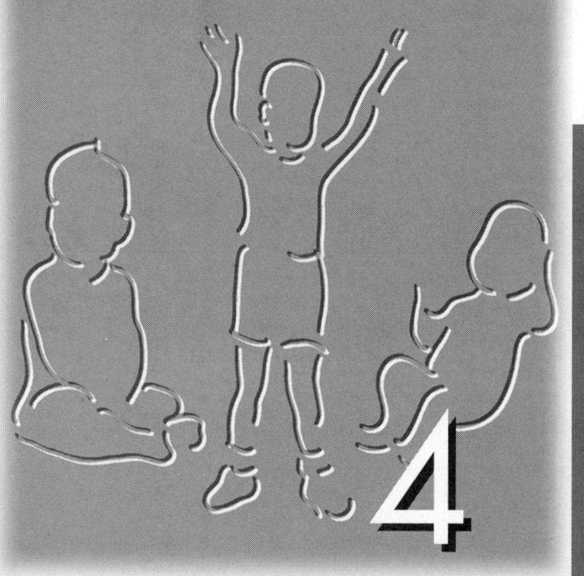

4 Children Are Different: Pediatric Differences and the Impact on Trauma

Lisa A. Rupp • Michael W. Day

In developed countries, traumatic injuries are the leading cause of death and disability in children older than 1 year. In children between the ages of 1 and 19 years, injuries cause more deaths than all diseases combined and are a leading cause of disability (National Center for Health Statistics, 1999). It is estimated that more than 30,000 children sustain permanent disabilities from injury every year in the United States (National Center for Health Statistics, 1999).

Even though the statistics are grim, the child has a significant potential for recovery. Therefore appropriate resuscitation begins as soon as possible after the injury. Successful evaluation and resuscitation of the pediatric trauma patient requires a thorough understanding of the anatomic and physiologic differences in children, an appropriately equipped and organized resuscitation area, and initial and ongoing education to maintain staff competency in caring for the critically injured child.

This chapter highlights key differences in pediatric anatomy and physiology, with emphasis on how these differences affect assessment and intervention. Second, this chapter proposes two possible strategies for equipping and organizing the pediatric resuscitation area. Specific recommendations are made for the initial and ongoing education of staff caring for pediatric trauma patients.

PEDIATRIC TRAUMA SCORING

Optimal care of the pediatric trauma patient depends not only on having knowledge of the important anatomic and physiologic differences in children but also on having established pediatric trauma criteria to activate an appropriate team response and identify the need for transport. The Pediatric Trauma Score (PTS), developed from data collected by the Pediatric Trauma Registry, has demonstrated accuracy in predicting injury severity (Tepas, Ramenofsky, Mollitt, Gans, & DiScala, 1988). The PTS scores six components, with a +2 for a minor injury and a −1 for a critical injury (Table 4-1). The component scores are added together and range from 12 to −6. Most sources recommend that children with a PTS of 8 or less be transported to a regional pediatric trauma center (Sabel & Bassuk, 1996).

Serious consideration is given to the transfer of the critically injured pediatric patient to a trauma center having comprehensive resources and expertise in treating children. These patients gain the benefit of the resources available in a tertiary intensive care unit. “Severely ill children are less likely to die when they are treated in a tertiary intensive care unit than in a community hospital” (Pollack, Alexander, Clarke, Ruttimann, Tesselaar, & Bachulis, 1991). Furthermore, in the first published study comparing the use of a specialized pediatric transport team with a nonspecialized transport team, it was concluded that the use of specialized pediatric transport teams can reduce transport morbidity (Edge, Kanter, Weigle, & Walsh, 1994).

ANATOMIC AND PHYSIOLOGIC DIFFERENCES BETWEEN CHILDREN AND ADULTS: ASSESSMENT AND INTERVENTION

Because children are not small adults, their injuries may be very different than those sustained by adults when the same

TABLE 4-1 Pediatric Trauma Score

Component	Category +2	+1	−1
Size (kg)	≥20	10-20	<10
Airway	Normal	Maintainable	Unmaintainable
Systolic blood pressure (mm Hg)	≥90	90-50	<50
Central nervous system	Awake	Obtunded/loss of consciousness	Coma/decerebrate
Open wound	None	Minor	Major/penetrating
Skeletal	None	Closed fracture	Open/multiple fractures
Sum total points			

From Tepas, J., Ramenofsky, M., Mollitt, D., Gans, B., & DiScala, C. (1988). The pediatric trauma score as a predictor of injury severity: An objective assessment. *Journal of Trauma, 28*(4), 427.

traumatic forces are applied. Blunt trauma is significantly more common in the pediatric patient. Because of the child's smaller size, traumatic forces are distributed over a larger area, making multisystem trauma the rule rather than the exception in the pediatric patient. Children also have lesser amounts of subcutaneous tissue and protective muscle; therefore blunt traumatic forces may cause significant injury to underlying organs, with little or no external trauma. The most commonly injured body areas are the head, musculoskeletal system, thorax, and abdomen. The genitourinary system and spinal cord are less commonly injured (Emergency Nurses Association, 2000).

The child with multisystem trauma may have both respiratory and circulatory compromise; therefore resuscitation with priority placed on airway, breathing, and circulation must begin immediately. Three common errors in a pediatric trauma resuscitation include failure to (1) open and maintain the airway, (2) provide adequate fluid resuscitation to the head-injured child, and (3) recognize and treat internal hemorrhage.

Effective management of the pediatric trauma patient requires not only knowledge of the anatomic and physiologic differences between children and adults but also recognition of the clinical significance of these differences and the appropriate interventions. In addition to recognizing and acting on these differences, caregivers should be aware of the age-related variations in children's vital signs and responsiveness (Tables 4-2 and 4-3). The clinical significance of anatomic and physiologic differences in children is reviewed in Table 4-4.

Text continued on p. 41

TABLE 4-2 Pediatric Vital Signs

Age	Heart Rate (beats/min)	Respirations (breaths/min)	Systolic Blood Pressure (mm Hg)
Newborn	100-160	30-60	50-70
1-6 wk	100-160	30-60	70-95
6 mo	90-120	25-40	80-100
1 yr	90-120	20-30	80-100
3 yr	80-120	20-30	80-110
6 yr	70-110	18-25	80-110
10 yr	60-90	15-20	90-120
14 yr	60-90	15-20	90-130

Data from Hudak, C. M., Gallo, B. M., & Morton, P. M. (Eds.). (1998). *Critical care nursing: A holistic approach* (p. 106). Philadelphia: Lippincott.

TABLE 4-3 Glasgow Coma Scale

Response	Adults and Children	Infants	Points
Eye opening	No response	No response	1
	To pain	To pain	2
	To voice	To voice	3
	Spontaneous	Spontaneous	4
Verbal	No response	No response	1
	Incomprehensible	Moans to pain	2
	Inappropriate words	Cries to pain	3
	Disoriented conversation	Irritable	4
	Oriented and appropriate	Coos, babbles	5
Motor	No response	No response	1
	Decerebrate posturing	Decerebrate posturing	2
	Decorticate posturing	Decorticate posturing	3
	Withdraws to pain	Withdraws to pain	4
	Localizes pain	Withdraws to touch	5
	Obeys commands	Normal spontaneous movement	6
Total score			3-15

TABLE 4-4 Clinical Significance of Anatomic and Physiologic Differences in Children

Assessment	Clinical Significance	Interventions
Airway Differences		
Smaller upper and lower airways	Foreign matter such as blood, mucus, vomit, and teeth easily obstruct small airways Small amounts of edema can obstruct the airway, markedly increasing airway resistance	Suction mouth and nose frequently Administer nebulized bronchodilators as indicated
Tongue is larger relative to the oropharynx	Airway is commonly obstructed by the tongue, especially in the patient with a depressed level of consciousness	In the trauma patient, open the airway using the jaw-thrust maneuver Repositioning often may be the only intervention needed to maintain a patent airway Oropharyngeal airways can be used in the unresponsive child
Cartilage of the larynx is softer	Hyperextension or hyperflexion of the neck can compress and obstruct the airway	Place child in "sniffing" position with chin-lift maneuver Use jaw thrust in the trauma patient
Larger head/body ratio	Neck may be in flexion when a child is immobilized on a backboard (Figure 4-1)	Place a small towel roll under the child's shoulders to maintain the "sniffing" position
Infants are obligate nose breathers for the first several months of life	Obstructed nasal passages can produce significant respiratory distress in the infant	Suction nares frequently Nasopharyngeal airway may be placed
Larynx is positioned more anteriorly and cephalad	There is an increased risk of aspiration Direct visualization of the vocal cords is more difficult during intubation	Use cricoid pressure to compress the esophagus against the spine during bag-mask ventilation to help prevent gastric insufflation and aspiration This maneuver also assists with visualization of the vocal cords during intubation attempts (Figure 4-2)
Shorter tracheal length	There is an increased chance of mainstem intubation Changes in head position will cause movement in endotracheal tube Flexion of the neck displaces the tube further into the trachea and extension of the neck moves the tube farther out of the trachea	Pay meticulous attention to initial endotracheal tube position (centimeter mark at the gum) Perform recurrent reassessment of tube placement with postintubation chest x-ray films Maintain head in midline position and prevent extension or flexion of the neck
Cricoid cartilage is the narrowest portion of the airway	Cricoid ring provides a natural seal for the endotracheal tube Cuffed tubes may cause airway damage in younger children	Use uncuffed endotracheal tubes in children age <8 yr
Respiratory Differences		
Cartilaginous ribs of the infant and small child are twice as compliant as those of an adult	Retractions are more common and reduce the infant's or small child's ability to maintain functional residual capacity or generate adequate tidal volume	Closely observe the child with continuous monitoring of heart rate, respiratory rate and effort, and pulse oximetry Deliver highest possible concentration of oxygen to infants and children in respiratory distress Provide nonthreatening environment and avoid noxious stimuli Allow alert child to maintain own position of comfort to optimize respiratory effort Allow parents to remain with child if their presence is comforting to the child
Intercostal muscles are poorly developed	Generation of tidal volume depends on diaphragmatic function Anything impeding diaphragm movement can lead to respiratory failure	If possible, maintain patient in upright position to support diaphragmatic function Avoid abdominal distention by inserting a nasogastric or orogastric tube to decompress the stomach

Continued

TABLE 4-4 **Clinical Significance of Anatomic and Physiologic Differences in Children— cont'd**

Assessment	Clinical Significance	Interventions
Respiratory Differences—cont'd		
The child's respiratory system has less compensatory reserve than the adult's respiratory system	The younger child may develop respiratory distress and failure more rapidly than an adult	Closely observe the child with continuous monitoring of heart rate, respiratory rate and effort, and pulse oximetry Deliver highest possible concentration of oxygen in a nonthreatening manner Consider blood gas analysis
Infants with respiratory distress often grunt during exhalation	Grunting is a result of premature glottic closure during exhalation Infants grunt to increase airway pressure, lung volume, and functional residual capacity	Provide high concentration of supplemental oxygen and consider ventilatory support
Infants and small children have less elastic and collagen tissue in their lungs	Liquid or air can enter an infant's pulmonary interstitium more easily than in the older child or adult, making the infant more susceptible to air leaks and edema	Maintain high index of suspicion for pneumothorax, pneumomediastinum, and pulmonary edema Obtain chest x-ray films as necessary
Infants and small children have thin chest walls	Breath sounds are easily transmitted across the chest wall and over the abdomen	Frequently reassess bilateral breath sounds with side-by-side comparison of differences in pitch and intensity Breath sounds should be auscultated over the anterior and posterior chest wall, and in the axillary areas, using a pediatric stethoscope Obtain chest x-ray films as necessary
Circulatory Differences		
Myocardium is less compliant and has less contractile tissue compared with that of an adult	Stroke volume is not easily adjusted; therefore children increase their heart rate in response to falling cardiac output	Provide continuous ECG monitoring with attention to trends in heart rate Tachycardia is the earliest clinical manifestation in compensated shock, but it also may be a result of anxiety, pain, fever, or increased activity If other signs of compensated shock are present (delayed capillary refill time, cool extremities, duskiness or mottling of the skin, diminished peripheral pulses, narrowing pulse pressure, tachypnea), rapid intravenous access is established and fluid resuscitation is initiated
There is a greater ability to compensate for falling cardiac output by increasing peripheral vascular resistance	Children may remain normotensive until 25% of their blood volume is lost Hypotension is a late and often sudden sign of cardiovascular decompensation (Figure 4-3)	Look for early indications of compensated shock as noted above Begin fluid resuscitation when compensated shock is present Even mild hypotension must be treated quickly and aggressively because hypotension indicates decompensated shock state and cardiopulmonary arrest may be imminent
Infants and children have a smaller overall blood volume	Although the child's circulating blood volume is greater per kilogram of body weight compared with an adult (child 80 ml/kg vs. adult 70 ml/kg), the circulating volume is significantly less Smaller amounts of blood loss can cause volume depletion (Table 4-5)	Carefully estimate blood loss, including blood drawn for laboratory analysis Serial hemoglobin and hematocrit analysis should be obtained Consider blood replacement therapy after 40-60 ml/kg of isotonic crystalloids in the pediatric trauma patient with signs of shock or when acute blood loss totals 5%-7% of the child's circulating blood volume (Hazinski, 1997)

TABLE 4-4 Clinical Significance of Anatomic and Physiologic Differences in Children—cont'd

Assessment	Clinical Significance	Interventions
Circulatory Differences—cont'd		
Most arrhythmias are clinically insignificant in the pediatric patient and do not require treatment	Bradycardia and SVT are the two most common significant arrhythmias in children	Provide continuous ECG monitoring Establish and maintain patent airway
Bradycardia is the most common terminal cardiac rhythm in children, whereas ventricular tachycardia or fibrillation is the usual terminal rhythm in the adult	Bradycardia is often a result of hypoxia and is not well tolerated in children because it significantly reduces cardiac output SVT usually is well tolerated in infants and children, but can lead to cardiovascular collapse	Provide adequate oxygenation and ventilation Establish intravenous access If severe cardiorespiratory compromise as evidenced by poor perfusion, respiratory distress, or hypotension is present, follow the Pediatric Advanced Life Support decision trees for bradycardia or tachycardia with poor perfusion (American Heart Association, 2000)
A greater percentage of total body weight is water in infants and children	Infants and young children will lose larger amounts of water through evaporation than will the adult	Calculate maintenance fluids based on each child's weight in kilograms and clinical condition
There is a larger surface area/volume ratio	Children have greater potential for dehydration Maintenance fluid requirements per kilogram of body weight are higher in children	Record all sources of fluid intake and fluid loss to calculate fluid balance and adjust fluid therapy accordingly
Infants and children have smaller, more difficult to cannulate veins	Rapid establishment of intravenous access is more difficult in infants and children	Establish a protocol that addresses obtaining intravenous and intraosseous access in critically ill or injured children For example, the Pediatric Advanced Life Support text recommends that during cardiopulmonary resuscitation, intraosseous access be established if venous access is not achieved rapidly (Figure 4-4)
Neurologic Differences		
The head of the infant and young child is larger and heavier in proportion to the rest of the body	If an infant or child falls or is thrown a significant distance, the initial impact more often will be to the head, which predisposes the child to head injury	Anticipate head injury in the traumatically injured child Suggest use of stress preventive measures, such as seat belts, car seats, and helmets, to patients and family members
The skull is thinner during infancy and childhood	The thin skull provides less protection for the brain Head trauma can result in severe brain injury in children	Same as above
Cranial sutures do not fuse until approximately age 16-18 mo	If intracranial volume increases during this time, head circumference may increase This ability to expand may better accommodate gradual increases in intracranial volume than in an adult Increased intracranial pressure may still develop, especially with acute increases in intracranial volume	Measure occipital frontal circumference with neurologic examinations in the child up to age 16-18 mo at risk for increasing intracranial pressure
Anterior and posterior fontanelles are open in infants	The anterior fontanelle is the junction of the coronal-sagittal and frontal bones and does not close until age 16-18 mo The posterior fontanelle is the junction of the parietal and occipital bones and closes at approximately age 2 mo The fontanelles will be tense or bulging in the event of increased intracranial pressure and will be sunken if the infant is dehydrated	Assess fontanelles for size and tension in the infant age 16-18 mo or younger

Continued

TABLE 4-4 Clinical Significance of Anatomic and Physiologic Differences in Children—cont'd

Assessment	Clinical Significance	Interventions
Neurologic Differences—cont'd		
Spinal cord injuries are less common in the pediatric trauma patient than in the adult trauma patient	The child's spine, especially the cervical spine, is more elastic and mobile When a child sustains a spinal cord injury, it is often present without radiographic abnormality, described as spinal cord injury without radiographic abnormality (SCIWORA)	Children with head and/or neck injuries should be presumed to have a spinal cord injury until proven otherwise Stabilize and immobilize the cervical spine with a hard cervical collar, long spine board, and either a commercial immobilization device or foam blocks, towel rolls, and tape Remember, the child's prominent occiput places the neck in flexion when lying flat on a spine board Place padding under the child's torso to elevate it approximately 2 cm, bringing the head into neutral position (see Figure 4-1)
Musculoskeletal Differences		
Children's bones are more flexible because of incomplete bone calcification	Significant force generally is necessary to break children's bones Underlying injury may be present without a fracture	Suspect injury to internal structures underlying fractures and areas subjected to significant forces as evidenced by contusions, swelling, and tenderness Obtain surgical consultation as necessary Monitor for signs of internal hemorrhage: Decreasing level of consciousness, poor peripheral perfusion, decreased urinary output, tachycardia, tachypnea, and narrowing pulse pressure Obtain hemoglobin and hematocrit analysis as necessary
There is increased elasticity and compliance of the chest wall because the ribs and sternum are more cartilaginous in infants and young children	There is a low incidence of rib or sternal fractures in children Increased chest wall compliance allows traumatic forces to be transmitted to underlying thoracic structures Pneumothorax is the most common result of thoracic trauma in children and may be more likely to progress to a tension pneumothorax due to the increased mobility of mediastinal structures	Suspect pneumothoraces and/or hemothoraces in the child who has significant chest trauma with or without rib fractures Monitor respiratory effort and oxygen saturation Obtain chest x-ray films as necessary Be prepared for needle thoracostomy or chest tube insertion in the event of a tension pneumothorax
Abdominal muscles are less developed in children	Children are at an increased risk of sustaining abdominal injuries The spleen and the liver are the most commonly injured abdominal organs in children (Emergency Nurses Association, 2000)	Obtain surgical consultation as necessary Monitor for signs of shock secondary to internal hemorrhage Obtain serial abdominal girth measurements Follow serial hemoglobin and hematocrit analysis
Pseudosubluxation of C2 on C3	This is seen in up to 40% of children age <7 yr and in <20% of children age <16 yr This is a normal variation caused by increased ligamentous laxity (Inaba and Seward, 1991)	Maintain cervical spine immobilization and suspect spinal cord injury in any child with head and neck injuries Perform thorough serial neurologic examinations Do not rule out cervical spine injury on the basis of negative radiographic studies only Neurosurgical consultation should be obtained Computed tomography scan and magnetic resonance imaging may be useful adjuncts in the evaluation of possible spinal cord injuries

TABLE 4-4 Clinical Significance of Anatomic and Physiologic Differences in Children—cont'd

Assessment	Clinical Significance	Interventions
Metabolic and Thermoregulation Differences		
Infants and young children have a larger body surface area/body mass ratio, and less insulating subcutaneous tissue and fat stores	A great deal of heat is lost to the environment through radiation and evaporation, especially from the child's proportionally large head Infants and children can become hypothermic very easily Hypothermia can cause metabolic acidosis, hypoglycemia, coagulopathies, central nervous system depression, respiratory depression, and myocardial irritability, making resuscitation more difficult	Monitor temperature frequently Cover children with warm blankets or place them under warming lights if they cannot be covered Use warmed intravenous fluids or blood for volume resuscitation Warm and humidify supplemental oxygen if possible Place warming pads, such as K pads, or chemically activated warming devices, such as porta warmers, under children Follow manufacturer's directions for the use of these devices
Infants <3 mo cannot produce heat by shivering and must burn their limited fat stores for thermogenesis	There is an increased risk of hypothermia in the small infant The burning of fat increases oxygen consumption, which can lead to hypoxia	Same as above Consider placing small infants in isolettes with overbed warmers Attach skin probe for continuous skin temperature monitoring to avoid underheating or overheating and thermal injury
Infants and young children have less glycogen stores than adults	The ill or injured child is at increased risk for developing hypoglycemia	Monitor glucose frequently during and after resuscitation Administer glucose as ordered
Children have higher metabolic rates than adults	Higher metabolic rates increase oxygen consumption The child's nutritional needs are higher per kilogram of body weight than in an adult	Provide supplemental oxygen to all seriously ill or injured children Consult with physician and dietitian to provide early, adequate nutritional support to the compromised child

ECG, Electrocardiograph; *SVT,* supraventricular tachycardia.

TABLE 4-5 Systemic Responses to Blood Loss in the Pediatric Trauma Patient

	Early Blood Loss (<25% Blood Volume Loss)	Prehypotensive (25%-40% Blood Volume Loss)	Hypotensive (>40% Blood Volume Loss)
Cardiac	Weak, thready pulse Increased heart rate	Tachycardia Positive tilt test	Hypotension Tachycardia to bradycardia
Central nervous system	Irritable, combative Confused, lethargic	Decreased consciousness Dulled response to pain	Comatose
Skin	Cool, clammy	Cyanotic, cold extremities Decreased capillary refill	Pale, cold
Renal	Decreased urine output	—	No urine output

From Jaimovich, D. G., & Vidyasagar, D. (1995). *Handbook of pediatric and neonatal transport medicine.* Philadelphia: Hanley & Belfus.

PREPARING THE RESUSCITATION AREA FOR PEDIATRIC PATIENTS

Few situations are as stress evoking as the initial moments after a center receives a report that a critically injured child is en route to the facility. These situations can be both clinically and emotionally challenging. Maintaining an appropriately equipped and well-organized pediatric resuscitation area may help reduce some of the stress in these situations. Because pediatric emergency care is delivered from rural and community hospitals to large medical centers with comprehensive pediatric services, all facilities responsible for treating critically ill or injured children require the appropriate equipment, medications, and skilled personnel available to resuscitate and initiate stabilization of these children.

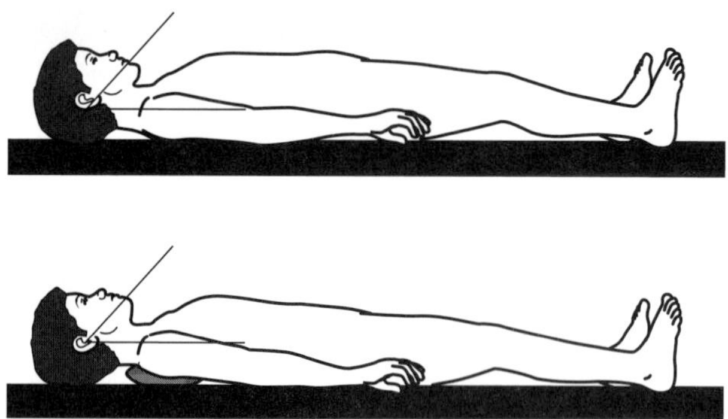

FIGURE 4-1 Child on backboard. (From Emergency Nurses Association. [2000]. Pediatric trauma. In B. Bennett-Jacobs [Ed.], *Trauma nursing core course provider manual.* Park Ridge, IL: Emergency Nurses Association.)

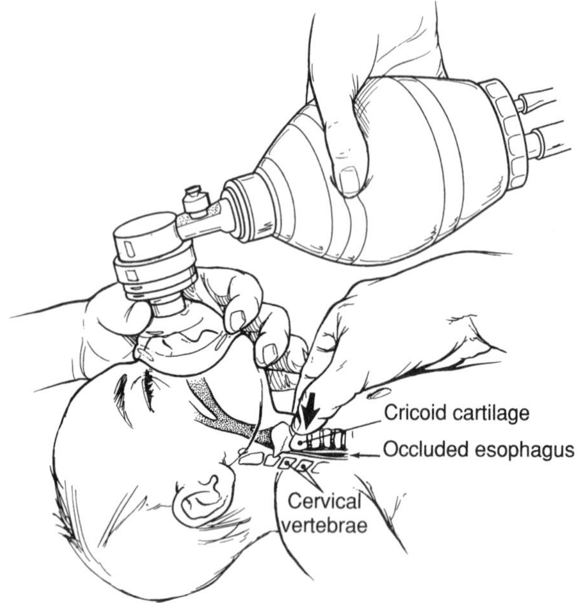

FIGURE 4-2 Bag-mask ventilation. (From Chameides, L., & Hazinski, M. F. [1997]. *Pediatric advanced life support.* Dallas: American Heart Association.)

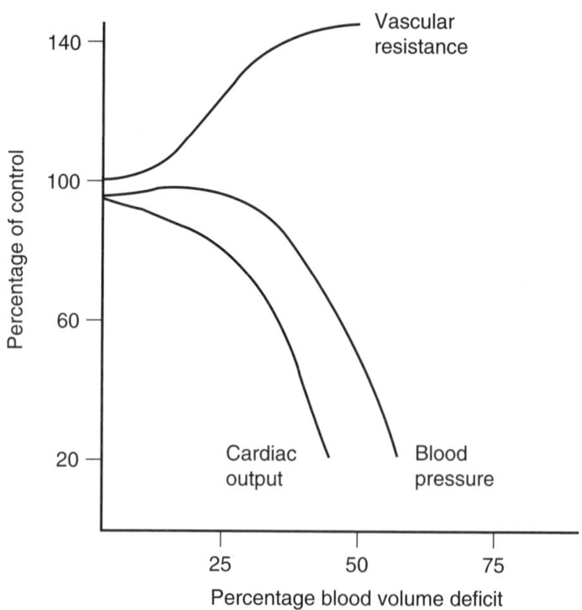

FIGURE 4-3 Hemodynamic response to hemorrhage. (From Chameides, L., & Hazinski, M. F. [1997]. *Pediatric advanced life support.* Dallas: American Heart Association.)

In a pediatric resuscitation, accessing age-appropriate equipment should be made as effortless as possible. Pediatric emergency supplies may be accessed more readily if they are stored separately from adult supplies. Organizing these supplies in a pediatric emergency cart or designated area facilitates ease of access. When children are being assessed and treated, equipment is selected considering the size of the patient—a factor that varies with age. Various charts are available with equipment size recommendations based on the patient's age. If such a resource is used, it should be attached to the pediatric supply cart for ease of reference in an emergent situation.

Basic Equipment Considerations

Stethoscope

Because the child has a more rounded chest wall, breath sounds can be auscultated more easily using a pediatric stethoscope with a smaller diaphragm and bell.

Blood Pressure Cuff

To obtain an accurate blood pressure in a child, the appropriate size cuff should be used. The cuff should cover two thirds to three fourths of the upper arm, and the cuff bladder should encircle the arm only once. If the cuff is too small, the blood pressure obtained may be falsely high; if the cuff is too large, it may reflect a falsely low blood pressure.

Resuscitation Masks

An appropriate-fitting mask should extend from the bridge of the nose to the cleft of the chin without putting pressure on the eyes. The mask should be clear to allow observation of vomitus and changes in lip color.

Resuscitation Bags

A self-inflating bag-valve device is the most appropriate choice in an emergent situation. These bags generally are available in three different sizes: 250, 500, and 1000 ml. To provide the highest concentration of oxygen possible, the resuscitation bag should have an oxygen reservoir and should be connected to an oxygen inflow of 10 to 15 L/min. Many self-inflating bags are equipped with popoff valves set to release around 35 to 45 cm H_2O; this prevents delivery of excessive pressure to the lungs. In a resuscitation situation in which lung compliance may be poor or airway resistance may be high, the popoff valve should be deactivated or manually occluded. A pressure manometer can be attached inline or directly to some bags to monitor peak airway pressure. However, the best indicator of adequate volume delivery is an observable rise and fall of the child's chest. Neonatal

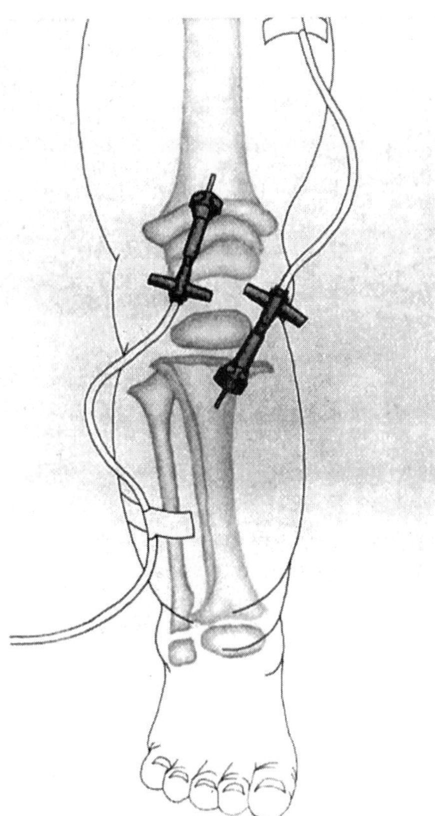

FIGURE 4-4 Intraosseous access. (From Manley, L., & Dick, M. [1988]. Intraosseous infusion: Rapid vascular access for critically ill or injured infants and children. *Journal of Emergency Nursing, 14,* 63-68.)

resuscitation bags (250 ml) are inadequate to ventilate children and infants beyond the neonatal period. Even some term infants require more volume than can be generated with a 250-ml bag. Therefore the half-liter and liter bags both should be available in a pediatric resuscitation area.

Oropharyngeal and Nasopharyngeal Airways

Both nasopharyngeal and oropharyngeal airways are available in a variety of sizes to accommodate the pediatric patient. An appropriate-fitting nasopharyngeal airway should be the same length as the distance from the tip of the child's nose to the tragus of the ear. If the airway is too long, it can irritate the vagus nerve, epiglottis, or vocal cords, causing coughing, gagging, or laryngospasm. An appropriate oropharyngeal airway should be used only in an unconscious child. To ensure an appropriate fitting oropharyngeal airway, one must measure the distance from the corner of the mouth to the angle of the jaw. The airway should equal this measurement.

Endotracheal Tubes

Endotracheal tubes ranging from 2.5 to 8.0 mm (internal diameter size in millimeters) should be available during a pediatric resuscitation. The appropriate-sized endotracheal tube may be determined by several different methods. One method is to choose a tube with an outside diameter approximately the diameter of the child's little finger. Another method is to use the child's age as a basis for selecting the tube size: Endotracheal tube size = (Age in years/4) + 4 (American Heart Association, 2000). However, length-based determination of endotracheal tube size (Broselow/Luten Pediatric Measuring Tape) has been found to be more accurate than age-based determination (Luten et al., 1992). Regardless of which method is used to select endotracheal tube size, endotracheal tubes 0.5 mm smaller and 0.5 mm larger than the predicted size should be immediately available when intubating a child.

Intravenous Catheters

Both over-the-needle catheters and butterfly needles are available in many sizes for infants and children. The catheter chosen should be large enough for the intended therapy but not so large as to impair blood flow around the catheter. In general, 24- to 22-gauge catheters should be used in infants, 22- to 20-gauge catheters in children, and 20- to 16-gauge catheters in adolescents.

Minimum Equipment

The amount of equipment and supplies available for treating children varies from facility to facility based on the facility's pediatric patient volume. However, all facilities that choose to offer emergency services to the community should have certain supplies available to meet the needs of children. Guidelines for the minimum equipment necessary to care for pediatric patients in an emergency department setting were determined by the Committee on Pediatric Equipment and Supplies for Emergency Departments, National Emergency Medical Services for Children Resource Alliance (1998). These guidelines represent the minimum equipment and supplies needed to care for children in an emergency department setting, not what is needed in a pediatric tertiary care facility. Routine equipment, such as oxygen blenders and tape, used in the care of patients of all ages is not included in the list (Box 4-1). In addition to equipment and supplies, the committee recommends that medications used in pediatric advanced life support be stocked in emergency departments caring for children (Table 4-6).

Organization and Accessibility

Pediatric emergency equipment should be organized in a logical manner that provides ease of accessibility. An optimally organized system of equipment and supplies should even prompt the clinician to consider certain aspects of a pediatric resuscitation. For example, placing a nasogastric tube close to airway and breathing supplies may prompt the caregiver to consider inserting an orogastric or nasogastric tube to avoid gastric distention in the child requiring bag-mask ventilation.

Once a system is implemented, the equipment and supplies should be checked routinely to ensure that all listed items are present and to assist staff in becoming more familiar with the pediatric cart contents. During a pediatric resuscitation,

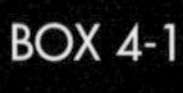

BOX 4-1 Guidelines for Minimum Equipment and Supplies for Care of Pediatric Patients in Emergency Departments

Essential Equipment and Supplies

Monitoring

Cardiorespiratory monitor with strip recorder
Defibrillator (0-400 J capability) with pediatric and adult paddles (4.5 and 8 cm)
Pediatric and adult monitor electrodes
Pulse oximeter with sensors, sizes newborn through adult
Thermometer/rectal probe[a]
Sphygmomanometer
Doppler blood pressure device
Blood pressure cuffs (neonatal, infant, child, adult, and thigh sizes)
Method to monitor endotracheal tube and placement[b]

Vascular Access

Butterfly needles (19- to 25-gauge)
Catheter-over-needle devices (14- to 24-gauge)
Infusion device[c]
Tubing for above
Intraosseous needles (16- and 18-gauge)[d]
Armboards (infant, child, and adult sizes)
Intravenous fluid/blood warmers
Umbilical vein catheters (size's 3.5 and 5 Fr)[e]
Seldinger technique vascular access kit (with pediatric sizes 3-, 4-, 5-Fr catheters)

Airway Management

Clear oxygen masks (preterm, infant, child, and adult sizes)
Nonrebreathing masks (infant, child, and adult sizes)
Oral airways (sizes 00-5)
Nasopharyngeal airways (12 to 30 Fr)
Bag-valve-mask resuscitator, self-inflating (450- and 1000-ml sizes)
Nasal cannulas (infant, child, and adult sizes)
Endotracheal tubes: uncuffed (sizes 2.5-8.5) and cuffed (sizes 5.5-9)
Stylets (pediatric and adult sizes)
Laryngoscope handle (pediatric and adult)
Laryngoscope blades, curved (sizes 2 and 3) and straight (sizes 0 to 3)
Magill forceps (pediatric and adult)
Nasogastric tubes (sizes 6 to 14 Fr)
Suction catheters: flexible (sizes 5 to 16 Fr) and Yankauer suction tip
Chest tubes (sizes 8 to 40 Fr)
Tracheostomy tubes (sizes 00-6)[f]

Resuscitation Medications

Medication chart, tape, or other system to ensure ready access to information on proper per kilogram doses for resuscitation drugs and equipment sizes[g]

Miscellaneous

Infant and standard scales
Infant formula and oral rehydrating solutions
Heating source[h]
Towel rolls/blanket rolls or equivalent
Pediatric restraining devices
Resuscitation board
Sterile linen[i]

Specialized Pediatric Trays

Tube thoracotomy with water seal drainage capability
Lumbar puncture (spinal needle sizes 20, 22, and 25 gauge)
Urinary catheterization with pediatric Foley catheters (sizes 5 to 16 Fr)
Obstetric pack
Newborn kit
  Umbilical vessel cannulation supplies
  Meconium aspirator
Venous cutdown
Surgical airway kit[j]

Fracture Management

Cervical immobilization equipment (sizes child to adult)[k]
Extremity splints
Femur splints (child and adult sizes)

Desirable equipment and supplies

Medical photography capability

From Committee on Pediatric Equipment and Supplies for Emergency Departments, National Emergency Medical Services for Children Resource Alliance. (1998). Guidelines for pediatric equipment & supplies for emergency departments. *Annals of Emergency Medicine, 31*(1), 54-57.
[a]Suitable for hypothermic and hyperthermic measurements with temperature capability from 25° to 44° C.
[b]May be satisfied by a disposable $ETCO_2$ detector, bulb, or feeding tube methods for endotracheal tube placement.
[c]To regulate rate and volume.
[d]May be satisfied by standard bone marrow aspiration needles, 13 or 15 gauge.
[e]Available within the hospital.
[f]Ensure availability of pediatric sizes within the hospital.
[g]System for estimating medication doses and supplies may use the length-based method with color codes, or other predetermined weight (kilogram)/dose method.
[h]May be met by infrared lamps or overhead warmer.
[i]Available within hospital for burn care.
[j]May include any of the following items: tracheostomy tray, cricothyrotomy tray, ETJV (needle jet).
[k]Many types of cervical immobilization devices are available.
These include wedges and collars. The type of device chosen depends on local preference and policies and procedures.
Whatever device is chosen should be stocked in sizes to fit infants, children, adolescents, and adults. Use of sandbags to meet this requirement is discouraged because they may cause injury if the patient has to be turned.

TABLE 4-6 PALS Medications for Cardiac Arrest and Symptomatic Arrhythmias

Drug	Dosage (Pediatric)	Remarks
Adenosine	0.1 mg/kg Repeat dose: 0.2 mg/kg Maximum single dose: 12 mg	Rapid IV/IO bolus Rapid flush to central circulation Monitor electrocardiogram during dose
Aminodarone for pulseless ventricular fibrillation/ ventricular tachycardia	5 mg/kg IV/IO Loading dose: 5 mg/kg IV/IO Maximum dose: 15 mg/kg/day	Rapid IV bolus IV over 20 to 60 min Routine use in combination with drugs
Aminodarone for perfusing tachycardias		prolonging OT interval is *not* recommended; hypotension is most common side effect
Atropine sulfate*	0.02 mg/kg Minimum dose: 0.1 mg Maximum single dose: 0.5 mg in child, 1.0 mg in adolescent; may repeat once	May give IV, IO, or ET. Tachycardia and pupil dilation may occur but *not* fixed dilated pupils
Calcium chloride 10% = 100 mg/ml (= 27.2 mg/ml elemental Ca)	20 mg/kg (0.2 ml/kg) IV/IO	Give slow IV push for hypocalcemia, hypermagnesemia, calcium channel blocker toxicity, preferably via central vein; monitor heart rate; bradycardia may occur
Calcium gluconate 10% = 100 mg/ml (= 9 mg/ml elemental Ca)	60-100 mg/kg (0.6-1.0 ml/kg) IV/IO	Give slow IV push for hypocalcemia, hypermagnesemia, calcium channel blocker toxicity, preferably via central vein
Epinephrine for symptomatic bradycardia*	IV/IO: 0.01 mg/kg (1:10,000, 0.1 ml/kg) ET: 0.1 mg/kg (1:1000, 0.1 ml/kg) First dose:	Tachyarrhythmias, hypertension may occur
Epinephrine for pulseless arrest*	IV/IO: 0.01 mg/kg (1:10,000, 0.1 ml/kg) ET: 0.1 mg/kg (1:1000, 0.1 ml/kg) Subsequent doses: Repeat initial dose or may increase up to 10 times (0.1 mg/kg, 1:1000, 0.1 ml/kg) Administer epinephrine every 3 to 5 min; IV/IO/ET doses as high as 0.2 mg/kg of 1:1000 may be effective	
Glucose (10%, 25%, or 50%)	IV/IO: 0.5-1.0 g/kg • 1-2 ml/kg 50% • 2-4 ml/kg 25% • 5-10 ml/kg 10%	For suspected hypoglycemia; avoid hyperglycemia
Lidocaine*	IV/IO/ET: 1 mg/kg	Rapid bolus
Lidocaine infusion (start after a bolus)	IV/IO: 20-50 μg/kg/min	1 to 2.5 ml/kg/hr of 120 mg/100 ml solution or use "rule of 6"
Magnesium sulfate (500 mg/ml)	IV/IO: 25-50 mg/kg; maximum dose: 2 g/dose	Rapid IV infusion for torsades or suspected hypomagnesemia; 10- to 20-min infusion for asthma that responds poorly to β-adrenergic agonists
Naloxone*	≤5 yr or ≤20 kg: 0.1 mg/kg >5 yr or >20 kg: 2.0 mg	For total reversal of narcotic effect; use small repeated doses (0.01-0.03 mg/kg) titrated to desired effect
Procainamide for perfusing tachycardias (100 and 500 mg/ml)	Loading dose: 15 mg/kg IV/IO	Infusion over 30-60 min; routine use in combination with drugs prolonging QT interval is *not* recommended
Sodium bicarbonate (1 and 0.5 mEq/ml)	IV/IO: 1 mEq/kg/dose	Infuse slowly and only if ventilation is adequate

Modified from American Heart Association (2000). Pediatric advanced life support. *Circulation, 102*(Suppl. I), I-308.
ET, Endotracheal; *IO*, Intraosseous; *IV*, intravenous.
*For endotracheal administration, use higher doses (2 to 10 times the IV dose); dilute medication with normal saline to a volume of 3 to 5 ml and follow with several positive-pressure ventilations.

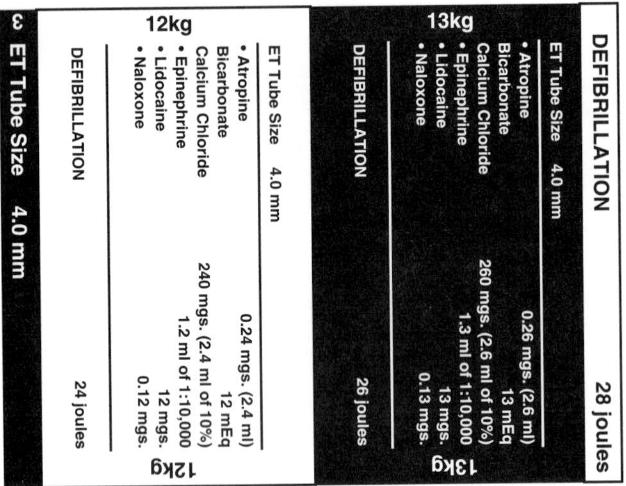

FIGURE 4-5 Broselow/Luten Pediatric Measuring Tape. (From Lubitz, D. S., Seidel, J. S., Chameides, L., Luten, R. C., Zaritsky, A. L., & Campbell, F. W. [1988]. A rapid method for estimating weight and resuscitation drug dosages from length in the pediatric age group. *Annals of Emergency Medicine, 17*[6], 576-581.)

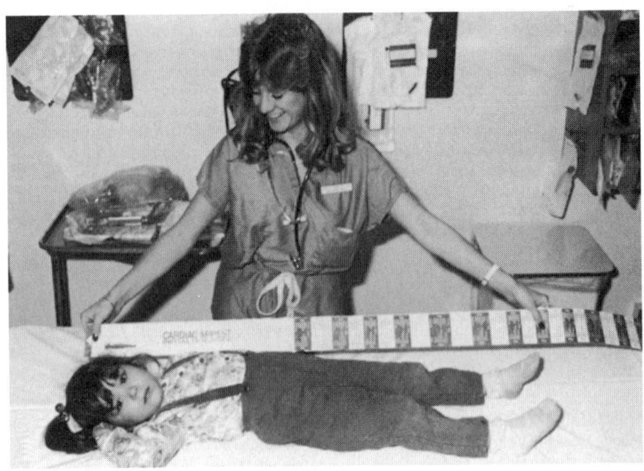

FIGURE 4-6 Measuring a child from head to toe. (From Lubitz, D. S., Seidel, J. S., Chameides, L., Luten, R. C., Zaritsky, A. L., & Campbell, F. W. [1988]. A rapid method for estimating weight and resuscitation drug dosages from length in the pediatric age group. *Annals of Emergency Medicine, 17*[6], 576-581.)

well-organized, easily accessible pediatric supplies may enhance the effectiveness of the resuscitative efforts. A variety of systems are available to organize pediatric equipment and supplies. Two systems are discussed in the following sections.

Color-Coded System

Broselow/Luten Pediatric Measuring Tape. In 1979 the National Center for Health Statistics published a new set of percentile curves for assessing physical growth of children in the United States (Lubitz, Seidel, Chameides, Luten, Zaritsky, & Campbell, 1988). James Broselow used this data to determine the 50th percentile weight for many lengths and heights. These determinations were used to produce a measuring tape with spaces representing weight in kilograms instead of units of length. Within each space representing a weight in kilograms are emergency drug dosages for that particular weight recommended by the American Heart Association (Figure 4-5). The tape is designed to measure the length of a child from head to toe and thereby determine the child's estimated weight in kilograms (Figure 4-6).

The first weight appearing on the tape (1998 version) is 3 kg. The spaces advance by 1-kg increments up to 20 kg and then by 2-kg increments up to 34 kg. On the reverse side of the tape, there are additional drug dosages per weight in kilograms, including vasoactive infusions and paralytic agents. Running along the side of the tape are color strips that correspond to a range of weight in kilograms. Inside these color strips, equipment sizes appropriate for children weighing within that range are listed. For example, the equipment sizes listed in the pink strip are appropriate for children weighing 6 to 7 kg.

In a study published in 1988, "the tape was found to be extremely accurate for children from 3.5 to 10 kg and from 10 to 25 kg" (Lubitz et al., 1988). However, the Broselow/Luten Pediatric Measuring Tape, like other published references, is only a guide. Clinical judgment should be used in determining drug dosages and equipment sizes on a patient-by-patient basis.

Broselow/Hinkle Pediatric Resuscitation System. The Broselow/Hinkle Pediatric Resuscitation System incorporates the Broselow/Luten Pediatric Measuring Tape to organize emergency supplies and equipment in colored pouches that correspond to the length-determined estimated weight in kilograms (Figure 4-7). When measured with the Broselow/Luten Pediatric Measuring Tape, the child's measurement will fall into a certain color range that corresponds to the estimated weight in kilograms. The appropriate-sized equipment can then be quickly obtained from that particular prestocked colored pouch. For example, equipment and supplies appropriately sized for a 6- to 7-kg infant is stored in a pink pouch. The Broselow/Hinkle Pediatric Resuscitation System lists recommend size-appropriate equipment and supplies for the various colored pouches. The system currently offers four different supply list modules: intravenous delivery (Box 4-2), oxygen delivery (Box 4-3), intraosseous delivery (Box 4-4), and intubation (Box 4-5). The contents of the pink and red pouches are identical.

This system allows quick access to emergency equipment and supplies without using time to reference age/equipment charts. This system is also valuable if the child's weight is already known. The Broselow/Luten Pediatric Measuring Tape can then be referenced to determine the color corresponding to that weight, and the appropriate-sized equipment can be obtained from that colored pouch. The Broselow/Hinkle Pediatric Resuscitation System, used in conjunction with the Broselow/Luten Pediatric Measuring Tape, is one effective method of quickly determining the estimated weight of a child and the appropriate equipment sizes based on that weight.

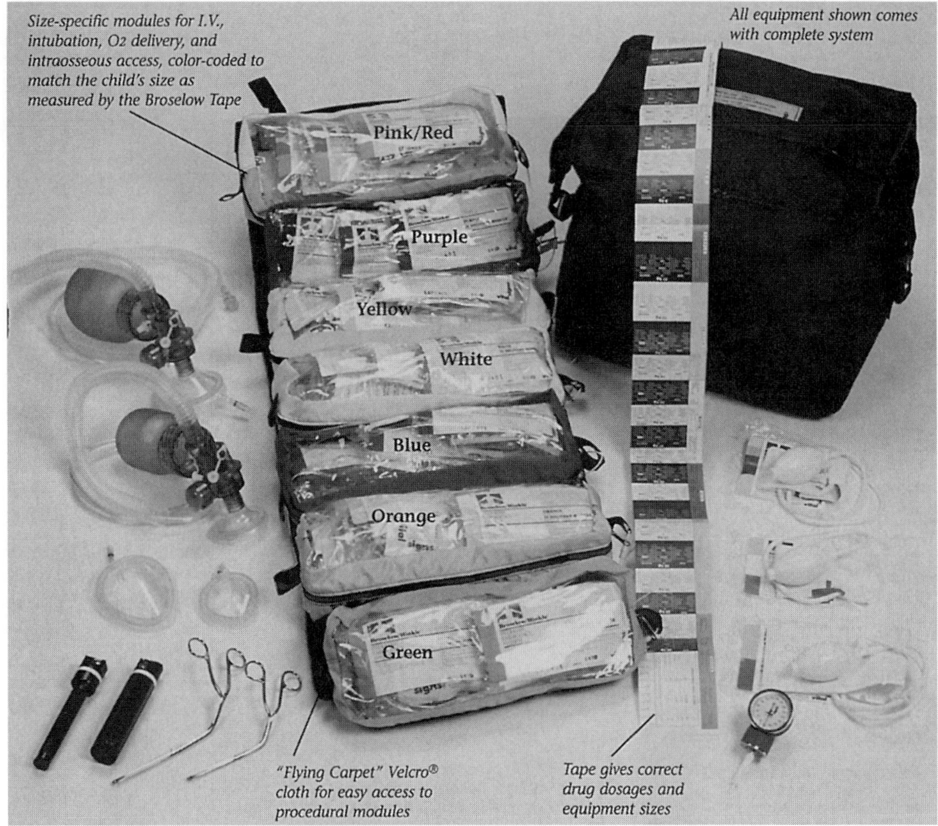

FIGURE 4-7 Pediatric resuscitation system. (Courtesy Armstrong Medical Industries, Inc., Lincolnshire, Ill.)

BOX 4-2 Broselow/Hinkle Pediatric Emergency System Intravenous (IV) Delivery Module Contents

Red/Pink

IV catheter/needle, 22-gauge × 1 inch, sterile—1
IV catheter/needle, 24-gauge × ¾ inch, sterile—1
IV prep kit, sterile—1
Extension set, sterile—1

Purple

IV catheter/needle, 22-gauge × 1 inch, sterile—1
IV catheter/needle, 24-gauge × ¾ inch, sterile—1
IV prep kit, sterile—1
Extension set, sterile—1

Yellow

IV catheter/needle, 20-gauge × 1¼ inch, sterile—1
IV catheter/needle, 22-gauge × 1 inch, sterile—1
IV prep kit, sterile—1
Extension set, sterile—1

White

IV catheter/needle, 22-gauge × 1 inch, sterile—1
IV catheter/needle, 20-gauge × 1 ¼ inch, sterile—1
IV catheter/needle, 18-gauge × 1 ¼ inch, sterile—1
IV prep kit, sterile—1
Extension set, sterile—1

Blue

IV catheter/needle, 20-gauge × 1 ¼ inch, sterile—1
IV catheter/needle, 18-gauge × 1 ¼ inch, sterile—1
IV prep kit, sterile—1
Extension set, sterile—1

Orange

IV catheter/needle, 20-gauge × 1 ¼ inch, sterile—1
IV catheter/needle, 18-gauge × 1 ¼ inch, sterile—1
IV prep kit, sterile—1
Extension set, sterile—1

Green

IV catheter/needle, 20-gauge × 1 ¼ inch, sterile—1
IV catheter/needle, 18-gauge × 1 ¼ inch, sterile—1
IV catheter/needle, 16-gauge × 1 ¼ inch, sterile—1
IV prep kit, sterile—1
Extension set, sterile—1

Courtesy Armstrong Medical Industries, Inc., Lincolnshire, Ill.

BOX 4-3 Broselow/Hinkle Pediatric Emergency System Oxygen Delivery Module Contents

Red/Pink

5-cm Berman oral airway—1
6-cm Berman oral airway—1
Infant nasal cannula with 7-foot crush-resistant oxygen tubing—1
Infant simple oxygen mask with 7-foot crush-resistant oxygen tubing—1

Purple

6-cm Berman oral airway—1
Pediatric nasal cannula with 7-foot crush-resistant oxygen tubing—1
Pediatric simple oxygen mask with 7-foot crush-resistant oxygen tubing—1

Yellow

7-cm Berman oral airway—1
Pediatric nasal cannula with 7-foot crush-resistant oxygen tubing—1
Pediatric simple oxygen mask with 7-foot crush-resistant oxygen tubing—1

White

7-cm Berman oral airway—1
Pediatric nasal cannula with 7-foot crush-resistant oxygen tubing—1
Pediatric simple oxygen mask with 7-foot crush-resistant oxygen tubing—1

Blue

7-cm Berman oral airway—1
8-cm Berman oral airway—1
Pediatric nasal cannula with 7-foot crush-resistant oxygen tubing—1
Pediatric simple oxygen mask with 7-foot crush-resistant oxygen tubing—1

Orange

7-cm Berman oral airway—1
8-cm Berman oral airway—1
Adult nasal cannula with 7-foot crush-resistant oxygen tubing—1
Adult simple oxygen mask with 7-foot crush-resistant oxygen tubing—1

Green

7-cm Berman oral airway—1
Adult nasal cannula with 7-foot crush-resistant oxygen tubing—1
Adult simple oxygen mask with 7-foot crush-resistant oxygen tubing—1

Courtesy Armstrong Medical Industries, Inc., Lincolnshire, Ill.

BOX 4-4 Broselow/Hinkle Pediatric Emergency System Intraosseous Module Contents

Red/Pink

18-gauge adjustable-length sternal/iliac aspiration needle—1
Povidone-iodine swabstick—1
Adhesive tape—1 roll
Extension set, sterile—1

Purple

18-gauge adjustable-length sternal/iliac aspiration needle—1
Povidone-iodine swabstick—1
Adhesive tape—1 roll
Extension set, sterile—1

Yellow

18-gauge adjustable-length sternal/iliac aspiration needle—1
Povidone-iodine swabstick—1
Adhesive tape—1 roll
Extension set, sterile—1

White

15-gauge adjustable-length sternal/iliac aspiration needle—1
Povidone-iodine swabstick—1
Adhesive tape—1 roll
Extension set, sterile—1

Blue

15-gauge adjustable-length sternal/iliac aspiration needle—1
Povidone-iodine swabstick—1
Adhesive tape—1 roll
Extension set, sterile—1

Courtesy Armstrong Medical Industries, Inc., Lincolnshire, Ill.

ABC System

Arranging pediatric supplies in a system that coincides with the airway, breathing, and circulation assessment sequence is another logical way to organize these supplies. To facilitate access, these supplies should be organized in a rolling cart capable of being moved from patient to patient. This pediatric supply cart, used in conjunction with a code cart equipped with a defibrillator and resuscitation medications, enhances resuscitative efforts by making pediatric equipment readily accessible. As with any equipment cart, a pediatric supply cart should be inspected frequently to ensure that all items are pres-

BOX 4-5 Broselow/Hinkle Pediatric Emergency System Intubation Module Contents

Red/Pink
Straight blade, size no. 1—1
3.5-mm endotracheal tubes, uncuffed—2
Pediatric endotracheal tube stylet—1
8-Fr suction catheter—1
5-Fr nasogastric tube—1
8-Fr nasogastric tube—1
36-inch adhesive tape—1 roll
Lubricating jelly packet, water soluble—1
3-×-3-inch gauze pad—1

Purple
Straight blade, size no. 1—1
4.0-mm endotracheal tubes, uncuffed—2
Pediatric endotracheal tube stylet—1
8-Fr suction catheter—1
10-Fr suction catheter—1
8-Fr nasogastric tube—1
10-Fr nasogastric tube—1
36-inch adhesive tape—1 roll
Lubricating jelly packet, water soluble—1
3-×-3-inch gauze pad—1

Yellow
Straight blade, size no. 2—1
Curved blade, size no. 2—1
4.5-mm endotracheal tubes, uncuffed—2
Pediatric endotracheal tube stylet—1
10-Fr suction catheter—1
10-Fr nasogastric tube—1
36-inch adhesive tape—1 roll
Lubricating jelly packet, water soluble—1
3-×-3-inch gauze pad—1

White
Straight blade, size no. 2—1
Curved blade, size no. 2—1
5.0-mm endotracheal tubes, uncuffed—2
Pediatric endotracheal tube stylet—1
10-Fr suction catheter—1
10-Fr nasogastric tube—1
12-Fr nasogastric tube—1
36-inch adhesive tape—1 roll
Lubricating jelly packet, water soluble—1
3-×-3-inch gauze pad—1

Blue
Straight blade, size no. 2—1
Curved blade, size no. 2—1
5.5-mm endotracheal tubes, uncuffed—2
Adult endotracheal tube stylet—1
10-Fr suction catheter—1
12-Fr nasogastric tube—1
14-Fr nasogastric tube—1
36-inch adhesive tape—1 roll
Lubricating jelly packet, water soluble—1
3-×-3-inch gauze pad—1

Orange
Straight blade, size no. 2-3—1
Curved blade, size no. 2-3—1
6.0-mm endotracheal tubes, cuffed—2
Adult endotracheal tube stylet—1
10-Fr suction catheter—1
14-Fr nasogastric tube—1
18-Fr nasogastric tube—1
10-ml syringe—1
36-inch adhesive tape—1 roll
Lubricating jelly packet, water soluble—1
3-×-3-inch gauze pad—1

Green
Straight blade, size no. 3—1
Curved blade, size no. 3—1
6.5-mm endotracheal tubes, uncuffed—2
Adult endotracheal tube stylet—1
12-Fr suction catheter—1
18-Fr nasogastric tube—1
10-ml syringe—1
36-inch adhesive tape—1 roll
Lubricating jelly packet, water soluble—1
3-×-3-inch gauze pad—1

Courtesy Armstrong Medical Industries, Inc., Lincolnshire, Ill.

ent and to increase staff familiarity with the contents. Box 4-6 depicts a pediatric supply cart list organized in an ABC system.

STAFF COMPETENCY

As with any situation in which skills are infrequently used, initial and ongoing education is essential for clinical staff to obtain and maintain competency. Many hospitals not only are resuscitating and stabilizing pediatric patients in their emergency departments but are also admitting these children to primarily adult critical care units for observation or stabilization. If these children become unstable or do not respond to the initial therapy, they should be transferred to a tertiary pediatric center (Paladichuk, 1998).

Adult intensive care unit staff caring for pediatric patients need to understand the anatomic differences between children and adults and how to adjust their interventions based on these differences. They also must be able recognize when a child is in trouble and how to deliver the therapies necessary to resuscitate and stabilize the child.

If a facility makes the decision to admit pediatric patients to an adult intensive care unit, it must make the commitment to provide staff with both initial and ongoing education about the resuscitation and stabilization of pediatric patients. Both the Pediatric Advanced Life Support Course (PALS) from the American Heart Association and the Emergency Nursing Pediatric Course (ENPC) from the Emergency Nurses Association are readily available as initial

BOX 4-6 Sample ABC Resuscitation Cart

Top of Cart

Broselow/Luten Pediatric Measuring Tape
Pediatric stethoscope
Infant and pediatric manual blood pressure cuffs
Doppler blood pressure device
Bolus kit: Liter bag of lactated Ringer's or normal saline, macrotubing, extension tubing, three-way stopcock, 30-ml syringe (placed together in a plastic bag)
One 500-ml and one 1-L self-inflating resuscitation bags with oxygen reservoirs

Airway and Breathing

Drawer 1

1 uncuffed endotracheal tube in each of the following sizes: 2.5, 3.0, 3.5, 4.0, 4.5, 5.0, 5.5
1 cuffed endotracheal tube in each of the following sizes: 6.0, 7.0, 7.5, 8.0
Small laryngoscope handle
Large laryngoscope handle
Size 0, 1, 2, and 3 straight blades
Size 2 and 3 curved blades
Pediatric stylets—2
Adult stylets—2
Pediatric Magill forceps
Various sizes of infant and pediatric nasopharyngeal airways
Various sizes of infant and pediatric oropharyngeal airways
Various sizes of infant and pediatric clear resuscitation masks
14-Fr over-the-needle catheter—1
10-ml syringe—1
ETCO_2 detector—1
Benzoin swabs
Cloth tape—1 roll

Drawer 2

6.5-Fr suction catheters—2
8-Fr suction catheters—2
10-Fr suction catheters—2
14-Fr suction catheters—2
Yankauer rigid suction tubes—2
Saline bullets—5
Pediatric nonrebreather mask—1
Oxygen tubing—1
Flow meter with nipple—1
Infant simple mask—1
Pediatric nasal cannula—1
Infant nasal cannula—1
Nebulizer set—1
Infant oximeter probe—1
Pediatric oximeter probe—1
ABG syringes—4
Capillary blood gas tubes—4
Betadine swabs
2 × 2s
Silk tape—1 roll

Circulation

Drawer 3

Tourniquet—1
Silk tape—1 roll
Alcohol swabs
Betadine swabs
2 × 2s
10-ml preservative normal saline vials—5
18-gauge 1 ½-inch needles—10
23-gauge 1-inch needles—10
25-gauge ⅝-inch needles—10
Filter needles—5
1-ml syringes—5
3-ml syringes—10
5-ml syringes—5
10-ml syringes—5
30-ml syringe—1
60-ml syringe—1
18-gauge short over-the-needle catheters—4
20-gauge short over-the-needle catheters—4
22-gauge over-the-needle catheters—4
24-gauge over-the-needle catheters—4
23-gauge butterfly needles—2
25-gauge butterfly needles—2
Pediatric T connectors—2
Three-way stopcocks—4
Small Tegaderm—2
Medium Tegaderm—2
Various sizes of infant and pediatric armboards—3

Drawer 4

500-ml normal saline bag—1
500-ml lactated Ringer's bag—1
Macrotubing—2
Pump tubing—1
Blood tubing—1
Single-line pressure tubing with transducer—1
15-gauge intraosseous needles—2
18-gauge intraosseous needles—2
Adult T connectors—2
2 × 2s
Silk tape—1 roll
Arterial catheter set with 22- and 20-gauge catheters—1
Pediatric T connector—1
Central line dressing kit—1
Surgical blades—2
Sterile gloves in sizes 6-8
Sterile towel—1
Various sizes of suture material

BOX 4-6 Sample ABC Resuscitation Cart—cont'd

Drawer 5: Nasogastric Tubes and Foley Catheters

Lubricating gel—10 packages
5-Fr feeding tube—1
8-Fr feeding tubes—2
10-Fr Salem sumps—2
12-Fr Salem sumps—2
16-Fr Salem sump—1
10-ml syringe—1
60-ml syringe with catheter tip—1
Pediatric urine bags—2
Sterile specimen cups—2
5-ml syringe—1
30-ml vials of sterile water—2
Betadine swabs
Foley catheter tray—1
6-Fr Foley catheter—1
8-Fr Foley catheter—1
10-Fr Foley catheter—1
12-Fr Foley catheter—1
Pink tape—1 roll

Drawer 6: Chest Tube Supplies and Central Line Kits

Sterile gown—1
Size 6-8 sterile gloves
Masks
Sterile towels—2
Pink tape—1 roll
5 : 1 connectors—2
Betadine—1 bottle
30-ml vials normal saline—2
Pediatric small instrument sets—2
Various sizes of suture
Vaseline gauze dressings—2
Packs 4 × 4s—2
4-Fr 12-cm central line kit—1
5-Fr 25-cm central line kit—1
7-Fr 20-cm central line kit—1
Surgical blades—2
Central line dressing kit—1
18-gauge over-the-needle catheter—1
14-gauge over-the-needle catheter—1
10-ml syringe—1
10-Fr chest tube—1
12-Fr chest tube—1
16-Fr chest tube—1
24-Fr chest tube—1
28-Fr chest tube —1

Bottom of Cart

Urometer—1
Peritoneal lavage kit—1
Infant lumbar puncture tray—1
Pediatric lumbar puncture tray—1
Chest drainage unit—1
500-ml bag normal saline—1
Pediatric cutdown tray—1
Pediatric cardiac/open chest tray—1
Umbilical catheter tray—1

education programs. Both programs provide thorough didactic content and "hands on" experience through simulated resuscitation situations.

PALS focuses on the immediate resuscitation of the pediatric patient. It also emphasizes identification of problems that could cause cardiopulmonary arrest and presents strategies to deal with these problems. The content is presented as a continuum of time, starting with preresuscitation care, through resuscitation, and ending with postresuscitation care. Activities inherent in the course include assessment, action, and reassessment of the response to the actions. The course should be completed successfully every 2 years for the participant to remain current with the standards.

ENPC provides a wider pediatric focus, incorporating both medical and trauma diagnoses. It provides information on the identification of problems and stabilization to transfer to a tertiary pediatric care center. Like PALS, ENPC uses both didactic and skills stations to provide information, allow practice, and build confidence. ENPC renewal is recommended every 4 years to maintain knowledge of current standards. Successful completion of PALS and ENPC indicates that the participant has passed both the written and skills examinations for the course. Neither course provides "certification" and should not be viewed as such.

In addition to remaining current in one or both of these courses, pediatric caregivers should regularly participate in organized "mock" pediatric resuscitation and stabilization scenarios. These "mock" scenarios will enable the caregiver to recall didactic material and apply it in a "hands-on" experience. The "mock" scenarios may be organized around a unit or shift and should include four elements at the minimum. The first element should include a review of the normal physiologic parameters for pediatric patients of various ages. The second element should include a review of the signs and symptoms associated with various types of both medical and trauma conditions that may affect pediatric patients admitted to the unit. The third element should review the procedures necessary for the resuscitation, stabilization, and transfer of pediatric patients. The fourth element should include a review of the equipment available for the resuscitation of pediatric patients.

Mock scenarios not only provide a review of previously acquired knowledge but can also provide a critique of existing procedures and protocols. They also can be used to identify specific staff education needs for the pediatric patient and the availability of specific resuscitation equipment (Bishop-Kurylo & Masiello, 1995).

The unit manager or educator, for review, should maintain documentation of initial and ongoing education by regulating agencies such as the Joint Commission on Accreditation of Healthcare Organizations (JCAHO). Copies of the PALS and/or ENPC cards should be documented. Mock scenarios not only provide documentation of various skills but also demonstrate age-specific competencies.

Development of a program of initial and ongoing education on the resuscitation and stabilization of pediatric patients in an adult setting is as important as having the necessary equipment available and should be seen as a priority. PALS and ENPC can provide the basics. Mock scenarios can provide ongoing development and refinement staff skills and policies and procedures related to pediatric patients.

SUMMARY

Providing optimal care for critically ill and injured children requires a coordinated, cohesive effort based on the recognition that children are different from adults. All clinicians caring for children, from prehospital providers to tertiary-level caregivers, should have a thorough understanding of the anatomic and physiologic differences in children. By understanding these differences and their clinical significance, caregivers can provide appropriate interventions.

Because the resuscitation and stabilization of a critically ill or injured child can create significant cognitive demand and emotional stress, especially for caregivers with limited pediatric experience, accessing appropriate-sized equipment should be made as simple as possible. Using tools such as the Broselow/Luten Pediatric Measuring Tape to determine an estimated weight in kilograms and the appropriate-sized equipment may facilitate a more effective resuscitation. Furthermore, by organizing pediatric equipment and supplies in a system such as the color-coded Broselow/Hinkle Pediatric Resuscitation System or the ABC system, clinicians can readily obtain resuscitation supplies.

Staff responsible for the care of the critically ill or injured child should receive initial and ongoing pediatric specific education. Both PALS and ENPC provide thorough didactic content and hands-on experience through simulated resuscitation situations. In addition to remaining current in one or both of these courses, pediatric caregivers should participate in organized mock pediatric resuscitation and stabilization scenarios. These mock scenarios will enable the caregiver to recall didactic material and apply it in a hands-on experience. These situations also provide the opportunity to practice accessing and using pediatric equipment and supplies.

BIBLIOGRAPHY

American Heart Association. (2000). Pediatric advanced life support. *Circulation, 102*(Suppl. I), I-291-I-342.

Bishop-Kurylo, D., & Masiello, M. (1995). Pediatric resuscitation: Development of a mock code program and evaluation tool. *Pediatric Nursing, 21*(4), 333-336.

Chameides, L., & Hazinksi, M. F. (1997). *Pediatric advanced life support.* Dallas: American Heart Association.

Committee on Pediatric Equipment and Supplies for Emergency Departments, National Emergency Medical Services for Children Resource Alliance. (1998). Guidelines for pediatric equipment and supplies for emergency departments. *Annals of Emergency Medicine, 31*(1), 54-57.

Edge, W. E., Kanter, R. K., Weigle, C., & Walsh, R. F. (1994). Reduction of morbidity in interhospital transport by specialized pediatric staff. *Critical Care Medicine, 22*(7), 1186-1191.

Emergency Nurses Association. (2000). Pediatric trauma. In B. Bennett-Jacobs (Ed.), *Trauma nursing core course provider manual* (pp. 249-264). Park Ridge, IL: Emergency Nurses Association.

Hazinski, M. F. (1997). Anatomic and physiologic differences between children and adults. In D. Levin & F. Morriss (Eds.), *Essentials of pediatric intensive care* (2nd ed., pp. 1112-1126). New York: Churchill Livingstone.

Hudak, C. M., Gallo, B. M., & Morton, P. M. (Eds.). (1998). *Critical care nursing: A holistic approach.* Philadelphia: Lippincott.

Inaba, A. S., & Seward, P. N. (1991). An approach to pediatric trauma unique anatomic and pathophysiologic aspects of the pediatric patient. *Emergency Medicine Clinics of North America, 9,* 523-548.

Jaimovich, D. G., & Vidyasagar, D. (1995). *Handbook of pediatric and neonatal transport medicine.* Philadelphia: Hanley & Belfus.

Lubitz, D. S., Seidel, J. S., Chameides, L., Luten, R. C., Zaritsky, A. L., & Campbell, F. W. (1988). A rapid method for estimating weight and resuscitation drug dosages from length in the pediatric age group. *Annals of Emergency Medicine, 17*(6), 576-581.

Luten, R. C., Wears, R. L., Broselow, J., Zaritsky, A., Barnett, T. M., Lee, T., Bailey, A., Vally, R., Brown, R., & Rosenthal, B. (1992). Length-based endotracheal tube and emergency equipment in pediatrics. *Annals of Emergency Medicine, 21*(8), 900-904.

National Center for Health Statistics. (1999). *Healthy People 2000—Review 1997.* Hyattsville, MD: U.S. Department of Health and Human Services.

Paladichuk, A. (1998). Children in the adult ICU: Preparation and practice. *Critical Care Nurse, 18*(6), 82-87.

Pollack, M. M., Alexander, S. R., Clarke, N., Ruttimann, V. E., Tesselaar, H. M., & Bachulis, A. C. (1991). Improved outcomes from tertiary center pediatric intensive care: A statewide comparison of tertiary and nontertiary care facilities. *Critical Care Medicine, 19*(2), 150-159.

Sabel, M. S., & Bassuk, A. B. (1996). Initial stabilization and transport of the pediatric trauma patient. In D. G. Jaimovich & D. Vidyasagar (Eds.), *Handbook of pediatric and neonatal transport* (pp. 327-346). Philadelphia: Hanley & Belfus.

Tepas, J., Ramenofsky, M., Mollitt, D., Gans, B., & DiScala, C. (1988). The pediatric trauma score as a predictor of injury severity: An objective assessment. *Journal of Trauma, 28*(4), 425-429.

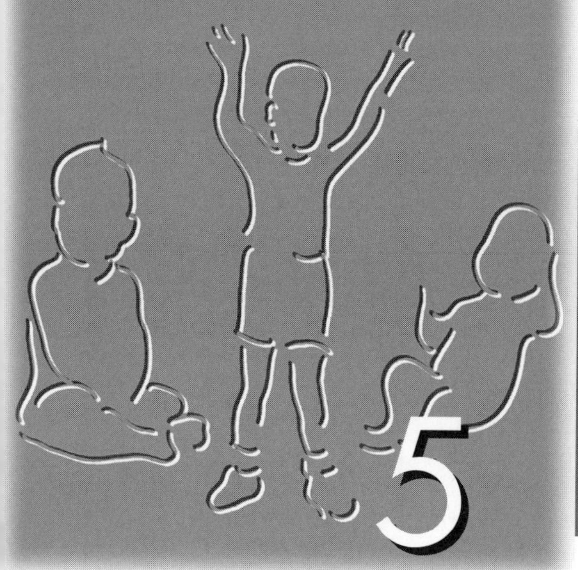

5 MECHANISM OF INJURY

Sally Jo Zuspan

HISTORY OF TRAUMATIC EVENT

Mechanism of injury (MOI) is often underestimated as an assessment tool in the injured child. Details about what has already transpired may seem trivial in the face of an active resuscitation. In reality, MOI can tell much about the trauma event and can provide important clues that help in detecting hidden injuries.

MOI refers simply to the manner in which a trauma victim is injured. Specifically, MOI describes how the impact of blunt or penetrating force affected a victim. Appreciation of differences in pediatric injury patterns is an essential part of nursing assessment of the injured child. In many circumstances the way in which children are injured is similar to that in the adult population. However, because of differences in size and development, patterns of injury in children can be different than those in adults. Research into traumatic events reveals that similar mechanisms result in predictable sets of injuries. Appreciation of pediatric mechanisms will help the clinical assessment proceed more efficiently and aid in the detection of injuries.

Understanding common injury patterns can help nurses anticipate clinical findings in the injured child and direct the plan of care. In fact, triage decisions may be made based largely on the MOI. For example, a child who fell 20 feet may appear alert and relatively uninjured; however, the nurse must recognize the potential for multisystem injury and proceed accordingly. Equally important is the nurse's ability to recognize an injury history that does not match the clinical presentation. A benign injury history that fails to explain major trauma is a red flag that suggests abusive injury. This concept is unique to pediatrics and can be easily missed. Even small wounds, such as contusions, abrasions, and simple fractures, accompanied by an insufficient explanation deserve special attention. Subtle signs, such as erythema or old bruises, may be the only external signs of child abuse. This is not to imply that every unusual history signals abuse. Pediatric MOI can be innovative and unusual. It is the nurse's job to discern injuries that resulted from inventive play, such as falling while trying to "fly like Superman," from trauma that may have been inflicted by an adult. Pediatric injuries are often occult and difficult to determine during initial assessment. Complete understanding of the MOI will alert the nurse to potential injuries so that appropriate interventions can be implemented.

A first step in assessment is to determine an exact injury history. A good history should include the details of the MOI. For example, a general history might be "child struck by car." Although this provides a basic idea of what happened, additional information is crucial to fully appreciate the potential injuries. A 2-year-old child who was run over by the wheels of a slow-moving car will have a very different set of injuries than a 7-year-old cyclist who was wearing a helmet, although both fit the description of having been struck by a vehicle. In this situation the nurse should determine and document the speed of the car, the location of vehicle impact, whether the child was thrown, the initial responsiveness of the child, and any protective devices that were in use. Although a detailed report may not always be available, obtaining the most complete description of the injury incident will prove invaluable in the assessment process.

BIOMECHANICS AND INFLUENCES ON INJURY

Motor vehicle crashes (MVCs), pedestrian and bike crashes, falls, and assaults continue to be the leading causes of blunt trauma in children (Cantor & Leaming, 1998). The primary manner in which children are injured has changed little throughout the years. Mechanisms of injuries do, however, reflect societal trends. Changes in attitudes, popular activities, and even legislation can influence injury patterns.

Recently, research in the epidemiology and MOI has implicated specific activities and devices that can result in pediatric morbidity and mortality. All-terrain vehicles, safety belts, infant walkers, shopping carts, and even window blinds have been identified as potentially fatal to children (Consumer Product Safety Commission, 2000). As public interests change or new devices become popular, unique injury patterns are likely to emerge. In recent years, reports of "new" pediatric injuries have begun to appear in the literature. Rice, Alvanos, and Kenney (2000) reviewed nearly a decade of pediatric snowmobile-related injuries and reported that head, neck, and face injuries were primarily associated with both nonfatal injuries and deaths. A study on snowboarding injuries in children suggested a possible predisposition to lumbar vertebral burst fractures in children and adolescents involved in this sport (Shorter, Mooney, & Harmon, 1999). Osberg, Schneps, DiScala, and Li (1998) found that skateboarding is a more dangerous activity than roller-skating or inline skating. Trampoline injuries have soared in recent years with the addition of trampolines to suburban backyards and play areas (Furnival, Street, & Schunk, 1999). The Committee on Sports Medicine and Fitness of the American Academy of Pediatrics (2000) has examined the sport of soccer. The number of injuries, including head injuries, has increased as the sport has grown in popularity. Soft tissue contusion is the most common type of nonfatal injury, and fatalities are associated with almost exclusively traumatic contact with goalposts. It is essential that nurses stay up-to-date with current injury patterns to recognize resultant injuries as they present to the emergency department. Ever-changing mechanisms also generate the need for new prevention programs and education activities.

Surprisingly, legislative initiatives aimed at preventing injury can lead to unique and unexpected injury patterns. Legislation regarding air bags and safety belts aim to save lives, but they also have been implicated in severe injuries to children. A study of pediatric injuries caused by air bags (Grisoni et al., 2000) concluded that passenger-side air bags lead to mortality or serious morbidity in properly and improperly restrained children. Marshall, Koch, and Egelhoff (1998) reported that air bag–related deaths and serious injuries were the direct result of neurologic injury. The authors also noted that injury patterns differed according to the child's age and type of restraint used. The lap belt is another protective device that can result in specific trauma. The *lap belt complex* refers to a pattern of injury in children that results in intraabdominal trauma and lumbar spine fractures (Rothrock, Green, & Morgan 2000). A study of children prematurely using safety belts found that these children were more likely to suffer significant injury than children in appropriate restraint systems (Winston, Durbin, Kallan, & Moll, 2000). An ever-changing legislative agenda can unwittingly create new MOIs. Close attention to new injury patterns and associated clinical findings will aid in identification and prevention of these injuries.

A review of MOI would not be complete without addressing rural pediatric trauma. Although urban mechanisms account for a larger volume of injury, farm trauma can be particularly devastating. In farming communities, children may operate heavy, dangerous equipment and are therefore at risk for both blunt and penetrating trauma. Zietlow and Swanson (1999) reported that mechanized equipment was responsible for half of the injuries in their study, and one third of the children sustained severe permanent disability. Injuries included amputations, head trauma, and soft tissue infections. Most deaths occurred in the field. In another study, Rivara (1997) examined fatal and nonfatal farm injuries and found that tractors, horses, and all-terrain vehicles were the primary mechanisms. Rural trauma continues to be a problem in children. This less common but potentially disabling activity should be recognized as an MOI in farming regions.

MOI can be described as the effect of energy on human tissue. Trauma can be caused by several types of energy. Chemical, thermal, electrical, and radiation energy cause cellular disruption that often results in burns (Templeton, 1993). *Kinetic energy* is the effect of external forces impacting the body during movement (Vardara, 1993). An impact is considered blunt trauma when the force strikes the external surfaces of the body. Penetrating trauma involves an object that directly enters the body, such as occurs with a stab or gunshot wound.

BLUNT TRAUMA

Blunt trauma is responsible for the majority of injuries to children. Blunt force produces crushing, shearing, or tearing of tissue both internally and externally. Assessment of blunt trauma can be difficult in children because there may be few signs even when significant injury has occurred. Consequently, frequent reassessment is vital to detect trauma to vital organs. Children with blunt force injury should be regarded with a high index of suspicion until injuries can be ruled out.

The severity of any blunt force injury is directly related to the following: (1) the mass of the victim, (2) the speed of the victim and/or the object, (3) the rate of change in velocity, and (4) the diffusion of the transfer of kinetic energy to the tissues (Templeton, 1993). Several unique features place children at greater risk for injuries based on these factors. Because of the small size of children, a blunt object that strikes a child will cover a larger percentage of body surface area than in an adult. In addition, energy is dissipated over a smaller area, often resulting in multisystem trauma. Other attributes of children include a relatively large head and weak neck that provide increased momentum and greater risk of head injury during falls and MVCs. Abdominal organs in children are larger and tend to be more exposed, making them more susceptible to injury. Less body fat and subcutaneous tissue also contribute to this effect (Ludwig & Loiselle, 1993). Children's bones tend to be more flexible than those of an adult. This greater compliance allows for more diffusion of energy and fewer fractures. However, because energy is transferred to deeper structures, there may be greater internal damage than in an adult patient (Templeton, 1993).

Although small stature clearly affects injuries seen in pediatric trauma, one well-known theory of childhood injury has been challenged in the literature. Waddel's triad has been used for many years to explain the etiology of multiple trauma. This theory described a predictable pattern, or triad, of trauma to the head, abdomen, and lower extremities as a consequence of a child being struck by a car. In a large review of pedestrian collisions, Orsborn, Haley, Hammond, and Falcone (1999) concluded that the incidence of this particular combination of injuries actually is low and should not be viewed as a predictive model of pedestrian injury. However, this study did validate multisystem trauma as a common finding in children. Nursing implications include maintaining a high index of suspicion for multiple trauma even in the child who presents with only one obvious system injury.

Age and development also play a role in understanding MOI. Each stage of childhood development is associated with common scenarios that result in injury. Familiarity with expected behaviors will help the nurse differentiate common patterns of injury from scenarios that suggest a child at risk for abuse or neglect. Infants and toddlers are totally dependent on adults and often sustain injuries when supervision has lapsed. Babies are at risk for rolling off surfaces while they are being bathed or while their diapers are being changed. Children who cannot walk may sustain injuries while learning to walk. Toddlers have a strong need to explore but lack sufficient judgment to recognize risk. At this stage, children may sustain head injuries from falls while they are climbing or suffer burns from touching hot objects. Older children have gained independence but still tend to be impulsive and often act without considering the consequences of their behavior. Thus they are more likely to dart into traffic or make sudden movements on a bicycle (Ludwig & Loiselle, 1993). These actions place them at greater risk for most injuries. Adolescents often take unnecessary risks that place them in harm's way. In this age group, a lack of common sense behavior often results in motor vehicle injuries, diving injuries, and assaults. Children of all ages will benefit from a detailed injury history combined with an appreciation of the child's developmental stage. Recognition of these factors will provide a more complete picture of a child's risk of injury and will promote early detection of serious trauma.

Child Abuse

Although most childhood injuries are unintentional, blunt trauma inflicted by adults is a reality in our society. The nurse's ability to differentiate accurate injury histories from those that are suspicious is an essential assessment skill. Any injury history that does not match the child's age or developmental stage should be questioned. Clinical signs and symptoms that contradict the story given by the caretaker should be investigated closely. Research suggests that infants who roll off household surfaces and fall short distances rarely sustain severe injuries. A very young child who presents with a severe head injury and a history of "falling off the couch" should be viewed with suspicion. Tarantino, Dowd, and Murdock (1999) evaluated infants who presented with a history of a short vertical fall (less than 4 feet). The most common mechanism was rolling off a bed. Fifteen percent had significant injuries. After suspected abuse cases were excluded, the authors found that no child suffered an intracranial hemorrhage as a result of this type of fall. Serious injuries from seemingly minor events should always be questioned. Unlikely or nonsensical scenarios should also be investigated. A toddler who is "always falling" and presents with multiple trauma or healing injuries should be evaluated for child abuse. Suspicion of abuse or neglect should always be considered when the MOI contradicts the clinical findings or the injury history is unexpected for the developmental stage of the child.

Head Injuries

As expected, a child's head and brain are extremely vulnerable to injury during a traumatic event. Patterns of injury are often related to the age and size of the child. During the first year of life, the child has a proportionately large head that comprises approximately 20% of body surface area (Haley & Baker, 1993). The resultant high center of gravity increases the likelihood of a head injury in a fall or collision. Suture lines are both protective and problematic. Energy is transferred to the brain, resulting in fewer skull fractures but greater intracranial damage (Cantor & Leaming, 1998).

The major mechanisms of childhood head injury tend to be age related. Children incur serious head injuries in falls, MVCs, and bicycle crashes. In children younger than 5 years, falls are the most common mechanism, with vehicular trauma becoming the most prevalent mechanism in older children (Luerssen, 1993; Reece & Sege, 2000). However, MVCs remain the leading cause of death for children older than 1 year (National Highway Traffic Safety Administration, 2000). With sudden deceleration in an MVC, the weight of the head leads the body and often becomes the first area to come into contact with a solid object, such as the interior of a vehicle. An unrestrained child involved in a 30-mph crash strikes the dashboard with the same intensity as in a fall from a three-story building (Templeton, 1993).

Serious injury head injury and death can occur even when protective devices are used. Passenger-side air bags can be lethal to children regardless of whether they are restrained or not buckled at the time of the crash (Grisoni et al., 2000). Despite increased use of child safety seats, many children are injured because of improper use of restraint systems, which contributes to serious injury. Winston et al. (2000) compared injuries in children protected by child restraint systems to those of children aged 2 to 5 years who used safety belts. Compared with the children in child restraint systems, the children in safety belts were more likely to suffer significant head injuries. Young children are too small to fit correctly in a lap belt. An improperly placed safety belt places the child at risk for sliding out of the lap belt during a crash and sustaining head injury. Clearly, the type of restraint must match the size and weight of a child in order to offer adequate protection against injury. The National Highway Traffic Safety Administration (1998) currently recommends that infants and children weighing less than 40 pounds be placed in child safety seats. Booster seats should be used for children weighing between 40 and 80 pounds to prevent injury related to inadequate fit of the lap belt. Although child restraint systems are complex, a history that includes information about restraint systems will form a clearer picture of the actual injury event. Facts regarding the type of restraint, age of the child, location of the child in the vehicle, and other pertinent information may be invaluable in identifying injuries.

Children also sustain head injuries as pedestrians or cyclists. An adult who is struck by a vehicle is likely to have a point of impact in the area of the pelvis and lower extremities. In a child of short stature, the impact more likely will involve the head and other areas of the body. In one study, nearly 50% of children involved in pedestrian vehicular incidents sustained head injury, and the majority had involvement of at least one other body system (Orsborn, Haley, Hammond, & Falcone, 1999). Driveway crush injuries occur primarily in children younger than age 6 years and result in head injuries, with a tenfold increase in mortality compared with other pedestrian incidents (Patrick, Bensard, Moore, Partington, & Karrer, 1998). Children commonly fall off bicycles; however, the majority of severe injury usually occurs as a result of collision with a vehicle (Puranik, Long, & Coffman, 1998). Helmets have been shown to significantly reduce pediatric head injury; consequently, an increase in the use of helmets will change the pattern of injuries that occur.

Falls are most common in younger age groups because of the immature judgment and lack of physical development in younger children. Very young children generally sustain a fall while rolling off a raised surface or climbing. Baby walkers have been identified as a cause of head trauma in children younger than age 2 years, with most injuries occurring in a fall down the stairs (Partington, Swanson, & Meyer, 1991). Older children are at risk for falling out of windows. Most household falls in young children result in minimal injury, and mortality from falls in children younger than 2 years appears to be low (Luerssen, 1993). Skull fractures, although often characteristic of inflicted injury, are common in children younger than 1 year as a result of accidental falls (Shane & Fuchs, 1997).

Controversy exists about whether fatal head injuries can result from short-distance falls. A widely held belief is that fatal falls from short heights actually represent inflicted trauma (Reiber, 1993). Tarantino, Dowd, and Murdock (1999) found that head injuries did occur when a child was accidentally dropped by a caregiver, but serious head injuries were attributed to child abuse. Falls from significant heights obviously raise suspicions of severe injury, but low falls may not trigger the same response. Because young children cannot relate the injury event, it is the responsibility of the medical professional to obtain a complete and accurate history of the injury event.

Infants and toddlers are especially vulnerable to mistreatment by adults in the form of shaking or hitting. A study by Dashti, Decker, Razzaq, and Cohen (1999) analyzed patterns of injury associated with child abuse. This study found that 32% of children younger than 2 years admitted for head trauma had an inflicted injury. In a similar study of children younger than 2 years, Duhaime et al. (1992) reported that 24% of injuries were presumed inflicted and an additional 32% were suggestive of abuse, neglect, or family problems. This study also confirmed that retinal hemorrhages remain highly suggestive of abuse. Reece and Sege (2000) described the mechanism of head injuries in children younger than 6.5 years. Unintentional injuries accounted for 81% of the injuries and 19% by definite abuse. In 56% of the abuse group, no history was given to explain the cause of the injury. A fall was given as the cause of injury in 17% of the abuse group. The children in the abuse group also had a higher incidence of subdural hematomas, subarachnoid hemorrhage, retinal hemorrhages, and associated cutaneous injury. A child who is suspected of having an inflicted injury should be examined closely for external signs of trauma. Gilliland and Folberg (1996) reported that most shaken babies present with impact injuries in the form of head injury and retinal hemorrhages, as well as with external evidence such as finger marks or rib fractures. When caring for a child with a head injury, the nurse must recognize an injury history that does not correlate with the physical presentation, complete a through physical assessment, and make appropriate referrals.

Spinal Injuries

The manner in which kinetic energy is transferred to the spine dictates the injuries that will occur. Cervical spine injury in children is primarily associated with flexion injuries, and thoracic and lumbar injuries are almost entirely flexion related (Templeton, 1993). Flexion injuries occur when the spine is bent forward beyond its normal range. In severe flexion injuries, the vertebral body is thrust forward, causing cord compression (Templeton, 1993). Rotational forces compound flexion injuries by placing additional stress on the spine. Hyperextension injuries cause posterior dislocation of upper vertebrae onto the lower vertebrae, as well as fractures of the vertebral body.

As with head trauma, the mechanisms of spinal injuries in children are related to age. Young children are more likely to be victims of vehicular trauma and falls, whereas older children more likely are injured in MVCs or sporting activities (Dickman & Rekate, 1993). Children who are unrestrained during an MVC are particularly vulnerable. Givens, Polley, Smith, and Hardin (1996) reviewed traumatic cervical spine injuries. MVC was the most common mechanism, and 80% of the children were incorrectly restrained or unrestrained altogether. Associated head injuries occurred in 53% of the patients. Lumbar spine injuries caused by lap belts are found largely in the pediatric population. Ill-fitting lap belts tend to ride up over the abdomen in children instead of being supported by the iliac spines. During a crash, momentum causes the body to be thrust forward, leaving the lumbar vertebral bodies to absorb the impact (Winston et al., 2000). The vertebrae are compressed by the lap belt, resulting in fractures or flexion distraction injuries (Dickman & Rekate,

1993). Compression fractures of the lumbar spine have also been documented secondary to lap belt use in children (Sturm, Glass, Sivit, & Eichelberger, 1995).

Active children are prone to falls that can lead to spinal injuries. Falls from the first floor or higher have been implicated as a leading cause of spinal cord paralysis in children (Peclet et al., 1990); however, low falls should not be excluded as a cause of vertebral trauma. Schwartz, Wright, Fein, Sugarman, Pasternack, and Salhanick (1997) identified eight children who sustained cervical spine injury after a fall from less than 5 feet. Injuries resulting from falls involving the trampoline have increased dramatically in recent years. Furnival, Street, and Schunk (1999) reviewed several hundred trampoline injuries. Twelve percent of patients sustained spinal injuries, and several thoracic and cervical spine fractures were noted. Although the popularity of recreational activities will change with time, falls will always be a consequence of playing. Clinical assessment must be combined with an injury history before spinal injury can be ruled out. A child with a history suggestive of spinal trauma should be triaged and evaluated immediately. Even a seemingly benign history can prove to be associated with a significant spinal injury.

Anatomic differences in younger children affect the presentation of spinal injury. The very young child's spine is more mobile than that of an adult. There is greater elasticity in the ligamentous structures of the spine, which allows more mobility during an injury event. The facet joints are more horizontal in children, allowing for more displacement during flexion (Luerssen, 1993). Less developed neck muscles and a disproportionately heavy head create an anatomic fulcrum in the upper cervical spine. Consequently, spinal cord injuries above C4 are most common in children younger than 8 years (Cantor & Leaming, 1998; Dickman & Rekate, 1993). Older children tend to incur injuries at the level of C5 to C6 (Luerssen, 1993). Interestingly, one study found "low" cervical spine injuries (below C4) in 50% of children with cervical spine injuries, challenging findings of previous studies. Although hypermobility of the spine acts as a protective mechanism by dissipating force throughout the spine, it is this momentum that causes serious damage to the spinal structures. In fact, spinal injuries cause permanent loss of function at a higher rate in pediatric populations than in any other age group (Dickman & Rekate, 1993). Around age 8 years, the anatomic characteristics change, and the spine begins to approximate that of an adult (Dickman & Rekate, 1993).

Flexibility of the vertebral bodies and more cartilaginous structures also contributes to a unique MOI found in children, known as *spinal cord injury without radiographic abnormality (SCIWORA)*. The term refers to an absence of bony disruptions on plain spine films and early computed tomography scans. The risk of SCIWORA is related to age and can account for nearly half of cervical spinal injuries. Dickman, Zabramski, Hadley, Rekate, and Sonntag (1991) reported that 16% of children with spinal injuries sustained SCIWORA, but in young children the frequency was 32%. Baker, Kadish, and Schunk (1999) reported that 32 of 70 cervical spine injuries in children younger than 15 years was SCIWORA. This subtle injury requires a high level of vigilance and attention from the nurse to avoid a missed spinal injury or a delay in diagnosis.

Thoracic Injuries

MOIs for thoracic trauma in children mimic the patterns described for other types of blunt trauma. Motor vehicle and pedestrian collisions constitute the most common causes of chest injuries. In a review of 25,000 children, Cooper, Barlow, DiScala, and String (1994) reported an 86% incidence of blunt thoracic injury. Blunt chest trauma is associated with high mortality and is accompanied by other significant injuries as often as 80% of the time (Allshouse & Eichelberger, 1993). Mortality rates as high as 50% are seen in serious injuries to vital thoracic structures (Cooper, 1995). As with other systems, abusive injuries must be considered in specific circumstances. Strouse and Owings (1995) found that rib fractures in infants and young children were a result of inflicted trauma in one third of cases.

Aspects of the child's anatomy that serve as protection also render the thoracic area more vulnerable to blunt impact. The flexible rib cage in children allows for greater dissipation of energy and fewer fractures, but this often results in more pulmonary contusions and other thoracic injuries (Allshouse & Eichelberger, 1993; Templeton, 1993). The presence of rib fractures suggests a force of great magnitude and should be regarded with high suspicion and rapid assessment. Traumatic pneumothorax occurs after a laceration by a fractured rib or by a sudden increase in intrathoracic pressure. Pulmonary contusions are common after blunt trauma and are generally caused by vehicular crashes. Neurologic injury, abdominal injury, and skeletal fractures often accompany the lung injury (Allen, Cox, Moor, Duke, & Andrassy, 1997). A more mobile mediastinum in infants and young children can result in a dramatic mediastinal shift after blunt trauma (Cantor & Leaming, 1998). In high-velocity mechanisms, rupture of the heart or severe myocardial contusion can occur. Tracheobronchial ruptures in blunt thoracic trauma are rare but can occur in high-velocity or crush injuries. Tracheobronchial tree disruption is insidious; children can have complete disruption of the airway with little external sign of injury (Grant, Meyers, Jaffe, & Johnson, 1998).

Thoracic trauma in children can be subtle. Multiple injuries, hemorrhage, or simply a screaming, frightened child may distract the nurse from a thorough assessment of the chest and respiratory system. In addition, life-threatening injuries may be present in the absence of any obvious external sign of trauma. A "well-appearing" child who has been struck by a car should be assumed to have thoracic injury until proven otherwise. Nursing implications include the need for a focused primary survey assessment and attention to the injury history to help reveal subtle signs of injury.

Abdominal Trauma

Serious abdominal injury is often overlooked in children. Unrecognized abdominal injuries can contribute to complications and extended recovery. As with other body areas, early assessments may reveal minimal external sign of trauma even when significant injuries are present. MOI data combined with subtle clinical cues can help prevent injuries from being missed.

Blunt trauma accounts for most abdominal injuries in children and usually results from falls, MVCs, and pedestrian and bicycle accidents (Rothrock, Green, & Morgan, 2000). Multiple organ injury is the usual pattern in children (Ascension & Torres, 1993). The spleen is particularly vulnerable and can sustain lacerations even at low impact during sporting injuries or short falls (Scorpio & Wesson, 1993). A review by Powell et al. (1997) found that MOI differed significantly between adults and children with spleen injury. Leading pediatric mechanisms were falls, MVCs, sports, and pedestrian injuries.

Kinetic forces affect vital organs in several ways. For example, sudden deceleration in an MVC results in shearing forces that can damage blood vessels as well as produce lacerations and contusions to solid organs. A burst injury is produced when a fluid-filled hollow organ, such as the bladder or stomach, is stretched to bursting by an increase in intraabdominal pressure (Newman, 1993). Crush injuries from traffic collisions or falls occur as a result of compression of the viscera against an unyielding object, such as adjacent ribs, spinal column, or abdominal wall. Rupture of the diaphragm can also occur after impact as a result of a massive increase in intraabdominal pressure (Templeton, 1993). Handlebars can cause serious abdominal injury in children as a result of a fall off a bike. Winston, Shaw, Kreshak, Schwarz, Gallagher, and Cnaan (1998) described splenic lacerations, liver lacerations, and kidney injuries that occurred as a result of sudden handlebar pressure to the abdominal wall. Straddle injuries occur with a direct blow to the perineum causing a crushing blow to the urethra.

Children have several unique aspects that predispose them to abdominal trauma. Solid abdominal organs are relatively larger, making them vulnerable to injury in blunt or penetrating trauma. A naturally protuberant abdomen creates a large "target area" that is vulnerable to impact. The bladder is an abdominal organ in children, thus increasing its susceptibility to injury. The rib cage offers less protection for the abdominal organs in children, and unlike in adults, the lower ribs expose the kidney (Allshouse & Betts, 1993). The liver and spleen in young children extend past the rib cage, making these organs more vulnerable to a sharp blow. Furthermore, less ossification of the rib cage results in a more flexible structure that allows energy transmission directly to the viscera (Scorpio & Wesson, 1993; Templeton, 1993). The child's abdomen also has weaker musculature and less protection from fat. These factors contribute to a vulnerable torso in the child. Constant vigilance and a high index of suspicion are essential when evaluating abdominal trauma in children.

Although vehicular trauma and falls cause most abdominal trauma, visceral injury can occur secondary to child abuse. With an inflicted injury, compression of abdominal organs occurs following a blow to the abdomen. A caretaker may report a fall or attribute the MOI to the actions of a sibling. Children presenting with significant abdominal trauma without a substantiated history or any apparent delay in seeking medical care should be investigated for possible abuse. A child who presents in extremis without a plausible MOI history should raise a red flag. Careful examination and reassessment of clinical signs combined with a high index of suspicion will help identify children who have been victims of child abuse.

Trauma resulting from the use of safety belts has been well described in the literature. Use of two-point restraints, or lap belts, has been linked to intraabdominal and lumbar spine injury in children. This injury occurs when focal energy is transmitted from the safety belt to internal structures during a crash. The child's body is thrust forward, and stress is concentrated at the level of the belt. Lap belts can also produce abdominal trauma in a crash when the child slides under the safety belt, forcing the belt against the abdomen. Typical injuries include small bowel contusions or lacerations and flexion distraction injuries to the lumbar spine (Newman et al., 1990; Sivit et al., 1991). Sivit et al. (1991) reviewed 61 restrained children who presented with abdominal ecchymosis from an MVC. Fifty-two had a combination or lumbar spine and/or intraabdominal injuries. A child with a history of being restrained in a MVC should prompt close evaluation for the presence of spinal and abdominal trauma.

Skeletal Injuries

Fractures are common in children and are generally caused by falls, MVCs, and recreational injuries. Increased interest in all-terrain and other motorized vehicles, inline skating, and trampolines are also responsible for an increasing number of skeletal injuries (Huurman & Ginsburg, 1997). Lillis and Jaffe (1997) found that upper extremity fractures were the most common injury requiring hospitalization after falls on the playground. The majority of trampoline injuries also involved the upper extremity fracture. A study that evaluated injuries secondary to all-terrain vehicle injuries in children indicated that orthopedic injuries were the most common, with the majority being open and comminuted (Lynch, Gardner, & Worsey, 1998).

Bony anatomic differences contribute to fractures in children. The periosteum is thicker and the cortex is more porous. A lack of ossification makes pediatric bones more compliant, with a greater ability to tolerate deformation than adults (Ludwig & Loiselle, 1993). Two bony injuries unique to children result from this flexibility. The torus fracture is a folding or buckling of the cortex without a fracture. A bending injury occurs when blunt trauma forces a bowing of the bone without breaking it. These fractures are common in toddlers and school-aged children and generally occur from falls. Shearing or bending from a variety of activities can damage the growth plate, a cartilaginous disc located between the epiphysis and metaphysis.

Open fractures can occur secondary to blunt trauma or penetrating trauma. Of pediatric patients with open fractures after blunt trauma, 30% have injuries to other body systems (Thomas, 1993). Gunshot wounds can also produce open fractures. Larger wounds or traumatic amputations in children result from farm trauma, crush injuries, or MVCs.

Active children are commonly brought to the emergency department from treatment of a fracture. The clavicle is the most frequently fractured bone in children, and this fracture is often associated with a fall (Ludwig & Loiselle, 1993). The specific mechanism of a forearm fracture, as well as the more complicated supracondylar fracture, is usually a fall on an outstretched hand. Oblique or "spiral" fractures are usually seen in the humerus or tibia and are often associated with abuse. These fractures result from the rotary force action required to break the bone (Huurman & Ginsburg, 1997). Spiral tibial fractures also occur by unintentional mechanisms (Mellick, Milker, & Egsieker, 1999). Femoral fractures are usually associated with traffic crashes and falls and are commonly seen in children older than 2 years. However, femoral fractures in infants and toddlers should raise suspicion of abuse, especially in the absence of a reasonable history (Templeton, 1993). Radial head subluxation, also called *nursemaid's elbow*, is generally seen in children younger than 6 years. The injury is often related to a sudden pull to the arms, which traps the annular ligament under the radial head (Huurman & Ginsburg, 1997). Although orthopedic trauma shares many aspects with adult injuries, those features unique to the pediatric population still must be recognized.

Penetrating Trauma

Although less common than blunt injury, penetrating trauma has become an increasing problem, especially in adolescents. Although penetrating trauma can be caused by guns, knives, and other objects, firearms pose the greatest risk. Firearms are the fourth leading cause of death in individuals 5 to 24 years old (National Safety Council, 1999). A Connecticut study found firearm injuries were second only to MVCs as a cause of mortality among children. Death rates were highest among children 15 to 19 year old (Zavoski, Lapidus, Lerer, & Banco, 1995). Another state study found guns, in particular, were responsible for the rising penetrating injury rates in children (Crandall, Olson, Fullerton, Sklar, & Zumwalt, 1997). Air guns, often perceived as toys by parents, are more common in pediatric penetrating injury. Bhattacharyya, Bethel, Caniano, Pillai, Deppe, & Cooney (1998) reported 16 of 42 patients with air gun injuries had serious long-term disability.

Although the incidence of penetrating trauma is lower than that of blunt trauma, gunshot and stab wounds are associated with higher mortality. Cooper et al. (1994) reported that abdominal trauma was the primary cause of mortality in only 22% of cases involving blunt visceral injury. Conversely, 67% of penetrating trauma deaths were attributed directly to the abdominal injury (Cooper et al., 1994). Thoracic trauma presents a similar scenario. Cooper (1995) demonstrated that in blunt trauma patients, 15% of deaths resulted directly from intrathoracic injuries, whereas penetrating trauma accounted for 100% of deaths from chest injuries.

As with blunt trauma, body mass plays a role in the severity of injury seen in penetrating mechanisms. Multiple organ injuries are more common because of the proximity of vital organs, especially within the abdominal and thoracic cavity. Associated injury to vital organs often results in an increased need for surgical intervention in pediatric patients (Dicker, Sartorelli, McBrids, & Vane, 1996). Peterson, Tepas, Edwards, Kissoon, Pieper, and Ceithaml (1994) reported similar findings in children with penetrating thoracic trauma. The small size of the pediatric airway renders it more vulnerable. An expanding hematoma after direct injury to the neck can quickly occlude a child's airway (Knudson, 1993). Although stab wounds generally cause less associated injury, factors such as the location and depth of the wound are important determinants of damage (Knudson, 1993). Less musculature and fatty tissue in children means that less penetration is required to reach vital structures. Any penetrating wound below the nipples can damage structures within both the thorax and the abdomen. Even shallow injuries in the precordial area can cause fatal injury (Templeton, 1993). A complete history that addresses the specific mechanism of the penetrating trauma is essential to recognizing serious injury in pediatrics.

TRAUMA SCORES

Scoring systems have been developed for the purpose of accurately describing the severity of traumatic injuries. Trauma scores have been used to predict mortality, compare populations of injured patients, perform quality assurance analyses, direct health care policy, and perform field triage. Most scores use a combination of physiologic values and injury sites to produce a numerical value that represents trauma severity. Adult scoring systems have been applied to the pediatric population without clear consensus as to their value in assessing injury to children. In response, pediatric experts have designed special scoring methods to evaluate injury effects in younger patients. A successful scoring system should be simple to apply in the clinical setting and demonstrate high interrater reliability. The score should also correlate with the desired outcome measure, such as death, disability, injury severity, or hospital length of stay (Furnival & Schunk, 1999).

A variety of scoring systems are available for use with the trauma patient. Several of the most popular methods are discussed. The Glasgow Coma Scale (GCS) is widely used as a measure of level of consciousness. It is based on the sum of three variables for responsiveness: eye opening, best verbal response, and best motor response. Pediatric modifications on the GCS have been developed to account for the lack of verbal abilities and capacity to follow directions in young children (Sacco, Copes, & Gotschall, 1993). The Trauma Score (TS) was originally designed to predict patient outcomes on the basis of physiologic indicators and uses values from the GCS. The Revised Trauma Score (RTS) simplified the TS by limiting the number of physiologic factors required and has been widely used as a field triage tool. The Injury Severity Score (ISS) was devised to assess multiple injuries and results in a numerical score between 1 and 75 based on the number and severity of body regions injured. The ISS does not include physiologic data and does not account for patient age or preexisting medical conditions (Furnival & Schunk, 1999). The TRISS methodology combines the physiologic values from the TS and the anatomic scores from the ISS to determine probability of survival after trauma. The TRISS can be used to identify patients with unexpected outcomes and is especially useful in quality assurance investigations (Furnival & Schunk, 1999). The Pediatric Trauma Score (PTS) was designed to predict injury severity of the traumatized child by using physiologic and anatomic aspects particular to the pediatric patient. Size is incorporated into this system by assigning a numerical value to the child's weight in combination with assessments of the airway, systolic blood pressure, neurologic status, and obvious external injuries to the skeleton and skin surface (Ramenofsky, Ramenofsky, Jurkovich, Threadgill, & Powell, 1988).

Extensive research regarding the effectiveness and use of trauma scoring in children has produced controversy. Experts have not unanimously accepted a single scoring system that is most appropriate in determining severity of injury in children. Ramenofsky et al. (1988) reported the PTS to be highly accurate, reliable, and predictable when used to triage injured children. Other research has indicated the PTS demonstrates no advantage over the RTS in evaluating outcome of children (Sacco, Copes, & Gotschall, 1993). Hannan, Farrell, Meaker, and Cooper (2000) evaluated several scoring systems and concluded that an alternative evaluation using a combination of specific aspects of other scoring systems was more reliable than the PTS or the RTS. Another study evaluated prehospital triage in the injured pediatric patient and found that the PTS and RTS missed 36% and 45% of major pediatric trauma victims, respectively (Engum et al., 2000). The study concluded that a combination of physiologic variables and anatomic injury contained within trauma scores, along with MOI, provides a sensitive and safe system of triage. Each of the major trauma scoring methods offers an advantage over the other in statistical research, field triage, regional comparisons, and as an outcome measure. Although experts disagree on which system is best, it is clear that consistent use of one or more of these tools will help identify the most critical patients. It is most important for health care professionals to find a tool that is simple, accessible, and works well in their clinical setting. Nurses who care for pediatric patients should be well trained in at least one of these tools and be able to easily integrate them into daily practice.

BIBLIOGRAPHY

Allen, G. S., Cox, C. S., Moor, F. A., Duke, J. H., & Andrassy, R. J. (1997). Pulmonary contusions: Are children different. *Journal American College of Surgery, 18*(3), 229-233.

Allshouse, M. J., & Betts, J. M. (1993). Genitourinary injury. In M. Eichelberger (Ed.), *Pediatric trauma: Prevention, acute care and rehabilitation* (pp. 503-519). St. Louis: Mosby.

Allshouse, M. J., & Eichelberger, M. R. (1993). Patterns of thoracic injury. In M. Eichelberger (Ed.), *Pediatric trauma: Prevention, acute care and rehabilitation* (pp. 437-450). St. Louis: Mosby.

American Academy of Pediatrics. Committee on Sports Medicine. (2000). Injuries in youth soccer: A subject review. *Pediatrics, 105*(3), 659-661.

Ascension, M. T., & Garcia, V. F. (1993). Hepatobiliary trauma. In M. Eichelberger (Ed.), *Pediatric trauma: Prevention, acute care and rehabilitation* (pp. 464-474). St. Louis: Mosby.

Baker, C., Kadish, H., & Schunk, J. E. (1999). Evaluation of pediatric cervical spine injuries. *American Journal of Emergency Medicine, 17*(3), 230-234.

Bhattacharyya, N., Bethel, C. A., Caniano, D. A., Pillai, S. B., Deppe, S., & Cooney, D. R. (1998). The childhood air gun: Serious injuries and surgical interventions. *Pediatric Emergency Care, 14*(3), 188-190.

Cantor, R. M., & Leaming, J. M. (1998). Contemporary issues in trauma: Evaluation and management of pediatric major trauma. *Emergency Medicine Clinics of North America, 16*(1), 229-256.

Consumer Product Safety Commission. (2000). Strategic plan revised 2000. Available at: http://www.cspc.gov.

Cooper, A. (1995). Thoracic injuries. *Seminars in Pediatric Surgery, 4*(2), 109-115.

Cooper, A., Barlow, B., DiScala, C., & String, D. (1994). Mortality and truncal injury: The pediatric perspective. *Journal of Pediatric Surgery, 29*(1), 33-38.

Crandall, C., Olson, L., Fullerton, L., Sklar, D., & Zumwalt, R. (1997). Guns and knives in New Mexico: Patterns of penetrating trauma. *Academy of Emergency Medicine, 14*(4), 263-267.

Dashti, S. R., Decker, D. D., Razzaq, A., & Cohen, A. R. (1999). Current patterns of inflicted head injury in children. *Pediatric Neurosurgery, 31*(6), 302-306.

Dicker, R. A., Sartorelli, K. H., McBrids, W. J., & Vane, D. W. (1996). Penetrating hepatic trauma in children: Operating room or not? *Journal of Pediatric Surgery, 31*(8), 1189-1191.

Dickman, C. A., & Rekate, H. L. (1993). Spinal trauma. In M. Eichelberger (Ed.), *Pediatric trauma: Prevention, acute care and rehabilitation* (pp. 362-377). St. Louis: Mosby.

Dickman, C. A., Zabramski, J. M., Hadley, M. N., Rekate, H. L., & Sonntag, V. K. (1991). Pediatric spinal cord injury without radiographic abnormalities: Report of 26 cases and review of the literature. *Journal of Spinal Disorders, 4*(3), 296-305.

Duhaime, A. C., Alario, A. J., Lewander, W. J., Schut, L., Sutton, L. N., Seidl, T. S., et al. (1992). Head injury in very young children: Mechanisms, injury types, and ophthalmologic findings in 100 hospitalized patients younger than 2 years of age. *Pediatrics, 90*(2), 179-185.

Engum, S. A., Mitchell, M. K., Scherer, L. R., Gomez, G., Jacobson, L., Solotkin, K., & Grosfelt, J. L. (2000). Pre-hospital triage in the injured pediatric patient. *Journal of Pediatric Surgery, 35*(1), 82-87.

Furnival, R. A., & Schunk, J. E. (1999). ABCs of scoring systems for pediatric trauma. *Pediatric Emergency Care, 15*(3), 215-223.

Furnival, R. A., Street, K. A., & Schunk, J. E. (1999). Too many pediatric trampoline injuries. *Pediatrics, 103*(5), e57.

Gilliland, M. G., & Folberg, R. (1996). Shaken babies—Some have no impact injuries. *Journal of Forensic Science, 41*(1), 114-116.

Givens, T. G., Polley, K. A., Smith, G. F., & Hardin, W. D. (1996). Pediatric cervical spine injury: A three-year experience. *Journal of Trauma, 41*(2), 310-314.

Grant, W. J., Meyers, R. L., Jaffe, R. L., & Johnson, D. G. (1998). Tracheobronchial injuries after blunt chest trauma in children-hidden pathology. *Journal of Pediatric Surgery, 33*(11), 1707-1711.

Grisoni, E. R., Srikumar, P. B., Volsko, T. A., Mutabagani, K., Garcia, V., Haley, K., Schweer, L., Marsh, E., & Cooney, D. (2000). Pediatric airbag injuries: The Ohio experience. *Journal of Pediatric Surgery, 35*, 160-163.

Haley, K. A., & Baker, P. (Ed.). (1993). Pediatric trauma. In *Emergency nursing pediatric course instructor manual* (pp. 109-152). Park Ridge, IL: Emergency Nurses Association.

Hannen, E. L., Farrell, L. S., Meaker, P. S., & Cooper, A. (2000). Predicting inpatient mortality for pediatric trauma patients with blunt injuries: A better alternative. *Journal of Pediatric Surgery, 35*(2), 155-159.

Huurman, W. W., & Ginsburg, G. M. (1997). Musculoskeletal injury in children. *Pediatrics in Review, 18*(12), 429-440.

Knudson, M. M. (1993). Penetrating injuries. In M. Eichelberger (Ed.), *Pediatric trauma: Prevention, acute care and rehabilitation* (pp. 332-342). St. Louis: Mosby.

Lillis, K. A., & Jaffe, D. M. (1997). Playground injuries in children. *Pediatric Emergency Care, 13*(2), 149-153.

Ludwig, S., & Loiselle, J. (1993). Anatomy, growth, and development: Impact on injury. In M. Eichelberger (Ed.), *Pediatric trauma: Prevention, acute care and rehabilitation* (pp. 39-59). St. Louis: Mosby.

Luerssen, T. T. (1993). General characteristics of neurologic injury. In M. Eichelberger (Ed.), *Pediatric trauma: Prevention, acute care and rehabilitation* (pp. 345-361). St. Louis: Mosby.

Lynch, J. M., Gardner, M. J., & Worsey, J. (1998). The continuing problem of all-terrain vehicle injuries in children. *Journal of Pediatric Surgery, 33*(2), 329-332.

Marshall, K. W., Koch, B. L., & Egelhoff, J. C. (1998). Air bag-related deaths and serious injuries in children: Injury patterns and imaging findings. *American Journal of Neuroradiology, 19*(9), 1599-1607.

Mellick, L. B., Milker, L., & Egsieker, E. (1999). Childhood accidental spiral tibial (CAST) fractures. *Pediatric Emergency Care, 14*(5), 307-309.

National Highway Traffic Safety Administration. (1998). *Child transportation safety tips (1-14).* Available at: www.nhtsa.cot.gov/people/injury/child/ps.

National Highway Traffic Safety Administration. (2000). *Buckle up America.* Available at: http://www.nhtsa.dot.gov/people/injury/airbags/buckleplan/buaweek/buaweekmobil/page06.htm.

National Safety Council. (1999). *Injury facts.* Available at: http://www.nsc.org.

Newman, K. D. (1993). Gastric and intestinal injury. In M. Eichelberger (Ed.), *Pediatric trauma: Prevention, acute care and rehabilitation* (pp. 475-481). St. Louis: Mosby.

Newman, K. D., Bowan, L. M., Eichelberger, M. R., Gotschall, C. S., Taylor, G. A., Johnson, D. L., & Thomas, M. (1990). The lab belt complex: Intestinal and lumbar spine injury in children. *Journal of Trauma, 30,* 1133-1140.

Orsborn, R., Haley, K., Hammond, S., & Falcone, R. (1999). Pediatric pedestrian versus motor vehicle patterns of injury: Debunking the myth. *Air Medical Journal, 18*(3), 107-109.

Osberg, J. S., Schneps, S. E., DiScala, C., & Li, G. (1998). Skateboarding. *Archives of Pediatric Adolescent Medicine, 152*(October), 985-991.

Partington, M. D., Swanson, J. A., & Meyer, F. B. (1991). Head injury and the use of baby walkers: A continuing problem. *Annals of Emergency Medicine, 20*(6), 652-654.

Patrick, D. A., Bensard, D. D., Moore, E. E., Partington, M. D., & Karrer, F. M. (1998). Driveway crush injuries in young children: A highly lethal, devastating, and potentially preventable event. *Journal of Pediatric Surgery, 33*(11), 1712-1715.

Peclet, M. H., Newman, K. D., Eichelberger, M. R., Gotschall, C. S., Guzzetta, P. C., Anderson, K. D., Garcia, V. F., Randolph, J. G., & Bowman, L. M. (1990). Patterns of injury in children. *Journal of Pediatric Surgery, 25*(1), 85-90.

Peterson, R. J., Tepas, J. J., Edwards, F. H., Kissoon, N., Pieper, P., & Ceithaml, E. L. (1994). Pediatric and adult thoracic trauma: Age-related impact on presentation and outcome. *Annals of Thoracic Surgery, 58*(1), 14-18.

Powell, M., Gardner, M., Lynch, J., Harbrecht, G. G., Udekwu, A. O., Billiar, T. R., Federle, M., Ferris, J., Meza, M. P., & Peitzman, A. B. (1997). Management of blunt splenic trauma: Significant differences between adults and children. *Surgery, 122*(4), 654-660.

Puranik, S., Long, J., & Coffman, S. (1998). Profile of pediatric bicycle injuries. *Southern Medical Journal, 91*(11), 1033-1037.

Ramenofsky, M. L., Ramenofsky, M. B., Jurkovich, G. J., Threadgill D., & Powell, R. W. (1988). The predictive validity of the Pediatric Trauma Score. *Journal of Trauma, 28*(7), 1038-1042.

Reece, R. M., & Sege, R. (2000). Childhood head injuries: Accidental or inflicted? *Archives of Pediatric Adolescent Medicine, 154*(1), 11-15.

Reiber, G. D. (1993). Fatal falls in childhood: How far must children fall to sustain fatal head injury? *American Journal of Forensic Medical Pathology, 14*(3), 201-207.

Rice, M. R., Alvanos, L., & Kenney, B. (2000). Snowmobile injuries and deaths in children: A review of national injury data and state legislation. *Pediatrics, 105*(3), 615-619.

Rivara, F. P. (1997). Fatal and non-fatal farm injuries to children and adolescents in the United States. *Injury Prevention, 3*(3), 190-194.

Rothrock, S. G., Green, S. M., & Morgan, R. (2000). Abdominal trauma in infants and children: Prompt identification and early management of serious and life-threatening injuries. Part I; Injury patterns and initial assessment. *Pediatric Emergency Care, 16*(2), 106-112.

Sacco, W. J., Copes, W. S., & Gotschall, C. S. (1993). Measurement and assessment of outcomes. In M. Eichelberger (Ed.), *Pediatric trauma: Prevention, acute care and rehabilitation* (pp. 641-654). St. Louis: Mosby.

Schwartz, G. R., Wright, S. W., Fein, J. A., Sugarman, J., Pasternack, J., & Salhanick, S. (1997). Pediatric cervical spine injury sustained in falls from low heights. *Annals of Emergency Medicine, 30*(3), 249-252.

Scorpio, R. J., & Wesson, D. E. (1993). Splenic trauma. In M. Eichelberger (Ed.), *Pediatric trauma: Prevention, acute care and rehabilitation* (pp. 456-464). St. Louis: Mosby.

Shane, S. A., & Fuchs, S. M. (1997). Skull fractures in infants and predictors of associated intracranial injury. *Pediatric Emergency Care, 13*(3), 198-203.

Shorter, N. A., Mooney, D. P., & Harmon, B. J. (1999). Snowboarding injuries in children and adolescents. *American Journal of Emergency Medicine, 17*(3), 236-263.

Sivit, C. J., Taylor, G. A., Newman, K. D., Bulas, D. I., Gotschall, C. S., Wright, C. J., & Eichelberger, M. R. (1991). Safety-belt injuries in children with lap-belt ecchymosis: CT findings in 61 patients. *American Journal of Roentgenology, 157*(1), 111-114.

Strouse, P. J., & Owings, C. L. (1995). Fractures of the first rib in child abuse. *Radiology, 197*(3), 763-765.

Sturm, P. F., Glass, R. B., Sivit, C. J., & Eichelberger, M. R. (1995). Lumbar compression fractures secondary to lap-belt use in children. *Journal of Pediatric Orthopedics, 15*(4), 521-523.

Tarantino, C. A., Dowd, M. D., & Murdock, T. C. (1999). Short vertical falls in infants. *Pediatric Emergency Care, 15*(1), 5-8.

Templeton, J. M. (1993). Mechanism of injury: Biomechanics. In M. Eichelberger (Ed.), *Pediatric trauma: Prevention, acute care and rehabilitation* (pp. 20-35). St. Louis: Mosby.

Thomas, M. D. (1993). Musculoskeletal injury. In M. Eichelberger (Ed.), *Pediatric trauma: Prevention, acute care and rehabilitation* (pp. 533-547). St. Louis: Mosby.

Vardara, D. R. (Ed.). (1993). *Taber's cyclopedic medical dictionary.* Philadelphia: FA Davis.

Winston, F. K., Durbin, M. D., Kallan, M. S., & Moll, E. K. (2000). The danger of premature graduation to seat belts for young children. *Pediatrics, 105*(6), 1179-1183.

Winston, F. K., Shaw, M. D., Kreshak, B. A., Schwarz, D. D., Gallagher, P. R., & Cnaan, A. (1998). Hidden spears: Handlebars as injury hazards to children. *Pediatrics, 102*(3) 596-601.

Zavoski, R. W., Lapidus, G. D., Lerer, T. J., & Banco, L. I. (1995). A population-based study of severe firearm injury among children and youth. *Pediatrics, 96*(2), 278-282.

Zietlow, S. P., & Swanson, J. A. (1999). Childhood farm injuries. *American Surgeon, 65*(7), 693-697.

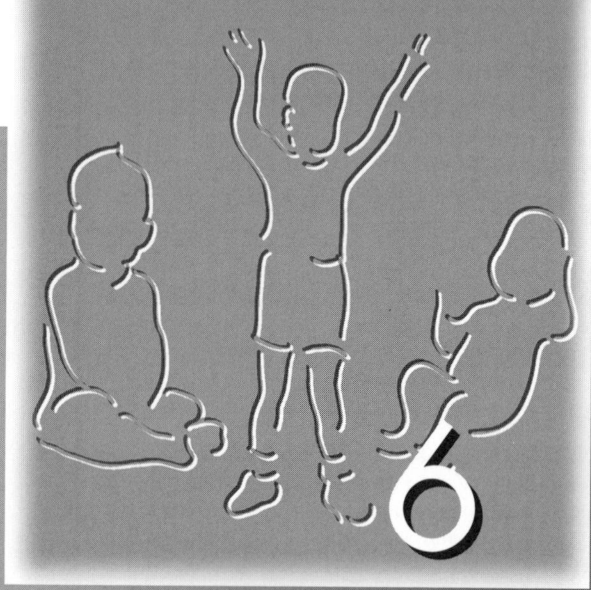

Initial Resuscitation of the Pediatric Trauma Victim

Monica Artiles Liebman

Trauma continues to be the leading cause of death and disability in children between the ages of 1 and 19 years (National Center for Health Statistics, 1999). The single largest cause of trauma-related death is motor vehicle crashes. Approximately 24% of pediatric motor vehicle–related deaths involve alcohol. Nonintentional injury is not the leading cause of death in children younger than 1 year; however, a recent study demonstrated 32.1 injury deaths per 100,000 infant years (Scholer, Hickson, & Ray, 1999). Other causes of death include homicides, suicides, drowning, burns, and falls.

INITIAL RESUSCITATION

The initial assessment and management of the critically injured child requires rapid assessment and prioritization of injuries. This systematic approach is similar to that of adults; however, children require special consideration due to their unique characteristics (see Chapter 4).

Primary Survey

The principles of the primary and secondary surveys guide the initial resuscitation of the pediatric trauma patient. The primary survey allows for the rapid identification of any life-threatening injuries and focuses on the initial stabilization of the cardiopulmonary system.

Airway

Airway assessment begins by determining airway patency. The child is assessed for trauma to the face or neck that may compromise the airway. Noisy respirations, such as stridor, may indicate airway obstruction. The child's mouth is examined for blood, loose teeth, and visible foreign objects.

The goals of airway management in the injured child are optimal oxygenation and ventilation, cervical spine protection, and minimal increases in intracranial pressure (Rice & Britton, 1993). Any child who sustains trauma is presumed to have a cervical spine injury until proven otherwise. A child's head is larger in proportion to the body and has less musculoskeletal support. This relatively larger head size makes the cervical section of the spine more vulnerable to injury and causes undesirable cervical flexion. All injured children require cervical spine management by inline immobilization with the head in a neutral position or by application of a rigid cervical collar (Rice & Britton, 1993).

If a cervical collar is being used, it is of utmost importance that a properly sized collar be placed on the child. An oversized collar can result in hyperextension of the neck, as well as limit access to the child's airway. This becomes very challenging when attempting to size the child who is 3 years or younger. Infants and toddlers have "no neck," which adds to the challenges of finding the proper fit. To determine the correct size, the collar is measured in width from the top of the shoulder to the chin with the head in neutral position.

While inline manual immobilization is maintained, the airway is opened using the jaw-thrust method. This maneuver alone may relieve airway obstruction by moving the tongue forward. However, if the child does not respond, vomit, blood, or broken teeth may be causing the obstruction. Severe maxillofacial injuries or injuries to the larynx and/or chest may produce airway obstruction. Foreign material, such as vomit or blood, can be removed by suctioning with a large, plastic, tonsil-tip suction catheter.

If positioning and suctioning do not relieve the child's respiratory distress, artificial ventilation is initiated with a bag and mask. A self-inflating bag capable of delivering 100% oxygen is preferred. While the bag is being compressed, care is taken not to deliver an excess amount of pressure and volume. Ventilation is limited to the amount that is necessary for the chest to rise. The mask should provide a good seal, and the fingers used to hold the mask in place should always rest on the bony prominences, not on the submandibular tissue.

An oral airway can be used as an adjunct to providing ventilation in the obtunded patient. To determine the correct size, the airway is placed next to the child's face with the flange at the corner of the mouth and the tip at the angle of the jaw (Manley, 1994). The airway is inserted by opening the child's mouth and lifting the tongue with a tongue depressor. The airway is slid into position, taking care to avoid pushing the tongue backward and thus obstructing the airway. The practice of inserting the airway in an inverted position and rotating it 180 degrees is not recommended in pediatric patients because trauma to the teeth or soft tissue may occur.

In the conscious child, gagging may occur with an oral airway, and it is generally tolerated poorly. A nasopharyngeal airway is indicated for these patients. To determine the correct size, the length should approximate the distance between the nares and the tragus of the ear. The diameter should be slightly smaller than the diameter of the nares (Fallon Smith & Lyons, 2001). The airway is lubricated and the tube inserted through the nostril and into the nasopharynx.

Endotracheal intubation is the intervention of choice for the injured child who cannot maintain an airway, has a Glasgow Coma Scale (GCS) score of 8 or less, or is demonstrating signs of shock. Table 6-1 provides guidelines for laryngoscope, endotracheal tube (ETT), and suction catheter sizes. Oral endotracheal intubation is preferred over nasotracheal intubation in the injured child. Rice and Britton (1993) report that nasotracheal intubation is contraindicated with injuries such as basilar skull fracture.

Endotracheal intubation is always preceded by the administration of 100% oxygen (American Heart Association, 2000). Uncuffed ETTs are used in pediatric patients up to age 7 years to prevent subglottic edema and stenosis. However, cuffed tubes are available for younger children in whom high inspiratory pressures may be present (American Heart Association, 2000). The appropriate interior diameter (ID) of the ETT for a particular child can be estimated by using the following formula:

$$\frac{16 + \text{Age in years}}{4} = \text{ID of ETT}$$

For example, for a 2-year-old child, the following calculation applies:

$$\frac{16 + 2}{4} = 4.5 \text{ mm}$$

This is an approximate rule, so it is recommended that tubes of the next higher and lower sizes also be readily available. Another approximate measure often used to determine ETT diameter is the size of the internal naris. If the tube will fit into one naris, it will probably fit comfortably down the trachea.

Once the child is intubated, correct placement is determined. This is initially done by providing positive-pressure ventilation, watching chest wall movement, and auscultating breath sounds over the peripheral lung fields. ETT placement should be confirmed by monitoring exhaled carbon dioxide (American Heart Association, 2000). If pulse oximetry is monitored, oxygen saturation generally increases after successful tube placement. Once the tube is secured, position is confirmed by chest radiograph.

Rapid-sequence intubation (RSI) is indicated for respiratory arrest, need for airway control, GCS score of less than 8, shock, and respiratory failure, or whenever there is a risk of aspiration of gastric contents (Fallon Smith & Lyons, 2001). All pediatric trauma patients are assumed to have a full stomach, and RSI minimizes the possibility of regurgitation (Tobias, Rasmussen, & Yaster, 1996). This technique also blunts the response of increased intracranial pressure that can be stimulated by intubation. RSI is done using a

TABLE 6-1 Recommended Resuscitation Equipment for the Infant and Child

Age	0-6 mo	6-12 mo	1 yr	18 mo	3 yr	5 yr	6 yr	8 yr	10 yr	12 yr	14 yr
Weight (kg)	3-5	7	10	12	15	20	20	25	30	40	50
Resuscitation mask	0-1	1	1-2	2	3	3	3	3	3	4	4-5
Laryngoscope (Miller/Mac)	0	1	1	1	2	2	2	2	2	2	3
ETT	3.0	3.5	3.5	4.0	4.5	5.0	5.5	6.0	6.0	6.5	7.0
Suction catheter (ETT/tracheal)	6	6	8	8	10	10	10	10	10	14	14
Suction (OP/NP)	10	10	10	10	14	14	14	16	16	16	16
Chest tube	10-12	10-12	16-20	16-20	16-20	20-28	20-28	20-28	28-32	28-42	32-42
NG/OG	8	8	8	8	10	10	10	10	12	12	14
Foley	5	5	8	8	10	10	10	10	12	12	12
Trach (pediatric)	00	1	1	1-2	2-3	3	3	4	4	5	6

Data from Widner-Kolberg, M. R. (1989). Maryland Institutes for Emergency Medical Services Systems.
ETT, Endotracheal tube; *NG*, nasogastric; *NP*, nasopharyngeal; *OG*, orogastric; *OP*, oropharyngeal.

BOX 6-1 Rapid-Sequence Induction Process

1. Organize equipment and personnel.
2. Administer 100% oxygen.
3. Administer premedications.
4. Administer sedatives and paralysis.
5. Intubate.
6. Confirm endotracheal tube placement.

From Curley, M. A. Q., & Moloney-Harmon, P. A. (2001). *Critical care nursing of infants and children* (2nd ed.). Philadelphia: WB Saunders.

sequence of preparation, preoxygenation, premedication, sedation, and paralysis as outlined in Box 6-1 and Table 6-2. Medications are based on the child's condition and institution-specific guidelines (Fallon Smith & Lyons, 2001).

The technique of cricoid pressure (Sellick maneuver) is used during RSI to prevent passive regurgitation of stomach contents into the pharynx. In this technique, the upper esophagus is compressed against the cervical vertebral column by applying anteroposterior pressure on the cricoid cartilage. Cricoid pressure must be maintained until correct placement of the ETT is confirmed.

In some uncommon instances the child will require a needle cricothyroidotomy. This technique is indicated in the child with an obstruction below the larynx or with a significant maxillofacial or airway injury. A 14- or 16-gauge needle is inserted through the cricothyroid membrane to establish the airway. If this is not possible, a surgical tracheostomy is performed.

Intubation needs to occur as soon as possible in the child who requires assisted ventilation. However, in the out-of-hospital setting, effective bag-mask ventilation may be preferable. A study conducted by Gausche et al. (2000) showed that scene time was lengthened and fatal complications more likely to occur when children were intubated in this setting. Gausche et al. recommend that training for prehospital providers focus on effective bag-mask ventilation with prompt transport. Endotracheal intubation should be deferred until the child reaches the hospital setting.

TABLE 6-2 Rapid-Sequence Intubation Medication Preparation Guidelines

Nonhead Trauma

1. Atropine (age <7 yr)—0.02 mg/kg/dose (min 0.1 mg/dose)
2. Rocuronium (0.6-1.2 mg/kg/dose) or succinylcholine (1-2 mg/kg/dose)
3. Pentothal (4-6 mg/kg/dose) or etomidate (0.3 mg/kg/dose)

Head Trauma/Increased ICP/No Hypotension

1. Atropine (<7 yr)—0.02 mg/kg/dose (min 0.1 mg/dose)
2. Lidocaine (1 mg/kg)
3. Pentothal (4-6 mg/kg)
4. Rocuronium (0.6-1.2 mg/kg/dose)

Asthma

1. Atropine (<7 yr)—0.02 mg/kg/dose (min 0.1 mg/dose)
2. Ketamine (0.5-2 mg/kg/dose)
3. Rocuronium (0.6-1.2 mg/kg/dose)

Hypotension

1. Atropine (<7 yr)—0.02 mg/kg/dose (min 0.1 mg/dose)
2. Etomidate (0.3 mg/kg/dose) or midazolam (0.05-0.1 mg/kg/dose)
3. Rocuronium (0.6-1.2 mg/kg/dose) or succinylcholine (1-2 mg/kg/dose)

Postintubation

1. Lorazepam (0.05-0.1 mg/kg/dose)
2. Pancuronium (0.1 mg/kg/dose)

Modified from Collaborative Practice Group, Emergency Department, Children's Hospital, Boston.

Breathing

The nurse should assess the breathing status of the child, observing for signs of respiratory distress (e.g., retractions, use of accessory muscles, seesaw breathing, rapid labored breathing, nasal flaring, and change in the child's mental status). The chest wall should be inspected for signs of contusions, lacerations, deformity of the rib structure, and unequal chest movement. The respiratory rate in the child decreases with age. An infant requires 40 to 60 breaths per minute, whereas the child between 1 and 8 years breathes 20 to 40 times per minute (American College of Surgeons, 1997). Systematic auscultation of breath sounds is performed at both apices and bases bilaterally.

Management of the injured child's respiratory status is achieved by the administration of 100% oxygen at a rate that is age and condition specific. Insertion of a nasogastric tube is mandatory in children who require intubation to prevent diaphragmatic compromise. If the child begins to show signs of respiratory distress, coupled with unequal breath sounds and unstable vital signs, several complications are considered. These include equipment problems, displacement of the ETT, and obstruction of the tube. If these complications are not causing the signs of respiratory and cardiovascular instability, a pneumothorax or hemothorax should be considered. The immediate treatment for a pneumothorax is needle decompression, which is performed by inserting a 14- to 20-gauge needle into the fifth intercostal space, anterior to the midaxillary line (American College of Surgeons, 1997). A syringe is used to temporarily decompress the pneumothorax, followed by placement of a chest tube. If a hemothorax is suspected, fluid resuscitation is required before evacuation of the hemothorax to prevent exsanguination (Moloney-Harmon & Adams, 2001).

Circulation

The injured child is assessed for any signs of active bleeding. Because of the child's small blood volume (80 ml/kg), a small amount of blood loss can quickly produce hypovolemic shock. The child also compensates effectively for blood loss and does not show a change in systolic blood pressure until 25% of the blood volume has been lost.

Assessment of the child for hypovolemic shock consists of close observation and monitoring of heart rate, systemic perfusion, and blood pressure. Symptoms of shock include tachycardia, capillary refill time greater than 2 seconds, cool and mottled extremities, pallor, narrowed pulse pressure, decreased urine output, and decreased level of consciousness. Table 6-3 shows the four classes of hemorrhage, with the clinical signs and treatment for each. As mentioned previously, a decrease in the systolic blood pressure is a late sign of shock.

If active bleeding is apparent, the nurse must maintain accurate records of blood loss and observe for signs of occult blood loss. Direct pressure should be applied to any bleeding wounds to prevent further blood loss. All critically injured children should have at least two functioning vascular access lines (peripheral, central, or intraosseous). Placement of the catheters in veins above and below the diaphragm is optimal (Table 6-4). The ideal situation is to be able to place the intravenous catheter upon the first attempt and obtain blood for laboratory studies at the same time. The American College of Surgeons (1997) recommends that if placement of vascular access into a peripheral vein is unsuccessful after two attempts, an intraosseous line should be considered, especially in children younger than 6 years, or a direct venous cutdown. Table 6-4 outlines sites ideal for venous access in children.

The most crucial aspect of treatment for the injured child is restoration of the circulating blood volume. As stated by the American College of Surgeons (1997), "the goal in fluid resuscitation in the child is to rapidly replace the circulating volume." The process begins with infusing 20 ml/kg of warm crystalloid solution as quickly as possible. The child's response to the fluid bolus is evaluated by assessing a decrease in heart rate and capillary refill time; an increase in pulse pressure, urine output, and temperature of the extremities; and an improvement in the level of consciousness. If the response to fluid resuscitation is inadequate, an second fluid bolus of 20 ml/kg is given. Generally, the rule of thumb is to administer 3 ml of crystalloid for every 1 ml of blood loss. If shock persists after the second fluid bolus, consideration should be given to the use of packed red blood cells (10 ml/kg) (American College of Surgeons, 1997). Refer to Table 6-3 for the treatment of hemorrhage.

If the child remains in shock after all interventions, other causes should be considered. These causes may include occult bleeding, which warrants immediate surgical intervention. Development of a tension pneumothorax may also cause continued signs of shock.

Once shock has been controlled, fluids can be delivered at the maintenance rate. Table 6-5 provides the calculations for maintenance fluid for a 24-hour period in children.

TABLE 6-4 Ideal Sites for Venous Access

Site	Comment
Percutaneous peripheral	Two attempts or <90 sec before attempting alternate method
Intraosseous	No age restriction
Saphenous vein at the ankle	Venous cutdown
Femoral vein	Percutaneous placement
Subclavian vein	Percutaneous placement
External jugular vein	Percutaneous placement
Internal jugular vein	Percutaneous placement

From American College of Surgeons. (1997). *Advanced trauma life support program for doctors: The instructor manual. First impression: The United States of America.* Chicago: The American College of Surgeons.

TABLE 6-3 Classes of Hemorrhage in Children

Class	Blood Loss	Signs	Treatment
I	≤15% 40-kg child = 500 ml of blood	Pulse: Slight ↑ BP: Normal Respiration: Normal Capillary refill: Normal Tilt test*: Normal	Crystalloids
II	20%-30% 40-kg child = 800 ml of blood	Pulse: Tachycardia >150 BP: ↓ systolic; ↓ pulse pressure Respiration: Tachypnea >35-40 Capillary refill: Delayed Tilt test: Positive Urine output: Normal (1 ml/kg/hr)	Crystalloids
III	30%-35% 40-kg child = 1200 ml of blood	BP: Decreased Narrow pulse pressure Urine output: Decreased	Crystalloids Packed red cells
IV	40%-50% 40-kg child = 1600 ml of blood	Pulse: Nonpalpable BP: Nonpalpable No response to verbal or painful stimuli	Crystalloids Packed red cells

From K. McQuillan, K. Von Rueden, R. Hartsock, M. Flynn, & E. Whalen (Eds.). (2002). *Trauma nursing: From resuscitation to rehabilitation* (3rd ed.). Philadelphia: WB Saunders.

BP, Blood pressure.

*A tilt test is done by sitting the child upright. The test result is normal if the child can stay up more than 90 seconds and maintain blood pressure.

TABLE 6-5 Calculation of Maintenance Fluids (Per 24 Hours) in Children

Weight (kg)	Kilogram Body Weight Formula
0-10	100-120 ml/kg
11-20	1000 ml for the first 10 kg and 50 ml/kg for each kilogram over 10 kg
21-30	1500 ml for the first 20 kg and 25 ml/kg for each kilogram over 20 kg

From Moloney-Harmon, P. A. (2002). Pediatric trauma. In K. McQuillan, K. Von Rueden, R. Hartsock, M. Flynn, & E. Whalen (Eds.), *Trauma nursing: From resuscitation to rehabilitation* (3rd ed., pp. 747-771). Philadelphia: WB Saunders.

BOX 6-2 AVPU Scale

A = Alert
V = Responds to verbal stimuli
P = Responds to painful stimuli
U = Unresponsive

Although volume is the intervention of choice for hypovolemia, some children may require resuscitation medications to restore cardiac output. Resuscitation medications indicated for cardiac arrest and symptomatic arrhythmias are discussed in Chapter 4.

DISABILITY

During the primary survey, the neurologic assessment consists of level of consciousness, pupil size and reaction to light, and motor response (Moloney-Harmon & Adams, 2001). Evaluation of the level of consciousness after a head injury is probably the single most important aspect of the neurologic assessment but often the most difficult to perform in an infant or young child. Because level of consciousness means different things to different people, a uniform system like AVPU (Box 6-2) or the GCS (see Table 4-3) should be used.

With children, as with adults, pupil reactivity, size, shape, and symmetry are responses used to assess brainstem function. When increased intracranial pressure develops, the oculomotor nerve is compressed by general expansion of the brain, an intracranial lesion, or herniation of the brain. The pupil dilates but does not constrict in response to light. Eye movements are also noted. Abnormal eye movements include deviation of one or both eyes from midline or back-and-forth movements.

Any difficulty in movement of the extremities is evaluated, and the nature of the movement is described as spontaneous or in response to pain. The extremity in which the response is elicited is recorded. The child with increased intracranial pressure will decreased motor function and abnormal posturing or reflexes. Babinski reflex is positive when the toes fan out and the great toe moves dorsally. The reflex is assessed by scratching the sole of the foot with an object such as the blunt tip of a tongue depressor. A positive reflex is normal in a child younger than 18 months but abnormal in any child who is walking and may indicate the presence of increased intracranial pressure.

The goals of management of a child with a neurologic injury are to control intracranial hypertension, maintain cerebral perfusion, and prevent hypoxia. Children who have sustained a severe head injury (GCS score of 8 or less) require intubation with proper sedation to prevent further increase in intracranial pressure. In patients with a head injury less than 72 hours old, computed tomography (CT) scanning remains the procedure of choice for several reasons, including the limited potential for magnetic resonance imaging (MRI) to diagnose acute subarachnoid hemorrhage or acute parenchymal hemorrhage, the ease of monitoring unstable patients during the CT scan procedure, and the short time frame required to complete the procedure (Grasso & Keller, 1998). MRI is a technique used to image intracranial structures and is superior for imaging the posterior fossa, spinal cord structure, small vascular lesions, and most brain tumors. Lengthy procedure time, difficulty in monitoring critically ill patients during the procedure, cost, and inability to visualize bone directly are among the limitations of this diagnostic procedure.

A secure airway is critical because hypoxia and hypercapnia must be avoided. If the child is hypotensive, fluids are given at the resuscitation dose, even if neurologic injury is present. However, an isolated head injury rarely causes shock. If shock is present, there should be a high index of suspicion for another source of bleeding.

If the child shows signs of intracranial pressure, hyperventilation may be initiated. By lowering the $Paco_2$, cerebral blood flow is decreased, which reduces intracranial pressure. The current recommendation is that this therapy be used only for acute increases in intracranial pressure resulting in acute neurologic deterioration or that is refractory to other methods of reduction (Allen & Ward, 1998). Mild hyperventilation ($Paco_2$ 30 to 34 mm Hg) is instituted to decrease cerebral blood flow but prevent cerebral ischemia associated with severe vasoconstriction (Allen & Ward, 1998). The child's head is kept in a midline position and, if not contraindicated, may be slightly elevated (15 to 30 degrees) to facilitate venous drainage from the brain.

If the child is not in hypovolemic shock, fluids may be restricted to one half to two thirds of maintenance levels. Hypotonic fluids are not given to prevent exacerbation of brain edema because of free water. Hypertonic saline may be used for resuscitation of the child with a severe head injury. A recent study demonstrated that hypertonic saline (3% sodium chloride [NaCl]) maintains blood pressure and cerebral oxygen delivery, decreases overall fluid requirements, and results in overall improved survival rates (Shackford, Bourguignon, Wald, Rogers, Osler, & Clark, 1998).

Osmotic diuretics, such as mannitol 0.25 g/kg, may be given to children with increased intracranial pressure who are not responsive to other forms of therapy. These agents should be used with caution, however, because mannitol can increase cerebral blood flow dramatically as a result of the shift of fluid from the cellular to the vascular space. When mannitol is used, boluses of 0.25 g/kg are recommended. Continuous administration of mannitol may result in a reverse osmotic shift, leading to increased brain osmolarity and increased intracranial pressure (Allen & Ward, 1998). Serum osmolality is monitored every 6 hours and should not exceed 320 mOsm.

Posttraumatic seizures, which can occur in the child as a result of a severe head injury (GCS score of 3 to 8), diffuse cerebral edema, or an acute subdural hematoma, must be pharmacologically controlled (Hahn, Fuchs, Flannery, Barthel, & McLone, 1988). Diazepam (0.1 to 0.3 mg/kg) or phenobarbital (20 to 30 mg/kg) may be given in the acute situation, with phenytoin (5 mg/kg/day) used for long-term control. Posttraumatic seizures may occur up to 1 to 2 years after injury.

Exposure

The child is completely exposed to determine the presence of other life-threatening injuries. However, this does place the child at risk for hypothermia. Hypothermia produces various physiologic consequences, such as metabolic acidosis and arrhythmias, and it can interfere with resuscitation efforts.

Hypothermia is treated by external and internal measures. External warming measures include radiant warmers, warm blankets and sheets, and the bear hugger. Internal warning measures include warmed intravenous fluids and warm humidification. The child's temperature should be measured every hour and document the child's response to interventions.

Secondary Survey

According to Advanced Trauma Life Support (ATLS) guidelines, the "secondary survey does not begin until the primary survey (ABCDE's) have been fully completed, resuscitative efforts have been fully established and the child is demonstrating normalization of vital functions" (American College of Surgeons, 1997). The secondary survey is a head-to-toe assessment that seeks to identify previously undetected injuries and allows for reassessment of primary survey findings at the same time. Additional information about each system injury is given in later chapters.

Head Trauma

Head injury is a common pediatric injury and the most common cause of traumatic death in children (Ghajar & Hariri, 1992). Each year in the United States, approximately 22,000 children with acute brain injuries die, and another 29,000 are left with a permanent disability. Mortality in children with severe head injuries is 6% to 10%, as opposed to 30% to 50% in adults with severe head injuries (Mansfield, 1997).

The head is inspected for lacerations, swelling, and depressions. Scalp lacerations can cause significant bleeding because of the vascularity of the area. The anterior fontanelle of the infant should be examined for bulging or depression. The face is examined for symmetry and the presence of injury, such as lacerations. The ears and nose are assessed for the presence of cerebral spinal fluid or blood, which may indicate a basilar skull fracture or a meningeal tear. Ecchymosis in the periorbital region and behind the ear are also indicative of a basilar skull fracture. The presence of maxillofacial fractures should be assessed, especially over bony prominences. The eyes are examined for pupil size and reaction and fundal appearance. If the child is conscious, vision should be assessed and motor response observed. Chapter 14 provides in-depth information about assessment and management of the child with a head injury.

Spinal Cord Injury

Spinal cord injury is relatively rare in children. Approximately 1100 children with spinal cord injury are reported annually (Cantor & Leaming, 1998). Motor vehicle crashes are the leading cause of spinal cord injury in children. The large head and weak cervical muscles of young children predispose them to cervical spine injury. Infants and toddlers are at risk for a degree of torque from forces transmitted along the cervical spine. The "anatomic fulcrum" in children younger than 8 years is at the C2 to C3 level, compared with adults, in whom it is located between C5 and C7. In addition, the ligaments and musculature of the pediatric spine are more elastic, especially in children younger than 8 years (Laskowski-Jones & Salati, 2000). These features all contribute to creating hypermobility of the neck and a tendency toward spinal cord injury without radiographic abnormality (SCIWORA), severe ligamentous injury, and upper cervical spine injuries (Dickman, Rekate, Sonntag, & Zabramski, 1989).

All pediatric trauma victims are initially assumed to have a cervical spine injury, especially children who experience facial or head trauma or who complain of pain in the neck or back. Clearance of the cervical spine requires anteroposterior, lateral, and open-mouth views of the cervical spine (Cantor & Leaming, 1998). It is critical that the cervical spine films include views of C7 and T1. These views are obtained by gently pulling the shoulders downward to visualize the seven cervical vertebrae.

Children younger than 8 years are prone to SCIWORA. A normal spine series can be seen in approximately two thirds of children with a spinal cord injury. When in doubt about the integrity of a child's cervical spine, the nurse should keep the child's head and neck firmly immobilized, obtain appropriate radiographic studies, and consult the appropriate subspecialty service. Methylprednisolone is the drug of choice for nonpenetrating spinal cord injury. The pediatric dose is 30 mg/kg administered over 15 minutes, followed in 45 minutes by a continuous infusion of 5.4 mg/kg/hr for 23 hours (Allen, Boyer, Cherney, & Tait, 1996).

Chest Trauma

Serious thoracic injury is most commonly the result of blunt trauma. Motor vehicle–related and bicycle-related injuries account for the majority of thoracic trauma (Cantor & Leaming, 1998). Falls and child abuse are other common causes of thoracic injury in children. The presence of serious thoracic injury increases the potential for mortality by a factor of 10.

The chest is observed for contusions, lacerations, abrasions, deformities, and abnormalities in chest wall movement. Assessment continues for signs and symptoms of respiratory distress. Breath sounds are auscultated, and the thorax is palpated for the presence of tenderness, swelling, and crepitus.

Management of the child with thoracic trauma is injury specific. Care is directed toward the final common pathways of respiratory failure and low cardiac output.

Abdominal Trauma

Abdominal injuries in children are not common; however, failure to promptly diagnose these injuries and successfully manage them accounts for increased mortality and morbidity. Usually, serious injury to the head or limbs is obvious, whereas serious abdominal injury tends to be subtle.

Most pediatric abdominal injuries occur as a result of blunt trauma, such as bicycle incidents and motor vehicle crashes. The primary goal of the management of pediatric abdominal injury is to prevent hemorrhage, sepsis, and overall organ dysfunction.

The abdomen is first inspected for lacerations, contusions, abrasions, puncture wounds, distention, and exposed internal organs. The abdomen is then assessed for tenderness and rigidity by using gentle palpation and percussion. Bowel sounds are auscultated; absence may indicate bleeding or perforation. A rapidly increasing abdominal girth is consistent with ongoing bleeding and warrants immediate diagnostic studies, such as a peritoneal lavage, CT scan, or exploratory laparotomy in the operating room.

Historically, diagnostic peritoneal lavage (DPL) and CT scanning have been considered the standard methods for evaluating blunt abdominal trauma. DPL is helpful for deciding whether laparotomy is indicated in hemodynamically unstable patients. CT scanning provides more precise information about the severity of injuries if the patient can tolerate the scanning procedure. More recently, another diagnostic tool, ultrasonography, has been used for evaluating blunt abdominal trauma (Yoshii et al., 1998). The decision as to which diagnostic method to apply is often controversial.

Genitourinary Trauma

The perineal area is examined for lacerations, abrasions, contusions, swelling, and bleeding. Palpating and applying gentle pressure over the iliac crests and symphysis pubis allow assessment of the stability of the pelvis. The urinary meatus is checked for the presence of blood; if blood is present, a urinary catheter is not inserted. A rectal examination is done to assess for hematomas or lacerations, and a stool sample is checked for blood. A rectal examination is not performed until after the cervical spine has been cleared.

Musculoskeletal Trauma

Injuries to the extremities are usually obvious or easily identified by roentgenogram. Extremities are assessed for pain, swelling, contusions, lacerations, and deformities. The neurovascular status of each limb is noted and documented; temperature, sensation, pulses, and color are checked. Range of motion for each limb is assessed. Soft tissues are thoroughly inspected for foreign bodies and dead tissue.

EMOTIONAL CARE OF THE FAMILY

An important aspect of the care of the pediatric trauma patient is care of the family. The family experiences the circumstances surrounding trauma as a crisis. Because trauma is unexpected, the parents do not have time to adjust to the possible death or disability of their child. Parents initially may experience shock and disbelief. Normal reactions include confusion, disorganized behavior, and increased tension and anxiety (Carnevale, 1999). Parents may have difficulty in accepting the situation as real. The normal coping mechanisms they have always used to deal with previous crises may no longer be effective. Decision-making abilities may be impaired. Parents often experience feelings of guilt that may be indicated by feelings of anger at themselves, each other, the child, or the health care team. These feelings of anger may occur immediately or later as the family passes through the shock and disbelief phase to the developing awareness phase (Boie, Moore, Brummet, & Nelson, 1999).

These families require compassionate support through their adjustment to this crisis in their lives, and they need to be informed. Too often, parents are in a waiting area left to wonder about what is happening. Parents require information from the health care team as soon as possible because they are often imagining the worst. An important priority is having them see their child as soon as possible. As the child's condition stabilizes, other concerns that the family members may have must be addressed.

Information about their child is given to parents in a simple, straightforward manner because it is often difficult for them to synthesize a lot of information at this time. Any misconceptions that the family may have about the situation and/or their child's injuries and treatment plan are addressed. When the family is being prepared to see the child, they are told about the change in their child's appearance and about the equipment and personnel that will be at the bedside. Parents are asked how the child appears to them, and explanations then can be given based on their perceptions.

An important consideration for the health care team is family presence during the resuscitation. Boie et al. (1999) determined that most parents whose children require resuscitation in the emergency department wish to be in attendance. Nurses take on the important responsibility of preparing families to stay with their child.

Response to the Death of a Child

Some children may not survive resuscitation efforts; care then shifts to the family. These parents need support from the nursing staff when the news about the death of the child is shared. The immediate reactions of the family are shock, numbness, and disbelief—a time when parents often feel out of touch with reality. Parents are often immobilized and unable to make decisions (Pearson, 1999). Guilt is another feeling that parents often experience when a child dies, especially if it is a nonintentional death.

After the initial shock of a child's death, the phase of intense grief begins. This may begin immediately or may be delayed for weeks. During this phase, parents may experience loneliness and an intense yearning for their child. They may feel extremely helpless, which often leads to feelings of anger and despair. At this time, they are at risk for developing physical symptoms such as loss of appetite, and they may experience sleep disturbances (Pearson, 1999).

The phase of reorganization follows. Parents report that they never recover completely from a child's death, but most are able to regain their previous level of functioning with the support and care from others. This is evidenced by a return to normal daily activities, more happy memories of the child, and a decrease in feelings associated with intense grief.

Nurses play a crucial role with parents who have lost their child. Initial interactions with the family usually occur as they experience the shock and numbness of their loss. At this time, it is important to let parents know that all extraordinary measures were taken to save the child. The family is often comforted to know that the child did not suffer. Further conversation is guided by the family's expressed need for more information. Quiet time is often needed and appreciated. The nurse's physical presence while the family begins to experience their loss is often helpful.

Some parents may feel a need to express their great pain and sorrow. Guilt feelings may surface as the family begins to grieve. Such feelings should not be negated because they are a significant part of the process to help families come to term with their loss.

Anger may be experienced at this time and is often directed toward hospital personnel. Such feelings usually pass, and the family members may become extremely confused by the various emotions that have overcome them. The most appropriate intervention at this time is for the nurse to listen, reinforce the positive aspects of their parenting role, and explain the normalcy of their feelings.

Parents may need assistance with problem solving as they face the many decisions that must be made during this time of great stress. Many families will benefit from the support offered through social service programs. Appropriate referrals should be made at this time. Clergy members and social workers may assist the family by providing guidance in making funeral arrangements and by offering emotional and spiritual support.

In addition, it is helpful if the nurse who cared for the child makes contact with the family shortly after the child's death. This conveys to the family that they have been remembered and provides them the opportunity to ask questions and express feelings that have surfaced since the child's death. Many parents need reassurance and continued support as they experience various aspects of their personal grief. Chapter 10 provides more in-depth information about family support.

SUMMARY

The care that the child receives during the initial resuscitation and stabilization of a life-threatening injury makes a difference in long-term outcome. Children who die as the result of a traumatic injury do so because of the complication of airway compromise, bleeding, or central nervous system injury. If these complications are prevented or treated early, the effects can possibly be reversed. The potential for a good outcome is maximized by expert nursing care, which includes rapid, accurate assessment and interventions during both the primary and secondary surveys. Family interventions are an important component of the expert care.

BIBLIOGRAPHY

Allen, E. M., Boyer, R., Cherney, W. B., & Tait, V. (1996). Head and spinal cord injury. In M. C. Rogers (Ed.), *Textbook of pediatric intensive care* (3rd ed., pp. 814-862). Baltimore: Williams & Wilkins.

Allen, C. H., & Ward, J. D. (1998). An evidence-based approach to management of increased intracranial pressure. *Critical Care Clinics, 14,* 485-495.

American College of Surgeons. (1997). *Advanced trauma life support program for doctors: The instructor manual. First impression: The United States of America.* Chicago: American College of Surgeons.

American Heart Association. (2000). Pediatric advanced life support. *Circulation, 102*(Suppl. I), I291-I342.

Boie, E. T., Moore, G. P., Brummett, C., & Nelson, D. R. (1999). Do parents want to be present during invasive procedures performed on their children in the emergency department? A survey of 400 parents. *Annals of Emergency Medicine, 34,* 70-74.

Cantor, R. M., & Leaming, J. M. (1998). Evaluation and management of pediatric major trauma. *Emergency Medicine Clinics of North America, 16*(1), 229-256.

Carnevale, F. A. (1999). Striving to recapture our previous life: The experience of families with critically ill children. *Journal of the Canadian Association of Critical Care Nursing, 10,* 16-22.

Chaimedes, L., & Hazinski, M. F. (1997). *Textbook of pediatric advanced life support* (pp. 41-5). Dallas: American Heart Association.

Dickman, C. A., Rekate, H. L., Sonntag, V. K. H., & Zabramski, J. M. (1989). Pediatric spinal trauma: Vertebral column and spinal cord injuries in children. *Pediatric Neuroscience, 15,* 237-256.

Fallon Smith, M., & Lyons, A. (2001). Resuscitation and transport of infants and children. In M. A. Q. Curley & P. A. Moloney-Harmon (Eds.), *Critical care nursing of infants and children* (2nd ed., pp. 1025-1053). Philadelphia: WB Saunders.

Gausche, M., Lewis, R. J., Stratton, S. J., Haynes, B. E., Gunter, C. S., Goodrich, S. M., Poore, P. D., McCollough, M. D., Henderson, D. P., Pratt, F. D., & Seidel, J. S. (2000). Effect of out-of-hospital pediatric endotracheal intubation on survival and neurological outcome. *JAMA, 283,* 783-790.

Ghajar, J., & Hariri, R. J. (1992). Management of pediatric head injury. *Pediatric Clinics of North America, 39*(5), 1093-1125.

Grasso, S. N., & Keller, M. S. (1998). Diagnostic imaging in pediatric trauma. *Current Opinions in Pediatrics, 10,* 299-302.

Hahn, Y. S., Fuchs, S., Flannery, A. M., Barthel, M. J., & McLone, D. G. (1988). Factors influencing post-traumatic seizures in children. *Neurosurgery, 22,* 864-867.

Laskowski-Jones, L., & Salati, D. S. (2000). Responding to pediatric trauma. *Dimensions of Critical Care Nursing, 19*(6), 2-12.

Manley, L. K. (1994). Procedures involving the respiratory system. In L. M. Bernardo & M. A. Bove (Eds.), *Pediatric emergency nursing procedures* (pp. 63-81). Boston: Jones and Bartlett.

Mansfield, R. T. (1997). Head injuries in children and adults. *Critical Care Clinics, 13*(3), 611-627.

Moloney-Harmon, P. A. (2002). Pediatric trauma. In K. McQuillan, K. Von Rueden, R. Hartsock, M. Flynn, & E. Whalen (Eds.), *Trauma nursing: From resuscitation to rehabilitation* (3rd ed., pp. 747-771). Philadelphia: WB Saunders.

Moloney-Harmon, P. A., Adams, P. (2001). Trauma. In M. A. Q. Curley & P. A. Moloney-Harmon (Eds.), *Critical care nursing of infants and children* (2nd ed., pp. 947-978). Philadelphia: WB Saunders.

National Center for Health Statistics. (1999). *Healthy people 2000—Review 1997.* Hyattsville, MD: U.S. Department of Health and Human Services.

Nichols, D., Yaster, M., Lappe, D., & Buck, J. R. (1991). In *Golden hour: The handbook of advanced pediatric life support* (p. 180.). St. Louis: Mosby.

Pearson, L. J. (1999). Separation, loss, bereavement. In M. E. Broome & J. A. Rollins (Eds.), *Core curriculum for the nursing care of children and their families* (pp. 77-92). Pitman, NJ: Jannetti Publications.

Rice, L. J., & Britton, J. T. (1993). Airway management. In M. R. Eichelberger (Ed.), *Pediatric trauma: Prevention, acute care, rehabilitation* (pp. 162-168). St. Louis: Mosby.

Scholer, S. J., Hickson, G. B., & Ray, W. A. (1999). Sociodemographic factors identify US infants at high risk of injury mortality. *Pediatrics, 103,* 1183-1188.

Shackford, S. R., Bourguignon, P. R., Wald, S. L., Rogers, F. B., Osler, T. M., & Clark, D. E. (1998). Hypertonic saline resuscitation of patients with head injury: A prospective, randomized clinical trial. *Journal of Trauma: Injury, Infection, Critical Care, 44,* 50-58.

Tobias, J., Rasmussen, G. E., & Yaster, M. (1996). Multiple trauma in the pediatric patient. In M. C. Rogers (Ed.), *Textbook of pediatric intensive care* (pp. 1467-1504). Philadelphia: WB Saunders.

Yoshii, H., Sato, M., Yamamoto, S., Motegi, M., Okusawa, S., Kitano, M., Nagashima, A., Doi, M., Takuma, K., Kato, K., & Aikawa, N. (1998). Usefulness and limitations of ultrasonography in the initial evaluation of blunt abdominal trauma. *Journal of Trauma: Injury, Infection, Critical Care, 45*(1), 45-51.

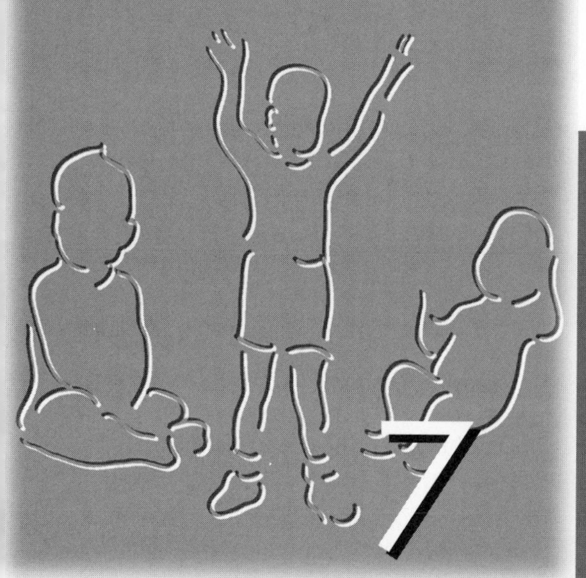

7 Transporting the Critically Ill Child

S. Louise Bowen

Pediatric trauma patients, ranging in age from infancy to adolescence, may be transported by the local emergency medical services system. Transport of these pediatric patients presents unique challenges. Because of children's anatomic differences, stature, body weight, age, and developmental stage, the mechanisms of injury and the stabilization techniques vary from those of adult trauma patients.

The transport team may be requested to transport the pediatric trauma patient from the scene of the injury or from a hospital, depending on the mission of the transport program. The scene focus is on immediate stabilization and transfer. The focus of interfacility transports is to provide transfer of a patient from one hospital to another. Interfacility transport systems expand the intensive care that is available at the tertiary or trauma center into the community or region.

DECISION TO TRANSPORT

Scene Calls

Each state, region, or local area may use different criteria in their decision to transport a patient to a designated trauma center or to the closest hospital. The decision usually is based on the first responder's assessment and local emergency medical services protocols. A number of factors are used to classify a critical trauma patient and determine how and where a patient is transported. These factors include type and location of injury, mechanism of injury, age of the patient, clinical condition, hemodynamic instability, and various measures of acuity or scoring systems (Furnival & Schunk, 1999; Hazinski, 1999). Additional factors are the location of the incident, distance to the trauma center, weather and traffic conditions, and resources available at the community hospitals (Wijngaarden, Kortbeek, Lafreniere, Cunningham, Joughin, & Yim, 1996). Protocols should be in place for prehospital personnel to use in triaging pediatric patients to a designated trauma center or to the closest hospital. These transports should be reviewed routinely to evaluate the protocols and the appropriateness of triage decisions.

Injury severity scoring systems are one of the tools used by prehospital providers to determine patient transport. Scoring methodology attempts to quantify the severity of the injury. The Pediatric Trauma Score (PTS) is a widely used scoring system in the prehospital triage of pediatric patients (Hazinski, 1999; Orr & Karr, 1995). The PTS takes into account the physiologic and anatomic differences unique to the pediatric patient. The PTS consists of six parameters that are assessed individually. A numeric score is given based on the assessment (Table 7-1). A score of 8 or less warrants transfer to a pediatric trauma center (Tepas, Ramenofsky, Mollitt, Gans, & DiScala, 1988). In addition to predicting severity of injury, the PTS identifies children who are at immediate risk of mortality. Tepas et al. (1988) found that a score less than 6 predicted mortality. Orliaguet et al. (1998) determined that a score less than 4 was associated with immediate risk of mortality.

Other scoring systems include the Trauma Score (TS); the Injury Severity Score (ISS); Circulation, Respiration, Abdomen, Motor, Speech (CRAMS) Scale; Revised Trauma Score (RTS); Abbreviated Injury Scale (AIS); Pediatric Risk of Mortality (PRISM); and Glasgow Coma Scale (GCS). These scores are used for field triage, quality assessment, scientific comparison of trauma patients, and epidemiologic research (Furnival & Schunk, 1999). The GCS is a neurologic scoring system widely used by both prehospital providers and interfacility transport teams. The GCS is not designed as a triage tool but rather as a means to rapidly and consistently evaluate the patient's neurologic status (see Chapter 14).

TABLE 7-1 Pediatric Trauma Score

Component	+2	+1	−1	Score
Weight (kg)	>20	10-20	<10	
Airway	Patent	Maintainable	Unmaintainable	
Systolic blood pressure (mm Hg)	>90	50-90	<50	
Pulses	Pulse palpated at radial or brachial	Pulse palpated at groin but not radial or brachial	Nonpalpable	
Central nervous system	Awake	Obtunded	Comatose	
Fractures	None	Closed or suspected	Multiple closed or open	
Wounds	None	Minor	Major, penetrating or burns >10% or involving hands, face, feet, or genitalia	
Total score 9-12: Minor trauma 6-8: Potentially life threatening 0-5: Life threatening <0: Usually fatal				

TABLE 7-2 Methods of Transportation for Pediatric Transport

Method of Transport	Advantages	Disadvantages
Local emergency medical services	• Fast mobilization time in transferring the child out of the referring hospital • Possible lower cost	• Limited training of emergency medical services personnel in transporting critically ill children • Equipment and supplies on the ambulance may not be appropriate for the pediatric population • Decreased coverage and response to emergency calls by the local ambulance service while they are engaged in interfacility transport
Transport by the referring hospital	• Fast mobilization time in transferring the child out of the referring hospital	• Lack of competency and expertise of the referring hospital staff in pediatric transport medicine • Equipment may not be manufactured for use in the transport environment • Decreased staffing at the referring hospital
Critical care transport team	• Varied expertise and training • Equipment and supplies may vary depending on the volume and expertise of the team	• Lack of expertise with pediatric patients if number of pediatric transports is limited
Pediatric transport team	• High level of expertise and training in caring for critically ill children	• Limited availability in all geographic regions • Increased response times

Interfacility Calls

The necessary equipment, supplies, ancillary departments, and trained personnel required to meet the needs of the critically ill pediatric patient may not be available at the community hospital. In this case the patient will need to be transported to a tertiary or trauma center. The referring hospital should have established protocols that outline how, where, and when a child should be transported. Names of hospitals, physicians, phone numbers, and transport systems equipped to care for critically ill and injured children are posted. The level of care during transport is required to be equal or better than that at the sending facility. Each method of transportation has advantages and disadvantages and is appropriate for specific patient populations (Table 7-2).

TRANSPORT REQUEST

Requests for transport vary depending on the origin of the call. Requests for interfacility transports are handled differently than scene requests. The call requesting dispatch of the transport team may come to the dispatch center or directly to the team through several mechanisms: prehospital providers, referring physician, or accepting physician.

The initial call is brief, and minimal information is obtained to decide on the team composition, mode of transport (ground, rotor-wing aircraft, fixed-wing aircraft), and any special equipment required. The initial call should take a maximum of 5 minutes. Box 7-1 lists the general information that is gathered in the initial request. The information is recorded in a transport computer database or on a specific form designated for transport request. This transaction is stored in a permanent file or as part of the patient's medical record.

Referring hospitals may be provided with a copy of the tertiary or trauma center's transport request form. This may expedite obtaining the information required by the tertiary or trauma center. Specialized hospitals, such as burn centers, may have an additional transfer checklist.

Once the transport team has been activated, further information is obtained. The follow-up call to the referring facility provides information on the estimated time of arrival of the team and mode of transportation. Additional patient information obtained during this time is outlined in Box 7-2. Consultation with a physician at the receiving facility should be available to the referring hospital at all times during the transfer process. Medical advice given by the receiving facility is recorded and communicated to the transport team.

BOX 7-1 Sample Information on an Initial Transport Request

Name of person calling
Name of patient
Location of patient/referring hospital
Scene response: Obtain exact information, especially if potential obstruction will prevent team from visualizing scene
Name of referring physician
Phone number of the person calling
Age of the patient, including date of birth—for interfacility transports
Weight—for interfacility transports
Reason for transfer/diagnosis
Pertinent clinical information

BOX 7-2 Sample Information to Obtain on the Follow-Up Call

Blood gas
Significant laboratory values
Vital signs
X-rays films
Intravenous access and fluids
Medications
Allergies
Further information on history and current clinical condition
Demographic data: parents' names, address, telephone number, insurance information

EQUIPMENT FOR TRANSPORT

The transport environment presents unique limitations and criteria. Because of limited space, weight restrictions, vibration, changes in barometric pressure, and extreme temperatures, the equipment used should be portable, compact, lightweight, durable, and capable of operating on AC and DC power; have a battery backup system; emit no electromagnetic interference; be easily secured in the vehicle; and meet federal and state guidelines for use in a ground ambulance, rotor-wing aircraft, or fixed-wing aircraft. The equipment designated for a specific transport program depends on the program's mission, patient population, geographic area, climate, and federal, state, and local regulations. Box 7-3 lists equipment to be considered when transporting a critically ill child. Each transport system identifies the equipment and supplies that meet its program's mission, scope of practice, patient population requirements, and federal, state, and local regulations.

Equipment designated for transport is dedicated to the transport program and is not borrowed or loaned to other departments within the hospital or from the referring facility. Obtaining equipment for transport from other departments decreases efficiency and delays mobilization time. In addition, the equipment must function at peak performance because of the limited resources in the transport environment. The equipment should be readily accessible to the team at all times. It should be maintained in a state of readiness and checked a minimum of every shift and after each transport.

Equipment and supplies may be stored on the vehicle or be available in bags or packs. Supplies may be organized into separate bags or packs to increase efficiency and ease of access. Transport bags may be categorized as respiratory, nursing/miscellaneous supplies, and medications. Packs may be organized for specific functions: trauma, burn, thoracic, and vascular access. Transport bags should not be too cumbersome or packed so that supplies are difficult to locate. Emergency and frequently used supplies are stored for fast access.

All equipment is secured in the vehicle. Any unsecured object may act as a missile in the event of an accident. Incubators and stretchers are secured in the vehicle by an approved locking mechanism. Configuration inside the transport vehicle should allow for easy loading and unloading of the patient and equipment. The environment within the vehicle should ensure unrestricted access to the patient and easy access to supplies and equipment. Monitors, ventilators, intravenous (IV) pumps, and defibrillators are

BOX 7-3 Transport Equipment

Vehicle
- Generator
- Inverter
- Appropriate medical gas source connectors
- Extra oxygen/air tanks
- Communication equipment (e.g., radios, cellular phones)

Monitoring Equipment
- Stretcher
- Incubator for infants <5-6 kg
- Cardiac monitor with recorder
- Ventilator
- Noninvasive blood pressure monitor
- End-tidal CO_2 monitor
- Pulse oximetry
- Transcutaneous O_2 and CO_2 monitors
- Defibrillator/cardioverter
- Invasive pressure monitoring
- Doppler
- Intravenous pumps capable of delivering from 0.1 ml to rapid infusions
- Suction
- Transilluminator
- Portable glucose analyzer
- Thermometer
- Portable blood gas analyzer
- Stethoscope—appropriate size
- Pressure bag
- Extra equipment batteries

General Supplies
- Backboard—various sizes
- Cervical collars—various sizes
- Towel or blanket rolls
- Femur splint designed for pediatric patients
- Burn pack
- Equipment sizing tape or age/weight chart
- Chemical heat packs
- Thermal blanket
- Cardiac arrest board
- Container to carry blood/blood products
- Broselow tape
- Parent information packet: consent forms, maps, booklet/pamphlet to receiving hospital

Respiratory/Airway Supplies
- Laryngoscope with extra batteries and bulbs
- Laryngoscope blades—sizes 0, 1, 2, 3; straight and/or curved (A straight blade is generally used in infants and toddlers and a curved blade is used in older children.)
- Oxygen
- Endotracheal tubes uncuffed—sizes 2.5, 3.0, 3.5, 4.0, 4.5, 5.0, 5.5
- Endotracheal tubes cuffed—sizes 6.0, 6.5, 7.0, 8.0 (6.0-6.5 may be cuffed or uncuffed)
- Lubrication (water soluble)
- Oral airways—various sizes: 00, 0, 1, 2, 3, 4, 5
- Magill forceps—small and large
- Yankauer—small and large
- Stylettes—pediatric sizes
- Tape
- Bag-valve ventilation device—various sizes (self-inflating bags should have an oxygen reservoir)
- Ventilation face mask—various sizes: infant, toddler, child/small adult, adult
- Suction catheters—various sizes
- Ventilator circuits—appropriate sizes
- Nasal trumpet—22, 24, 26, 28, 30
- Heimleich valves
- Aerosol nebulizer
- Aerosol mask—adult and pediatric sizes
- Nasal cannula

Nursing/Miscellaneous Supplies
- Blood pressure cuffs—various sizes
- Sphygmomanometer
- Penlight
- Pacifier
- Gastric tubes—various sizes
- Foley catheters—8 Fr, 10 Fr
- Blood sample tubes
- Tape
- Gauze sponges
- Elastic bandages
- Protective eyewear, gloves, and masks
- Biohazard disposal

Vascular Access
- Intravenous catheters—various sizes
- Intraosseous needles—various sizes
- Syringes—various sizes
- Medication and IV fluid access devices: needles, needleless system
- Antiseptic wipes, tourniquet, tape—various sizes
- Medication labels
- IV tubing to infuse from IV bags and syringes
- IV fluids—D_5W, $D_{10}W$, normal saline (NS), Ringer's lactate, D_5 0.45% NS, D_5 0.25% NS
- IV boards—various sizes
- Three-way stopcocks
- Needles/needle system devices

Medications
- Acetaminophen
- Adenosine
- Albumin 5%
- Albuterol for inhalation therapy
- Antibiotics—broad spectrum
- Amrinone
- Atropine sulfate
- Calcium chloride 10%
- Calcium gluconate
- Dexamethasone
- Dextrose 50%
- Diazepam
- Digoxin
- Diphenhydramine (Benadryl)
- Dobutamine
- Dopamine
- Epinephrine 1:1000
- Epinephrine 1:10,000

BOX 7-3 Transport Equipment—cont'd

- Furosemide
- Isoproterenol
- Heparin
- Lidocaine
- Mannitol
- Methylprednisolone sodium succinate
- Naloxone
- Narcotics
- Normal saline vials
- Paralytics and reversals
- Phenobarbital
- Phenytoin (Dilantin)
- Phenylephrine
- Potassium chloride
- Procainamide
- Prostaglandin E_1
- Racemic epinephrine
- Regular insulin
- Sedation and reversals
- Sterile water for injection
- Sodium bicarbonate 4.2% and 8.4%
- Sodium chloride vials
- Vecuronium

IV, Intravenous.

BOX 7-4 Sample Information to Obtain on the Follow-Up Call

Scene versus interfacility
Distance
Ground ambulance*—range from base of operation up to a 100-mile radius
Helicopter*—range from base of operation up to 180- to 200-mile radius
Fixed-wing*—consider for transports more than 150 to 200 miles from base of operation
Geographic considerations:
A. Is egress to the scene impeded or limited by selection of a particular vehicle?
B. Weather conditions?
C. Traffic conditions?
D. Landing zone requirements of helicopter or fixed-wing aircraft?
Transit time
Diagnosis
Clinical status of the patient
Access to specific surgical or medical interventions
Resources available at the referring hospital
Number of patients
Crew configuration
Cost/insurance/managed care
Altitude and pressurization considerations
Specialized treatment or equipment required during the transport

*Will also depend on type of vehicle or aircraft.

secured appropriately. Packs and bags containing supplies and medications must be secured either on the incubator or stretcher or in a designated compartment in the vehicle.

VEHICLE SELECTION

Vehicle selection for transport varies depending on a variety of clinical, diagnostic, and geographic variables; trauma criteria; insurance; cost; and state or local regulations. Modes of transport include ground or surface ambulances, rotor-wing aircraft, and fixed-wing aircraft. Transport programs may use one type or a combination of vehicles. No one type of vehicle is appropriate for all transports. Each state or local region may have specific criteria to classify pediatric trauma patients. These criteria usually specify the mode of transport. Box 7-4 outlines criteria that may be used in vehicle selection.

MANAGEMENT DURING TRANSPORT

Optimal patient outcomes during the transport require organization, skilled and knowledgeable staff, and procedures/protocols in place. Each team member has designated responsibilities but also functions in a variety of roles within his or her scope of practice.

During transit to the hospital, the team discusses the injury, possible mechanisms, individual team member's role, and any special considerations. Emergency drugs and fluids are calculated based on the patient's weight (Table 7-3). During a long-distance interfacility transport, the referring hospital is contacted en route by the transport team for a patient update and to notify the referring hospital personnel of any change in the estimated time of arrival. Medications, IV fluids, and equipment may be prepared during transit.

Upon arrival to a scene call, the team evaluates the overall situation for any potential safety or environmental hazards, such as fire, smoke, toxic fumes, live wires, or falling debris. A general assessment of the scene provides information regarding the mechanism of injury by noting details such as the location and condition of the motor vehicle or bicycle and the location and injuries of the other victims.

Team members identify themselves and receive an up-to-date report of the patient's condition upon arrival. An identification band is placed on the patient to prevent any errors.

TABLE 7-3 Sample of Emergency Drugs and Fluids Calculation Worksheet

Weight (kg):___

Drips

Drug	Dispensed	Mixture	Milliliters	Dilution
Dopamine	40 mg/ml	(Pedi) ___ kg × 1.5 = ___ mg	___ ml/25 ml	1 ml/hr = 1 μg/kg/min
		(Neo) ___ kg × 15 = ___ mg	___ ml/25 ml	1 ml/hr = 10 μg/kg/min
Dobutamine	12.5 mg/ml	(Pedi) ___ kg × 1.5 = ___ mg	___ ml/25 ml	1 ml/hr = 1 μg/kg/min
		(Neo) ___ kg × 15 = ___ mg	___ ml/25 ml	1 ml/hr = 10 μg/kg/min
Epinephrine	1 mg/1 ml	} ___ kg × 0.15 = ___ mg	___ ml/25 ml	} 1 ml/hr = 0.1 μg/kg/min
Isuprel	0.2 mg/ml		___ ml/25 ml	
Neo-Synephrine (phenylephrine)	10 mg/ml		___ ml/25 ml	
Fentanyl	50 μg/ml	___ kg × 50 = ___ μg	___ ml/25 ml	1 ml/hr = 2 μg/kg/hr
Midazolam	5 mg/ml	___ kg × 2.5 = ___ mg	___ ml/25 ml	1 ml/hr = 0.1 mg/kg/hr
Morphine	10 mg/ml	___ kg × 2.5 = ___ mg	___ ml/25 ml	1 ml/hr = 0.1 mg/kg/hr
Prostaglandin E_1	500 μg/ml	___ kg × 0.15 × 1000 = ___ μg	___ ml/25 ml	1 ml/hr = 0.1 μg/kg/min
		___ kg × 0.15 × 500 = ___ μg	___ ml/25 ml	2 ml/hr = 0.1 μg/kg/min

Regular insulin drip: 3 × ___ kg = ___ units to add to 30 ml (1 ml/hr = 0.1 units/kg/hr)

Paralytics

Drug	Dispensed	Dose
Pavulon (Pancuronium)	2 mg/ml	0.1 mg/kg × ___ kg = ___ mg = ___ ml
Norcuron (vecuronium)	1 mg/ml	0.1 mg/kg × ___ kg = ___ mg = ___ ml
Succinylcholine (Anectine)	20 mg/ml	1.0 mg/kg × ___ kg = ___ mg = ___ ml

Reversals

Narcotic Reversal

Naloxone	0.4 mg/ml	0.1 mg/kg × ___ kg = ___ mg = ___ ml (includes fentanyl, morphine, Demerol)

Pancuronium/Vecuronium Reversals

Atropine	Varies	0.15 mg for every baby = ___ ml
Neostigmine	0.25 mg/ml	0.07 mg/kg × ___ kg = ___ mg = ___ ml
Flumazenil	0.1 mg/ml	0.01 mg/kg × ___ kg = ___ mg = ___ ml

Intubation

Valium (diazepam)	5 mg/ml	0.1-0.5 mg/kg × ___ kg = ___ mg = ___ ml
Atropine	Varies	0.02 mg/kg × ___ kg = ___ mg (0.1 mg is minimum) (maximal single dose = 0.5 mg for child; 1.0 mg for adult)

Sodium Bicarbonate Correction

$NaHCO_3$	(Neo) 0.5 mEq/ml	___ kg × ___ base deficit × 0.3 = ___ mEq = ___ ml
	(Pedi) 1 mEq/ml	___ kg × ___ base deficit × 0.3 = ___ mEq = ___ ml

IV Rates

Neo		___ ml/kg/day × ___ kg v 24 = ___ ml/hr
Pedi:	0-10 kg = 4 ml/kg	___ kg × 4 ml = ___ ml/hr
	10-20 kg = 2 ml/kg	___ kg × 2 ml = ___ ml/hr
	>20 kg = 1 ml/kg	___ kg × 1 ml = ___ ml/hr
		Add for total IV rate ___ ml/hr

IV, Intravenous; *Neo,* neonatal; *Pedi,* pediatric; *PGE,* prostaglandin E.

Initial Assessment

Upon arrival of the transport team, the primary and the secondary surveys take place (see Chapter 6). The initial focus is on performing rapid assessment for any life-threatening conditions, focusing on airway, breathing, and circulation. Prompt respiratory and cardiovascular assessment with initiation of effective ventilation, oxygenation, and perfusion are essential for a successful outcome. Because of the need for rapid assessment and intervention, it is very easy to cause or exacerbate hypothermia. Maintenance of core body temperature is difficult in infants and small children because of their larger ratio of body surface area to weight. Hypothermia causes increased hypoxia, metabolic acidosis, increased metabolic demands, increased oxygen consumption, vasoconstriction, and pulmonary hypertension. Appropriate measures to conserve body heat and maintain the child's temperature within a normal range during transport are critical. Interventions include the use of chemical heat packs/mattresses, warm IV fluids, warm humidified oxygen and air, external heat lamps, and radiant warmer/transport incubators for infants. Only the body surface area being assessed should be exposed, and exposed areas should be covered with blankets, plastic wrap, or commercially available warming blankets. The external environment can also be warmed. Water-filled gloves or items heated in a microwave are never used as warming devices because of the risk of burns.

Hypothermia may be caused by rapid administration of cold blood products. This can lead to inadequate citrate clearance and subsequent ionized hypocalcemia and myocardial dysfunction. Blood products are warmed during or before administration.

In some cases it may be impossible to maintain normothermia because of the presence of severe hypoxic ischemic brain injury. Interventions are then taken to stabilize and maintain the temperature in as normal a range as possible and proceed with the transport.

The secondary survey continues the assessment process with a more thorough physical examination. Vital signs and any abnormal findings identified during the primary survey are reassessed a minimum of every 15 minutes. The extent of the secondary survey is limited in the transport environment because of the need to stabilize as quickly as possible and transfer the child to the tertiary center for more definitive care. Information determined during assessment and data on interventions, the condition of the patient, the equipment required upon admission to the hospital, and the estimated time of arrival of the patient to the hospital are communicated by the transport team to the receiving unit before departure to ensure a smooth transition and continuity of care.

Serum Glucose

Serum glucose measurement is indicated in the critically ill child with cardiorespiratory instability or traumatic injury. Hypoglycemia may occur in small infants and toddlers because limited glycogen stores are depleted by stress. Severe hypoglycemia may lead to central nervous system damage and myocardial dysfunction. High serum glucose levels may increase serum lactic acid and create an osmotic diuresis, leading to further hypovolemia and hypoperfusion. This may worsen central nervous system damage (Tobias, 1999). Glucose screening is performed using a portable monitoring device in the transport environment.

Blood and Blood Products

Administration of blood or a blood product may be required to resuscitate a severely injured child. Blood and blood products may be routinely carried by the transport team for scene response. For interfacility transports, arrangements are made with the referring hospital before the team's arrival to prepare blood products for transport with the child if the condition warrants. This will decrease stabilization time at the referring hospital and expedite patient transfer to the tertiary center.

Stabilization Time

Stabilization of the pediatric trauma patient before transport is critical. The concept of stabilization is defined within the framework of the diagnosis, scene versus interfacility transport, distance/time to the tertiary center, and mode of transport. Two methodologies commonly used are *swoop and scoop*, which involves rapid transport of the patient, versus *stay and resuscitate*, in which case increased time is directed toward stabilizing the patient for transfer (Task Force on Interhospital Transport, American Academy of Pediatrics, 1999). However, at times there may be a fine line between the need to rapidly transport the patient to a trauma center versus continued attempts at stabilization at the scene or in a referring facility.

Follow-Up

Follow-up and feedback are provided by the tertiary hospital to the referring physician to identify any problems encountered during the stabilization and transport process. Information regarding the patient's outcome may be requested by the referring physician and referring hospital. The tertiary/trauma center should have a mechanism in place for responding to these requests to ensure that patient confidentiality is maintained while providing valuable information to the referring institution.

TRANSPORT REGULATIONS

The transport program must be in compliance with local, state, and federal regulations related to the transport of critically ill children. Regulations involving certificate of need (CON), county/state/federal licensure, emergency medical services, Consolidated Omnibus Budget Reconciliation Act (COBRA), Health Care Financing Administration (HCFA), Medicaid, Federal Aviation Regulations (FARs), and the Federal Aviation Administration (FAA) affect the transport, documentation requirements, team composition, equipment, protocols, and transport/transfer consent forms. Not only does the program director need to be knowledgeable of these regulations, but the transport staff also needs to understand the regulations that influence the operation of the program.

PSYCHOSOCIAL IMPACT OF THE TRANSPORT

Transport of a child may create feelings of anxiety, fear, guilt, helplessness, or loss of control in the parents and family. The injured child may be transported many miles from home, to a town the family has never visited and to an unknown hospital by people they have just met. The possibility of death, disability, or disfigurement may increase the family's anxiety. In critical situations or during the resuscitation process, the environment may appear chaotic, which may exacerbate anxiety. The reactions of the patient and family will vary based on the condition of the patient, perception of the situation, past experiences, support systems, and coping mechanisms. Cultural and religious beliefs also play a role in how the family copes with the situation. The transport team is pivotal in recognizing crisis, anticipating further issues, and intervening and assisting the family through the transport process and admission to the hospital. This often is a difficult and challenging role for the team. The team not only has to care for a critically ill child but also has to provide psychosocial support to the family in a limited span of time. However, psychosocial support can be provided through effective communication; by providing opportunities to the family to bond with their child; and by giving information to the parents and family on the stabilization, transport, and transfer process.

Communication is essential in the intervention process. Having unfamiliar personnel caring for their child increases the family's stress. Upon arrival to the referring facility, the team members introduce themselves to the patient and family. The transport team may be the first contact the family has with the receiving hospital. This initial interaction may have a lasting impact. The transport team should refer to the patient by name when talking to both the patient and family. In critical situations the team initially may have time only to introduce themselves and then later may return to speak with the family.

One of the greatest needs of the parents is to be informed of their child's condition. The parents should be kept informed of the current patient status, stabilization process, and treatment plans. This may be done by the referring hospital staff if the team is unable to leave the patient's bedside. At some point during the transport process, the team should speak with the parents and family to discuss management and the transport process and to provide general information about the receiving hospital. The parents are informed of any changes in their child's condition. In critically ill or unstable children, the receiving or trauma physician may speak with the family by phone. If possible, allowing the parents to remain in the room as their child is being prepared for transport may help decrease the anxiety of both the parents and child and increase their trust in the team (Lewis, Holditch-Davis, & Brunssen, 1997).

The parents should be informed of the mode of transport back to the receiving facility and whether they are allowed to accompany their child. Information is provided to the parents and family on the location of the referring hospital, including directions and maps, name of receiving physician, name and location of the admitting unit, phone numbers, visiting policy, and where the parents can stay while their child is hospitalized. A photograph of the tertiary center and informational letters or pamphlets are helpful. The family may be so overwhelmed that only a portion of the information is heard and an even smaller portion is understood. Often, it is necessary to repeat information multiple times to help the parents comprehend. Information is communicated both verbally and in writing.

The parents are encouraged to express their emotions. This not only assists the parents through the crisis situation but also allows the team to assess the parents' needs and level of understanding. The team may need to contact social services or a chaplain to meet the family upon arrival to the tertiary facility. Before the injured child is transported, it is important that the parents see and touch their child.

SUMMARY

Optimal care during initial resuscitation and stabilization is needed to ensure the best possible outcome for the critically injured child. Transporting the child to a pediatric tertiary care center enhances the ability to decrease mortality and morbidity. Transport requires specialized knowledge and skill and specific training and equipment. Transport care includes both the child and the family.

BIBLIOGRAPHY

Furnival, R. A., & Schunk, J. E. (1999). ABCs of scoring systems for pediatric trauma. *Pediatric Emergency Care, 15*(3), 215-223.

Hazinski, M. F. (1999). *Manual of pediatric critical care.* St. Louis: Mosby.

Lewis, M. M., Holditch-Davis, D., & Brunssen, S. (1997). Parents as passengers during pediatric transport. *Air Medical Journal, 16*(2), 38-43.

Orliaguet, G. A., Meyer, P. G., Blanot, S., Jarreau, M. M., Charron, B., Buisson, C., & Carli, P. A. (1998). Predictive factors of outcome in severely injured children. *Anesthesia and Analgesia, 87,* 537-542.

Orr, R. A., & Karr, V. A. (1995). Assessing severity of illness before transport. In K. McCloskey & R. Orr (Eds.), *Pediatric transport medicine* (pp. 123-131). St. Louis: Mosby.

Task Force on Interhospital Transport, American Academy of Pediatrics. (1999). *Guidelines for air and ground transport of neonatal and pediatric patients* (2nd ed.). Elk Grove, IL: American Academy of Pediatrics.

Tepas, J. J., Ramenofsky, M. L., Mollitt, D. L., Gans, B. M., & DiScala, C. (1988). The pediatric trauma score as a predictor of injury severity: An objective assessment. *Journal of Trauma, 28*(4), 425-429.

Tobias, J. D. (1999). *Pediatric critical care: The essentials.* Armonk, NY: Futura Publishing Company.

Wijngaarden, M., Kortbeek, J., Lafreniere, R., Cunningham, R., Joughin, E., & Yim, R. (1996). Air ambulance trauma transport: A quality review. *Journal of Trauma: Injury, Infection, and Critical Care, 41*(1): 28-31.

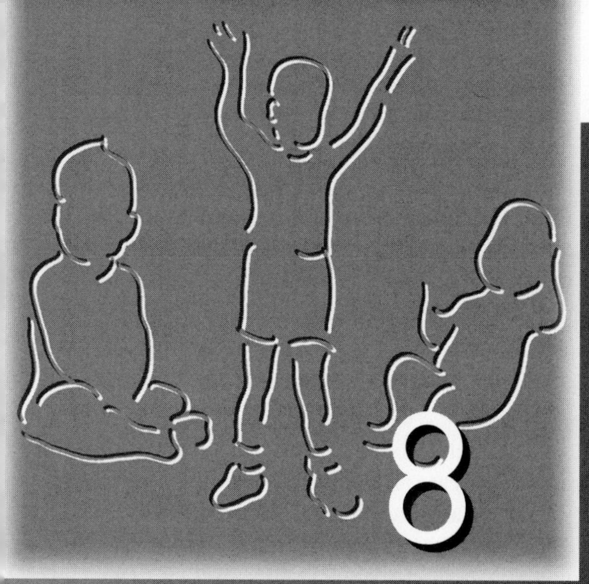

8 PEDIATRIC TRAUMA REHABILITATION

Teresa Beck • Naomi Higuchi

Rehabilitation is "the process of providing those comprehensive services deemed appropriate to the needs of persons with disabilities in a coordinated manner in a program designed to achieve objectives of improved health, welfare, and realization of the persons' maximum physical, social, psychologic, and vocational potential for useful and productive activity" (Commission on Accreditation of Rehabilitation Facilities [CARF], 1998). This is a dynamic process that should maintain dignity and self-respect in a person's life that is as independent and self-fulfilling as possible. Habilitation differs from rehabilitation because *habilitation* "refers to the process that involves individuals who need to acquire particular skills and/or functional abilities they did not possess previously . . . while rehabilitation refers to the process that involves individuals who need to require or maximize lost skills and/or functional abilities" (CARF, 1998). A widely accepted framework within rehabilitation was developed from the World Health Organization (WHO). WHO included simple terminology that needs to be fully understood. The WHO model definitions state the following:

Impairment is "a loss or abnormality of a psychological, or anatomical structure and function" (WHO, 1980). A person may consider impairment on the organ level. An example of an impairment is a spinal cord injury located at the cervical region of C5.

Disability is a "restriction or lack (resulting from an impairment) of ability to perform an activity in the manner or within the range considered normal for a human being" (WHO, 1980). One may view a disability on the person level. The person with a C5 injury is unable to independently perform all of his or her activities of daily living (ADLs) (e.g., eating, grooming, dressing, toileting).

Handicap is "a disadvantage for a given individual resulting from impairment or disability that limits or prevents fulfillment of a role that is normal for that individual" (WHO, 1980). Therefore a handicap is based on the societal barriers and places the disadvantage on the disabled person. An example is when the individual who uses a wheelchair for mobility cannot enter and access public buildings where ramps are not available.

PEDIATRIC REHABILITATION

Pediatric rehabilitation is a specialty practice that takes into consideration the growth and development of the child. A developmental or life span approach is taken that considers the "fluid and evolving nature of child and adolescent growth and the particular age or stage of the individual child's current physical, cognitive and sociopsychological status" (Harper, 1990). This approach helps guide the treatment program plan so that the child's evolving needs and continuing growth are considered.

Pediatric rehabilitation nurses are committed to improving the quality of life for children and adolescents with disabilities and their families. Their mission is to provide a continuum of care from the point of injury and diagnosis to productive adulthood in collaboration with an interdisciplinary team (Association of Rehabilitation Nurses, 1992). Pediatric rehabilitation nursing uses developmental theory as a cornerstone. Nurses must have an understanding of the theories of growth and development to realize the impact an injury has on the child and family. They also need to recognize the importance of the family's role in the care of the child.

Pediatric trauma rehabilitation is a growing specialty as a result of advances in medical technology. More children are surviving extremely devastating injuries than in the past. These children require more care and support from their family and community. Some of the typical diagnoses associated with pediatric trauma rehabilitation include traumatic brain injury, spinal cord injury, burns, amputations, and complex trauma.

Pediatric rehabilitation nurses play an important role in the lives of children with disabilities and their families. One can see pediatric rehabilitation nurses in a variety of settings, including hospitals, rehabilitation facilities, and home settings. These nurses serve in various roles. The primary role as an educator/teacher is most important. The key to rehabilitation, as described by Brillhart and Stewart (1989), is education. The nurse as educator gives the child and his or her family the essential information they need to continue to care for child and grow with the child's disability. The nurse shares the needed information and skills that are required to adequately care for the children. The nurse not only teaches the family but shares critical information with insurance companies, schools, and the community where the family lives.

The most familiar role of the nurse is probably that of caregiver. As the caregiver, the nurse provides the "hands-on" care and implements the treatment plan instituted by the interdisciplinary team. According to CARF, rehabilitation nursing services must be provided 24 hours per day, 7 days a week (CARF, 1998). Following the nursing process, the nurse cares for the child and thoroughly documents the care given.

The nurse also functions as the advocate and coordinator of care for the child and family. These roles begin during inpatient admission and continue throughout the outpatient phase. As the coordinator, the nurse brings together the knowledge of the health care team and integrates the interdisciplinary team's plan. The fulfillment of this plan may require the nurse to be an advocate for the child in the school reentry process and throughout the long-term follow-up that addresses the rehabilitation and habilitation process. The pediatric rehabilitation nurse may function in the additional roles of case manager, life care planner, counselor, researcher, legal consultant, and expert witness.

Goals of Pediatric Rehabilitation

"The goals of rehabilitation are to limit secondary damage, relearn lost skills, and learn new skills that will be needed to compensate for disabilities. Rehabilitation begins almost immediately after vital signs are stabilized, often while the child is still in a coma" (Michaud & Duhaime, 1992). These goals should remain function oriented, measurable, and obtainable. With pediatric rehabilitation, the child and family are at the hub of the wheel. Family-centered care is critical for a successful plan of treatment. When developing a pediatric rehabilitation plan of care, one must keep in mind the immediate results and long-term effects on the overall growth and development of the child.

NURSING CONSIDERATIONS

Disability as a functional impairment is a concept important to the understanding of rehabilitation. The history and physical examination reflect this concept by paying particular attention to neuromuscular, cognitive, and functional status. In addition, the child's developmental history, general health, family history, and school, behavioral, and psychosocial history are explored. Family and discharge needs are also determined.

The pediatric rehabilitation nurse must be able to address many aspects of patient care. These include, but are not limited to, skin care, eating and swallowing, vision, hearing, respiratory care, elimination, mobility, functionality, and psychosocial issues.

Skin

Skin breakdown can interfere with or delay achievement of rehabilitation goals. It can threaten the health of the child, increase the length of stay (LOS) and cost of care, and restrict daily activities. Identifying the patient who is at risk for the development of skin problems is the first step.

Assessment

Physical Assessment. Skin assessment is included as part of the admission assessment. Areas of focus are skin color, pigmentation, texture, temperature, moisture, turgor, lesions, and masses. Lesions are assessed for location, stage, size, sinus tracts, undermining, tunneling, exudate, necrotic tissue, and granulation tissue (Cooper, 1992). Risk assessment tools, such as the Braden Scale or Norton Scale, may be used to assess a patient's risk for impaired skin integrity. Both are validated risk assessment tools that provide a systematic approach to evaluating individual risk factors (Agency for Health Care Policy and Research [AHCPR], 1992). The frequency with which reassessments should occur is unknown; however, the clinical practice guideline, *Pressure Ulcers in Adults: Prediction and Prevention,* recommends daily systematic skin inspection (AHCPR, 1992).

Pressure Sores. A *pressure sore* can be defined as "any lesion caused by unrelieved pressure resulting in damage of underlying tissue" (AHCPR, 1992). Pressure sores usually occur over bony prominences where the pressure applied exceeds the normal capillary pressure of 32 mm Hg, which is considered the usual capillary closing pressure (Quigley & Curley, 1996). This results in a decreased blood supply to the area, causing cell death. Other factors that may contribute to the development of pressure sores are excessive moisture, shearing forces, friction, and poor nutrition (Quigley & Curley, 1996).

Progression of Tissue Breakdown. Tissue breakdown advances through the stages of tissue ischemia, normal reactive hyperemia, and abnormal reactive hyperemia, resulting in an open pressure sore. *Tissue ischemia* is the localized absence of blood or major reduction of blood flow resulting in blanched appearance. *Normal reactive hyperemia* occurs after ischemia has lasted a few minutes to approximately 2 hours. The skin can appear pink or light red and blanches when pressure is applied with the fingertips. Normal reactive hyperemia lasts less than 1 hour. *Abnormal reactive hyperemia* or *nonreactive hyperemia* occurs when tissue ischemia occurs for more than 2 hours. It is the body's normal response of vasodilation to repair the damage caused by ischemia. The tissue appears pink to dark red or purplish and does not blanch when pressure is applied with the fingertips. This is an indication that there is damage to the capillary bed. Nonreactive hyperemia lasts more than 1 hour. Induration may be present, indicating extensive tissue damage (Maklebust, 1987).

An open pressure sore is characterized by a broken skin surface that is surrounded by edema and erythema. Necrotic tissue and eschar are present and must be removed before the sore can be staged. Pressure sores are classified using a grading scale (Box 8-1). All other wounds are identified by anatomic depth. The recommended grading scale is consistent with the recommendations of the National Pressure Ulcer Advisory Panel (1989).

There are recognized limitations to the staging definitions. Stage I pressure sores may not be easily recognized in patients with darkly pigmented skin. Accurate staging of a wound cannot occur if eschar is present. Either the wound must be debrided or the eschar must be sloughed from the wound.

Severe complications may develop from the presence of a pressure sore. These complications can include wound infection, septicemia, osteomyelitis, negative nitrogen balance, anemia, pain, and altered body image. All of these complications have the potential to increase the cost of treatment, prolong hospitalization, or both.

Treatment of Pressure Sores. Treatment of pressure sores focuses on prevention of impaired skin integrity and management of wounds once they occur. Preventive measures include daily skin assessments, proper positioning and support surfaces to promote pressure relief, frequent repositioning or weight shifts, decreased or eliminated exposure to friction and shearing forces, maintenance of good body alignment, and promotion of optimal nutrition (AHCPR, 1992). If the child experiences impaired skin integrity, preventive measures should continue so that normal skin is protected. Wounds should undergo a thorough initial assessment as described earlier. Reassessments should occur at least weekly (AHCPR, 1992). Progress must be monitored regularly. A clean pressure sore with adequate innervation and blood supply should show evidence of some healing within 2 to 4 weeks. Wounds may need to be debrided to promote healing. This can be accomplished through mechanical, surgical, enzymatic, or autolytic debridement. The use of an appropriate wound-cleansing solution further optimizes wound healing. This is done with a minimum of chemical and mechanical trauma to the wound. Normal saline can be used to clean most pressure sores. The wound requires a dressing to maintain a physiologic environment. When a dressing is being selected, the following criteria must be considered and met: maintaining a moist wound bed, keeping the surrounding skin dry, controlling exudation, and respecting the caregiver's schedule restrictions or availability (AHCPR, 1992). Many products are available for use in wound management. Table 8-1 lists some of these products.

BOX 8-1 National Pressure Ulcer Advisory Panel Grading Scale

Stage I: Nonblanchable erythema of intact skin; the heralding lesion of skin ulceration

Stage II: Partial-thickness skin loss involving epidermis and/or dermis. The ulcer is superficial and presents clinically as an abrasion, blister, or shallow crater.

Stage III: Full-thickness skin loss involving damage or necrosis of subcutaneous tissue that may extend down to, but not through, underlying fascia. The ulcer presents clinically as a deep crater with or without undermining of adjacent tissue.

Stage IV: Full-thickness skin loss with extensive destruction, tissue necrosis, or damage to muscle, bone, or supporting structures, such as tendon or joint capsule.

Head, Eyes, Ears, and Throat

Disorders of the head, eyes, ears, and throat can affect the daily functions of the child. Vision and hearing impairments affect communication, academic performance, and the ability to perform ADLs. Neuromuscular and neurologic disorders or structural problems in the oral cavity, pharynx, larynx, or esophagus may affect eating and swallowing. Impaired eating and swallowing may result in poor mastication, pocketing of food in the sides of the mouth, uncoordinated swallowing, aspiration, nasal regurgitation of undigested food, or inadequate nutritional intake.

Assessment

Assessment starts with a history from the patient or caregiver. This may include information about changes in vision, such as blurred or double vision; difficulty seeing near or far objects; the need for glasses or contact lenses; hearing difficulties; the use of hearing aids; ear infections; pain; dizziness or ringing in the ears; adequacy of the patient's diet; difficulties eating; and loss of appetite. Questions about the patient's ability to smell should also be asked. Neurologic injury can result in altered olfactory perception and taste. The physical examination should include vision and hearing testing, in addition to inspection of the external and internal structure of the eyes, ears, nose, mouth, and throat. All of the cranial nerves should be tested.

Chewing and Swallowing. Chewing and swallowing impairments may exist in patients who have neurologic or

TABLE 8-1 Wound Dressings

Type	Characteristics	Advantages	Disadvantages	Indications	Examples
Gauze dressing	Made of cotton or synthetic fiber that is absorbent and permeable to water, water vapor, and oxygen	• Absorbs wound exudate • Protects wound • Can be used with a variety of solutions to maintain a moist environment	• Bulky • When left to dry, it may remove viable tissue	• Stage II, III, and IV pressure sores • Wound packing	• Gauze sponge • Sof-Wick • Kling • Bulky bandage • Nu-gauze • Bioclusive • Tegaderm
Polyurethane transparent film	Synthetic, permeable to oxygen, moisture and vapor permeable, impermeable to bacteria, nonabsorptive	• Moisture retentive • Allows for easy wound inspection • Maintains physiologic environment • Conforms to the wound • Water resistant	• Adhesive may damage new wound epithelium or fragile skin surrounding the wound • If wound exudate pools, it may cause maceration of the surrounding skin.	• Superficial abrasions • Stage I and II pressure sores • Stage III pressure sores with eschar	
Hydrocolloid	• Contains hydroactive, absorptive particles that interact with the wound fluid to form a gel and provide a moist environment • Minimal to moderate absorption of wound exudate • Impermeable to environmental contaminants • Less permeable to oxygen	• Moisture retentive • Provides a barrier to external bacteria • Protects from reinjury • Fosters autolytic debridement • Waterproof • Nonadhesive to healing tissue • Molds well	• "Melt out" occurs, resulting in residue in the wound bed • May soften and lose shape with heat and friction • Not effective for heavily exudating wounds	• Used to absorb wound exudate • Stage I pressure sores • Partial- or full-thickness wounds • Stage II or III pressure sores	• Restore extra thin • DuoDERM CGF • DuoDERM hydroactive granules
Hydrogel	• Nonadherent, water-based polymer • Oxygen permeable • Maintains a clean, moist wound • Has the ability to cool a wound • Translucent • Maintain a physiological wound environment	• Moisture retentive • Cooling, soothing effects relieve pain	• Can macerate surrounding skin • Requires a cover dressing to secure in place	• Stage I pressure sores • Partial-thickness or stage II pressure sores • Full-thickness or stage III pressure sores • Abrasions	• Carrington gel • Restore hydrogel
Foam dressing	• Made from a spongelike polymer • Hydrophobic, nonadherent outer surface generally covers the foam dressing on one side	• Moisture retentive • Moderately absorbent • Insulating • Provides padding • Permits some autolytic debridement	• Poor barrier • Nontransparent	• Stage I, II, and III pressure sores • Secondary dressing to provide additional absorption of excess secretions	• LYOfoam • Hydrosorb

facial injuries. These impairments must be detected early to prevent choking or aspiration. Swallowing is a complex process that is composed of three phases: oral, pharyngeal, and esophageal. In the oral phase, food is chewed using the mastication muscles and mandibular muscles. Tongue movements move the food to the back of the oral cavity. The soft palate rises and occludes the nasal passageway, thus preventing nasal regurgitation. The food bolus is then propelled into the pharynx by posterior tongue movements.

During the pharyngeal phase of swallowing, the food bolus travels down the pharynx. There is laryngeal elevation and vocal cord closure, which protects the airway. The epiglottis closes, which inhibits food from entering the trachea. The food bolus then enters the esophagus and is propelled to the stomach via peristalsis and gravity. This begins the esophageal phase of swallowing. The cricopharyngeal sphincter remains in a tonic state, preventing the contents of the esophagus from refluxing into the pharynx. The reflux of gastric contents into the esophagus is avoided by the lower esophageal sphincter maintaining a tonic state (McCourt, 1993).

A neurologic injury could interfere with any of the phases of swallowing. The cranial nerves provide both motor and sensory input. It may be difficult to identify which phase of swallowing is affected. Cognitive impairments may also be present, especially if the patient has either an acquired brain injury or an underlying neurologic condition such as cerebral palsy.

Sensory Perception. Neurologic injuries are common causes of sensory and perceptual dysfunction. Impairments of vision, hearing, smell, touch, proprioception, and taste may occur. This can put the child at risk for developmental delays, learning problems, and behavioral problems. Unlike adults, children may not be able to compensate for sensory and perceptual deficits because they lack previous experiences to draw from.

Impaired Vision and Hearing. Impaired vision and hearing may result from a neurologic or structural injury. Damage to the internal structures of the eye may be difficult to detect because they usually do not cause pain to the patient (Janelli, 1989). Changes in vision, such as blurred vision, may be the only sign of damage. Hemianopsia, the loss of half of the visual field on the same side of each eye, is commonly associated with hemiplegia; this condition may result from a brain injury. Hemianopsia results in blindness on the same side as the hemiplegia. Patients are usually not aware of this deficit until it is brought to their attention (Janelli, 1989). New onset of blindness can result from either a structural or neurologic injury. The child's ability to adapt depends on his or her personality, the child's family, and the existence of other sensory deficits.

Hearing loss can be attributed to trauma, infection, or injury to cranial nerve III. The nurse should be concerned if the child demonstrates signs of hearing loss. These signs may include absent startle reflex, inattention to the environment, the need to increase the volume on the television, requests to have information repeated, and the inability to follow directions. The child should undergo testing to determine whether there is hearing loss and what the cause of the loss is.

INTERVENTIONS

Impaired Swallowing. A child with impaired swallowing may need interventions that are general or phase specific. Some general interventions that may be implemented are supervision during meals, oral motor exercises, and reinforcement of recommendations from other members of the therapy team. The services of a speech therapist, feeding therapist, or occupational therapist may be needed to address issues related to chewing and swallowing.

Sensory Deficits. Sensory deficits may require the services of a specialist who has experience in treating patients with blindness and hearing loss, depending on the deficits present in the child. Adaptive devices may need to be used to improve vision or hearing. Alterations to the environment, such as better lighting, contrasting colors, accentuated visual cues, and reduction in background, should be implemented as appropriate (McCourt, 1993).

RESPIRATORY

Respiratory problems can have a significant impact on the child's recovery from trauma. Sequelae from the trauma, such as the need for an artificial airway, mechanical ventilation, traumatic brain injury, and spinal cord injury, may affect a child's respiratory status. Exercise intolerance, shortness of breath while eating or performing ADLs, difficulty swallowing, poor air exchange, and disruption of sleep patterns may result from impaired breathing. The child may not be able to clear secretions from the airway if he or she has an ineffective cough. The child may also have decreased lung capacity as a result of muscle weakness. Recognizing the potential for respiratory complications is important in the development of the plan of care. The prevention and early treatment of respiratory problems may reduce the risk of complications and long-term sequelae.

ASSESSMENT

Assessment includes a complete health history and physical examination. Inquiring about the child's health history and conducting a review of systems can assist in identifying potential problems that will need to be addressed. Patients with preexisting neuromuscular, neurologic, or respiratory diseases that affect the respiratory system should be identified. Complaints of increased work of breathing, shortness of breath, pain, and cough should increase the nurse's awareness of an underlying condition. If the child has a neurologic injury, the nurse must be aware of the impact of that injury. Patients with spinal cord injuries may be at high risk for respiratory complications, depending on the level of injury. Immobility also puts a child at risk for developing alterations in respiratory status. A physical examination that includes inspection, palpation, percussion, and auscultation will provide objective data to use in assessing the patient.

A functional assessment done at the time of admission will provide information that can alert the nurse to underlying functional deficits. Some of the areas to be examined are the patient's ability to conserve energy while performing ADLs, the ability to perform pulmonary hygiene activities, the ability to handle secretions, and the ability to endure specialized equipment (e.g., suction catheters, tracheostomy tubes, ventilators). If deficits exist, they must be addressed so that the patient's independence can be maximized.

INTERVENTIONS

Mobilization of Secretions. Neuromuscular impairments, fatigue, and infections may result in problems related to ineffective airway clearance. A child who has difficulty clearing secretions from his or her airway is at risk for airway obstruction, atelectasis, or other respiratory problems. Nursing interventions that promote effective clearance include providing the child with adequate hydration, encouraging the patient to cough, applying chest physiotherapy, promoting energy conservation, and controlling environmental factors. Adequate hydration is necessary to keep the secretions thin. Thick or dried secretions may obstruct small airways or tracheostomy tubes, or they may be difficult for the patient to clear by coughing. The child should be encouraged to drink fluids that do not contain caffeine, which tends to act like a diuretic.

Many environmental factors may cause dryness or irritation of the airways. Interventions that minimize these effects should be implemented. Adequate humidity can be provided through various delivery systems, including mist tents or humidification devices that are part of an oxygen delivery system. Room humidifiers can also be used. Contact with irritants, such as cleaning substances, aerosols, powders, and paints, should be avoided (Moody-Szymanski & Scherer, 1989).

Coughing is an important mechanism used to clear secretions from the respiratory tract. One or two forceful coughs are more effective than multiple weak coughs. To facilitate an effective cough, the child should sit or be in Fowler's position. Hugging a toy or pillow can provide physical support during a cough. Deep breathing can stimulate an effective cough. Some methods that can be used to encourage children to take deep breaths include blowing bubbles, using incentive spirometers, moving small items by blowing through a straw, and blowing through party horns (Whaley & Wong, 1991).

Patients with obstructive lung disease or spinal cord injury may not be able to produce an effective cough (Moody-Szymanski & Scherer, 1989). An alternative method, such as an assisted cough, should be used. To perform an assisted cough, the child is encouraged to take a deep breath and then forcefully exhale or cough. When the patient coughs, the nurse quickly pushes in and up on the upper abdomen. This helps increase abdominal pressure and the upward movement of the diaphragm (Moody-Szymanski & Scherer, 1989). Alternatively, the nurse can encircle the child's chest and compress the sides of the lower chest as the child coughs (Whaley & Wong, 1991).

Postural drainage is used to drain secretions from the various segments of the lungs by gravity. Postural drainage takes advantage of the effects of gravity and assists in moving secretions into the larger airways. It usually is performed three to four times a day and is performed before meals to decrease the risk of vomiting. Respiratory treatments should be performed before postural drainage to increase effectiveness. Most patients will not need to be placed in all the positions used in postural drainage. The patient's health history should be checked because some positions may be contraindicated. Often, chest percussion and vibration are performed in association with postural drainage to encourage the movement of secretions into the upper airways, where they can be suctioned or expectorated.

Breathing Retraining. Breathing exercises are used to strengthen the muscles used for respiration. They are mostly commonly used in patients with high spinal cord injuries and chronic obstructive airway disease. The goals of breathing exercises are to decrease dyspnea and to make more effective use of the diaphragm. The most commonly used techniques are pursed-lip breathing and abdominal-diaphragmatic breathing (Moody-Szymanski & Scherer, 1989). Both techniques use the diaphragm instead of the accessory muscles while the person is breathing, and each can be performed with the patient in a semisitting or supine position.

ELIMINATION

Dysfunction in bowel and bladder elimination can result from traumatic injury, such as a spinal cord injury or brain injury. Losing control of these processes can result in feelings of powerlessness, dependency, embarrassment, shame, and isolation. School-age children and adolescents may be subjected to ridicule and therefore limit their social contacts. Understanding the causes and manifestations of the various types of neurogenic bowel and bladder disorders will assist in the development of appropriate interventions. Other alterations in bowel function that need to be addressed are constipation and diarrhea.

NEUROGENIC BLADDER

Neurogenic bladder results from a disruption in the integrity of the neuroanatomy of the lower urinary tract. Any disruption in the sensory or motor pathways can result in problems with voluntary retention or voiding. Most neurogenic bladders result from a combination of motor and sensory impairments (Dittmar, 1989). The cause of traumatic neurogenic bladder is determined after spinal shock has subsided (Vogel & Pontari, 1997). Neurogenic bladders are generally classified as upper motor neuron, or spastic, and lower motor neurons, or flaccid. Serious complications such as autonomic dysreflexia, detrusor sphincter dyssynergia, hydronephrosis, vesicoureteral reflux, urinary tract infections, and urinary calculi may occur (Dittmar, 1989).

NEUROGENIC BOWEL

Neurogenic bowel is caused by interruption in the motor and sensory pathways of the autonomic and somatic nervous systems. This results in altered bowel function and voluntary control, such as incontinence or constipation. It is commonly associated with central nervous system vascular disorders, traumatic injury, and neurologic diseases. Diet, mobility, hydration, cognition, activity, and medication affect neurogenic bowel. There are three common types of neurogenic bowel: uninhibited, reflex, and areflexic or autonomous.

An uninhibited neurogenic bowel is associated with injuries such as traumatic brain injury, trauma, and stroke. There is damage to upper motor neurons located in the cerebral cortex, brainstem, or spinal cord. Bowel sensation and the lower motor neurons are intact, as are the internal and external sphincters (Dittmar, 1989). Sensory impulses from the bowel continue to be sent to the brain. However, the brain is unable to interpret these impulses, resulting in impaired voluntary bowel control. Involuntary elimination occurs suddenly when the sacral reflex is stimulated.

Reflex neurogenic bowel occurs in patients with spinal cord injuries above the T12 to L1 vertebral level. The upper motor neuron and sensory tracts are affected, but the lower motor neurons are intact. There may be partial or complete loss of voluntary sphincter activity. Sensation may be either decreased or absent. There is no voluntary control of bowel elimination; instead, there is a sudden mass reflex emptying of the rectal vault when it becomes full. Incontinence usually does not occur between episodes of mass reflex emptying because anal sphincter tone is maintained (McCourt, 1993).

Areflexic neurogenic bowel function occurs in patients with spinal cord lesions below the T12 to L1 vertebral level. The lower motor neurons and the sacral reflex are damaged. The extent of the damage depends on whether the spinal cord injury is partial or complete (McCourt, 1993). There is decreased or absent sensation in the perineum and rectum. Both the internal and external anal sphincters lack tone; thus there is frequent incontinence.

DIARRHEA

Diarrhea results from the rapid transit of stool through the colon. There is frequent emptying of the bowel, and the stools are either very loose or liquid. Diarrhea can be caused by disorders of digestion, absorption, and secretion. Something may be interfering with bowel absorption or causing the bowel to secrete fluid instead of absorbing it (Whaley & Wong, 1991). Common causes of diarrhea are gastritis caused by bacteria, virus or protozoa in the gastrointestinal tract, psychosomatic factors, food, and medications.

CONSTIPATION

In contrast to diarrhea, constipation is characterized by dry, hard stools resulting from delayed passage of stool through the colon. The frequency of bowel movements may or may not be decreased. There may be bleeding, pain, or abdominal distention. The patient may need to strain to have a bowel movement. Constipation may be caused by changes in activity, medications, diet, fluid intake, psychosocial factors, and disorders of the central nervous system or autonomic nervous system.

ASSESSMENT

A comprehensive assessment must be performed before appropriate bladder and bowel programs are implemented. Factors that must be considered include traumatic injuries, past surgeries, preexisting gastrointestinal disorders, medications, mental status, functional status, developmental level, age, nutrition, fluid intake, and premorbid bowel and bladder habits and patterns. A physical examination should include an abdominal examination, inspection of the genitalia and the perianal and peritoneal areas, rectal examination, and a neurologic examination. The neurologic examination should include tests for saddle sensation (paresthesia in the buttocks), bulbocavernosus reflex (anal sphincter contraction in response to squeezing the glans penis or putting slight pulling pressure on the urinary catheter), and anal reflex (ability of the anus to contract in response to stimulation). Saddle sensation is an important indicator of the integrity of sensory function at the sacral level of the spinal cord. The bulbocavernosus reflex is an indicator of an intact reflex of the sensory and motor components of S2, S3, and S4. Another sign of intact sacral roots is the anal reflex or anal wink. If the bulbocavernosus reflex and anal reflex are present, there will be a return of reflex bowel function (Dittmar, 1989). The patient's ability to use a bathroom and to perform toileting skills are objective data that can be used in developing a bowel and bladder program. Developmentally, children may not be able to perform these tasks. Laboratory and diagnostic tests may provide additional information.

INTERVENTIONS

Elimination programs are developed to meet the needs of children with neurologic insults that affect elimination. The programs usually are not elaborate, but they require consistency and patience. The programs may need to be modified when the patient is ill or if there are other changes in the patient's health status.

Neurogenic Bladder. The goals of a bladder program are to promote complete emptying of the bladder, prevent complications, preserve renal function, decrease urinary incontinence, maintain skin integrity, and provide minimal interference in daily activities. In the acute phase of injury, bladder overdistention is a concern. An indwelling catheter may be placed to keep the bladder drained so that urine does not reflux into the ureters and possibly cause damage to the upper urinary tract. Once this phase passes, intermittent catheterization is initiated.

Intermittent Catheterization. Intermittent catheterization may be used to manage any type of neurogenic bladder. The goals of this procedure are to retrain the bladder, simulate a "normal" voiding schedule, provide a catheter-free state, decrease or eliminate the risk for infection and complications associated with indwelling urinary catheters, and reduce the inconvenience of an indwelling catheter (Dittmar, 1989). Catheterization is performed at regular intervals, usually every 2 to 4 hours at the initiation of a program, to prevent the bladder from overdistending (Carendas, 1992). The procedure usually is performed with aseptic technique in the hospital, but it may be done using clean technique in the home setting. Studies investigating the use of clean intermittent catheterization support the method as being safe and effective. The frequency of the procedure may be more important than the sterility of the catheter (Rainville, 1994). Prophylactic antibiotics are not recommended because of the risk of antibiotic-resistant organisms (Vogel & Pontari, 1997).

The nurse should monitor the urine output and fluid intake. The volume of urine obtained at each catheterization and the amount of residual urine after each episode of incontinence are recorded. These volumes will help determine the frequency with which catheterization needs to occur. In some cases, intermittent catheterization may be stopped if there is a return of spontaneous voiding and a decrease in the volume of residual urine. Residual urine volume should not exceed bladder volume. A formula to determine bladder volume in children 2 to 11 years is as follows:

$$\text{Bladder capacity (ml)} = [\text{Age (in yr)} + 2] \times 30$$

For older children, the bladder volume is 300 to 350 ml (McCourt, 1993).

The amount and pattern of fluid intake are also important in a bladder program. Most bladder programs monitor the pattern of fluid intake and correlate it to the amount of catheterized urine. The patient's fluid intake is usually restricted so that urine volume does not exceed bladder volume (Dittmar, 1989). In some cases, caffeinated drinks are not allowed after lunch and fluids are withheld after dinner so that the patient does not need to be catheterized during the night to prevent bladder overdistention.

Medications. Medications may be used in a bladder program to promote emptying of the bladder. The drugs may be used either individually or in combination, depending on the patient's needs. Anticholinergics and antispasmodics depress the smooth muscle of the bladder, which allows for increased bladder capacity. If used alone, anticholinergics will inhibit bladder contraction by inhibiting acetylcholine, thus increasing bladder capacity (McCourt, 1993). Oxybutynin (Ditropan) and propantheline bromide (Pro-Banthine) are examples of an antispasmodic with anticholinergic properties and an anticholinergic, respectively, that are commonly used in bladder programs (Dittmar, 1989). If the bladder is hypotonic, bethanecol, which is a cholinergic, may be used to increase bladder tone and contractility, which facilitates emptying (Dittmar, 1989).

In patients with detrusor sphincter dyssynergia, dantrolene and phenoxybenzamine may be used. Dantrolene is a skeletal muscle relaxant that decreases the contractility of skeletal muscle, including the external urinary sphincter. Phenoxybenzamine is an α-adrenergic blocking agent that has been shown to be effective in decreasing the tone of the internal sphincter, causing decreased resistance of the bladder neck (Rivas, Abdill, & Chancellor, 1996). Baclofen, a centrally acting skeletal muscle relaxant, may be used to decrease external urinary sphincter spasticity. Some studies show that intravenous baclofen is more effective than oral baclofen but may put the patient at higher risk for side effects (Rivas, Abdill, & Chancellor, 1996).

Constipation. The cause and severity of the patient's constipation should be determined before a bowel program is developed. If a pathologic process is not found, a bowel program may be established. Dietary fiber and fluid intake are important factors to consider in the treatment of constipation. Fiber increases the bulk of the stool and, through its osmotic properties, softens the stool by increasing water retention. This, however, has not been proven consistently in clinical studies (Weingarden, 1992). Increased fluid intake may contribute by increasing the water content of stool, thus making stools easier to pass.

Fiber is commonly defined as a "plant component that is not digested in the upper gastrointestinal tract" (Weingarden, 1992). There are many sources of dietary fiber, such as fruit, vegetables, and grains. Wheat bran is a practical, inexpensive, and easily obtained source of fiber. Fiber should be added gradually to a patient's diet to prevent untoward side effects, such as bloating, cramps, diarrhea, and flatulence. The patient's food preferences, ability to chew, age, and cognition must also be considered. Creative ways of adding fiber to a child's diet include oatmeal chocolate chip cookie with wheat germ, popcorn, fruit pies, and fruit with dips. Cereals with bran may be used in baking. There is disagreement as to how much dietary fiber is necessary to manage constipation. High-fiber diets vary from 5 to 30 g of dietary fiber (Dittmar, 1989; Weingarden, 1992).

Medications may be used to treat constipation. These include bulk laxatives, stool softeners, and stimulants. Laxatives are not recommended for long-term use; however, they may be beneficial for the acute treatment of constipation. These medications are discussed in detail later in the chapter.

Bowel Management. Neurogenic bowel is associated with neurologic insults, usually spinal cord injury. Bowel programs are developed according to the type of neurologic injury and the needs of the patient. The objectives of a successful bowel program are continence; regularity; and the absence of complications such as constipation and nausea. Bowel management is started soon after injury as long as there are no contraindications, such as acute ileus. The bowel is cleaned out before initiation of a bowel program. It is recommended that the bowel program be done 30 to 45 minutes after the patient eats to take advantage of the gastrocolic reflex. This reflex, though, is absent in patients with cervicothoracic lesions. The rectal vault is cleared of stool before a suppository is inserted. Digital stimulation may be performed to stimulate the anorectal reflex in patients with reflex neurogenic bladder (Dittmar, 1989). Initially, results are variable. Diarrhea and incontinence may occur. If possible, the patient should sit on a commode or toilet so that gravity can assist. If suppositories or mini-enemas are used, the patient should wait 15 to 20 minutes before sitting (McCourt, 1993).

The bowel program is monitored and altered as needed. Changes should not be made before a 1-week trial period. The results of the changes may not be fully appreciated if frequent changes are made. A typical bowel program may take 30 to 45 minutes to complete. If the patient requires more than 1 hour to complete the program, the program should be evaluated for improvement (Kirshblum, Gulati, O'Conner, & Voorman, 1998). The patient should have a bowel movement at least three times a week. Most patients will use an alternate-day program, which is performed in the morning.

A combination of diet, oral medications, suppositories, mini-enemas, and digital stimulation may be used. The most commonly used medications are Colace, Senokot, Metamucil, and Dulcolax (Kirshbaum, Gulati, O'Conner, & Voorman, 1998). Stool softeners directly decrease stool firmness. They may also cause fluid accumulation in the intestine. Stimulant laxatives, such as Senokot, cause local irritation of the mucosa, which enhances bowel motility. When given orally, the agents should be given 6 hours before the planned time for the bowel program. Bulking or fiber agents increase bulk, decrease stool softness, and are used for all types of neurogenic bladder. They usually begin to work in 12 to 24 hours. Some patients may choose not to use these agents because of taste and texture. Rectal suppositories and mini-enemas usually contain a contact stimulant laxative that has a direct effect on the smooth muscle of the intestine. Most laxative suppositories contain bisacodyl powder that is either in a hydrogenated vegetable oil or polyethylene glycol base. The mini-enema Therevac SB contains a combination of glycerin and docusate sodium in a polyethylene glycol base. It has been shown that polyethylene glycol–based suppositories and mini-enemas decrease the duration of bowel care (Dunn & Galka, 1994; House & Stiens, 1997).

Physical Mobility

A child with a traumatic injury may experience problems with mobility depending on the cause of the injury or as a result of prolonged immobilization. Physical mobility encompasses bed mobility, transfers, wheelchair mobility, and ambulation. Physical factors that influence mobility are range of motion (ROM), strength, balance, endurance, tone, and proprioception (McCourt, 1993). Complications of immobility include loss of muscle tone, strength, and mass; contractures; thromboembolism; bowel dysfunction; and pressure sores. The child's ability to perform ADLs may become severely impaired, resulting in a loss of independence, social isolation, regression of developmental stages, and behavioral issues. The nurse, in combination with the physical and occupational therapists, should implement interventions for maintaining or improving mobility.

Assessment

Assessment of mobility is not limited to the patient's physical body, but rather includes functional mobility and home environment. The physical assessment includes ROM, muscle strength and tone, balance, endurance, proprioception, and gait. The presence or absence of age-appropriate fine and gross motor movements is noted. Deficits in visual and auditory acuity are identified because they may influence the patient's ability to function. Cognitive status should also be assessed. Concerns about safety may arise if the patient is disoriented, has memory deficits, is impulsive, or is unable to communicate. Psychologic factors such as fear, anxiety, depression, and motivation may affect mobility. The patient's home environment is assessed for accessibility, lighting, and safety (McCourt, 1993). The child's ability to maneuver within the home may raise concerns about safety. Concerns include use of throw rugs; stairs; and location of furniture, bedside rails, and doorways. Safety issues are reassessed as the child progresses to the next stage of development.

Functional Assessment. The patient's ability to perform tasks is assessed. The nurse determines whether the child is able to perform age-appropriate tasks, such as feeding, bathing, dressing, toileting, and walking. The child may need to relearn some of these tasks as part of his or her rehabilitation program. Adaptive equipment, splints, and modifications to clothing, utensil handles, and other tools used in daily activities may be necessary to accomplish everyday tasks. Children should be encouraged to perform tasks that are normal for their developmental age and within their capabilities (Hoeman, 1992).

Interventions

Remobilization of the child after a traumatic injury occurs as soon as possible to prevent complications from immobility. Physical and occupational therapists may be involved in the child's care. They can each provide knowledge from their area of expertise related to exercise, assistive devices, orthotics, seating, positioning, and ambulation. Children who were in a prone or reclined position for a prolonged period or who have a spinal cord injury will need to be gradually raised to an upright position to allow the body to adjust. Otherwise, the child may experience orthostatic hypotension as a result of pooling of blood in the lower extremities. Abdominal binders and elastic stockings may be used to prevent pooling of blood. Thigh-high elastic stockings or elastic bandages wrapped from groin to toes can be used to prevent venous stasis and decrease the risk for deep vein thrombosis.

Passive ROM exercises and positioning are important interventions to prevent contractures and promote function. Contractures limit functional ROM, thus reducing the child's ability to perform functional tasks such as eating, grooming, and dressing. Passive ROM is performed in patients who are not able to perform active ROM to maintain joint mobility. Resting splints are used to maintain extremities in a functional position to prevent deformity. Other types of splints are used during functional activity to provide support (Blanchet & McGee, 1996). The child's body and extremities are positioned to prevent contractures and skin breakdown and to maximize the child's performance in daily activities.

Mobility and ambulation are addressed. The child and caregivers are taught transfer techniques and general safety precautions for performing transfers. Appropriate wheelchairs and seating systems are obtained for the child who requires a wheelchair for mobility. Ambulation aids, such as walkers and crutches, are used to assist with mobility. Orthotics and braces are used to provide proper alignment. The child and caregivers are taught how to properly use the equipment to ensure the child's safety.

Home visits are performed by the rehabilitation team to assess the home environment. Accessibility to the home, physical layout, lighting, and safety are evaluated. Potential adaptations to the home include ramps, stair glides, enlarged doorways, additional lighting, and grab bars. Independent mobility, safety, and independence are the desired outcomes of the modifications. In most rehabilitation programs, arrangements are made for the child to visit his or her home before discharge. This provides the child with the opportunity to learn how to maneuver and function in the home environment.

FUNCTIONAL ASSESSMENT

The Functional Independence Measure for Children (WeeFIM System Clinical Guide, Version 5.0) is a discipline-free tool used to assess the consistent and usual performance of what a child does. It evaluates the functional skills in children ages 6 months to 18 years. It measures disability as defined by the WHO's Disablement Model (WHO, 1980). This tool measures the child's need for additional or future assistance, and documents the outcomes of pediatric rehabilitation and habitation programs.

This instrument uses a 7-point ordinal scale that measures 18 types of essential daily functional skills across three domains: self-care, mobility, and cognition. Under the self-care domain, a child's level of independence in eating, grooming, bathing, upper-body dressing, lower-body dressing, toileting, bladder management, and bowel management is evaluated. Chair/wheelchair transfers, toileting, tub/shower transfers, walk/wheelchair/crawl mobility, and stairs are assessed in the mobility domain. The cognition domain addresses the child's level of comprehension, expression, social interaction, problem solving, and memory. Figure 8-1 shows an example of the WeeFIM.

Test-retest and interrater reliability have been found to be excellent and equivalent to the reliability of phone interviews. The WeeFIM ratings for 205 children (ages 11 months to 87 months) with developmental disabilities who participated in outpatient developmental rehabilitation centers, in school programs, and in the children's homes found consistent interrater agreement and stability of the WeeFIM (Ottenbacher, Msall, Lyon, Duffy, Granger, & Braun, 1997). Sperle, Ottenbacher, Braun, Lane, and Nochajski (1997) describe a study that showed the equivalence reliability of the WeeFIM. This study involved 30 children between the ages of 19 and 71 months with identified developmental disabilities.

Direct observation and interview methods were randomly administered to each subject within a 3-week period. Direct observation of the children was completed in the schools, and the WeeFIM interview was obtained either by conducting an in-person interview or by interviewing the child's parent over the phone. The results showed a good agreement for ratings when the WeeFIM was administered by direct observation and by interview with a parent.

The Pediatric Functional Outcomes measure (PEDI) is another well-known discriminative measure for assessment of functional limitations in children ages 6 months to 7.5 years. It can be used for older children if their functional abilities are below that of a 7.5-year-old child with no disabilities. This is a discipline-free tool that assesses the child's capability and performance in the domains of self-care, mobility, and social function.

Each PEDI scale is self-contained and can be used separately or in combination with the other scales. For example, an evaluator can administer the self-care scale without completing the mobility section. This entire instrument is composed of 210 test items that can be administered by observation or by parent interview. It requires 45 to 60 minutes to complete. The PEDI uses a 6-point ordinal scale for caregiver assistance and modification items. There is dichotomous scoring of self-care, motor, and social domains (Haley, Coster, Ludlow, Haltiwanger, & Andrellos, 1992).

TEAM PROCESS

There are three different types of team models in most rehabilitation settings: multidisciplinary, interdisciplinary, and transdisciplinary (McCourt, 1993).

Multidisciplinary Team

A multidisciplinary team (Figure 8-2) is composed of individuals from different disciplines. Each discipline (e.g., nursing, occupational therapy, physical therapy) has efforts that are parallel and discipline-oriented. Members of the team tend to work alone and establish their own plan. Good communication often is lacking. There is not much group responsibility, but rather individual discipline responsibility. During team conferences, each therapist reports the child's progress. The team leader decides the plan and treatment of the child's care.

WeeFIM® instrument

LEVELS		
	7 Complete Independence (Timely, Safely) 6 Modified Independence (Device)	**No Assistance**
	Modified Dependence 5 Supervision (Subject = 100%) 4 Minimal Assist (Subject = 75%+) 3 Moderate Assist (Subject = 50%+) **Complete Dependence** 2 Maximal Assist (Subject =25%+) 1 Total Assist (Subject = less than 25%)	**Assistance**

		ASSESSMENT		GOAL
Self-Care				
.1	Eating			
.2	Grooming			
.3	Bathing			
.4	Dressing - Upper			
.5	Dressing - Lower			
.6	Toileting			
.7	Bladder			
.8	Bowel			
	Self-Care Total		***Quotient***	
Mobility				
.9	Chair, Wheelchair			
.10	Toilet			
.11	Tub, Shower			
.12	Walk/Wheelchair		W Walk C wheelChair L crawL B comBination	
.13	Stairs			
	Mobility Total		***Quotient***	
Cognition				
.14	Comprehension		A Auditory V Visual B Both	
.15	Expression		V Vocal N Nonvocal B Both	
.16	Social Interaction			
.17	Problem Solving			
.18	Memory			
	Cognitive Total		***Quotient***	
	WeeFIM Total		***Quotient***	

NOTE: Leave no blanks. Enter 1 if patient not testable due to risk

FIGURE 8-1 WeeFIM instrument (Functional Independence Measure for Children). (From Uniform Data System for Medical Rehabilitation, a Division of UB Functional Activities, Inc.)

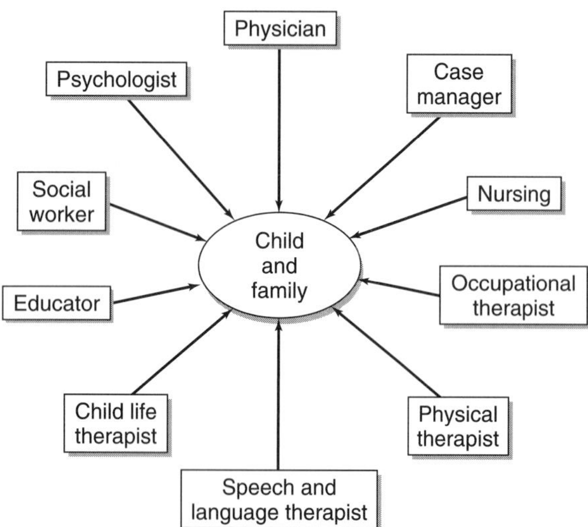

FIGURE 8-2 Multidisciplinary team diagram.

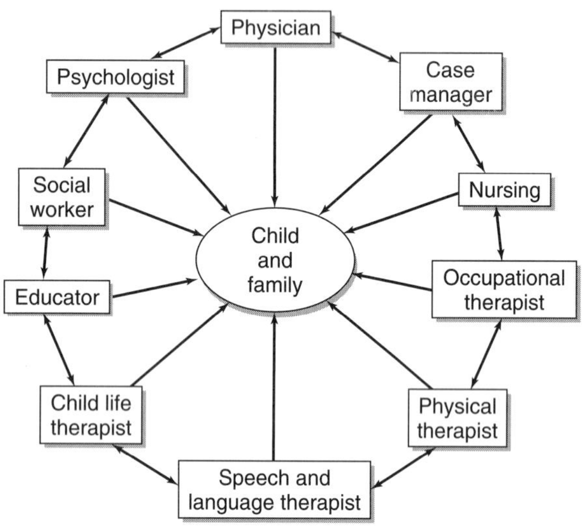

FIGURE 8-3 Interdisciplinary team diagram.

Interdisciplinary Team

An interdisciplinary team (Figure 8-3) includes members who work as a group to develop team goals and intervention strategies. The team meets as a whole and works together to problem solve each particular case. This team produces coordinated goals to produce a comprehensive plan of care.

Transdisciplinary Team

A transdisciplinary team model (Figure 8-4) has members who all are involved collaboratively in treatments, but usually one member acts as "primary therapist." The other members exchange information and advice with regard to management through the primary therapist. This primary therapist implements the treatment. The transdisciplinary model is more cost effective and can work well with individuals who have traumatic brain injuries.

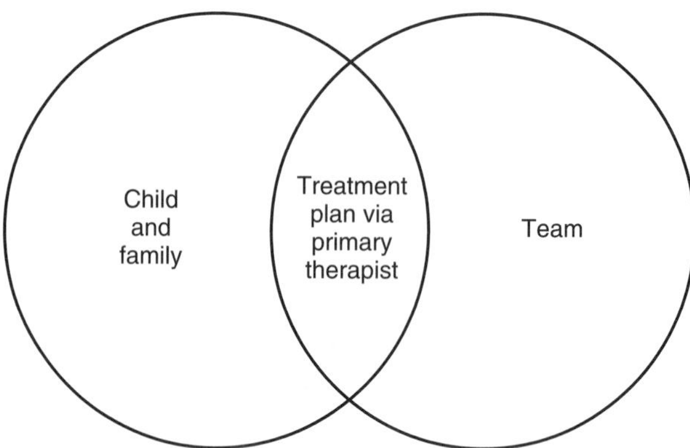

FIGURE 8-4 Transdisciplinary team diagram.

Rehabilitation Team

A "typical" inpatient pediatric rehabilitation model consists of the interdisciplinary team. The team consists of members from various disciplines, including a physician, nurse, physical therapist, occupational therapist, speech and language therapist, social worker, child life therapist or recreational therapist, psychologist and/or neuropsychologist, and educator. The team may include other members, such as a rehabilitation counselor and a cognitive, art, or music therapist.

An interdisciplinary admission assessment form (see Appendix A) may be used to collect patient and family information. The assessment is completed within the first 24 hours of admission and is designed to collect routine clinical information. This single document reduces redundant questions asked of the child and family. Communication is facilitated among the disciplines in a legible and standard format.

MASTER PROBLEM LIST/PLAN OF CARE

Master Problem List

A master problem list (Figure 8-5) is developed to design an individual plan of care with functional, measurable, and attainable goals. These goals are established in conjunction with the child and his or her family. The problems that are identified can be viewed as barriers to discharge. The functional goals are documented in the plan of care and continually assessed to update and revise the plan according to the progress of the child. The master problem list includes the following domains: physiologic, mobility, ADLs, communication, cognition, psychosocial, and discharge plan.

Case Management

Upon admission, each child and his or her family are assigned to a case manager, who is a certified rehabilitation registered nurse. According to CARF, a *case manager* is "an individual who is responsible for collaboration with the team and external entities to assess, coordinate, implement, and evaluate all services required to meet the needs of the persons served to promote quality and cost effective outcomes" (CARF, 1998). Case managers review daily therapy notes and continually assess the progress or lack of progress

CHILDREN'S SEASHORE HOUSE

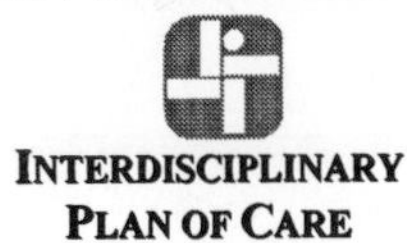

INTERDISCIPLINARY PLAN OF CARE

Addressograph

	AREAS ADDRESSED	✓	INPATIENT & DAY HOSPITAL GOALS	ESTIMATED TIME FRAME	INITIALS
PHYSIOLOGICAL	Pain				
	Cardio-Pulmonary				
	Skin				
	Elimination				
	Nutrition				
	Swallowing/PO Feeding				
	Sensory				
	Vision/Hearing				
	Neuromuscular				
MOBILITY	Transfers				
	Ambulation				
	Stairs Wheelchair				
MOBILITY	Endurance				
ADLS	Self-feeding				
	Bathe				
	Dressing				
	Grooming				
	Toileting				
COMMUNICATION	Receptive Language				
	Expressive Language				
	Oral-Motor/Speech				

Continued

FIGURE 8-5 Interdisciplinary plan of care. (Courtesy Children's Seashore House of the Children's Hospital of Philadelphia.)

CHILDREN'S SEASHORE HOUSE

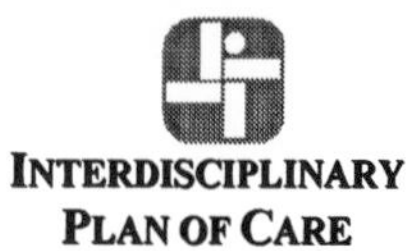

INTERDISCIPLINARY PLAN OF CARE

Addressograph

	AREAS ADDRESSED	✓	INPATIENT & DAY HOSPITAL GOALS	ESTIMATED TIME FRAME	INITIALS
COGNITION	Orientation				
	Attention				
	Memory				
	Critical Thinking				
	Visual Perception				
	Safety Awareness/Judgement				
PSYCHOSOCIAL	Social Interaction				
	Individual Coping				
	Family Coping				
	Leisure				
DISCHARGE PLAN	Pt./Family Education				
	Equipment				
	Discharge Disposition / Home Assessment				
	School Re-entry				
	Community Re-entry				
	Aftercare				

ACCORDING TO THIS INITIAL EVALUATION, I AM RECOMMENDING:

DISCIPLINE	FREQUENCY OF TREATMENT	SIGNATURE	DATE	INITIAL

FIGURE 8-5, cont'd

toward the attainment of goals. The case manager, in conjunction with the whole team, facilitates reentry to family, home, school, and community by focusing on the needs of the family. Weekly team meetings and family meetings are held to keep the team (including the family) abreast of the child's progress, discharge needs, and discharge planning.

The average number of hospital days has decreased dramatically over the last several years. Primarily, the LOS has been shortened because of the restrictions imposed by the insurance companies on hospital facilities. One positive result of the oversight by third-party insurance carriers is efficiency of care. In turn, there is less disruption of family time and earlier transition to family, school, and community. However, health care professionals must study the effects of the decreased LOS on patient outcomes.

Morrison and Stanwyck (1999) studied the difference in LOS and functional status at the time of discharge from inpatient rehabilitation and 2 months after discharge, and they examined the patients with postdischarge complications admitted to Shepherd Center in Atlanta, Georgia, in 1991 and 1995. The study involved 127 persons with traumatic spinal cord injuries. "Even with the LOS decreasing significantly, performance of functional skills did not appear to be affected. What seemed to be most affected were medical complications and employment status. It appeared that the decreased amount of time for inpatient rehabilitation may have reached the point of becoming detrimental to individuals receiving rehabilitation for spinal cord injury" (Morrison & Stanwyck, 1999). Further research is necessary to study the long-term effects of medical complications and psychosocial issues.

DISCHARGE PLANNING

Discharge planning is essential for successful outcomes and smooth reentry to home, school, and community. The rehabilitation team must determine to whom and where the child will be discharged. Factors that may influence disposition of the child include type and severity of the injury, complexity of the child's care, the caregivers' ability to provide care, the home environment, and social issues. The parents may not be able to care for the child if they also were victims of the trauma. Alternative placement may need to be considered. Potential options should be explored as soon as possible (Beck & Spoltere, 1996).

The rehabilitation team assesses the child and designs an individualized plan of care. After the team meets, a goal-oriented family meeting occurs and an estimated date of discharge is established. The discharge plan should address family/caregiver education related to the child's care; the caregiver's ability to provide care; accessible and safe housing; home nursing needs; therapy needs; and equipment issues, such as wheelchairs, orthotics, and splints.

School Reentry

Early school involvement in the school reentry process is necessary for a smooth transition. Communication among the family, hospital staff, and school officials should be established as soon as possible. Some critical factors that must be assessed include the accessibility of the school, availability of an elevator for child with impaired mobility, transportation needs, and education of the teachers and school nurse regarding the child's needs.

For example, successful school reentry for a child with a spinal cord injury includes the distribution and review of pertinent literature and education of the school staff that will have contact with the child. The rehabilitation team should provide the information needed to properly care for the child. This may include, but is not limited to, information about the child's medical condition, such as the child's functional ability, neurogenic bladder and bowel, autonomic dysreflexia, medications, thermoregulation, and spasticity.

A child with a traumatic brain injury may have no physical impairments; however, cognitive and behavioral problems may be present. The school staff, especially the teaching staff and school nurse, need to know about these issues before the student's return. This will allow time for behavioral interventions and adaptive strategies to be developed, implemented, and taught to the school personnel. This will assist in the development of an appropriate individual education plan.

LEGISLATION RELATED TO CHILDREN WITH DISABILITIES

Historically, the United States has discriminated against children with disabilities within the education system. In the 1970s, "one million children with disabilities had been excluded from the public school system" (Lewis & Doorlag, 1999). Many of the disabled children who were admitted to school were not provided with an appropriate education. Recent legislation has sought to correct this. In 1975, Public Law (PL) 94-142, The Education for All Handicapped Children Act, was enacted. This law mandated that all states make available to all children "free and appropriate education." PL 94-142 was later renamed the Individuals with Disabilities Education Act (IDEA). IDEA provides federal money to state and local educational agencies to help them provide education to children. IDEA defines *special education* as specially designed instruction that meets the unique needs of a student with a disability. The education is inclusive and addresses daily living skills, community living skills, and prevocational and transitional services to prepare the child for citizenship. This instruction is free, is provided in various settings, and includes related services. Box 8-2 lists some of the potential related services. The school district is required to provide the disabled child's education in the least restrictive environment. This includes placing disabled children in the same class as nondisabled children. Box 8-3 lists the least restrictive to most restrictive environments. If the parents or guardians for the child do not think the school district's actions are in the best interest of the child, they have a right to procedural due process. This provides safeguards for the child against a school district's action, including a right to sue in court.

PL 94-142 has undergone many revisions since its inception. The most updated amendment to IDEA is PL 105-17, The Individuals with Disabilities Education Act Amendments of 1997. Several modifications were added that placed emphasis on what is educationally best for disabled children rather than the required paperwork. PL 105-17

BOX 8-2 Related Services Available From the School for the Child With a Disability

- Audiology
- Counseling services
- Early identification and assessment of disabilities in children
- Medical services
- Occupational therapy
- Physical therapy
- Speech therapy
- Recreation
- School health services
- Rehabilitative counseling services
- Psychology services
- Parent counseling and training
- Social work services in schools
- Transportation
- Assistive technology

BOX 8-3 Scale of the Least Restrictive to Most Restrictive Environment

- Full-day regular class placement with consultation services for the teacher
- Full-day regular class placement with instruction delivered in regular class by specialist
- Part-day regular class placement and part-day resource or itinerant services
- Part-day regular class placement and part-day special class placement
- Full-day placement in special class and social integration with general school population
- Full-day placement in special class
- Full-day placement in special school
- Full-time placement in residential facility
- Homebound or hospital placement

requires students with disabilities to participate in statewide and districtwide assessments, with accommodations as necessary, or in alternative assessments. This law enhances the input of parents of children with disabilities in the decision making that affects their child's education.

CIVIL RIGHTS LEGISLATION

The American with Disabilities Act of 1990 (ADA) (PL 101-336-ADA) extends civil rights protection to individuals who have special needs, including cognitive and sensory disabilities. This act protects both children and adults. It prohibits discrimination against people with disabilities in employment, public accommodations (e.g., movie theaters, hotels, restaurants), transportation, state and local government services, and telecommunication services. The ADA is the most significant law protecting the rights of all individuals with disabilities.

The Developmental Disabilities Bill of Rights Act Amendment of 1987 (PL 100-146; reauthorized in 1990 and 1994) provides financial means to enable those who have special needs to achieve their maximum potential. This law serves individuals who have severe and chronic physical and/or mental disabilities.

The Rehabilitation Act of 1973 Section 504 (PL 93-112) applies the civil rights protection to individuals of all ages with disabilities or special needs. It states, "no otherwise qualified handicap in the United States . . . shall, solely by reason of his handicap, be excluded from the participation in, be denied the benefits of, or be subjected to discrimination under any program or actively receiving federal financial assistance." Often, this act has been used to assist with services for children who do not meet the criteria for special education.

FOLLOW-UP AND LONG-TERM NEEDS

Follow-up care and long-term need assessments are essential to help provide continual successful outcomes. This can be accomplished through follow-up telephone calls to the family and follow-up appointments with the rehabilitation specialists. The child's care is reviewed and plan of care revised as needed. If additional services are required, the rehabilitation team will help facilitate their acquisition. Life care planners may be involved in coordinating the child's care. They can assist in developing a plan of care that will take into account the anticipated needs spanning the child's lifetime. A child with a disability will have long-term needs across the continuum of the life span. As the child continues to grow and develop, his or her needs will continue to change. For example, when a toddler sustains a spinal cord injury, the issue of sexuality is not a priority. When the child becomes an adolescent and young adult, however, the issue of sexuality becomes important.

SUMMARY

The goal of rehabilitation is to provide a better quality of life for the child and to return the child to maximum potential within the family and community. All efforts during the resuscitation process are taken to assist the child and family in adapting to the life changes resulting from the trauma experience. Early recognition of available or lack of available support systems for the pediatric patient and family can facilitate the process of rehabilitation planning as assistance is offered from appropriate resource programs.

BIBLIOGRAPHY

Agency for Health Care Policy and Research. (1992). *Pressure ulcers in adults: Prediction and prevention* (AHCPR Publication No. 92-0047). Rockville, MD: Author.

American Spinal Injury Association. (1996). *International standards for neurological and functional classification of spinal cord injury* (rev. ed.). Chicago: Author.

Association of Rehabilitation Nurses. (1992). *Pediatric rehabilitation nursing* [Brochure]. Skokie, IL: Author.

Beck, T., & Spoltere, T. (1996). Processes involved in discharge planning. In R. R. Betz & M. J. Mulcahey (Eds.), *The child with a spinal cord injury* (pp. 557-566). Rosemont, IL: American Association of Orthopedic Surgeons.

Blanchet, D., & McGee, S. M. (1996). Principles of splint design and use. In L. A. Kurtz, P. W. Dowrick, S. E. Levy, & M. L. Batshaw (Eds.), *Handbook of developmental disabilities: Resources for interdisciplinary care* (pp. 465-480). Gaithersburg, MD: Aspen.

Brillhart, B., & Stewart, A. (1989). Education as the key to rehabilitation. *Nursing Clinics of North America, 24,* 675-680.

Carendas, D. D. (1992). Neurogenic bladder: Evaluation and management. *Physical Medicine and Rehabilitation Clinics of North America, 4,* 751-733.

Commission on Accreditation of Rehabilitation Facilities (CARF). (1998). *Medical rehabilitation standards manual.* Tucson, AZ: Author.

Cooper, D. M. (1992). Wound assessment and evaluation of healing. In R. A. Bryant (Ed.), *Acute and chronic wounds: Nursing management* (pp. 69-104). St. Louis: Mosby.

Dittmar, S. S. (1989) Bladder elimination. In S. S. Dittmar (Ed.), *Rehabilitation nursing: Process and application* (pp. 150-195). St. Louis: Mosby.

Dunn, K. L., & Galka, M. L. (1994). A comparison of the effectiveness of Theravac SB(and bisacodyl suppositories in SCI patients' bowel programs. *Rehabilitation Nursing, 19,* 334-338.

Haley, S. M., Coster, W. J., Ludlow, L. H., Haltiwanger, J. T., & Andrellos, P. J. (1992). *Pediatric Evaluation of Disability Inventory (PEDI): Development, standardization and administration manual.* Boston: New England Medical Center Hospital PEDI Research Group.

Harper, D. C. (1990). Children and rehabilitation: A new frontier [guest editor's perspective]. *Journal of Rehabilitation, 56,* 10.

Hoeman, S. P. (1992). Pediatric rehabilitation nursing. In G. E. Molnar (Ed.), *Pediatric rehabilitation* (2nd ed., pp. 202-219). Baltimore: Williams & Wilkins.

House, J. G., & Stiens, S. A. (1997). Pharmacologically initiated defecation for persons with spinal cord injury: Effectiveness of three agents. *Archives of Physical Medicine and Rehabilitation, 78,* 1062-1065.

Janelli, L. M. (1989). Eating and swallowing. In S. S. Dittmar (Ed.), *Rehabilitation nursing: Process and application* (pp. 334-359). St. Louis: Mosby.

Kirshblum, S. C., Gulati, M., O'Conner, K. C., & Voorman, S. J. (1998). Bowel care practices in chronic spinal cord injury. *Archives of Physical Medicine and Rehabilitation, 79,* 20-23.

Lewis, R. B., & Doorlag, D. H. (1999). *Teaching special students in general education classrooms* (5th ed.). Upper Saddle River, NJ: Prentice Hall.

Maklebust, J. (1987). Pressure ulcers: Etiology and prevention. *Nursing Clinics of North America, 22,* 359-377.

Maklebust, J. (1996). Using wound care products to promote a healing environment. *Critical Care Clinics of North America, 8,* 141-158.

McCourt, A. E. (Ed.). (1993). *The specialty practice of rehabilitation nursing: A core curriculum* (3rd ed.). Skokie, IL: Rehabilitation Nursing Foundation.

Michaud, L. J., & Duhaime, A. C. (1992). Traumatic brain injury. In M. L. Batshaw & Y. M. Perret (Eds.), *Children with disabilities* (pp. 527-546). Baltimore: Paul H. Brookes.

Moody-Szymanski, E. A., & Scherer, Y. K. (1989). Breathing. In S. S. Dittmar (Ed.), *Rehabilitation nursing: Process and application* (pp. 82-119). St. Louis: Mosby.

Morrison, S. A., & Stanwyck, D. J. (1999). The effect of shorter lengths of stay on functional outcomes of spinal cord injury rehabilitation. *Topics in Spinal Cord Injury Rehabilitation, 4*(4), 44-55.

National Pressure Ulcer Advisory Panel. (1989). Pressure ulcer prevalence, cost, and risk assessment: Consensus development conference statement. *Decubitus, 2*(2), 24-28.

Ottenbacher, K. J., Msall, M. E., Lyon, N. R., Duffy, L. C., Granger, C. V., & Braun, S. (1997). Interrater agreement and stability of the Functional Independence Measure for Children (WeeFIM): Use in children with developmental disabilities. *Archives of Physical Medicine and Rehabilitation, 78,* 1309-1315.

Quigley, S. M., & Curley, M. A. Q. (1996). Skin integrity in the pediatric population: Preventing and managing pressure ulcers. *Journal of the Society of Pediatric Nurses, 1,* 7-18.

Rainville, N. C. (1994). The current nursing procedure for intermittent urinary catheterization in rehabilitation facilities. *Rehabilitation Nursing, 19,* 330-333.

Rivas, D. A., Abdill, C. A., & Chancellor, M. B. (1996). Current management of detrusor sphincter dyssynergia. *Topics in Spinal Cord Injury Rehabilitation, 1*(3), 1-17.

Sandor, M. K., Copeland, D., & Robinson, S. Team-building interventions for interdisciplinary teams: A case study of a pediatric client. *Rehabilitation Nurse, 23,* 290-294.

Sperle, P. A., Ottenbacher, K. J., Braun, S. L., Lane, S. J., & Nochajski, S. (1997). Equivalence reliability of the Functional Independence Measure for Children (WeeFIM) administration methods. *American Journal of Occupational Therapy, 51,* 35-41.

WeeFIM System Clinical Guide (Version 5.0). (1998). Buffalo, NY: Uniform Data System for Medical Rehabilitation.

Vogel, L. C., & Pontari, M. A. (1997). Pediatric spinal cord injury issues: Medical issues. *Topics in Spinal Cord Injury Rehabilitation, 3*(2), 20-30.

Weingarden, S. I. (1992). The gastrointestinal system and spinal cord injury. *Physical Medicine and Rehabilitation Clinic of North America, 4,* 765-781.

Whaley, L. F., & Wong, D. L. (1991). *Nursing care of infants and children* (4th ed.). St. Louis: Mosby.

World Health Organization (WHO). (1980). *International classification of impairments, disabilities and handicaps: A manual of classification relating to the consequences of disease.* Geneva: Author.

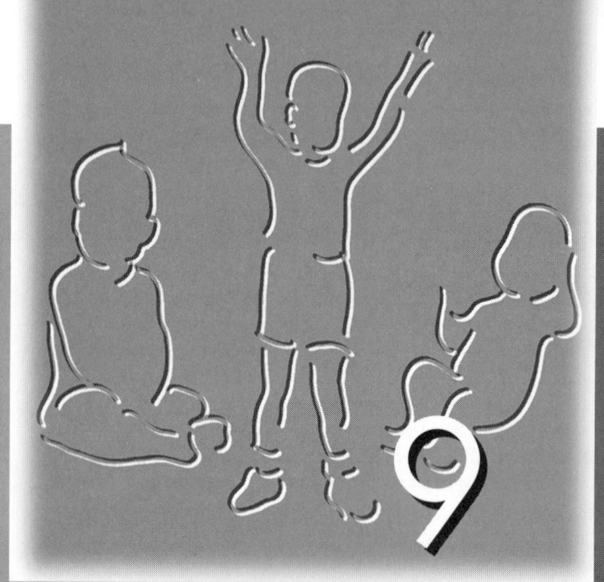

9 IMPACT OF TRAUMA ON GROWTH AND DEVELOPMENT

Ruth M. Lebet

Pediatric trauma victims come in all ages, and each child who experiences physical injury has many unique characteristics. These children have different temperaments, are at different developmental levels, have a variety of previous life experiences, and come from various cultural backgrounds. Each of these factors plays an important role in shaping the child's response to the traumatic event. These children are cared for in a variety of settings by clinicians, ranging in experience from those with limited pediatric experience to pediatric experts who care only for children. A health care system staffed by clinicians who are able to recognize the child's unique age and stage and respond appropriately assists the child in moving through the injury experience in a way that results in a positive developmental outcome. This is important in allowing the child to move on to further developmental tasks.

Knowledge of normal growth and development is crucial in understanding each child's response to traumatic events. This knowledge permits the clinician to facilitate a child's coping mechanisms and provide a developmentally appropriate environment. In the following discussion, information is presented that will assist the caregiver in providing a positive environment for the pediatric trauma victim. Specific points of discussion include developmental tasks and coping behaviors of each age group, factors that promote successful coping, and the effects of stressors experienced by the injured child on normal growth and development. The discussion concludes with strategies that are useful in minimizing potential negative effects of hospitalization.

It is crucial to recognize that caring for a child is, in fact, caring for a family. However, this discussion focuses on the child's developmental tasks and responses. For a discussion of the effects of trauma on the family, see Chapter 10.

NORMAL GROWTH AND DEVELOPMENT

Children go through very specific stages of development in a precise sequence. The stages are generally discussed in terms of age groups, although each child progresses through the specific sequence on an individual timeline (Table 9-1). Certain tasks must be accomplished in each stage to provide a framework that will allow the child to advance to the next stage and successfully accomplish subsequent tasks. It is important to note that there are times in the child's developmental sequence when he or she may be more affected by negative events that occur.

Generally, each stage of development is discussed in terms of several factors, including language acquisition, moral development, learning theories, and psychosocial and cognitive development (Freiberg, 1992). For the purposes of this discussion, two primary factors are considered: psychosocial and cognitive development. Psychosocial development is discussed using the theory developed by Erikson (1963). Erikson's theory of personality development describes a core conflict that must be resolved at a specific developmental level for the child to progress to the next level. Successful resolution of these conflicts ultimately results in a healthy personality. Erikson's theory consists of eight stages. For the purposes of this discussion, the five stages occurring in childhood are discussed.

Cognitive development in children often is discussed in terms of the work of Piaget (1969). Piaget's theory describes ways of learning about the world and stages of reasoning that a child moves through until the he or she arrives at the level of adult reasoning and logical thinking. These theories are summarized briefly for each stage and linked to concrete ways to help the child master the environment, which is more likely to result in a positive developmental outcome. For more in-depth discussion, the reader is referred to Dixon

TABLE 9-1 Developmental Considerations

	Infant (0-1 yr)	Toddler (1-3 yr)	Preschool Child (3-6 yr)	School-Age Child (6-12 yr)	Adolescent (12-18 yr)
Developmental task (Erikson)	Trust vs. mistrust	Autonomy vs. shame and doubt	Initiative vs. guilt	Industry vs. inferiority	Identity vs. role confusion
Cognitive development (Piaget)	Sensorimotor knowing	Preoperational thought	Preoperational thought (late phase)	Concrete operations	Formal operations
Communication	Cries, facial expressions, motor activity	Simple phrases, cries, physical activity	Sentences, crying, physical activity Very literal Does not comprehend cause and effect	Well-developed vocabulary Thinks in specifics, not abstract or hypothetical	Abstract thinker Generally seeks/desires information
Stresses/fears	Disruptions in routine	Separation, pain	Separation, abandonment, pain, mutilation	Loss of control, bodily injury, death, separation, pain	Disfigurement, separation from peers, loss of control
Illness concept	None	None	Illness as feeling state Depends on visual cues	Understands various aspects of illness, some basic anatomy	Understands anatomy and physiology
Preparation		Simple, honest explanation just before the event, using sensory information Medical play with equipment	Simple, honest explanation just before the event, using sensory information Medical play with equipment	Explanation before the procedure, using concrete and specific information Medical play with equipment Encourage questions Allow child to have some control if possible	Explanation before the procedure Provide enough time for the adolescent to formulate questions Explain why the procedure is necessary

and Stein (1992), Freiberg (1992), and DiVito-Thomas (1999).

Infants (Birth to About 1 Year of Age)

Erikson (1963) describes the major conflict to be resolved in infancy as trust versus mistrust. Successful resolution of this conflict results in the development of trust and the ability of the infant to look to parents and caregivers for care and support. One of the most important factors that promotes this outcome is the provision of a stable, predictable environment with a consistent primary clinician. It is important that the child's basic needs for food, warmth, and comfort be met consistently. The infant requires a sense of physical safety, which is often achieved by providing boundaries to the infant's environment through bundling or swaddling.

Piaget (1969) described the infant's cognitive development as progressing through the stage of sensorimotor knowing, which consists of six substages. Throughout the sensorimotor period, infants learn about their environment through exploration and touch, the interaction of the senses and motor activity. The infant progresses from reflex activity to repetition of behaviors, to imitation of the behaviors of others. Early in infancy, objects and people exist for the infant only when the infant is aware of them in the environment. In late infancy, the infant develops object permanence, something or someone exists even when it is out of the environment. The development of object permanence is what allows the infant to demonstrate separation anxiety. Also in late infancy, the child begins to make associations between objects and events. For instance, the infant comes to know that the presence of a bottle usually means food.

Toddlers (About 1 to 3 Years of Age)

The developmental conflict for toddlers as described by Erikson is autonomy versus shame and doubt. Successful resolution of this conflict results in a child who has some control of his or her body and environment. Toddlers acquire autonomy as they master skills such as walking, basic language (including frequent use of "No!"), and potty training.

Piaget describes this stage of development as preoperational thought. During this stage the child is developing the ability to remember things. A toddler has a mental picture of an object not immediately present, such as a bottle, blanket, or parent. The child is acquiring language skills and has words to describe the mental pictures. Toddlers are egocentric; they can conceive of and understand all events in their world only in direct relationship to themselves. In this early stage of preoperational thought, physical sensations guide how a child comprehends the world. The preoperational child experiences the present and cannot understand or imagine the future. As a child comes to the end of toddlerhood, universal and magical thinking often are used. Universal thinking is generalization of one person's behavior to all similar people. Clinicians often experience this when a toddler becomes very frightened at the sight of a person in a laboratory coat. In magical thinking, the toddler gives powers to inanimate objects, such as monitors or x-ray machines. It is important to remember that toddlers are rapidly acquiring language and the child understands much more than he or she can convey.

Preschool Children (About 3 to 6 Years of Age)

Erikson's conflict that must be resolved for the preschool child is initiative versus guilt. The child who successfully completes this developmental stage will have a sense of initiative. This is achieved through the acquisition of motor skills, beginning interactions with others outside the family, further development of language skills, and use of imagination and role-playing.

In Piaget's schema the preschool child is in the late phase of preoperational thought. The preoperational child believes the world is purposive, that is, that there is a reason for everything that happens. However, the preoperational thinker has a limited understanding of causation. At this stage the child believes that two events that occur together (e.g., riding in the car and having a sore finger); that is, they cause each other to happen. When an attempt is made to correct this misinterpretation, the child cannot understand and therefore may not accept the accurate information. The preschool child tends to focus on one aspect of an object, for example, its size or the noise it makes. Language skills progress rapidly, but in this stage children are very literal and concrete. Careful choice of words when describing events or procedures to preschoolers (e.g., a "CT scan") is critical. It is important to be aware of what children may have overheard. Words that have more than one meaning or sound alike may be heard and interpreted by the child in a very different way than was intended.

In this late stage of preoperational thought, children still are unable to conceptualize things they cannot see or feel. Also, they cannot conceptualize something of which they have not had sensory experience. For example, it is difficult for a child at this stage to understand the concept of internal organs. For this reason, teaching with props such as dolls or simple models that the preoperational child can manipulate is likely to be successful. Volume concepts are not clear in this stage. Early in this stage the preschool child may be able to count, but he or she will not be able to correctly identify which number is greater.

School-Age Children (About 6 to 12 Years of Age)

For the school-age child, industry versus inferiority is the developmental challenge described by Erikson. The child who meets this goal will have developed industry through the acquisition of knowledge and the ability to complete tasks. Achievement and success are important to this age group, and the child begins to develop peer relationships, which become more important as the child moves through this stage. Rules are very important to the school-age child, and the child expects that everyone will abide by the rules.

At this age the child moves into Piaget's stage of concrete operations. The school-age child is able to use logical thinking, but he or she remains very concrete. The concrete thinker is able to consider several aspects of a situation at once, a view that greatly expands the child's abilities to correctly interpret events in his or her world. Although this child can consider another person's point of view, he or she will be unable to discuss a hypothetical situation. The school-age child still interprets and understands the world through characteristics experienced by the senses. At this stage a child will be able to learn concepts such as basic anatomy, but physiology, which involves abstract concepts, will be difficult to understand.

Adolescents (12 to 18 Years of Age)

In adolescence, children enter Erikson's stage of identity versus role confusion. Successful development of a strong sense of identity is achieved primarily through peer group interactions. A key concern for adolescents is how they appear to others. Clothes, hairstyles, and other means of body ornamentation are daily preoccupations for the adolescent. Egocentrism again is a factor. An adolescent thinks that everyone in the environment is always watching and judging him or her. A small blemish not noticeable to others will seem the size of a quarter to the adolescent. In this stage the adolescent is taking steps away from the family, working toward a place in society and developing a self-image. Adolescents tend to classify themselves and their peers in categories, and adolescents may try on several of these roles in their search for identity.

In terms of Piaget's stages of cognitive development, the adolescent enters formal operations. Less trial-and-error learning takes place. In this stage the child can think in abstract terms, which allows the adolescent to consider and discuss hypothetical situations and to use them as learning experiences. Causal relationships are identified correctly, and the adolescent begins to develop a personal values system.

Additional Factors

In addition to psychosocial and cognitive development theories, other areas may be helpful to clinicians in understanding how a particular child will integrate a traumatic injury experience into his or her further development. Understanding the development of a child's concept of illness allows the clinician to understand the child's framework for the events occurring during the child's interaction with the health care system. In addition, the individual's temperament and resilience influence how he or she will respond to traumatic events.

Child's Concept of Illness

As might be expected, beliefs about, and understanding of, illness develop in parallel with conceptual development (Bibace & Walsh, 1980; Perrin, Sayer, & Willett, 1991). Children who sustain a traumatic injury will develop their own explanation of what caused the injury. This explanation may contain several misconceptions. It is important to ask children about what they believe happened and why they became ill.

Preshool Children. A concept of health or illness is first seen in the preschool-age group. For this developmental level *illness* is defined as a feeling state that is not well differentiated. It is difficult for a preschooler to tell you what exactly hurts, just that it does hurt. They may be able to point to an area of pain, but they are unable to describe the pain. For the preschooler, an "either/or" state exists; a person is well, or a person is sick. The preschooler does not understand that, with time, the person will usually heal or get better. For instance, if a child has a femur fracture and receives a cast, he or she may believe that the cast will never be removed. Children in this age group have a good understanding of their external body but little or no understanding of internal organs (Vessey, Braithwaite, & Wiedmann, 1990). At this stage the child uses visual cues, such as Band-Aids, incisions, and blood, to indicate illness. The preschool child often uses magical thinking to describe how he or she became ill. It is also common for the preschool child to think that hospitalization is a punishment for bad behavior (Bibace & Walsh, 1980). Petrillo and Sanger (1980) asked preschool children who had been hospitalized why they came to the hospital. Answers such as, "My mommy doesn't want me anymore because she has a new baby" or "My sister hit me so I had to come here" illustrate the preschool child's use of illogical but developmentally appropriate reasoning.

School-Age Children. The school-age child views health and illness in more precise and concrete terms. Health is identified as a construct with several aspects, and the child is able to understand a basic difference between diseases (Hester, 1987). The school-age child can be specific in describing pain and injuries and is able to differentiate areas that hurt a little from those that hurt a great deal. At this level the child can understand that a hospitalization will end, a fracture will heal, and medical devices such as IVs will eventually be removed. At this stage the child has a limited understanding of some anatomy. The child may be able to identify organs such as the brain, bones, lungs, and heart, but he or she may not be able to understand how the organs are interrelated (Jones, Badger, & Moore, 1992).

Adolescents. Adolescents have a more abstract and hypothetical understanding of health and illness. Adolescents are able to comprehend not only anatomy but some physiology as well (Whitt, 1982). Adolescents believe that they have some control over whether or not they are healthy. They are specific in describing injuries and can describe experiences, such as pain, in great detail. They are able to understand how procedures or treatments are necessary for identifying problems or allowing them to return to a previous state of health.

Temperament

The temperament theory of Thomas and Chess (1977) describes temperament as the way in which an individual behaves in response to his or her environment and the people in it. Based on temperament type, if there is excessive stress in the child's environment, the child may be unable to master developmental tasks. By observing children at various ages and through parent interview, the authors developed nine attributes of temperament.

- *Adaptability* refers to how easy or difficult it is for a child to adjust to a new situation.
- *Intensity of reaction* refers to the child's energy level of reaction, whether the reaction is positive or negative.
- *Threshold of responsiveness* describes the amount of stimulation needed to produce a response in a child, for example, the child who wakes to a barking dog versus the child who sleeps through a thunderstorm.
- *Attention span and persistence* refers to how long and against what obstacles a child will pursue an activity.
- *Rhythmicity* describes a child's patterns or consistency in daily behaviors.
- *Approach-withdrawal* refers to the way in which a child initially responds to a new situation.
- *Mood, distractibility,* and *activity* are the other attributes.

Based on these nine attributes, Thomas and Chess developed three categories of temperament. The *easy* child is even tempered and predictable, has an approach (positive) response to new stimuli, generally has a positive mood, and is adaptable. About half of the children studied by Thomas and Chess fell into this category. The *difficult* child is active, lacks rhythmicity (e.g., regular patterns of sleeping and eating), usually demonstrates a withdrawal response, and adapts slowly to new situations. This child usually is intense and often is negative. About 10% of the children studied fell into this category. The *slow-to-warm-up* child is fairly predictable and has a low level of activity. This child generally reacts in a negative way to new situations; however, the reaction is fairly low energy. About 15% of the children studied met the criteria for this temperament type. Children in these categories differ in terms of amount of crying, soothability, and capacity for self-comforting behaviors. Not all children fit one of these three categories, but there is some indication that children who fit the slow-to-warm-up and difficult categories may be more likely to develop behavior problems when they encounter a significant stress. Parents should be asked to describe their child's temperament and how the child best handles new situations. Knowledge of a child's temperament type provides information on the best way to interact with the child and how best to present information. For example, the difficult child may have an increased fear of strangers. The slow-to-warm-up child may need additional time before he or she is ready for a procedure to start. This information should be used not only in developing an individualized plan of care but also in identifying the child more at risk for problems with further development after his or her interaction with the health care system.

Resilience

In the 1970s researchers involved in the identification of children at risk for impaired development found that some of their subjects, who were expected to have extremely abnormal development, were actually at a normal developmental level. These children came to be labeled by a variety of terms, including *resilient, resourceful,* and *stress resistant* (Garmezy, 1987). Stewart, Reid, and Mangham (1997) define *resilience* as the "capacity to 'bounce back' in spite of significant stress or adversity." Hospitalization for a traumatic injury is certainly a significant stress, and knowledge about characteristics of resilient children is useful in identifying children who may be more at risk for a negative developmental outcome. Stewart, Reid, and Mangham (1997) specify three groups of factors that influence the resilience of children in a positive or negative way.

Individual risk factors that may influence a child's resilience in a negative way include male gender, minority racial status, chronic illness, and difficult temperament. *Protective factors* of the individual may include helpfulness, problem-solving abilities, optimism, and social competence. Easy temperament, creativity, reading skills, and progress in school also may be protective factors. *Family risk factors* that may have a negative impact on a child's resilience include separation from parents, parental illness, exposure to violence, large family size, and poverty. Family factors that may be protective include strong parent-child attachment, an effective extended family network, and a family dynamic that includes rules and responsibilities for the child. Risk factors within the community may include poverty, a violent neighborhood, and a high-risk peer group. Protective factors in the community include positive relationships with adults outside of the family network and positive school experiences.

Many children who sustain traumatic injuries will have one or more of these risk factors. The clinician can use this information to identify children most at risk for negative developmental outcomes as a result of hospitalization and to promote resilience in the child.

DEVELOPMENTAL CHALLENGES OF TRAUMA

The experience of hospitalization for trauma and traumatic injuries is a developmental challenge to the child, especially the child younger than 7 to 8 years (Rollins, 1999). The child will attempt to master this challenge by using coping skills. A child's repertoire of coping skills increases and develops over time as the child is exposed to various developmental experiences and challenges. It is important for the clinician to understand coping strategies available to the child at various developmental levels, as well as the fears and concerns most prominent at each level. This knowledge will facilitate development of a plan of care that allows the child to successfully move through and master the experience, resulting in a positive developmental outcome. Stewart, Reid, and Mangham (1997) note that "successful coping in one situation strengthens the individual's competence to deal with adversity in the future." Promoting the child's use of coping skills assists him or her in mastering the experience of hospitalization.

Coping Skills

Coping can be defined as "any attempt to manage stress through either cognitive or behavioral efforts" (Bossert, 1994). The ability to cope with a stressful situation develops over the life span. Multiple factors affect how the child will be affected by a stress such as a traumatic experience. These factors include the nature and severity of the illness, the child's previous life experiences, parental response to the event, gender, the attitudes and responses of the members of the health care team, and prior experiences with the health care system and hospitalization. In addition, to manage a stress, the child must have energy available to expend on coping. Bossert (1994) points out that a child may use different coping strategies at different points during the hospitalization, depending on factors such as current physiologic state and the presence or absence of parents.

The health care team can manage some elements of situation to facilitate effective coping (Kavanaugh, 1989). First is presentation of an unambiguous stimulus. An example is telling the child that something will hurt. Awareness of a threat also helps facilitate effective coping. Inform the child before beginning a procedure that it will hurt or upset him or her. The appropriate time to present this information varies with the child's developmental level. A toddler or preschooler should be told just before the procedure. A school-age child or adolescent should have some time before the procedure to recruit coping strategies. Next, attribution of cause, or knowledge of what caused the stress, promotes coping. This may be difficult or impossible with the toddler or preschooler in the preoperational thought stage. However, the child may attempt to manage this through universal or magical thinking. Finally, the use of active coping skills promotes successful coping. To facilitate the child's use of coping skills, one must know what those skills are and allow the use of all that are appropriate.

It is important to remember that each child is unique, and events or procedures that are most stressful to one child may not be for another. Something seen as benign by members of the health care team may, in fact, be the most stressful event for a particular child. Kavanaugh (1989) indicates that it is not the intensity of an aversive stimulus that determines its stressfulness, but rather the ability of the individual to predict and control the stimulus. An injured child who has no experience with hospitalization may cope fairly well with the first few procedures. As the trauma workup progresses and more procedures are performed on the child, the child may feel a total lack of control and an inability to predict the next event. This child might then find a fairly painless procedure, such as a blood pressure measurement, to be extremely stressful.

Specific Fears and Coping Skills of Various Developmental Levels

Coping skills are primarily emotion focused until late childhood (Kavanaugh, 1989). Young children with limited verbal skills are unable to find words to express their emotions; they must instead demonstrate them. By school age, children generally have developed and are able to use internalized coping skills. Ryan-Wegner (1996) evaluated 32 studies that examined coping strategies used by ill children. She concluded that whether children are healthy or ill, they tend to use the same strategies to cope with stress. Questioning parents about a child's usual repertoire of coping skills will aid the clinician in developing a plan of care that will promote the child's use of preferred coping strategies.

Infants. For infants, the greatest stress initially is disruption in routine and not having basic needs met. Later in infancy, separation from parents or the primary caregiver becomes the greatest stressor. Infants exhibit behaviors that indicate they are stressed or overstimulated by their environment. These cues include changes in skin color; disorganized, often flailing movements; an irregular respiratory rate; avoidance of eye contact or gaze aversion; and hiccuping. Infants have a limited number of coping strategies available. Coping behaviors include motor activity, crying, and sucking as a tension release or self-soothing behavior. Head rocking may also be seen as a self-soothing behavior. In late infancy the presence of parents or the primary caregiver becomes an important coping strategy, especially during procedures or other threatening events.

Toddlers. The most significant stress for toddlers is separation from parents. The presence of parents is the primary source of security for toddlers, and this is their main coping strategy. During procedures, parental presence is very comforting to toddlers, but parents should not participate in the procedure. Rather, parents should provide comfort and reassurance, especially at the completion of the procedure. Although toddlers have developed additional coping strategies, their ability to use these strategies is decreased in an unfamiliar environment. Another commonly used coping strategy is the use of motor activity. Toddlers often attempt to remove themselves from an unpleasant experience. The presence of security objects and the use of rituals and repetition help facilitate effective coping for toddlers.

Preshool Children. The most significant fears for preschool children include abandonment, fears of mutilation, and pain. Parental presence, allowing self-expression (for instance, permitting loud crying when a procedure hurts), and encouraging the use of fantasy promote successful coping. Other coping skills include regression, motor activity, self-comforting behaviors such as thumb sucking or playing with the hair, cuddling with parents, and projection of feelings. The preschool child often uses aggression (e.g., pinching, hitting, biting, spitting), and it is important to recognize that this is a normal behavioral response from a child who feels threatened.

School-Age Children. School-age children, who are developing peer relationships and learning to abide by rules, are fearful of loss of control (not following rules or acting wrong in front of other children), bodily injury, death, and separation from family. Hart and Bossert (1994) looked at fears reported by hospitalized school-age children and found "being away from family," "getting a shot," and "having to stay a long time" were the top three fears reported.

Children in this age group still derive security from the presence of their parents, but they begin to use internalized coping strategies as well. These strategies include use of a support person or "coach"; cooperation; attempts to control aspects of a procedure, such as timing; and emotionally removing themselves from a situation. Children in this age group may also regress. Vessey, Farley, and Risom (1991) describe behaviors such as reverting to fantasy, apathy toward favorite activities, increased dependency, and increased self-centeredness as examples of regressive behaviors. In a study of 82 school-age children, Bossert (1994) found that acutely ill children could identify 69 coping strategies that fell into six categories: cognitive processing, cognitive restructuring, cooperation, countermeasures (avoidance), control, and seeking support. Using countermeasures and seeking support were the first choice of more than half of the subjects.

Adolescents. For adolescents the biggest fear is often disfigurement or looking different. Other concerns for children in this age group are loss of control, loss of identity, and separation from their peer group. Adolescents may have a wide range of coping skills, including attempting to predict or control events; using physical activity an as outlet for tension; attempting to maintain self-control at all costs; and using denial, regression, and withdrawal. Often, adolescents use intellectualization as a coping strategy, asking for a great deal of information and attempting to seem detached and unemotional. For some adolescents, maintaining contact with peers may be a very important coping strategy. For others, this may be a stressor, especially if they perceive that they are "abnormal."

Any hospitalized child will undergo multiple procedures, and this is a specific instance where coping skills will be called into play. There is substantial nursing literature about the appropriate preparation of children for procedures, mainly dealing with children in a hospital or clinic setting (Brennan, 1994). Children with traumatic injuries may be introduced to medical procedures in the field when they are immobilized and an IV is started. The manner in which this initial encounter is managed will have an effect on how the child attempts to manage further procedures. It is beneficial to the child if all members of the health care team have the ability to provide developmentally appropriate care.

When working with a child and developing a plan of care, one must consider several factors. First, what coping skills do children in this age group usually use? Next, which coping skills has this child successfully used in the past? Finally, which of these skills can be used given the child's medical condition, the environment of the child, and the presence or absence of individuals the child usually looks to as a support system? It may be necessary to help the child learn new coping skills and strategies, but as much as possible the child should be allowed to use skills that have been successful in the past.

DEVELOPMENTALLY APPROPRIATE CARE

Regardless of the child's age and developmental level, certain elements of the hospital experience must be acknowledged for all children. Whether care is provided in an emergency department, general care unit, or intensive care unit (ICU), the child is placed in a very foreign environment that generally provides a great deal of sensory overstimulation. The child usually is sleep deprived, must undergo many procedures that are threatening or painful to the child, and is experiencing pain from injuries. There are also periods when the child is separated from his or her parents. All of these stressors may contribute to a negative developmental outcome. Bar-Mor (1997) reports that more than 50% of children followed for 1 month after hospitalization demonstrated behavioral and/or emotional changes during that period. Jones, Fiser, and Livingston (1992) studied children hospitalized in either an ICU or a ward. They found that any hospitalization, whether or not an ICU stay was required, is a stress for the child. When these two groups were evaluated for anxiety, depression, agitation, and withdrawal, they found few differences between the two groups and many similarities.

Developmentally appropriate care seeks to prevent potentially negative developmental effects of this experience. The pediatric trauma victim moves through several phases of the health care delivery system, which may include prehospital, emergency department, ICU, general care unit, and rehabilitation care. In each of these areas, the environment must be assessed to identify factors that block the delivery of developmentally appropriate care that is child and family centered. Petrillo and Sanger (1980) noted in their classic text, *Emotional Care of Hospitalized Children:*

> Despite our present sophistication regarding the psychological response of children to illness and hospitalization, and the impressive body of knowledge in child development, it is striking to note the discrepancies between what we know and what we do in the hospital environment.

In 1998 Ahmann noted that this discrepancy still exists. Limited visiting hours, lack of provisions for a parent to room in with the child, and nursing assessment and documentation routines that do not routinely consider growth and development history or pain are examples of factors that do not facilitate developmentally appropriate care.

Aspects of Care to Consider for Various Developmental Levels

From previous discussion, it is clear that parental presence is crucial to all pediatric patients, because the parents provide support and promote the use of coping skills. An assessment tool should be in place that allows the clinician to obtain information about the child's usual coping skills, temperament style, and developmental level. Hospitalization is often especially difficult for children who have recently obtained a new developmental milestone, particularly if they cannot use it in the hospital setting. The child who has recently been potty trained and must wear a diaper while in the hospital or the child who just started walking and now must be confined to bed becomes very frustrated.

An important aspect of caring for the child who is hospitalized and who will undergo painful or frightening procedures during that time is the provision of a safe area (Rollins, 1999). This is especially important for the toddler, preschooler, and school-age child. The safe area is an area where the child knows that no bad things can happen. In many hospitals the playroom and the child's bed are considered safe or off-limit areas for procedures such as drawing blood, inserting a nasogastric (NG) tube, and starting IVs. Use of a treatment room for these procedures provides the child with cues as to when the procedure will stop and start. Once the child can leave the room, he or she knows that the painful experience is over.

Excellent pain management is crucial to promoting a positive developmental outcome. The child in prolonged or undertreated pain will focus energies on the pain being experienced and will not have resources for positive coping. (For further discussion of this important issue, see Chapter 11.) The environment should promote therapeutic play, which will provide the child with opportunities to express feelings and concerns related to the hospitalization. Both nursing and child life are in an ideal position to facilitate this. In addition to general environmental issues, there are aspects of care specific to each age group that should be considered.

Infants

For infants, significant effects of the hospital environment are disruption in the child's normal sleep/wake patterns, lack of stability in the environment, and for the older infant, separation from parents. Often, this is seen as sleeping or feeding problems (Stein, 1992). Minimizing the number of individuals who provide care to the infant promotes stability. Those individuals should be sensitive to the infant's cues that he or she is being overstimulated. Cares should be grouped, when possible, to provide blocks of uninterrupted sleep. The environment should be conducive to sleep, with decreased lighting and minimal noise. Some infants will have difficulty sleeping once they are back in their home environment, and parents should be aware of this. Parents often need to provide infants with background noise when they sleep for the first few days at home. They should also provide opportunities for the infant to release tension and engage in self-soothing behaviors, such as thumb or hand sucking. If this is not possible, use of a pacifier is appropriate (assuming the infant will accept one). Parental presence should be promoted and parents allowed to hold the child and participate in the child's care. When possible, the infant should be fed on demand. Boundaries to the infant's environment should be established by swaddling the infant or using towel or blanket rolls to cocoon the infant. Verbal stimulation through playing music or speaking to the infant in a soft tone is important.

Toddlers

Toddlers are most affected by separation from parents. Toddlers use physical activity as a stress outlet and as a means of communication, so the restrictions on activity that are required during hospitalization are especially difficult for children in this age group. Toddlers are beginning to make attempts to control the world around them, and the loss of opportunities to assert their independence is very stressful. For children in this age group, as well as for infants, disruption of the toddler's sleep/wake patterns, as well as total disruption of normal routines and roles of their parents, is very upsetting. Behavioral changes seen during a hospitalization include temper tantrums, apathy, sleep problems, and poor feeding (Stein, 1992).

Care for children in this age group should focus on involving parents in care and attempting to preserve some home routines. Recreating bedtime rituals in the hospital or having the bath done by the parent who usually bathes the child at home provides some stability and comfort for the child. Transitional objects, such as a blanket or stuffed animal, are important for toddlers. Toddlers should be given some opportunities to be active while remaining safe. Restraint of toddlers should be avoided if possible. If the toddler requires more than a day or two of hospitalization, an attempt should be made to develop a consistent structure and routine for the child's day because this will promote feelings of security. For older toddlers, simple explanations should be given just before the procedures and, if possible, the child allowed to manipulate equipment. Explanations should be very simple and should focus on what the child will see, hear, feel, or smell. Children in this age group tends to focus on one aspect of an experience, so it is helpful to prepare them for what will be the most actively involved sense (e.g., the loud noise of a cast cutter). After a painful or threatening procedure, it is important to allow toddlers some recovery time, with comfort provided by a parent if possible. Separation anxiety is at its peak in this age group, and parents need to be aware that it is "normal" for a toddler to start to cry when he or she sees the parents. Children in this age group still depend on "acted-out emotions," and they are accustomed to showing their parents their feelings. Leaving a parent's object, such as a watch, keys, or article of clothing, may help the toddler tolerate the separation when parents must leave the bedside.

Preschool Children

For preschool children, separation from parents remains the major issue of hospitalization. Children in this age group, who are just starting to develop a concept of time based on the family's usual routine, lose these cues, which they depend on to order the world. Another issue for these children is the fear of mutilation. IVs and other invasive lines give preschoolers the sense that they have been mutilated. Fear of pain is significant in this age group, and it is important to be honest with the children about what will hurt. Like toddlers, preschoolers use physical activity as a coping mechanism, so activity restriction is very difficult for them. Regression is common; regressive behaviors include requesting to wear a diaper, wanting a bottle, sucking their thumbs, hitting, biting, and eating poorly (Stein, 1992). Bedwetting may be seen, and it is important to reassure the child that this is not seen as bad behavior.

Parental presence is a key requirement in helping preschoolers cope with the stress of hospitalization. Many of the strategies useful in assisting toddlers are also appropriate for preschoolers, such as maintaining routines, providing transitional objects, allowing time for physical activity, and giving information in very simple terms that involve the senses just before a procedure. It is crucial to be honest with children about whether something will hurt. It is also important that sleeping children be woken before painful procedures are performed. Children who wake because of a painful event may be apprehensive about going to sleep. Medical play is very appropriate for children in this age group and permits the clinician to identify fears or misperceptions these children may have developed using their very active and well-developed imaginations. Because these children are in the preoperational thought stage and are not logical thinkers, it is not always appropriate to try to correct their misperceptions using logic (Whitt, 1982).

Preschool children have a much more extensive vocabulary than toddlers but have very literal interpretation of words. It is important for clinicians to consider the specific words and phrases used when talking to children or to others at the bedside in children's hearing. "Contrast dye" may be heard and understood as "die." Preschool children would "draw" blood with a crayon, not a needle, and would "stick" someone with a piece of wood. Preschoolers are learning which behaviors are acceptable and which are not, and limit setting is appropriate for this age group. It is essential that all members of the team be consistent in enforcing limit settings, so it must be clear to everyone what the limits are. Praise is important to the preschooler, but it should be focused on the child's accomplishment rather on the child. "You did a great job holding still" is supportive of positive development. "You were a good girl" sends a very different message.

School-Age Children

School-age children are likely to suffer negative developmental effects as a result of hospitalization. Children in this age group fears separation from parents, loss of physical and emotional control, and bodily injury. Children in this age group are beginning to have an understanding of the concept of death, and they may fear that they will die as the result of their injuries. School-age children are developing a sense of self-worth through accomplishments at home and at school, and hospitalization will be stressful for children who have limited opportunities to accomplish tasks or be successful. In addition, parents who are concerned for their injured child often treat the child as more dependent during a hospitalization.

Modesty is a key issue for school-age children, and privacy can be very difficult to maintain in the hospital. Regression is often seen during the hospitalization of the school-age child. Stein (1992) notes "Children of all age groups can be expected to demonstrate a loss of some developmental milestones during and after a hospitalization." It is reassuring for parents to know this, and it helps the parent accept the behavior as a normal response to a significant stressor.

When caring for the school-age child, the clinician must recognize the importance of providing the child with opportunities for accomplishment. The school-age child should be encouraged to participate in cares such as dressing changes. The clinician should work with the child to set goals, for instance, volume to be achieved with the incentive spirometer. Modest goals should be set initially, and lots of positive feedback should be given when the goal is met. The goal should be gradually increased and the child's progress noted. Tangible rewards, such as stickers, special Band-Aids, or posters charting progress, are very effective and provide objects the child can show to others.

Protect the child's privacy and ensure that other members of the team also respect the child's need for privacy. It is not inappropriate to ask a school-age girl if she would like her father to step out of the room while she uses the bed pan or has her bath. Routine is also helpful to children this age group, as is parental presence. Both provide these children with feelings of safety and security. Parents should be encouraged to allow the child some independence whenever possible. The child should be allowed to participate in decisions, such as ordering of cares, which arm to have blood drawn from, or which reward will be given after the procedure is completed. Remember that this age group still needs to have limits set for them.

Opportunities for play with other children and play activities or tasks that result in a "product," such as a craft activity, provide children with opportunities for achievement while they interact with peers. Often, school-age children worry about the other children who are hospitalized with them, and opportunities to interact productively are useful. School-aged children are still very literal in their use of words, so what they hear is very important. Medical play is useful for identifying the child's understanding of events and the concerns the child has.

Boyd and Hunsberger (1998) asked school-age children with chronic illness to describe what they believed were the biggest stressors and which interventions they found helped them most while in the hospital. The top three stressors were IVs, needles or invasive procedures, and surgery. Activities of clinicians that the children believed promoted coping included talking with and listening to the child, explaining and providing information, allowing the child some control, being patient, providing consistency in caregivers, and having a positive mood. Although the sample size was small, these findings generally support recommendations for caring for the hospitalized school-age child.

Parents of the school-age child should have information on behaviors that may be seen at home several days to several weeks after the child's discharge. Whitt (1982) describes several behaviors, including eating difficulties; sleep problems, such as fear of the dark or nightmares; social or behavioral regression; bedwetting; anxiety; and depression. If these problems persist, it is important for the family to follow up with the pediatrician.

Adolescents

Adolescents are less likely to have significant negative developmental outcomes from a hospitalization. Adolescents are able to comprehend and interpret correctly more about what is happening to them. Disfigurement is one of the biggest fears of adolescents because appearance and outer image are key to their self-concept. Loss of control is also an important issue. Separation from the peer group, loss of independence, and lack of privacy are additional issues.

Adolescents cope well when they are provided with information, but they usually provide the care team with cues as to when they are ready and how much information can be handled at a time. Information should include what is presently happening and what is likely to happen in the future. The adolescent should be included in all decisions about the plan when possible. Material that the adolescent can read and later ask questions about is helpful in allowing the adolescent time to incorporate the large amount of new information.

For many adolescents, visits from friends are vitally important and provide a link with their "real life." Some adolescents will not want many visitors, especially if they are concerned about their appearance because of physical injuries, invasive lines, or equipment that must be used. It is important to ask the adolescent if visitors other than family are desired. It is also important to provide access to friends and family via phone if the adolescent does not want many visitors.

Intensive Care Unit Care

The previous paragraphs discussed hospitalization in general. Many children who sustain traumatic injuries require evaluation at an emergency department. A subset of that group will require inpatient hospitalization. An even smaller group will require an ICU admission. Although all of the interventions and stressors previously discussed apply to all of these settings, the child who is admitted to the ICU may be subjected to stressors not experienced by children on general care wards.

Smith and Martin (2001) note that children in the ICU are exposed to additional stressors, such as an excessive noise level, awareness and concern for other patients in their immediate vicinity who may be undergoing painful procedures, and excessive visual stimulation. In addition, the highly technical ICU setting may lead to what they describe as emotional deprivation resulting from loss of stimulation, immobilization, and interpersonal isolation. Children of all ages who are intubated will be frustrated by an inability to communicate effectively. Toddlers or preschoolers may fear that they will not be able to speak after the endotracheal tube is removed or that the tube may never be removed.

The interventions previously discussed are appropriate in this setting to the extent that they can be implemented. Supplying the child's important transitional object, allowing parental presence, giving explanations at an appropriate level and with appropriate timing, allowing play when possible, and limiting immobilization are crucial. Providing the child with a means of communication is an important intervention that is instituted early on for the intubated child. Use of pictures, a communication board, or even a simple yes/no hand signal can be developed. Whatever means is selected should be communicated to, and used by, all members of the team, including the family.

SUMMARY

Any encounter with the health care system is a developmental challenge to the child. Traumatic injuries, which occur suddenly and allow no time for preparation, present even more of a challenge. There may be circumstances such as injury to other family members or the need to rapidly transport the child to a specific trauma center that decrease or limit the child's usual coping mechanisms. A knowledgeable clinician, aware of developmentally appropriate care and functioning in an environment that facilitates such care, can assist the child in working toward a positive developmental outcome. Despite developmentally appropriate care, some children will experience prolonged setbacks (see Chapter 23). For most children treated for traumatic injuries, however, developmentally appropriate care will have a profound and positive effect on their outcome.

BIBLIOGRAPHY

Ahmann, E. (1998). Examining assumptions underlying nursing practice with children and families. *Pediatric Nursing, 23*(5), 467-469.

Bar-Mor, G. (1997). Preparation of children for surgery and invasive procedures: Milestones on the way to success. *Journal of Pediatric Nursing, 12*(4), 252-255.

Bibace, R., & Walsh, M. (1980). Developmental concepts of illness. *Pediatrics, 66*(6), 912-917.

Bossert, E. (1994). Factors influencing the coping of hospitalized school-age children. *Journal of Pediatric Nursing, 9*(5), 299-306.

Boyd, J. R., & Hunsberger, M. (1998). Chronically ill children coping with repeated hospitalizations: Their perceptions and suggested interventions. *Journal of Pediatric Nursing, 13*(6), 330-342.

Brennan, A. (1994). Caring for children during procedures: A review of the literature. *Pediatric Nursing, 20*(5), 451-458.

DiVito-Thomas, P. A. (1999). Growth and development in children. In D. L. Wong, M. Hockenberry-Eaton, D. Wilson, M. L. Winklestein, E. Ahmann, & P. A. DiVito-Thomas (Eds.), *Whaley and Wong's nursing care of infants and children* (6th ed., pp. 117-167). St. Louis: Mosby.

Dixon, S. D., & Stein, M. T. (Eds.). (1992). *Encounters with children: Pediatric behavior and development* (2nd ed.). St. Louis: Mosby.

Erikson, E. H. (1963). *Childhood and society* (2nd ed., rev. ed.). New York: W. W. Norton.

Freiberg, K. L. (1992). *Human development: A life-span approach* (4th ed.). Sudbury, MA: Jones and Bartlett.

Garmezy, N. (1987). Stress, competence, and development. *American Journal of Orthopsychiatry, 57,* 159-174.

Hart, D., & Bossert, E. (1994). Self-reported fears of hospitalized school-age children. *Journal of Pediatric Nursing, 9*(2), 83-89.

Hester, N. O. (1987). Health perceptions of school-age children. *Issues in Comprehensive Pediatric Nursing, 10,* 137-147.

Jones, E. G., Badger, T. A., & Moore, I. (1992). Children's knowledge of internal anatomy: Conceptual orientation and review of research. *Journal of Pediatric Nursing, 7*(4), 262-268.

Jones, S. M., Fiser, D. H., & Livingston, R. L. (1992). Behavioral changes in pediatric intensive care units. *American Journal of Diseases of Children, 146,* 375-379.

Kavanaugh, C. (1989). The critically ill pediatric patient. In B. Reigel & D. Ehrenreich (Eds.), *Psychological aspects of critical care nursing* (pp. 257-276). Rockville, MD: Aspen.

Perrin, E. C., Sayer, A. G., & Willett, J. B. (1991). Sticks and stones may break my bones...reasoning about illness causality and body functioning in children who have a chronic illness. *Pediatrics, 88*(3), 608-619.

Petrillo, M., & Sanger, S. (1980). *Emotional care of hospitalized children: An environmental approach.* Philadelphia: JB Lippincott.

Piaget, J. (1969). *The theory of stages in growth and development.* New York: McGraw-Hill.

Rollins, J. A. (1999). Family-centered care of the child during illness and hospitalization. In D. L. Wong, M. Hockenberry-Eaton, D. Wilson, M. L. Winklestein, E. Ahmann, & P. A. DiVito-Thomas (Eds.), *Whaley and Wong's nursing care of infants and children* (6th ed., pp. 1139-1201). St. Louis: Mosby.

Ryan-Wegner, N. A. (1996). Children, coping, and the stress of illness: A synthesis of the research. *Journal of the Society of Pediatric Nurses, 1*(3), 126-138.

Smith, J. B., & Martin, S. A. (2001). Caring practices: Providing developmentally supportive care. In M. A. Q. Curley & P. A. Moloney-Harmon (Eds.), *Critical care nursing of infants and children* (2nd ed., pp. 17-46). Philadelphia: WB Saunders.

Stein, M. T. (1992). Children's encounters with illness: Hospitalization and procedures. In S. D. Dixon & M. T. Stein (Eds.), *Encounters with children: Pediatric behavior and development* (2nd ed., pp. 401-409). St. Louis: Mosby.

Stewart, M., Reid, G., & Mangham, C. (1997). Fostering children's resilience. *Journal of Pediatric Nursing, 12*(1), 21-31.

Thomas, A., & Chess, S. (1977). *Temperament and development.* New York: Brunner/Mazel.

Vessey, J. A., Braithwaite, K. B., & Wiedmann, M. (1990). Teaching children about their internal bodies. *Pediatric Nursing, 16*(1), 29-33.

Vessey, J. A., Farley, J. A., & Risom, L. R. (1991). Iatrogenic developmental effects of pediatric intensive care. *Pediatric Nursing, 17*(3), 229-232.

Whitt, J. K. (1982). Children's understanding of illness: Developmental considerations and pediatric interventions. *Advances in Developmental and Behavioral Pediatrics, 3,* 163-201.

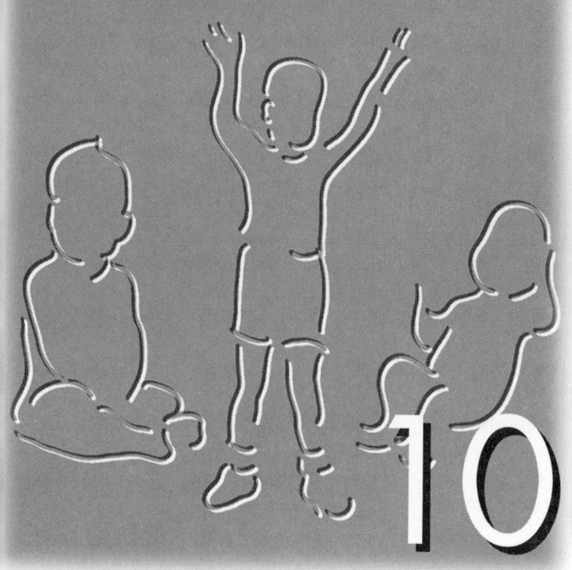

10 THE INJURED FAMILY

Franco A. Carnevale

The traumatic injury of a child gives rise to a traumatic injury of the child's family as well. Families consist of a web of interdependent relationships, such that the injury of one member affects the whole family and the consequent afflictions of the family affect the injured family member. Thus attending to the needs of the family of a traumatized child is important not only for the well-being of the family but also for the wellness of the traumatized child.

This chapter discusses the nursing care of the family with a traumatized child. It presents a conceptual framework for family nursing, an outline of the principal concerns of families of traumatized children, and a discussion of the nursing implications for the care of these families. Finally, this chapter discusses family nursing in the context of pediatric trauma at an advanced level, moving beyond a description of fundamental issues and delving into an in-depth examination of family nursing assessment and intervention of these highly vulnerable families presenting with complex needs.

UNDERSTANDING FAMILIES

A significant body of literature discussing the care of families has emerged within the field of nursing. The family nursing models developed by Lorraine Wright and her associates articulate a conceptual framework for family nursing (Wright & Leahey, 1994). This group (based in Calgary, Canada) has developed a comprehensive, cohesive, sustained, and well-documented family nursing framework that can provide a sophisticated orientation to the care of families of traumatized children. Wright and associates have developed the Calgary Family Assessment Model (CFAM) and the Calgary Family Intervention Model (CFIM). For the purposes of this discussion, these models are referred to jointly as the *Calgary Model.*

The Calgary Model is based on systems, cybernetics, communication, and change theories. The model recognizes the family as a system of interdependent relationships wherein (Wright & Leahey, 1994):

- The family is part of a larger "suprasystem."
- The family is composed of many subsystems (e.g., parental and sibling subsystems).
- A change in one family member affects all family members.
- All nonverbal communication is meaningful.
- All communication consists of two levels: content and relationship.
- Change is dependent on context, the perception of the problem, and coevolving goals for treatment.
- Change does not necessarily occur equally in all family members.

In addition to serving as an effective nursing assessment tool, the CFAM provides a framework for conceptualizing the multiple dimensions of family life. In turn, this provides a valuable orientation toward understanding the experience of a family of a traumatized child.

THE CALGARY FAMILY ASSESSMENT MODEL

The CFAM is composed of three major categories. These categories are each further subdivided into structural assessment, developmental assessment, and functional assessment (Figure 10-1).

STRUCTURAL ASSESSMENT

A structural assessment of a family consists of an examination of the family's internal structure, external structure, and context. The *internal structure* refers principally to who are the members of the family, their gender, how everyone is related to one another, and subsystem arrangements (e.g., sibling, parental, blended family, male and/or female subsystems, and boundaries). The *external structure* refers to how the family is related to an extended family and larger social systems that may be meaningful for the particular family. *Context* consists of the sociocultural background of the family (e.g., ethnicity, race, social class, religion, and community environment).

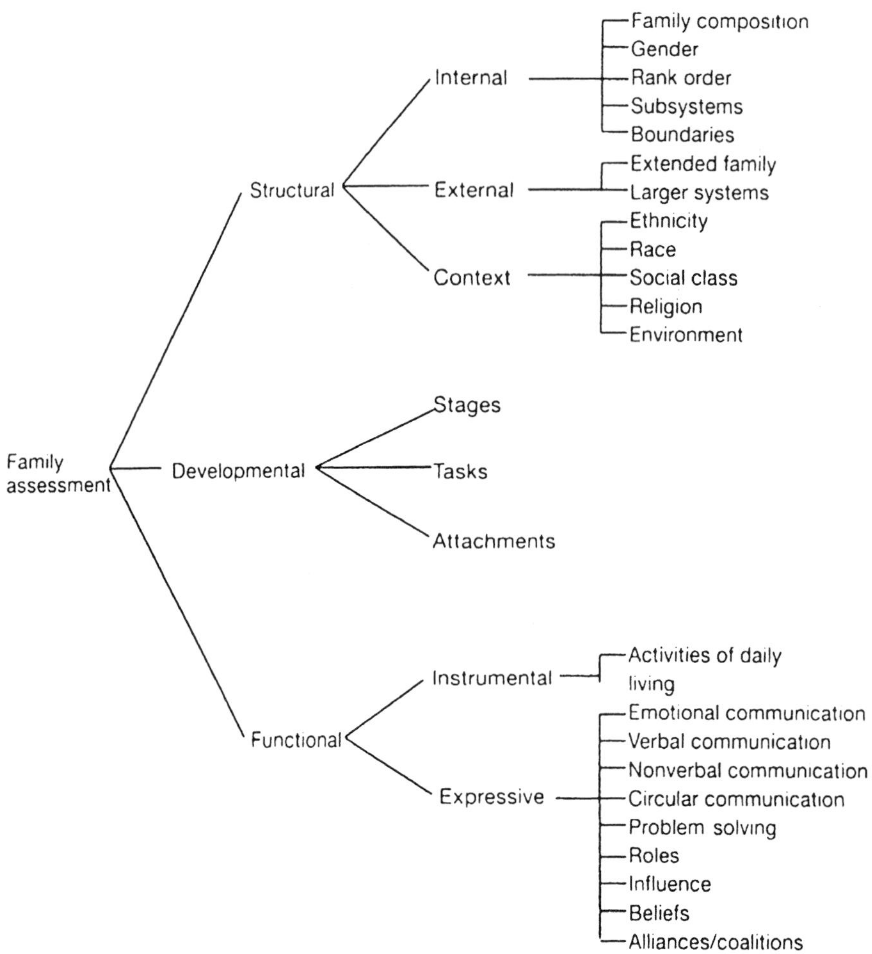

FIGURE 10-1 Branching diagram of the Calgary Family Assessment Model. (From Wright, L. M. & Leahey, M. [1994]. *Nurses and families: A guide to family assessment and interventions* [2nd ed., p. 38]. Philadelphia: FA Davis.)

The genogram is a structural assessment tool that is commonly used to visually represent the structure of a family constellation. Figure 10-2 outlines the symbols that are generally used in genograms.

DEVELOPMENTAL ASSESSMENT

A family developmental assessment requires an understanding of the family's *developmental life cycle* and associated *family tasks,* as well as an analysis of the family's patterns of *relational attachments.* Every particular family constellation (e.g., middle-class North American, adoptive, or remarried families) will undergo a trajectory of normative transitions characterized by developmentally related family tasks, such as the joining of families through marriage, development of a parental identity with childbirth, differentiation of an autonomous identity among adolescents, launching of (adult) children and moving on, and restructuring of parent-child relationships in the context of marital separation.

Attachment assessments involve a qualitative analysis of family relationships. This consists of a determination of the strength, symmetry, and quality (positive or negative) of relationships within the family system. Figure 10-3 illustrates a family attachment diagram. In the diagram the number of straight lines between members indicates the strength of their positive attachment, and the number of irregular lines signifies the intensity of their negative attachment.

FUNCTIONAL ASSESSMENT

Functional assessment of a family refers to how family members behave in relation to each other. This consists of an assessment of instrumental and expressive functioning. *Instrumental functioning* relates to "who does what" in the tasks and routines of daily living. *Expressive functioning* refers to patterns of communication (emotional, verbal, nonverbal, and circular), problem solving, roles, influence, beliefs, and alliances among family members. An assessment of expressive functioning in a family requires interviewing the family together.

By interviewing family members together, the nurse can observe how they spontaneously interact and influence each other. Furthermore, the nurse can ask questions about the impact family members have on one another and on the health problem. Reciprocally, the nurse can enquire about the impact of the health problem on the family. If the nurse thinks "interactionally" rather than "individually," then each individual family member's behavior will not be seen in isolation but rather will be understood in context (Wright & Leahey, 1994).

THE IMPACT OF PEDIATRIC TRAUMA

STRESS AND CRISIS IN THE FAMILY

The Calgary Model provides a rich framework for family nursing that can be applied across a diversity of contexts. This can be complemented by the work of Hamilton McCubbin and Charles Figley and their associates, who discuss the impact of various specific stressors on families (Figley & McCubbin, 1983; McCubbin & Figley, 1983). They developed the Double ABCX Model of family adaptation, which critically examines family adaptation to particular commonly occurring and catastrophic stressors. This model construes family adaptation as a balance of responses to demands with available capabilities. Family stress typically involves a "pile-up" phenomenon whereby the demands faced by a family are believed to surpass their capabilities. A family's capacity to manage these demands is affected by the three types of resources that the family can draw on: (1) family members' personal resources, (2) the family system's internal resources, and (3) social support.

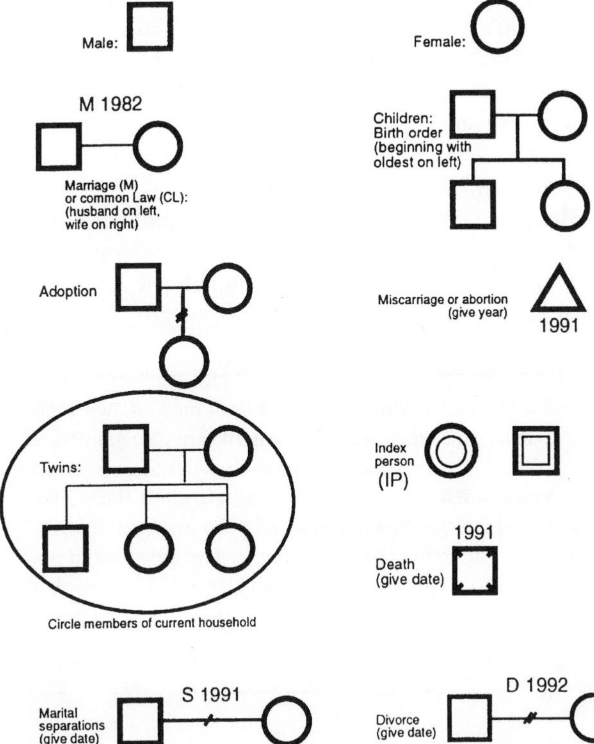

FIGURE 10-2 Symbols used in genograms. (From Wright, L. M., & Leahey, M. [1994]. *Nurses and families: A guide to family assessment and interventions* [2nd ed., p. 52]. Philadelphia: FA Davis.)

When confronted with a stressor or transition, a family will commonly "make adjustments in its pattern of interaction, with minimal change or disruption of the family's established patterns of behavior and structure. These efforts can best be described as family resistance to change" (McCubbin & Patterson, 1983). When faced with excessive demands and depleted resources, families enter into crisis and then adapt through a process of restructuring of family roles, rules, goals, and patterns of interaction in an attempt to achieve some functional stability. This framework has been further elaborated into the Resiliency Model of Family Stress, Adjustment, and Adaptation (McCubbin & McCubbin, 1993; McCubbin, Thompson, & McCubbin, 1996).

Figley (1983) identifies 11 characteristics that differentiate functional from dysfunctional family coping:

1. Ability to identify the stressor
2. Viewing of the problem as a family problem rather than merely a problem of one or two of its members
3. Adoption of a solution-oriented approach to the problem rather than simply blaming
4. Show of tolerance for other family members
5. Clear expression of commitment to and affection for other family members
6. Open and clear communication among members
7. Evidence of high family cohesion
8. Evidence of considerable role flexibility
9. Appropriate use of resources inside and outside of the family
10. Lack of overt or covert physical violence
11. Lack of substance abuse

THE EXPERIENCE OF FAMILIES WITH CRITICALLY ILL CHILDREN

Given that pediatric trauma is often life threatening, an insight into the particular needs and stressors confronted by

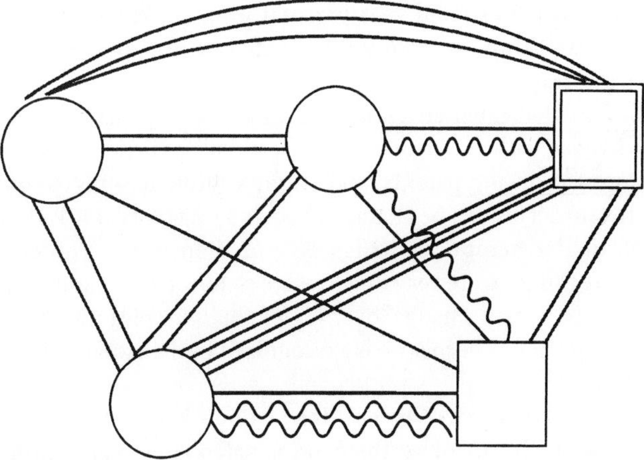

FIGURE 10-3 A family attachment diagram. The number of straight lines between family members indicates the strength of their positive attachment, and the number of irregular lines between family members indicates the intensity of their negative attachment. (From Carnevale, F. A. [1999]. Striving to recapture our previous life: The experience of families with critically ill children. *Official Journal of the Canadian Association of Critical Care Nurses, 10*[1], 16-22.)

families of traumatized children can be derived from studies of families in the pediatric intensive care setting.

Parents

A number of studies have highlighted that parents of critically ill children need (Fisher, 1994; Kirschbaum, 1990; Rennick, 1987) the following:

- To feel hopeful
- To know the child's prognosis
- To know how and why the child is being treated
- To trust that the child is getting the best possible care

Some studies have examined the principal sources of stress (i.e., stressors) reported by parents of children in a pediatric intensive care unit (PICU). These stressors include the following (Carnevale, 1990; Carter & Miles, 1989):

- *Parental role conflict:* thoughts and feelings related to an inability to parent
- *Concern for the child:* concern for the child's physical and emotional well-being
- *PICU environment:* activities, noises, lights, and people in the PICU
- *Relationships:* with health caregivers, friends, and family
- *Concern for other children in the family:* concern for the fears and feelings of the other children

Critical Illness and the Family System

Parents

In a follow-up study of families of critically ill children (including traumatized children), Carnevale (1999) traced the course of parental experiences throughout the child's critical illness, from the PICU to the child's home (for the children who survived). In the context of the complex constellation of parental needs and stressors outlined earlier, this study illustrated that parental preoccupations are not static and thus are poorly represented by lists of needs and stressors.

Parental experiences involve ongoing negotiations and struggles with the demands of the child's afflictions, superimposed on the parents' and family's "ordinary" needs and stressors. This can be characterized as a trajectory marked by particular temporal struggles and transitions (indeed, whereas nurses are very much aware of how patient and family experiences change over time, this complex temporal dimension has been scarcely recognized in the research literature).

The experience of parents throughout their child's course in the PICU involves three principal phases: (1) putting everything else aside and relying on the experts, (2) experiencing discouragement or excitement over the child's course, and (3) reconciling the changes and rebuilding their lives.

Putting Everything Else Aside and Relying on the Experts. The early phase is characterized by a "rallying" of all parental resources to attend to the critically ill child, such as taking time off from work, hiring a baby-sitter for the other children, and giving up on sleeping and eating. This also includes an obligatory, yet comforting, reliance on the expert health caregivers to meet the child's total needs. In effect, being "a good parent" for a critically ill child involves ensuring the child gets the best possible care.

Experiencing Discouragement or Excitement Over the Child's Course. A process of discouragement and/or excitement follows the initial period of rallying over the child's course. Parents experience profound rises and/or drops in their hopes as the child's condition improves or declines. They consume an enormous amount of mental and physical energy staying "on guard," fearing that things could change at any time.

Reconciling the Changes and Rebuilding Their Lives. Over time, acute fluctuations in the child's condition stabilize toward an eventual outcome. This outcome can vary widely in that the child (1) may have a full recovery to his or her preinjury state, (2) may have a partial recovery with significant limitations/changes but with a hope of continued significant improvement throughout the course of ongoing rehabilitative therapy, (3) may have a partial recovery with significant limitations/changes but with no hope of further improvement, or (4) may die. This situation requires parents to reconcile these profound changes with the way life was before the injury and to rebuild their life.

The Critically Ill Child

A central determinant of the family's experience is the course of the child's condition. Critical illness in children causes significant bodily and social disruptions that give "rise to a process of personal 'unmaking' whereby most aspects of the child's personal identity (are) traumatized. This (is) followed by a process of 'remaking' that (is) fundamentally shaped by the family's involvement" (Carnevale, 1999).

This personal unmaking involves (transient or persistent) changes in the child's disposition and mental function that are attributable to complex neurologic, psychologic, and social factors (Carnevale, 1997a):

> Typically, these children were amnesic of most of their PICU experience and exhibited mild to significant changes in their cognitive function, long-term memory, attention span, self-esteem, and self-confidence.... For most families, their child's critical illness resulted in unfavorable bodily, mental or dispositional afflictions (or even death). This gave rise to new care requirements, or a caregiving 'burden,' as well as changes in the relationships and functionality of the family as a whole (Carnevale, 1999).

The Experience of Siblings

Initially, the siblings of critically ill children typically express concern about their afflicted sibling. They are also commonly stressed by seeing their parents in profound distress.

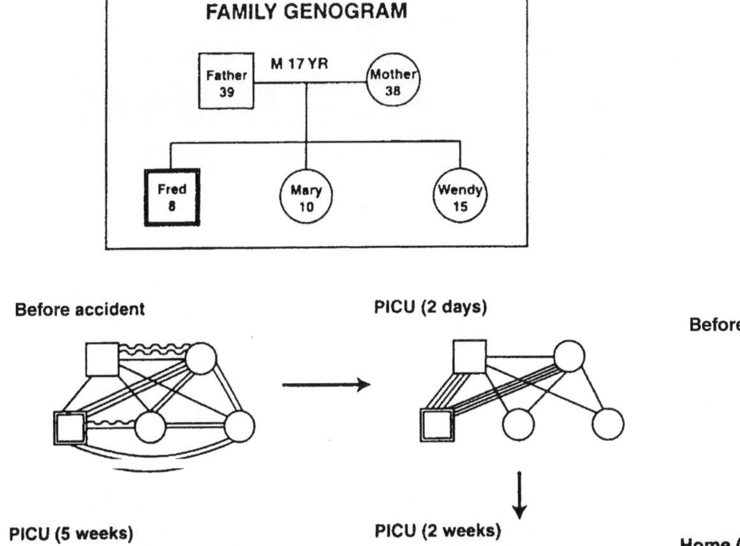

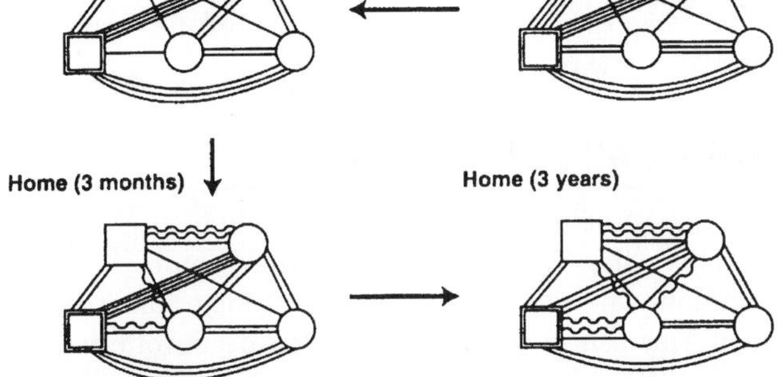

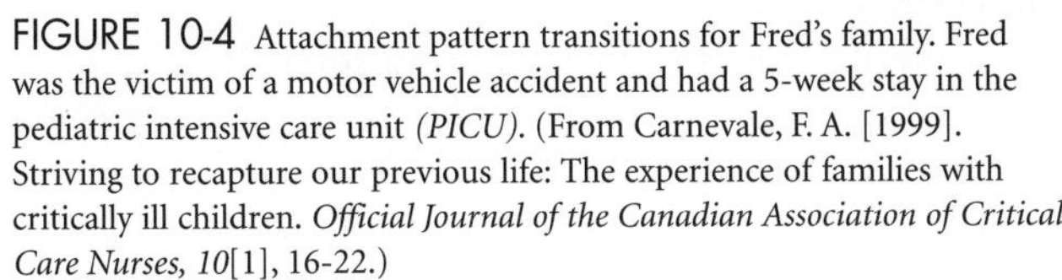

FIGURE 10-4 Attachment pattern transitions for Fred's family. Fred was the victim of a motor vehicle accident and had a 5-week stay in the pediatric intensive care unit *(PICU)*. (From Carnevale, F. A. [1999]. Striving to recapture our previous life: The experience of families with critically ill children. *Official Journal of the Canadian Association of Critical Care Nurses, 10*[1], 16-22.)

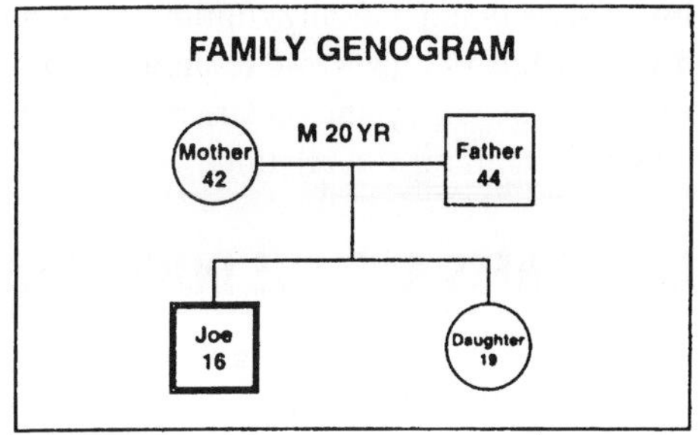

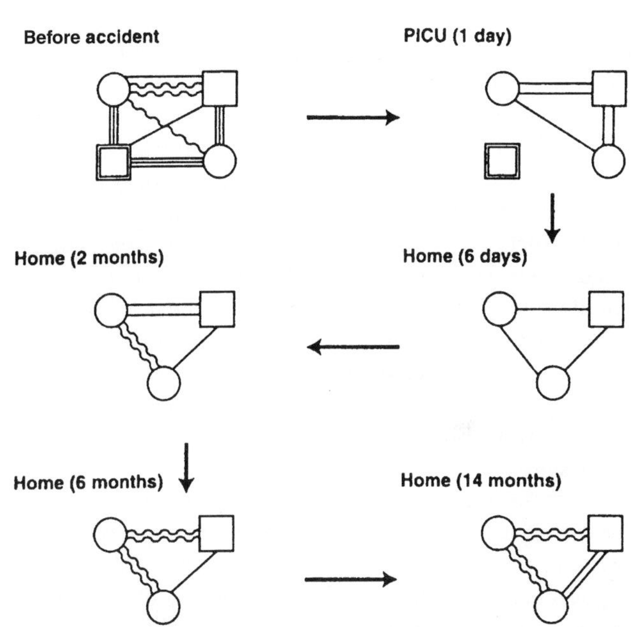

FIGURE 10-5 Attachment pattern transitions for Joe's family. Joe died in the pediatric intensive care unit *(PICU)* 3 days after he was in a motor vehicle accident. (From Carnevale, F. A.[1999]. Striving to recapture our previous life: The experience of families with critically ill children. *Official Journal of the Canadian Association of Critical Care Nurses, 10*[1], 16-22.)

Indeed, the sources of order and stability in the siblings' lives are deeply disrupted. Over time, if the injured child's hospitalization persists beyond a few days, many siblings report sentiments of isolation and relative insignificance in relation to the sick child. "In most prolonged cases, these children eventually developed a sense of resentment toward the disproportionate amount of attention the sick child was receiving, compared to themselves" (Carnevale, 1999).

Family System Transitions

The many issues encountered by family members (described earlier) must coexist and be managed within the context of the family's strengths and limits. This results in significant shifts in family roles, attachments, and patterns of interaction. Figures 10-4 and 10-5 illustrate how these shifts were manifested in two families with a traumatized child (the child died in the latter case).

When this multitude of family responses is examined collectively, a central "striving to recapture life as it was" before the critical illness emerges as a central phenomenon. Families are required to "move on" and adjust to the changes that confront them. Thus they are thrown into a struggle between "holding on" to their (cherished) view of life as it was and "letting go" of much of this as the reality of the child's injuries imposes significant changes (Carnevale, 1999). Most families undergo some form of mourning for their child, who may never be as he or she was, and the consequent losses in their family way of life.

These profound transitional experiences correspond with the findings of a study of families of patients with severe brain injuries, which reported that "such patients and their families find themselves in socially ambiguous and isolated positions which can best be described through the anthropological concept of liminality" (Mwaria, 1990). *Liminality* refers to a "betwixt and between" state of transition that characterizes major sociocultural life events that transform the identities of the persons involved, commonly referred to as *rites of passage* (van Gennep, 1960). Patients with severe brain injuries are trapped in a state in which they are "neither fully alive nor truly dead" (Mwaria, 1990). The patient enters into a state that drastically ruptures the family's identity and way of life and gives rise to an ambiguous state of limbo to which the family and its larger social circle has no means of understanding and relating.

MORAL DISTRESS AND THE INJURED FAMILY

Traumatic injury in children can give rise to moral questions about the extent to which interventional measures ought be pursued, in the context of treatments that impose significant burdens on the child with a limited outlook for recovery. The family and caregivers can be faced with dilemmas about what quality of life is worthy of "rescue." Ethical analyses of treatment decisions for children have been addressed elsewhere in the literature (American Academy of Pediatrics, 1994; Carnevale, 1996), as well as in this book. These analyses highlight that, in the case of a minor, such decisions should be made on the basis of the child's best interests, whereby the benefits of treatment should outweigh the burdens. Typically, the determination of which treatment option is best for the child is judged by the child's legal guardian (usually the parents) after a detailed discussion of the implications of each option with the caregiver team.

Despite the significant proliferation of conceptual analyses of these ethical issues, clinical studies of these dilemmas have been scarce, with the exception of a couple of reports from the pediatric intensive care setting. In an examination of life support decisions made by 39 parents of critically ill children, Kirschbaum (1996) identified eight key themes related to the values at issue for them:

1. *Life:* Preserving their child's life was an ultimate good.
2. *Pain and suffering:* Parents sought to protect the child from pain and suffering and did not always seek life at any cost for the child.
3. *Quality of life:* The child's life was valuable not only in terms of its length but also in relation to the quality of "the child's current and anticipated existence."
4. *Not self:* Parents regarded a change in the child's behavior or character as a diminished quality of life.
5. *Respect for person or best interest:* Parents respected the individuality of the child and tried to make decisions based on a projection of what the child would have wanted.
6. *Family:* The support and expectations of the parents' families affected their perceived stress and support in relation to particular decisions.
7. *Faith and nature:* Parental strategies were strongly related to whether they relied on supernatural/spiritual or natural explanations of their child's current condition.
8. *Technology:* Technological interventions (and advances) were universally viewed as favorable.

In a prospective study of 10 cases in a PICU involving life support decisions, Carnevale (1997b, 1997c) characterized ethical dilemmas in terms of a disparity of moral and explanatory frameworks. Critical illness in children obliges parents, nurses, and physicians to arrive at agreements about complex treatment plans, typically within a very limited amount of time and under ambiguous prognostic circumstances. Commonly, these various advocates for the child's interests hold disparate moral values (regarding what constitutes a "good enough life" and the lengths to which it ought to be pursued) and explanatory frameworks (relating to their own personal integration of scientific knowledge, traditional beliefs, and spiritual views that interpret the child's condition and prognosis, and associated parental obligations). The convergence of this disparity of moral and explanatory frameworks among the people involved in making treatment decisions for the child sets the stage for significant (and sometimes irreconcilable) disagreement and conflict.

This study also reported that ethical dilemmas commonly involved significant *relational conflicts over respect, trust, and power* among and between parents and caregivers. This highlights that conceptual analyses of ethical dilemmas need to be complemented by an examination of the corresponding relational issues.

DYING AND BEREAVEMENT

Sometimes the trauma endured by a child is so severe that the child dies. Children who die from traumatic injury commonly die within hours or days of the traumatic incident. This can be a relatively sudden death, offering the family little or no time to prepare for this profoundly disruptive loss.

Carnevale (1992) has documented some of the central themes reported by bereaved families after the unexpected death of a child in a PICU. The principal difficulties described by parents included *conflicts with their spouse; concern for the surviving siblings;* and *feelings of emptiness, guilt, and frustration.* They also reported feelings of anger and hurt toward their extended family and friends. These feelings resulted from some of the statements of "consolation" made by the family members or friends (e.g., "At least he won't be suffering anymore") or their withdrawal from regular contact with the parents, leading to a sense of abandonment. Issues identified by siblings included *feeling unimportant, alone, guilty, negatively (compared with the deceased sibling),* and *concerned for the parents' marriage.*

On a family systems level the death of a child resulted in immense familial disorganization. Family roles, functions, and routines that previously served the various needs of the family members were profoundly ruptured. Families underwent a series of transitions lasting months or years whereby members struggled to reconcile their needs to maintain their family life as it was before the traumatic incident with the current reality that their family composition has changed drastically.

Eventually, every family established a new way of life that was qualitatively diverse across families. Some families achieved a systemic reorganization whereby every member felt included and nurtured, despite the loss. Other families reacted to their grief in a manner whereby their loss resulted in changes that caused persistent strain on family life (e.g., one parent blamed the other for the fatal accident).

Brain Death

In the context of brain death, some families are faced with the news that their child's life cannot be saved in conjunction with a request for organ procurement for the purposes of transplantation. Many families regard organ transplantation as an opportunity to salvage some sense of meaning from the tragedy of their child's death, knowing that their child "lives on" in another person or has "courageously saved the life of another" by relinquishing his or her own life. On the other hand, many families cannot accept having organs removed from their child because of a complex mix of cultural, religious, and personal convictions. The context of the declaration of brain death and the procurement of organs for transplant give rise to deeply sensitive sociomoral questions that have been scarcely examined in the pediatric setting (Fox & Swazey, 1992; Lock, 1995).

HELPING THE INJURED FAMILY

A Framework for Family Intervention

The CFIM outlines a framework for family nursing intervention at basic and advanced levels. The "CFIM is focused on promoting, improving, and/or sustaining effective family functioning in three domains: cognitive, affective, and behavioral"(Wright & Leahey, 1994). Although an intervention can be directed primarily to any one of these domains, this will likely also have an impact on the other domains.

Interventive Questions

The CFIM regards *interventive questions* as highly effective nursing interventions. In particular, *circular questions* are presented as strategies that can affect all three domains of family functioning. Circular questions such as "What do you do when your son cries following his treatments?" or "Who's the best in the family in getting John to take his medication on time?" (Wright & Leahey, 1994) involve a cycle of questions and answers between family members and the nurse, seeking out "relationships between individuals, events, ideas, and beliefs" (Wright & Leahey, 1994). These questions are intended to facilitate change by helping family members to see their family, their problems, and their respective roles in a new light.

Other aspects of the framework include the following:

- *Commending family and individual strengths:* The commendation of demonstrated family competence and strengths can help counter family demoralization and foster change by helping families acquire a new (more favorable) opinion of themselves.
- *Offering information/opinions:* In light of the significant informational needs of families, nurses can facilitate family coping by offering information and opinions about the child/family's current and anticipated problems, available resources, and the merits and limits of potential coping strategies.
- *Offering education:* Nurses can help families by teaching them about the physical, emotional, and cognitive characteristics of the health problems confronting them.
- *Reframing:* Reframing involves a shift in the family's cognitive and/or emotional view of the situation in a way that favorably changes its meaning for the family.
- *Externalizing the problem:* Externalization involves a shifting of a problem from inside the person's identity to outside of the person. Viewing the problem (outside of oneself) in the context of one's life or various external factors can render the problem less personally threatening.
- *Validating/normalizing emotional responses:* The validation of intense feelings can help family members derive comfort from seeing themselves in relation to their current situation and the ways in which they can manage it.
- *Storying the illness:* A family's experience can be comforted through a process of validation and legitimization by encouraging family members to narrate their own account of the experience.
- *Drawing forth family support:* Nurses can facilitate communication among family members and foster deeper listening, understanding, and support among them.
- *Encouraging family members to be caregivers:* Nurses can help family members overcome their fears of providing direct care by encouraging and facilitating their involvement.
- *Encouraging respite:* Nurses can help families deal with guilt feelings associated with respite care by legitimizing its merits for the family's overall health.
- *Devising rituals:* Families can benefit from an encouragement to devise family rituals to help counter the chaos and confusion resulting from the disruptions of the illness.

The Caregiver-Family Relationship

Whereas most of the family nursing literature discusses problems within families and therapeutic strategies that can help families manage them, Robinson and Thorne (1984) examined the "therapeutic relationship" between families and health caregivers as a focus of problems. Their work outlines that these relationships evolve through three predictable stages, particularly when they are long-term engagements. These stages begin with a stage of *naive trust* whereby the family is highly impressed and reliant on the expertise and resources of the health caregivers. Over time, as some (unrealistically elevated) expectations are unfulfilled, the family enters into a stage of *disenchantment* with the caregivers whereby the caregivers are no longer regarded as unfailingly impressive and trustworthy. Over time, a *guarded alliance* is crafted between the family and the health caregivers whereby agreements are formed through a process of reciprocal negotiations and checks. Sensitization toward these developmental phenomena, which are inherent in complex family-nursing relationships, can help nurses become better attuned to the dynamics involved in their family interventions.

Specific Interventions for the Injured Family

Care for the Parents

Given the fundamental role of parents in maintaining family health, parents are necessarily a central focus of nursing for the family with a traumatized child. In light of the inescapable adversities confronted by parents of seriously ill children, family nursing should ensure the minimization of additional stresses resulting from the family's encounter with health care systems.

"Visiting" Policies. Most important, attention should be devoted toward ensuring that hospital "visiting" policies are sensitive to the enormous strains family relationships undergo in these circumstances, and they should seek to foster family intactness rather than impede it. In particular, it is important to recognize that families are not visitors. Family members are enacting their respective family functions (they are being parents, grandparents, aunts and uncles, brothers and sisters), they are not visiting. Hospital policies and practices that regard families as visitors serve to marginalize the vital importance of families. In light of the earlier discussion of how the child's distress is mediated by disruptions in the child's relational life and how the child's afflictions give rise to significant family distress, family presence and participation in the child's care is important in fostering the child's well-being, as well as that of the family.

Family Supports. Settings that provide care for injured children should develop flexible family policies whereby families can arrange to be as involved with their child's care as their circumstances permit. This would require physical facilities for overnight sleeping, access to low-cost food and parking, ease of access by public transportation, and the sensitization and commitment of health caregivers toward recognizing the importance of families in pediatric trauma care. Although family nursing has become increasingly valued, the corresponding demands and workload that this presents to nurses has been largely underrecognized and invisible. Nurses need to be provided with the supports they require to work with families having such complex needs. These supports can include the following (Carnevale, 1991):

- Workload management that ensures nurses have time to devote to family nursing
- Access to experts in family nursing to consult with for difficult cases and who are also available to intervene directly with families when required, using the advanced interventions described in the CFIM
- Assurance of regularly scheduled breaks to help prevent "fishbowl feelings" that some nurses report when parents are continuously present and watching
- Educational workshops on how to work effectively with families
- Staff meetings to discuss current issues in providing family nursing

Parent Informational Resources. The earlier discussion of parental needs and stressors highlighted the significance of information for parents of traumatized children. The most effective informational resources in this setting are expert health caregivers. Nurses are commonly well-suited sources of information, given their comprehensive knowledge of the biomedical and psychosocial aspects of pediatric trauma.

Parents should receive information on the child's current condition and have an opportunity to ask questions several times a day. The opportunity to ask questions should exist from the moment of admission to a critical care setting until the child's condition has stabilized and the child is transferred to an intermediate or "regular hospital unit" setting, where informational updates should be available on a daily basis until discharge.

This "live" informational resource can be complemented with informational tools, such as parent booklets. These booklets outline information about relevant unit policies, resources available to families, descriptions of the various members of the caregiver team, monitoring and interventional technology the family will likely encounter, and common emotional reactions reported by other families in this setting. The "hard copy" form of a parent booklet can serve to complement and reinforce the information provided by the health caregivers. Attention should be paid toward ensuring that the literacy level required to use such resources does not exceed the capabilities of the population served. In general, these could be targeted toward a grade-school education level of literacy.

Care for the Siblings. The effect of pediatric trauma on siblings and on parental concerns about the siblings necessitates the development of sibling-oriented interventions. Families and siblings vary widely in the types of concerns they express. Caregivers can help orient parents to the common stresses experienced by the siblings and discuss possible (developmentally appropriate) strategies that can offer some comfort to them, such as arranging for the siblings to spend time with the injured sibling in hospital, even in the critical care setting. A child life specialist or a nurse with advanced expertise in this area can help parents prepare the siblings for these activities and help the children process their consequent feelings. Play, art, or storybooks can serve as engaging media for facilitating the child's expression of feelings and concerns. As a general practice, the well-being of the siblings should be discussed with parents regularly.

Individualized Family Approach. Because of the unique needs and strengths that each family presents and the complex communication and relational processes involved in a family's coping with a child's traumatic injury, an individualized approach to family nursing is necessary. Whereas the broad strategies described earlier aim to foster a supportive environment for families on a general level, they need to be complemented with interventions tailored to the specific needs and strengths of each family. This "requires a comprehensive, individualized approach whereby technological biomedical care is blended with psychosocial interventions that are attentive to the issues identified in this [chapter]. In particular, strategies that minimize or prevent (family) disintegration and/or foster re/integration of family members, as well as the family as a whole, need to be promoted" (Carnevale, 1999).

This tailored approach is optimally achieved through the assurance of one or two principal caregivers (e.g., a primary nurse, a primary physician, and/or a primary social worker) throughout the course of the child's acute and long-term care. These primary caregivers should be attuned to the common issues confronting families in this setting (e.g., the issues described in this chapter) and skilled in advanced family assessment and intervention to help families identify their particular needs and enable them to enact the adaptive changes required by the situation.

The complexity of the biomedical and psychosocial needs of these children and their families will require the involvement of a multidisciplinary team. The primary caregivers will need to meet with and coordinate the activities of a comprehensive team of nurses and physicians working in collaboration with a child life specialist, social worker, pastoral worker, physiotherapist, occupational therapist, dietitian, psychologist, psychiatrist, and ethicist. This team "can offer a rich mix of expertise that can help address the wide range of needs that these children and families can present" (Carnevale, 1999). Members of the team can provide guidance to the primary caregivers for special problems that may arise and accept a referral to become directly involved when their expertise is particularly required.

Extended Family and Friends. The extended family and friends of a family with a traumatized child can be a source of comfort and distress. It is widely recognized that a family's social network can serve as a precious resource for tangible help (e.g., baby-sitting the siblings, caring for the home, financial assistance) and for emotional support. Indeed, families commonly expect to rely on this network for support. On the other hand, given that pediatric trauma gives rise to problems and demands with which the family's social network is unfamiliar, the family's requests for support are sometimes met with awkwardness and reluctance that often harm the quality of their relationships. Thus, in addition to encouraging families to draw upon their social resources to help them deal with their needs, caregivers can offer guidance and orientation to parents on how to manage the relational changes that they will need to depend on.

For example, grandparents are commonly a resource for various familial needs. Yet in addition to dealing with their own reactions to their grandchild's injury, as well their own child's pain as a parent, they commonly lack the specific capabilities required to readily adapt to their new role as the grandparent of an injured child. They are immediately confronted with the possibility of losing their grandchild, as they knew him or her. Caregivers can help sensitize parents to foreseeable malaises in their social network and discuss strategies for addressing them. For example, grandparents can be invited to a family meeting with the principal health caregivers to offer them an opportunity to express their own concerns and participate in the development of a cohesive family support plan.

Facilitating the Traumatized Child's Return to Family Life at Home. The return of the child into the home involves a readjustment into the family's daily life from that of a hospitalized child whose dependencies were partly (if not largely) met by health caregivers to that of a survivor of trauma who may have been partly (if not largely) altered by the injury. This results in significant shifts in family roles and functions. The child/family's primary health caregivers can facilitate this process by meeting with the family regularly before, during, and after the transfer home. This enables the family to proactively discuss and plan family changes that can ensure every member's needs are optimally met throughout the course of this demanding transition.

Care for the Bereaved Family. Sometimes pediatric trauma results in death. Pediatric trauma services should be prepared to provide care for the bereaved family. This should involve a recognition that grief is experienced in an individual way and is highly affected by each person's individual history, life values, and beliefs. The expression of grief and mourning can be shaped by culture, religion, gender, age, and the particular circumstances of the loss, among many other factors (Rando, 1986). This renders it difficult for a caregiver to evaluate the health of a family's coping.

Crosby and Jose (1983) examined family adjustment to loss and identified three forms of coping as "dysfunctional," that is, coping strategies that impede recovery. These coping strategies are avoidance, obliteration, and idolization.

Avoidance involves a "keeping busy" that distracts the person's thoughts and feelings away from his or her painful loss. Although this can be helpful in some measure, a profound and sustained avoidance can impede the personal transformation to the new reality that bereavement necessitates.

Obliteration "involves the attempt of total erasure of the deceased person's prior existence. This may involve disposal of all personal effects, belongings, collections, hobbies, pictures, and other possessions" (Crosby & Jose, 1983).

Idolization involves the endowment of the deceased with a "superhuman" quality of perfection. This creates a standard of splendor that is particularly difficult for the surviving siblings to compare favorably with.

Crosby and Jose (1983) recommend that families learn how to be permissive of feelings and commit to a process of communication that is accepting and supportive of all members, such that the actual loss is experienced collectively and individually by family members.

The surviving children particularly need (Crosby & Jose, 1983) the following:

1. Space and time to absorb the fact of the loss
2. Help in labeling and identifying the finality of death
3. Models who themselves are able to grieve and express the range of emotional response
4. Attention and respect when speaking
5. The opportunity to express themselves by giving their own individualized account of what happened

Family bereavement profoundly disrupts family organization and functioning. In addition to attending to whatever particular needs arise for each family, individual family members are faced with managing the consequent changes in family roles, patterns of authority and decision making, channels of communication and support, family routines and rituals, and relationships with the family's broader social network.

In the context of a dying child, caregivers can assist families by orienting them to the enormous transformations that this will require and helping them participate actively in adapting the experience as much as possible to the particular needs of the entire family. For example, in the context of an anticipated withdrawal of life support, arrangements can be made to foster the inclusion of the siblings, grandparents, and other significant persons during this extremely difficult moment.

All bereaved families should be offered bereavement follow-up tailored to their specific needs. Through the use of advanced family nursing skills, a nurse can offer to meet with each family regularly to help the family adapt to its loss, drawing on the resources that are available within the family, within the family's larger social network, and from local community resources. For example, some parents may benefit from involvement in a bereaved parents group.

Structured interventions include the use of play, art, or storybooks to foster children's expressions of grief and books or videos to help older children and parents gain insight into their particular reactions to their loss. Family activities, such as the production of family drawings or family mobiles, can help families acquire a collective insight into the shifts that are taking place within the family as a whole.

Many parents express some comfort from reading and discussing the book *The Bereaved Parent* by Harriet Sarnoff Schiff (1977), a bereaved parent herself. Of particular comfort is the closing passage:

> As long as I live I will be sorry Robby is dead. That is fact. That is something I carry always. There are times, especially the good times, when I miss him still. But there are still good times. We share joys as a family that he did not live to share and I am sorry. But we still have joys. That is as it should be for us. That is as it should be for you (Schiff, 1977).

SUMMARY

Because trauma is unexpected, parents do not have time to adjust to the possible death or disability of their child. Caring for the families of critically injured children requires expert nursing assessment and intervention. A variety of frameworks exist that help the nurse to provide appropriate interventions that will result in the best possible outcome for the child and family.

BIBLIOGRAPHY

American Academy of Pediatrics. (1994). Guidelines on forgoing life-sustaining medical treatment. *Pediatrics, 93*(3), 532-536.

Carnevale, F. A. (1990). A description of stressors and coping strategies among parents of critically ill children. *Intensive and Critical Care Nursing, 6*, 4-11.

Carnevale, F. A. (1991). Promoting family nursing in an intensive care unit. *Canadian Nursing Management, 37*, 38-42.

Carnevale, F. A. (1992). Family transitions following the death of a critically ill child. *Journal of Palliative Care, 8*(3), 68-69.

Carnevale, F. A. (1996). "Good" medicine: Ethics and pediatric critical care. In D. Tibboel & E. van der Voort (Eds.), *Intensive care in childhood: A challenge to the future* (pp. 491-503). Berlin: Springer-Verlag.

Carnevale, F. A. (1997a). The experience of critically ill children: Narratives of unmaking. *Intensive and Critical Care Nursing, 13*, 49-52.

Carnevale, F. A. (1997b). Life-support decisions for critically ill children: Challenging the utility of futility. *Proceedings from the 7th World Congress of Intensive & Critical Care Medicine* (p. 91), Ottawa, Canada.

Carnevale, F. A. (1997c). *Ethics and pediatric critical care: A conception of a "thick" bioethics*. Unpublished master's thesis, McGill University, Montreal, Canada.

Carnevale, F. A. (1999). Striving to recapture our previous life: The experience of families with critically ill children. *Official Journal of The Canadian Association of Critical Care Nurses, 10*(1), 16-22.

Carter, M. C., & Miles, M. S. (1989). The parental stressor scale: Pediatric intensive care unit. *Maternal-Child Nursing Journal, 18*(3), 187-198.

Crosby, J. F., & Jose, N. L. (1983). Death: Family adjustment to loss. In C. R. Figley & H. I. McCubbin (Eds.), *Stress and the family: Volume II. Coping with catastrophe* (pp. 76-89). New York: Brunner/Mazel.

Curley, M. A. Q. (1988). Effects of the nursing mutual participation model of care on parental stress in the pediatric intensive care unit. *Heart & Lung, 17*, 682-688.

Figley, C. R. (1983). Catastrophes: An overview of family reactions. In C. R. Figley & H. I. McCubbin (Eds.), *Stress and the family: Volume II. Coping with catastrophe* (pp. 3-20). New York: Brunner/Mazel.

Figley, C. R., & McCubbin, H. I. (Eds.). (1983). *Stress and the family: Volume II. Coping with catastrophe*. New York: Brunner/Mazel.

Fisher, M. D. (1994). Identified needs of parents in a pediatric intensive care unit. *Critical Care Nurse, 14*(3), 82-90.

Fox, R. C., & Swazey, J. P. (1992). *Spare parts: Organ replacement in American society.* New York: Oxford University Press.

Kirschbaum, M. S. (1990). Needs of parents of critically ill children. *Dimensions of Critical Care Nursing, 9,* 344-352.

Kirschbaum, M. S. (1996). Life support decisions for children: What do parents value? *Advances in Nursing Science, 19*(1), 51-71.

Kleiber, C., Montgomery, L. A., & Craft-Rosenberg, M. (1995). Information needs of the siblings of critically ill children. *Children's Health Care, 24*(1), 47-60.

Leahey, M., & Wright, L. M. (1987). *Families and life-threatening illness.* Springhouse, PA: Springhouse.

Lock, M. (1995). Contesting the natural in Japan: Moral dilemmas and technologies of dying. *Culture, Medicine and Psychiatry,* 19, 1-38.

McCubbin, H. I., & Figley, C. R. (Eds.). (1983). *Stress and the family: Volume I. Coping with normative transitions.* New York: Brunner/Mazel.

McCubbin, M. A., & McCubbin, H. I. (1993). Families coping with illness: The resiliency model of family stress, adjustment, and adaptation. In C. B. Danielson, B. Hamel-Bissell, & P. Winstead-Fry (Eds.), *Families, health, & illness: Perspectives on coping and intervention* (pp. 21-63), St. Louis: Mosby.

McCubbin, H. I., & Patterson, J. M. (1983). Family transitions: Adaptation to stress. In H. I. McCubbin & C. R. Figley (Eds.), *Stress and the family: Volume I. Coping with normative transitions* (pp. 5-25), New York: Brunner/Mazel.

McCubbin, H. I., Thompson, A. I., & McCubbin, M. A. (1996). *Family assessment: Resiliency, coping and adaptation.* Madison, Wisconsin: University of Wisconsin System Publishers.

Mwaria, C. B. (1990). The concept of self in the context of crisis: A study of families of the severely brain-injured. *Social Sciences & Medicine, 30*(8), 889-893.

Rando, T. A. (1986). *Parental loss of a child.* Champaign, IL: Research Press.

Rennick, J. (1987). *The needs of parents with a child in a pediatric intensive care unit.* Unpublished master's thesis, University of Toronto, Toronto, Canada.

Robinson, C. A., & Thorne, S. (1984). Strengthening family "interference." *Journal of Advanced Nursing, 9*(6), 597-602.

Schiff, H. S. (1977). *The bereaved parent.* New York: Penguin Books.

van Gennep, A. (1960). *The rites of passage.* Chicago: University of Chicago Press.

Wright, L. M., & Leahey, M. (1994). *Nurses and families: A guide to family assessment and intervention* (2nd ed.). Philadelphia: FA Davis.

Youngblut, J. M., & Lauzon, S. (1995). Family functioning following pediatric intensive care unit hospitalization. *Issues in Comprehensive Pediatric Nursing, 18,* 11-25.

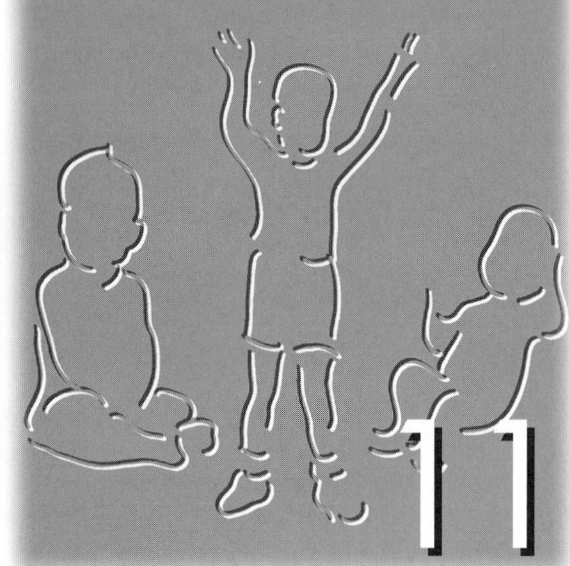

11 PAIN MANAGEMENT

Debbie Brinker

Managing pain in children presents special challenges to the health care team for many reasons. Traumatic injuries compound those challenges. *Pain* has been defined as whatever the person experiencing it says it is, existing whenever the person says it does (McCaffery & Beebe, 1989). This definition emphasizes the point that pain is both a physical and emotional event.

Children admitted to the hospital after a traumatic event experience varying degrees of pain, discomfort, distress, and anxiety. Lack of preparation, limited coping mechanisms, a foreign environment filled with loud noises and bright lights, and sometimes not having a parent or familiar adult present are all factors that contribute to increased anxiety and distress. In addition, the child experiences pain and distress from obvious sources, such as tissue injury, invasive procedures, and surgery, as well as from less obvious sources, such as tubes that pull, backboard and cervical collar immobilization, airway suctioning, and removal of tape and electrodes. There are many unpredictable caregiving events that are potential sources of aversive stimuli affecting the child physiologically and behaviorally. Anxiety and pain are assessed and managed as a "package" to optimize care of the pediatric trauma patient.

On admission to the emergency department, pain management is secondary to initial assessment and stabilization. Pain management may be delayed further because of the need to perform a full neurologic evaluation, which may be affected by narcotic administration. The challenge is to provide adequate analgesia and symptomatic pain relief as soon as possible while not compromising evaluation and stabilization or accepting unnecessary pain and suffering.

MISBELIEFS AND OBSTACLES REGARDING CHILDREN'S PAIN

Although appropriate reasons for suboptimal pain control in the trauma patient exist, there are obstacles that prevent optimal pain relief. Important among these obstacles are misbeliefs regarding children's perception of pain, although many other personal and professional issues may exist. Numerous studies have demonstrated that pain is consistently undertreated in children compared with adults undergoing similar medical or surgical treatments (Beyer, 1984; Eland & Anderson, 1977; McGrath, 1990; Schechter, Allen, & Hanson, 1986). In the last two decades, much attention in the literature has been given to disputing the myths regarding pain in children. Some of these myths include the following:

- *Infants cannot feel pain because of incomplete myelinization of peripheral sensory nerves.* This myth has been proven groundless. Several studies have demonstrated that the density and neurophysiologic properties of nociceptive nerve endings are similar to those found in adults (Anand, 1996).
- *Infants and children are more sensitive to the respiratory depressant effects of narcotics.* Infants younger than 6 months have been noted to be more sensitive to narcotics. However, analgesia can still be administered safely when appropriate dosing and intervals are used (Anand & Shapiro, 1993). Children have not been found to be any more sensitive to the respiratory depressant effects of morphine (Schecter, 1989).
- *If children do not look like they are in pain, they are not in pain.* Children use positive coping mechanisms, such as play, to deal with distress and pain. These behaviors may be misinterpreted, and nurses may withhold pharmacologic support for children who are experiencing pain.

These misbeliefs, along with other obstacles, such as personal, professional, and social biases, lead to inadequate recognition and treatment of pain. Clinicians may still believe that a given stimulus always results in a given level of pain. For example, the clinician may believe that once a fracture is set, the patient should not have much pain.

ANATOMY AND PHYSIOLOGY

The anatomy and physiology of pain are actually based on nociception, which is normal pain transmission. There is not a one-to-one relationship between a noxious stimulus and an individual's response to the pain because pain is a subjective experience.

Stages of Nociception and the Pain Response

Nociception involves responses of the peripheral nervous system, the autonomic and skeletal motor systems, and the central nervous system (CNS). The four stages are (1) transduction, (2) central processing abstraction, (3) modulation, and (4) development and plasticity.

Transduction

Transduction is the conversion of stimulus energy into neural activity. With tissue damage from injury, mediators such as histamine, bradykinin, substance P, prostaglandin E, and potassium are released from the damaged cells. These mediators depolarize the specialized receptors called *nociceptors,* which start an action potential that leads to the dorsal horn of the spinal cord. Peripheral afferent neurons responsible for nociception include the A delta fibers and the C polymodal fibers. The A delta fibers are thinly myelinated fibers that conduct impulses at a rapid speed and have a low threshold for firing. These fibers are associated with sharp, brief, and well-localized "first pain" sensation. The C polymodal fibers are unmyelinated, conduct impulses at a slower speed, and have a higher firing threshold. The C fibers are associated with a longer-lasting, dull, burning, aching, "second pain" sensation.

Both fibers share the properties of sensitization. They become more sensitive and more reactive with repeated episodes of noxious stimulation. Injuries such as burns and bruising are often accompanied by hyperesthesia (increased sensitivity to mild stimuli) or hyperalgesia (increased sensitivity to painful stimuli) (Oakes, 2001). As the threshold to sensory stimulation decreases, even innocuous stimulation is experienced as painful.

Peripheral nociceptors remain unmyelinated or thinly myelinated throughout life from birth to adulthood. Lack of myelination implies slower conduction, not absence of conduction or perception. The lack of myelination of peripheral nerves in the infant does not support the myth that infants cannot appreciate pain. Actually, the slower conduction may well be offset by the shorter distances that the nerve impulse travels in a small infant (Anand & Hickey, 1987; Oakes, 2001).

Central Processing Abstraction

Central processing abstraction is the processing of nociceptive neural signals by the CNS to extract relevant information. Nociceptive and other sensory input travel via afferent fibers to the dorsal horn of the spinal cord. The dorsal horn activates several central mechanisms that are involved in response to painful stimuli. Some neurons initiate a protective spinal reflex in response to pain (pulling one's hand away from a hot object before the heat and burning are consciously realized). Other dorsal horn neurons are involved with inhibition of further incoming nociceptive input. If these cells become damaged from nerve injury, inhibition is removed, more input is received, and pain sensation increases. Most important, dorsal horn neurons send peripheral input via central transmission tracts to the cortex.

Modulation

Modulation is the adaptation of nociceptive activity to changes in environment and needs of the individual. Nociceptive impulse transmission travels from the spinal cord to the cortex via the spinothalamic and spinoreticular tracts. The spinothalamic tracts travel to and synapse in the lateral thalamus, then continue to and terminate in the somatosensory cortex. These tracts map information onto the cortex, allowing one to identify and localize pain. The spinoreticular tracts ascend to either the somatosensory cortex or the limbic system and frontal cortex. These higher cortex areas are where pain is modulated. The responses include the appreciation of pain intensity, the presence of anxiety that accompanies pain, and the need to withdraw from pain. These areas of the cortex create an individual's perception and response to pain based on past pain experiences, emotion, culture, gender, personality, and the meaning of the pain.

Both the spinothalamic and spinoreticular tracts are completely myelinated by 30 weeks of gestation (Anand & Carr, 1989). Maturation of the nerve pathways that link the higher brain centers has not been studied, but it is believed to occur during early infancy and childhood.

The CNS also acts as a modulation system for endogenous opiates and opiate receptors. Endogenous compounds are identical pharmacologically to morphine in their action on opiate receptors. Opiate receptors are present throughout the body and are highly concentrated in the CNS. Action of endogenous opiates and opioid analgesics on the central receptors is believed to provide analgesia. Opiate receptors not involved with analgesia are responsible for many side effects and complications from narcotic administration, such as respiratory depression.

The gate control theory (Melzack & Wall, 1965) is the most widely accepted theory of pain. The premise of the theory is that a "gate" exists in the spinal cord that modulates the perception of pain, either by inhibiting impulses or by "opening" and allowing impulses to reach the higher brain centers. This "gate" modulates pain perception and the response to pain. The theory explains the physical aspects of pain and the psychologic factors, which influence one's experience of pain.

Development and Plasticity

Development and plasticity are the long-lasting and permanent changes in the neural mechanisms that mediate nociception in response to development and experience with injury. Perception of sensory stimuli is not consistent.

TABLE 11-1 **Children's Developmental Concepts of Pain**

Cognitive Stage (Age)	Concept of Pain
Sensorimotor period (newborn to 2 yr)	• Undifferentiated response to pain • Generalized responses to pain that are difficult to distinguish from responses to other distress-causing stimuli; crying and agitation may be the result of pain, hunger, separation anxiety, or respiratory insufficiency
Preoperational thought (2-7 yr)	• Conceives of pain primarily as physical, concrete experience • Focus on external physical cues to define pain (e.g., blood, needles, tubes) • Thinks in terms of magical disappearance of pain • May view pain as punishment for wrongdoing • Tends to hold someone accountable for own pain and may strike out at a person
Concrete operational thought (7-10+ yr)	• Conceives of pain physically (e.g., headache, fractures) • Able to perceive psychologic pain (e.g., someone dying) • Fears bodily harm and annihilation (body destruction and death) • May view pain as punishment for wrongdoings
Formal operational thought (13+ yr)	• Able to give reason for pain (e.g., fell and hit nerve) • Perceives several types of psychologic pain • Has limited life experiences for coping with pain despite mature understanding of pain • May vacillate between adult responses and regression to immature responses to pain

Data from Hurley, A., & Whelan, E. G. (1988). Cognitive development and children's perception of pain. *Pediatric Nursing, 14*(1), 21-24; and Wong, D. L., & Hess, C. S. (2000). *Wong and Whaley's clinical manual of pediatric nursing* (5th ed., p. 272). St. Louis: Mosby.

Perception changes in response to development, environmental experience, and the disease/injury state.

COGNITIVE DEVELOPMENT: INFLUENCE OF CHILDREN'S PAIN CONCEPT

Several authors have described the influence of cognitive development on children's concept of pain (Gaffney & Dunne, 1987). Piaget's theory of development provides the framework used by these authors. Children's developmental concepts of pain are summarized in Table 11-1.

Past Experiences

Children's past experiences with pain, including management and coping mechanisms, influence their responses to current pain. Parental presence also influences children's response to pain. Children who have had past painful experiences may have developed useful coping strategies. If memories of pain are difficult or frightening, anxiety may be increased and the pain may be exacerbated. Children may be able to draw on other situational (nonpain) coping strategies. The hospital environment, with its equipment, loud noises, and unfamiliar people, increases anxiety and may modulate the child's response to pain.

Culture

Cultural expectations and background are important to assess because they may dictate emotional responses to pain. These factors need to be evaluated individually because they are not descriptive of all children.

Disease/Injury

The disease/injury state also modifies children's response to pain. The neural mechanisms may not be intact because of spinal cord injuries, burns, or other trauma. Neurologic impairment may modify children's responses, and nociception (tissue injury) should be used to evaluate and treat children for pain. Pharmacologic interventions such as sedation and neuromuscular blockade obliterate or blunt the pain response. Again, nociception should be the guiding principle for pain management.

PAIN ASSESSMENT

Accurate pain assessment is the cornerstone for optimal pain management in the pediatric trauma patient. A variety of assessment strategies are used to provide information regarding the multidimensional aspects of pain. Pain can be measured by self-report (best), biologic markers (physiologic responses), and behavior (what children do). One approach described by Wong and Hess (2000) is QUESTT:

Question the child.
Use pain rating scales.
Evaluate behavior.
Secure parents' involvement.
Take cause of pain into account.
Take action.

Question the child. A description of pain is the most important factor in assessment of children who are able to communicate verbally. Children as young as toddler age can usually locate pain on a drawing of their body (Figure 11-1). Children use a variety of words for pain and may need help describing pain in familiar language. Children may deny pain because of their developmental level or fear, or they may do so in anticipation of receiving an injection for pain. However, these same children may readily tell a parent. A pain experience history gathered from a child and/or parent

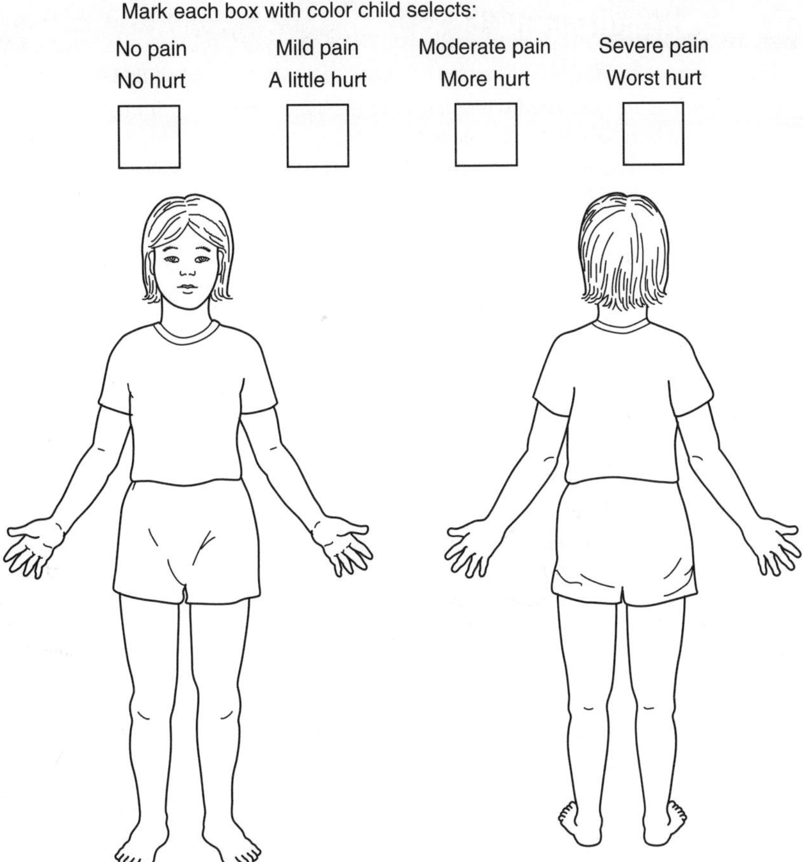

FIGURE 11-1 Eland color scale. (With permission from Joann M. Eland.)

BOX 11-1 Pain Experience History

Child Form

Tell me what pain is.
Tell me about the hurt you have had before.
Do you tell others when you hurt? If yes, who?
What do you do for yourself when you are hurting?
What don't you want others to do for you when you hurt?
What helps the most to take your hurt away?
Is there anything special that you want me to know about you when you hurt? (If yes, have child describe.)

Parent Form

What word(s) does your child use with regard to pain?
Describe the pain experiences your child has had before.
Does you child tell you or others when he or she is hurting?
How do you know when your child is in pain?
How does your child usually react to pain?
What do you do for your child when he or she is hurting?
What does your child do for himself or herself when in pain?
What works best to decrease or take away your child's pain?
Is there anything special that you would like me to know about your child and pain? (If yes, describe.)

Modified from Hester, N. O., & Barcus, C. S. (1986). Assessment and management of pain in children. *Pediatric Nursing Update 1,* 2-8; and Wong, D. L., & Hess, C. S. (2000). *Wong and Whaley's clinical manual of pediatric nursing* (5th ed.). St. Louis: Mosby.

will help with assessment and individualized pain management (Box 11-1).

Use pain rating scales that are developmentally appropriate for the child. Pain rating scales provide a subjective quantitative measure of pain intensity. Table 11-2 provides a summary of pain rating scales.

Select a scale that is suitable to the child's age, abilities, and preference. Scales that use numbers require an understanding of numerical value. When possible, self-report is the best pain assessment method, as opposed to merely evaluating behavior and physiologic responses. Self-report scales include the Oucher, faces, and numerical scales, as summarized in Table 11-2.

Practically speaking, select a few scales as the standard for caregivers to use, that is, one scale for each age/developmental range. This increases the likelihood of appropriate use

TABLE 11-2 Pain Rating Scales for Children

Pain Scale	Description	Comments
Chips scale	Uses plastic chips that are compared with pieces of hurt: One chip means "little hurt," and all chips mean "most hurt," with other chips representing intermediate amounts of hurt. Child chooses number of chips that most nearly describes his or her pain (Hester, 1979).	Recommended for children as young as 4 yr, although children who cannot count may have difficulty with the concept.
Color scale	Uses crayons in various colors. Child creates own scale by choosing color that is like "worst or worst hurt," then another color that is like "little less pain," until last color represents "no hurt." Child chooses color that most nearly describes his or her pain (Eland, 1983).	Recommended for children as young as 4 yr provided children know their colors and are not color blind.
Faces scale	Consists of series of drawn faces ranging from a very happy, smiling face for "no pain" to a sad, tearful face for "worst pain." Child chooses face that most nearly describes his or pain (see Figure 11-2).	Can be used with children as young as 3 yr.
FLACC scale	Consists of specific distress behaviors and scoring to determine postoperative pain rating (see Table 11-3) (Merkel, Voepel-Lewis, Shayevitz, & Malviya, 1997).	Age: 2 mo to 7 yr 0 = no pain, 10 = most pain
Numerical scale	Uses a straight line with end points identified as "no pain" and "worse pain" and divisions along the line market in units from 1 to 10 (high number may vary). Child chooses number that best describes his or her pain.	May be appropriate for children as young as 5 yr, although children who cannot count may have difficulty with the concept.
Oucher scale	Consists of six photographs of a child's face representing "no pain" to "biggest hurt you could ever have." Child chooses face that most nearly describes his or her pain. Also consists of vertical numerical scale with number from 0 to 100. Child chooses number that best describes his or her pain (Beyer, 1984).	Recommended for children approximately 3 to 15 yr; if children can count to 100, they can use numerical scale, otherwise, they should use photographic scale.
Simple descriptive scale	Uses descriptive words (no pain, mild, moderate, quite a lot, very bad, and worst pain) to denote varying intensities of pain. Child chooses word that most nearly describes his or her pain.	May be appropriate for children as young as 5 yr, although words may need explanation.

TABLE 11-3 FLACC Scale

Categories	0	1	2
Face	No particular expression or smile	Occasional grimace or frown, withdrawn, disinterested	Frequent to constant quivering chin, clenched jaw
Legs	Normal position or relaxed	Uneasy, restless, tense	Kicking or legs drawn up
Activity	Lying quietly, normal position, moved easily	Squirming, shifting back and forth, tense	Arched, rigid or jerking
Cry	No cry (awake or asleep)	Moans or whimpers, occasional complaint	Crying steadily, screams or sobs, frequent complaints
Consolability	Content, relaxed	Reassured by occasional touching, hugging, or being talked to; distractible	Difficult to console or comfort

From Merkel, S. I., Voepel-Lewis, T., Shayevitz, J. R., & Malviya, S. (1997). The FLACC: A behavioral scale for scoring postoperative pain in young children. *Pediatric Nursing, 23,* 292-297.
Each of the five categories—face (F), legs (L), activity (A), cry (C), and consolability (C)—is scored from 0 to 2, resulting in a total score range of 0 to 10.

with pediatric patients. Selection should be based on validity, reliability, ease of use, and availability. Examples of standardized assessment tools are as follows:

- *FLACC Scale:* This scale can be used in children 2 months to 7 years to score postoperative pain. The scores are determined by observation of specific distress behaviors (Table 11-3).
- *Children's Hospital of Eastern Ontario Pain Scale (CHEOPS):* CHEOPS is useful in children from 1 to 3 years. Behaviors are rated, and the total score may range from 3 to 13. A score of 8 indicates pain (Table 11-4).
- *Faces Scale:* This scale is useful in patients from age 3 years to adulthood. The child selects the face that represents pain. The faces range from a happy face (no pain) to a sad face (most pain) (Figure 11-2).

- *0 to 10 numerical scale:* The numerical scale may be used in patients from age 7 years to adulthood. The child rates pain from 0 (no pain) to 10 (most pain) (Figure 11-3).

Additional rating scales should be referenced in a pain management protocol and made available for individual patient use. These scales include the Oucher scale for children ages 3 to 15 years (Beyer, 1984), the Poker Chip Tool for children ages 4 years and older (Hester, 1979), and the Color Scale for children ages 4 years and older (Eland, 1983). For example, a 6-year-old who likes to draw may prefer the Color Scale to the Faces Scale, and this should be noted on the plan of care and used by all caregivers.

Pain intensity scales provide a means for communication between the child and caregiver and between caregivers. Trending ratings over time and with various activities, such as ambulating, give more information regarding the child's experience. Pain should be assessed a minimum of every 4 hours and after pharmacologic and nonpharmacologic interventions during the acute pain period.

Evaluate behavior and physiologic responses because these changes are common indicators of pain and are especially valuable with evaluation of nonverbal patients. Boxes 11-2 and 11-3 provide specific examples of behavioral and physiologic responses.

The child who has chronic pain from trauma (more than 3 to 6 months) will have blunted physiologic changes and may not demonstrate overt behavioral indicators. The child may sleep more than usual, have a decreased appetite, and appear depressed and withdrawn.

When the infant or child is unable to communicate information regarding pain, nurses rely solely on physiologic and behavioral changes for assessment. These signs may indicate another source of distress, such as fear or anxiety. All causative factors must be assessed to determine the cause of the distress. Observation for improvement in

TABLE 11-4 Behavioral Definition and Scoring of the Children's Hospital of Eastern Ontario Pain Scale (CHEOPS)

Item	Behavior	Rating	Definition
Cry	No crying	1	Child is not crying
	Moaning	2	Child is moaning or quietly vocalizing silent cry
	Crying	2	Child is crying but the cry is gentle or whimpering
	Scream	3	Child is in a full-lunged cry; sobbing may be scored with complaint or without complaint
Facial	Composed	1	Neutral facial expression
	Grimace	2	Score only if definite negative facial expression
	Smiling	0	Score only if definite positive facial expression
Child verbal	None	1	Child not talking
	Other complaints	1	Child complains but not about pain (e.g., "I want to see mommy" or "I am thirsty")
	Pain complaints	2	Child complains of pain
	Both complaints	2	Child complains about pain and other things (e.g., "It hurts, I want mommy")
	Positive	0	Child makes any positive statement or talks about other things without complaint
Torso	Neutral	1	Body (not limbs) is at rest; torso is inactive
	Shifting	2	Body is in motion in a shifting or serpentine fashion
	Tense	2	Body is arched or rigid
	Shivering	2	Body is shuddering or shaking involuntarily
	Upright	2	Child is in a vertical or upright position
	Restrained	2	Body is restrained
Touch	Not touching	1	Child is not touching or grabbing at wound
	Reach	2	Child is reaching for but not touching wound
	Grab	2	Child is grabbing vigorously at wound
	Restrained	2	Child's arms are restrained
Legs	Neutral	1	Legs may be in any position but are relaxed; includes gentle swimming or serpentine-like movements
	Squirming/kicking	2	Definitive uneasy or restless movements in the legs and/or striking out with foot or feet
	Drawn up/tensed	2	Legs tensed and/or pulled up tightly to body and kept there
	Standing	2	Standing, crouching, or kneeling
	Restrained	2	Child's legs are being held down

From McGrath, P., Johnson, G., Goodman, J. T., Schillinger, J., Dunn, J., & Chapman, J. (1985). CHEOPS: A behavioral scale for rating postoperative pain in children. *Advances in Pain Research and Therapy, 9*, 395-402.

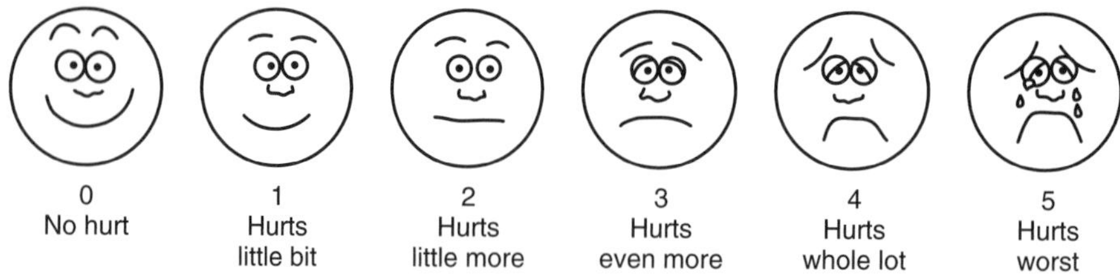

FIGURE 11-2 Faces rating scale. Explain to the child that each face is for a person who feels happy because he or she has no pain (hurt) or sad because he or she has some or a lot of pain. Face 0 is very happy because there is no pain at all. Face 1 hurts just a little bit. Face 2 hurts a little more. Face 3 hurts even more. Face 4 hurts a whole lot, but Face 5 hurts as much as you can imagine, although you don't have to be crying to feel this bad. Ask the child to choose the face that best describes how he or she is feeling. Rating scale is recommended for persons 3 years and older. (From Wong, D. L., & Hockenberry-Eaton, M. [2001]. *Wong's essentials of pediatric nursing* [6th ed.]. St. Louis: Mosby. Copyrighted by Mosby-Year Book, Inc. Reprinted by permission. The Wong-Baker Faces Pain Scale may be reproduced for clinical and research use, provided the copyright information is retained with the scale.)

Number scale:
(patient self-rating)
Appropriate age: Older than Age 7

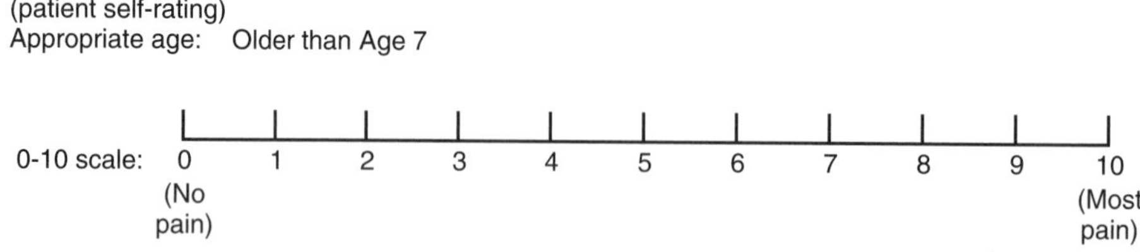

Explain to the patient that the numbers between 0 and 10 represent pain. Zero means no pain; 10 means the very worst pain that could be. Ask the patient to tell you the number that most represents his or her pain.

FIGURE 11-3 Pain intensity scale instructions.

behavior assists with evaluating efficacy of analgesics. Conversely, no change in behavior may mean that pain still exists and that the pain regimen is inadequate. Children who are asleep may still be in pain; they may be exhausted, or the medications may cause sedation without adequate analgesia.

Secure parents' involvement because they know their child best. Have a parent complete a parent form of the pain history (see Box 11-1). Encourage parents to participate in assessing their child's pain and give them instruction on how to use the appropriate pain scale. Realize that parents may have never seen their child in moderate to severe pain. Demonstrate to parents how to use the pain assessment flow sheet to record the ratings.

Take cause of pain into account because the mechanism of injury, tissue damage, and other pathologic condition may give clues to expected intensity and type of pain. Wong's golden rule of pain assessment is "Whatever is painful to an adult is painful to an infant or child, until proven otherwise" (Wong & Hess, 2000). Nurses are key advocates for appropriate analgesic dosing, especially when the patient's subjective pain assessment is not possible.

Take action to meet the child's established pain management goal. The only reason to assess pain is to optimize pain management for achievement of pain relief.

Additional Considerations

Additional considerations in pain assessment of the pediatric trauma patient include assessing the nonverbal, sedated child and assessing the child for agitation. The sedated intubated child still may have pain but may have blunted responses that are inconsistently interpreted by caregivers. When other pain scales are not appropriate, a modified Ramsey Sedation Scale may be used to set a sedation goal and consistently evaluate the child for adequate sedation (Box 11-4). Other sedation scales include the Comfort Scale (Table 11-5) and the Modified Motor Activity Assessment Scale (Table 11-6).

Agitation is a very common problem with critically ill trauma patients. Inadequate oxygenation and/or ventilation, poor tissue perfusion, or pain can cause agitation. A systematic approach to the assessment and management of agitation is critical (Figure 11-4). Assessment and management are essential because critically injured children can rarely tolerate the physiologic stress and consumption of calories that result from agitation.

Pain should always be considered with repeated episodes of agitation, after airway, breathing, and circulation have been managed. A trial of analgesics in trauma patients should be considered in the systematic approach to managing agitation in critically ill children.

PAIN MANAGEMENT

This section summarizes pain management considerations that are critical for the pediatric trauma patient. Acute and chronic pain management strategies are discussed in greater

BOX 11-2 Behavioral Indicators of Pain

Infant

- Facial expression: brow lowered and drawn together, broadened nasal root, eyes tightly closed and an angular, squarish mouth with a taut tongue
- Irritability
- Restlessness
- Continuous crying/whimpering
- Crying when the stimulus is applied
- Intense crying
- Knees drawn to chest
- Clenched fists
- Refusal to eat
- Hyperalertness
- Restless sleep/inability to sleep
- Hypersensitivity to touch
- Muscle tension

Toddler

- Says he or she "hurts" or has an "owie"
- Intense or continuous crying
- Aggressive behavior toward nurses, parents, or any available person
- Rubbing, pulling, guarding, or touching of the affected body part
- Inability to be comforted
- Regressive behavior
- Resistance to being held
- Irritability/restlessness
- Nightmares, inability to sleep
- Decreased activity tolerance
- Lowered frustration tolerance
- Change from usual play behavior
- Seeking of comfort objects (e.g., blanket, stuffed toy)
- Seeking of comfort from parents, caregivers

Preschool-Age Child

Generally similar to those of the toddler with the following additions:

- Denies pain in the presence of other behavioral cues and a physical injury
- Repetitive verbalizations such as "It hurts, it hurts, it hurts."
- Refusal to allow nurse/parent to touch the affected body part

School-Age Child

- Denial of pain in the presence of behavioral cues
- Resistance of movement
- Facial expression: grimacing
- Nightmares
- Low frustration tolerance
- Guarding
- Emotional withdrawal
- Irritability/restlessness/thrashing

Teenager

- Muscle tension
- Guarding of painful area
- Change in activity level
- Nightmares
- Change in eating pattern
- Irritability/restlessness/thrashing
- Increased sleeping in the absence of pain control measures
- Lowered frustration tolerance
- Facial grimacing

Nonverbal/Neurologically Damaged

- Facial grimacing
- Facial flushing
- Increased muscle tension
- Hypersensitivity to the environment
- Grinding of the teeth
- Seizure activity
- Clenched fists
- Hypersensitivity to touch
- Inability to be comforted
- Continuous crying
- Spasms of extremities (leg "jumps")
- Vomiting
- Inability to tolerate lying in the same position

Sources: Johnston, C. C., & Strata M. E. (1986). *Pain management in children.* Milwaukee, WI: MaxiShare Corp; and Wong, D. L., & Hockenberry-Eaton, M. (2001). *Wong's essentials of pediatric nursing* (6th ed.). St. Louis: Mosby.

BOX 11-3 Physiologic Responses to Pain

- Increased pulse, blood pressure, respiratory rate
- Increased blood pressure
- Increased respiratory rate
- Increased depth of respirations
- Flushing or pallor
- Diaphoresis
- Dilated pupils
- Decreased oxygen consumption; decreased oxygen saturation
- Muscle tension, especially in the painful area
- Nausea and/or decreased gastric motility

In addition, infants can have the following physiologic responses:

- Apnea
- Color changes
- Seizures
- Stooling
- Hiccoughing

depth in specific pediatric pain references (Agency for Health Care Policy and Research [AHCPR], 1992; American Pain Society, 1999; Yaster, Krane, Kaplan, Cote, & Lappe, 1997).

The child admitted after a traumatic incident does not have the benefit of anxiety-reducing preparation. Instead, the child is emergently thrust into the trauma system of care. Although initial approach to the trauma patient focuses, by necessity, on rapid cardiopulmonary assessment and stabilization, pain assessment and management need to be addressed immediately after this phase. Analgesics may be withheld pending a full neurologic evaluation, which is less than optimal because children will often cooperate for the evaluation if pain is relieved. A systematic sequential approach for pain assessment and management will assist in preventing inadequate pain relief.

BOX 11-4 Clinical Sedation Scale

1 Anxious, agitated, or restless
2* Cooperative, accepting ventilation; oriented and tranquil
3* Asleep; brisk response to three light strokes to the cheek
4* Asleep; sluggish response to three light strokes to the cheek
5 No response to above; responds to nail bed pressure
6 No response to nail bed pressure

Modified from Ramsey, M. A. E., Savege, T. M., Simpson, B. R., & Goodwin, R. (1974). Controlled sedation with alphaxalone-alphadolone. *British Medical Journal, 2,* 656-659.
*Desired level of sedation.

TABLE 11-5 Comfort Scale

Criteria/Descriptor	Score
Alertness	
Deeply asleep	1
Lightly asleep	2
Drowsy	3
Fully awake and alert	4
Hyperalert	5
Calmness/Agitation	
Calm	1
Slightly anxious	2
Anxious	3
Very anxious	4
Panicky	5
Respiratory Response	
No coughing and no spontaneous respiration	1
Spontaneous respiration with little or no response to ventilation	2
Occasional cough or resistance to ventilator	3
Actively breathes against ventilator or coughs regularly	4
Fights ventilator; coughing or choking	5
Physical Movement	
No movement	1
Occasional, slight movement	2
Frequent, slight movement	3
Vigorous movement limited to extremities	4
Vigorous movement including torso and head	5
Blood Pressure (Mean Arterial Pressure) Baseline _____	
Blood pressure below baseline	1
Blood pressure consistently at baseline	2
Infrequent elevations 15% or more (1-3)	3
Frequent elevations 15% or more (>3)	4
Sustained elevation ≥15%	5
Heart Rate Baseline _____	
Heart rate below baseline	1
Heart rate consistently at baseline	2
Infrequent elevations ≥15% above baseline (1-3) during observation period	3
Frequent elevations ≥15% above baseline (>3)	4
Sustained elevation ≥15%	5
Muscle Tone	
Muscles totally relaxed; no muscle tone	1
Reduced muscle tone	2
Normal muscle tone	3
Increased muscle tone and flexion of fingers and toes	4
Extreme muscle rigidity and flexion of fingers and toes	5
Facial Tension	
Facial muscles totally relaxed	1
Facial muscle tone normal; no facial muscle tension evident	2
Tension evident in some facial muscles	3
Tension evident throughout facial muscles	4
Facial muscles contorted and grimacing	5
Total Score = _______	

From Marx, C. M., Smith, P., Lowrie, L. H., Hamlett, K. W., Ambuel, B., & Yamashita, T. S. (1994). Optimal sedation of mechanically ventilated pediatric critical care patients. *Critical Care Medicine,* 22, 163-170.

Pain and anxiety are managed as a package to provide comfort and decrease a child's distress. The combination includes pharmacologic and nonpharmacologic strategies individualized for each child.

PHARMACOLOGIC MANAGEMENT

The AHCPR has published pain management guidelines in a flowchart (Figure 11-5). These guidelines are useful because, compared with adults undergoing similar procedures, fewer analgesic regimens are usually prescribed and administered to children (Foster, 1996). When used, opioid doses and intervals of administration are often inadequate. When a physician's order includes a selection of one or more analgesics, the tendency is to choose the least potent drugs (AHCPR, 1992; Yaster et al., 1997). Nurses need to be knowledgeable about principles of analgesic pain management, drug pharmacokinetics, appropriate dose ranges, titration side effects and antidotes, and appropriate assessment/monitoring requirements so that they can provide optimal pain and anxiety relief. The AHCPR guidelines provide the sequence of activities for pain management that can optimize pain relief for the child.

ANALGESIC STRATEGIES

Some types of acute trauma pain respond well to nonopioid analgesics alone. The nonopioid analgesics include nonsteroidal antiinflammatory drugs (NSAIDs) and acetaminophen. Other types of trauma pain, such as lacerations, respond well to mild opiates, such as codeine with an NSAID or acetaminophen. Many trauma patients who experience severe pain require higher-dose opiates with an NSAID (Table 11-7). This three-step approach to treatment of pain, progressing from nonopioid, to mild opioid, to potent opioid analgesics has been identified by the World Health Organization Expert Committee (1990).

Nonopioids. Nonopioids, such as acetaminophen and the NSAIDs (ibuprofen, naproxen, ketorolac) are useful for alleviating pain caused by trauma. The key is to administer the drugs on an around-the-clock regimen, not on an as-needed (prn) basis, for optimal analgesic effect. Because the nonopioids inhibit peripheral pain pathways differently than opioids do, an additive analgesic effect is achieved when nonopioids

TABLE 11-6 Modified Motor Activity Assessment Scale

Score	Description	Definition
−3	Unresponsive	Minimal or no response to noxious* stimulus; does not communicate or follow commands.
−2	Responsive only to noxious stimuli	Opens eyes or raises eyebrows or turns head toward stimulus or moves limbs with noxious stimulus.
−1	Responsive to touch or name	Opens eyes or raises eyebrows or turns head toward stimulus or moves limbs with touch or when name is spoken; drifts off after stimulation; follows simple commands.
0	Calm and cooperative	No external stimulus is required to elicit movement; calm, awakens easily, and follows commands.
+1	Restless and cooperative	No external stimulus is required to elicit movement; picking at tubes but consolable.
+2	Agitated	No external stimulus is required to elicit movement; attempting to sit or move limbs to get up and inconsolable despite frequent attempts; requires physical restraint, biting ETT.
+3	Dangerously agitated, uncooperative	No external stimulus is required to elicit movement; patient unsafe—attempting to pull at ETT/catheters; desaturating; thrashing side-to-side; climbing over the rail; striking at staff.

Modified from Devlin, J. W., Boleski, G., Mlynarek, M., Nerenz, D. R., Peterson, E., Jankowski, M., Horst, H. M., & Zarowitz, B. J. (1999). Motor activity assessment scale. *Critical Care Medicine* 27, 1271-1275, 1999, via personal communication from M.A.Q. Curley, 1999.
ETT, Endotracheal tube.
*Noxious stimulus, suctioning, or 5 sec of nail bed pressure.

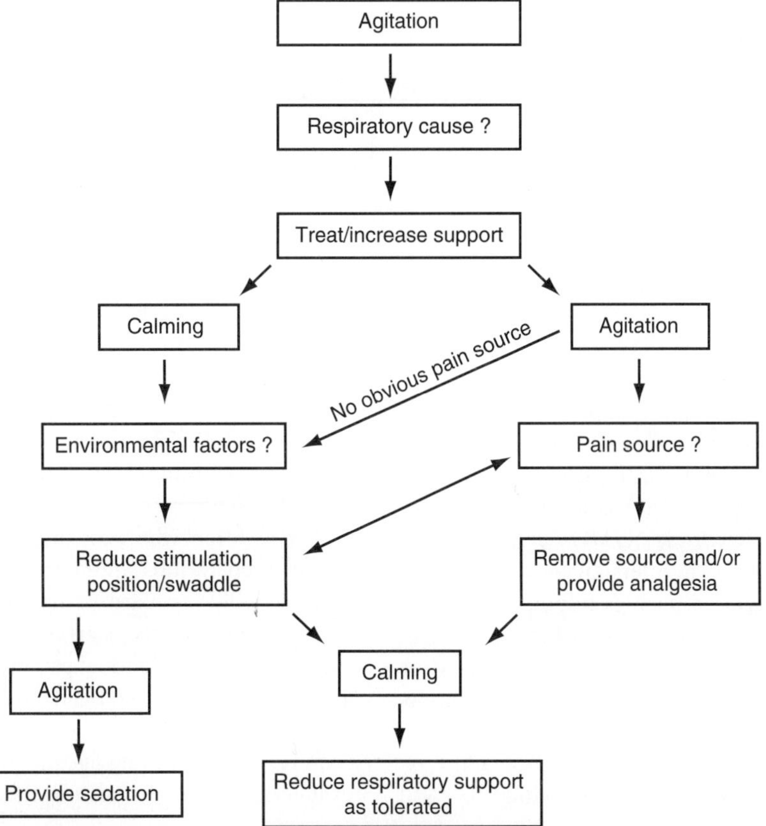

FIGURE 11-4 Agitation flowchart. (Modified from Gordin, P. C. [1990]. Assessing and managing agitation in a critically ill infant. *MCN American Journal of Maternal Child Nursing, 15,* 26-32.)

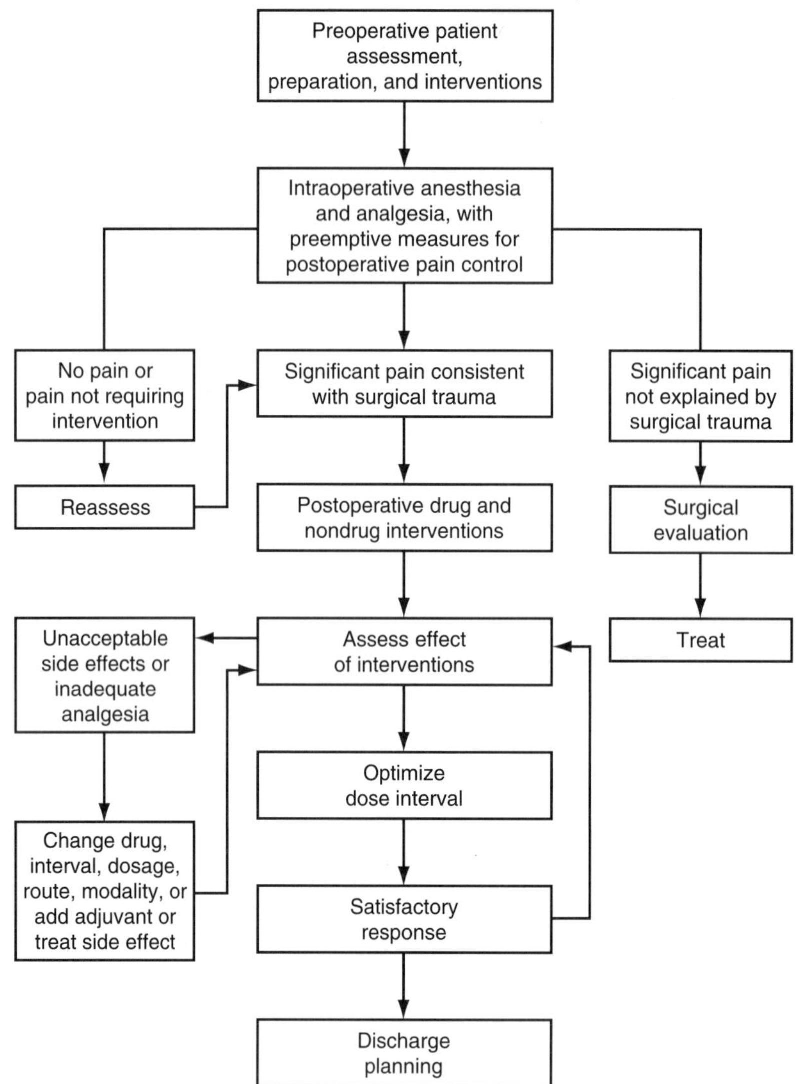

FIGURE 11-5 Abbreviated pain management flowchart for infants, children, and adolescents. (From Agency for Health Care Policy and Research. [1992]. *Acute pain management in infants, children, and adolescents. Quick reference guide for clinicians* [AHCPR Publication No. 92-0020]. Rockville, MD: U.S. Department of Health and Human Services.)

and opioids are given concurrently. Nonopioids exhibit a ceiling effect (a maximum level of analgesia) despite increasing dosages. Because NSAIDs interfere with platelet functioning, they should not be used in patients at risk for bleeding.

Ketorolac is the only injectable NSAID currently available. Intravenous (IV) ketorolac offers analgesia similar to opioids without the side effects, such as respiratory depression. Equianalgesic doses are cited as 30 mg ketorolac intramuscular (IM) or IV equivalent to 12 mg morphine IM or IV (O'Hara, Fragen, Kinzer, & Pemberton, 1987). Patients are monitored for side effects of NSAIDs, which include signs and symptoms of gastrointestinal upset (oral administration), ulcers, and platelet dysfunction (bleeding).

Opioids. Opioids (see Table 11-7) are necessary for most trauma patients. For moderate pain an opioid such as codeine should be considered for the child who can tolerate oral agents. Codeine, hydrocodone, and oxycodone are usually prescribed in fixed combination with acetaminophen. Care must be taken not to exceed the maximum recommended acetaminophen dosage (15 mg/kg/dose repeated every 4 to 6 hours, not to exceed 4 g/day).

For children who need more potent analgesia, stronger opioid preparations are given. Morphine sulfate is considered the gold standard of narcotics. For all narcotic analgesics, recommended starting dosages are guidelines, not rigid standards. Individual patients vary in their responses to analgesics. The key is to titrate to clinical effect, which is adequate analgesia with manageable side effects. Safe titration requires understanding agents' peak actions and timing for evaluating maximal analgesic effect and complications.

Guiding Principles for Safe Administration of Opiates

Nurses need current references to identify peak action time of opiates and other pharmacokinetics and pharmacodynamic

TABLE 11-7 Pharmacologic Management of Pain and Agitation

Drug Action	Dosage	Approximate Equianalgesic Dose	Route	Onset of Action	Duration of Action
Nonsteroidal Antiinflammatory Drugs (NSAIDs)					
Ibuprofen (Motrin)	10 mg/kg q6-8h		PO	30-60 min	4-6 hr
Ketorolac	0.5 mg/kg q6h		IM, IV	30-60 min	4-6 hr
Narcotic Analgesics					
Morphine	Neonates and infants: 0.03 mg/kg Children: 0.1 mg/kg *Continuous infusion:* Neonates and infants: 15 μg/kg/hr Children: 20 μg/kg/hr *Epidural:* 0.03-0.05 mg/kg q6-12h Infusion 3 μg/kg/hr	10 mg q3-4h	IV, IM, SC	IV: 10-15 min IM: 20-30 min	4 hr
Fentanyl	1-5 μg/kg *Continuous infusion:* 1-3 μg/kg/hr	0.1 mg (100 μg)	IV, IM	3-5 min	30-60 min
Methadone	0.1 mg/kg	10 mg q6-8h 20 mg (oral)	PO, IM, SC	1 hr	IM: 3-4 hr PO: 6-12 hr
Codeine	0.6-1.0 mg/kg	75-90 mg q3-4h	PO	1 hr	4-6 hr
Meperidine	1 mg/kg	100 mg q3h	IV, IM, SC, PO	IV: 10 min IM: 15-20 min PO: 20 min	2-4 hr 3 hr
Benzodiazepines					
Diazepam	0.1-0.2 mg/kg	NA	IV, PO	IV: 15 min PO: 30-60 min	IV: 4-6 hr PO: 6-8 hr
Lorazepam	0.05-0.1 mg/kg	NA	IV, IM, PO	IV: 15 min PO: 30-60 min	8-12 hr
Midazolam	0.05-0.15 mg/kg	NA	IV, IM, PO	IV: 2-5 min IM: 20-30 min PO: 10-30 min	2 hr
Barbiturates					
Phenobarbital	2-5 mg/kg	NA	IV, PO	IV: 5 min PO: 20-60 min	8-12 hr
Pentobarbital	2 mg/kg	NA	IV, IM, PO, PR	IV: <5 min IM: <20 min PO: 20-60 min PR: 20-60 min	4-6 hr
Hypnotics					
Chloral hydrate	*Sedative:* 25-50 mg/kg *Hyponotic:* 75-100 mg/kg	NA	PO, PR	30-60 min	6-8 hr

IM, Intramuscular; *IV,* intravenous; *NA,* not applicable; *PO,* orally; *PR,* per rectum; *SC,* subcutaneous.
Anxiolytics and sedatives do not provide analgesia.

properties. Route, dosage, and schedule of administration need to be individualized for each child and type of trauma pain.

There are several key points to consider when choosing the route of administration. IM injections should be avoided in children because of the psychologic trauma of shots. IV bolus opiates achieve the most rapid effect. Continuous IV infusions achieve a steady blood level, more effective analgesia, and fewer side effects than boluses alone (Yaster et al., 1997). In trauma patients with severe pain, repeated IV boluses are required to load concentrations, which provide pain relief, followed by a maintenance infusion. Patient-controlled analgesia has been used effectively in children older than 7 years and in younger children if they were assessed to be developmentally capable (Berde, Lehn, Yee, Sethna, & Russo, 1991). Epidural administration of preservative-free morphine or fentanyl has been used to control pain postoperatively with less sedation than IV administration. A local anesthetic, such as bupivacaine, may be added to potentiate the analgesic effect and allow for a lower dosage of narcotic (Yaster et al., 1997). Epidural opioids can be delivered as a single dose, bolus, or continuous infusion.

Dosage of the narcotic is another important consideration (see Table 11-7). When changing to another opioid or changing route (IV to orally), one must use equianalgesic dosing references (American Pain Society, 1999). As mentioned, the key to appropriate dosing is titration to clinical effect. A change to oral opioids (equianalgesic dose) should take place as soon as the child can tolerate oral intake.

When an administration schedule is being developed, consideration should be given administering opiates regularly (around the clock, not prn) if pain is present most of the day. The prn doses are important for intermittent or breakthrough pain, such as in trauma patients who have increased pain with ambulation.

Nurses need to recognize and treat side effects. The most common side effects are nausea, vomiting, constipation, sedation, pruritus, and respiratory depression. If side effects are not managed easily, a change to a different opioid may benefit the patient.

Respiratory depression is rare, but nurses should monitor closely for this complication. Critical judgment and careful assessment of the sedated child include monitoring respiratory rate, chest excursion, breath sounds, and if indicated, oximetry. Oxygen saturation should be monitored in all infants younger than age 6 months who are receiving IV opiates (AHCPR, 1992). Oximetry for older infants and children receiving opiates depends on clinical judgment and institutional policy. Naloxone is the drug of choice to treat respiratory depression. Naloxone should be diluted (0.1 mg in 10 ml of normal saline) and given in 1-ml increments titrated to reverse respiratory suppression, without causing total obliteration of analgesic effect.

Nurses should be knowledgeable regarding key concepts related to the use of opioids. Misunderstanding of these concepts often leads to suboptimal pain management. *Physical tolerance* is a characteristic of opioids when increasing dosages of medication are required to attain the same effect. This is normal in a patient with acute pain. *Psychologic dependence* or *addiction* is the use of narcotics or other drugs for psychologic effect, not for pain relief. *Physical dependence* is a withdrawal syndrome after sudden discontinuation of opioids. This is an expected outcome when opioids are used for 5 to 7 days.

When a patient has been taking opiates for 5 to 7 days, a weaning schedule should be followed to prevent withdrawal. Weaning is accomplished by reducing the baseline opioid dose by 10% to 20% per day (Yaster et al., 1997). Assessment for withdrawal with an abstinence scoring system should be used to quantify symptoms and base tolerance to weaning on ratings that do not increase (Finnegan et al., 1975). This scoring system has been adapted for use in pediatric patients by deleting the motor reflex responses, but further validity and reliability testing need to occur before its use in the older infant and child.

ADJUNCTIVE MEDICATIONS FOR SEDATION

Because anxiety and agitation contribute to the pain experience, sedatives are commonly used to modify the child's response, normalize sleep/wake cycles, facilitate mechanical ventilation, decrease intracranial pressure (ICP), and make procedures more tolerable. Nurses need to critically assess children to advocate for appropriate pain and sedation management. Sedatives alone do nothing to ease the distress of a patient in pain. Conversely, the disoriented child with a head injury who is receiving large doses of opiates could benefit from adjunctive sedatives. Because there is minimal research regarding a standardized plan for pain and agitation management, nurses should be experienced at evaluating the patient's response and advocating for appropriate pharmacologic management.

BENZODIAZEPINES

Benzodiazepines are useful sedatives that have powerful CNS effects, which include sedation, sleep, anxiolysis, amnesia, and reversal of seizures. Some patients may have a paradoxical excitatory effect. Commonly used benzodiazepines are listed in Table 11-7.

Benzodiazepines and opioids are often combined for analgesic and sedative effects. For the trauma patient, opioids should be the first-line medication, followed by benzodiazepines to help ease distress. The narcotic should be titrated according to recommended guidelines, and the benzodiazepine should be dosed at half the recommended guideline (Oakes, 2001). Both should be titrated to therapeutic effect.

BARBITURATES

Barbiturates exert a CNS depressant effect that ranges from mild sedation to deep anesthesia. The half-life of this class of drugs is usually greater than 24 hours. Barbiturates are used for procedural sedation but rarely as an infusion for the critically ill trauma patient. Occasionally, a barbiturate is ordered for a patient with severe head injury refractory to sedation/anticonvulsant management with benzodiazepines.

CHLORAL HYDRATE

Chloral hydrate is a hypnotic used to produce mild sedation and immobility for nonpainful procedures such as computed tomography. It is occasionally ordered for sedation in the hospitalized child, but caution needs to be exercised with long-term use because of accumulation of a toxic metabolite.

NEUROMUSCULAR BLOCKADE AGENTS

Neuromuscular blockade agents are often administered to intubated patients to facilitate mechanical ventilation and decrease oxygen requirements. These drugs do not provide analgesia or sedation; they merely block the patient's neuromuscular response. The patient feels pain but cannot move. Nurses advocate for the administration of appropriate analgesia and sedation in the patient receiving these agents. Nurses have to intervene based on the *potential* for pain and agitation because the only evaluation available is changes in vital signs and pupil size.

Other Adjunctive Medications

Other classes of drugs may be included in the pain regimen for trauma patients. Tricyclic antidepressants, such as amitriptyline, have been used to treat neuropathic pain. Anticonvulsants have been used to treat posttraumatic neuralgias (American Pain Society, 1999).

Sedation for Procedures

Children who experience trauma are subject to many painful procedures. Sedation combined with developmentally appropriate nonpharmacologic comfort measures has become the standard of care for children. The American Academy of Pediatrics (1992) has published guidelines regarding safe administration of sedation for children. Medications now are given routinely before pediatric patient procedures (Curley et al., 1992). An extensive review of procedural sedation for procedures can be found in the *Pediatric Pain Management and Sedation Handbook* (Yaster et al., 1997).

Analgesics and/or anesthetics are the foundation for pharmacologic management of painful procedures. Sedatives are used for anxiety reduction (see Table 11-7). Nurses require competency to administer sedation/analgesic agents, with appropriate assessment and monitoring for the level of sedation. Nurses are also key in evaluating the recovery from the effects of these agents.

Local Anesthetics

Local anesthetics are used primarily to prevent or treat pain, rarely as a motor blockade in the child with traumatic injuries. They are administered topically, subcutaneously into peripheral nerves, or centrally (epidural). Epinephrine may be added for laceration repair because of its vasoconstrictive property. Assessment for systemic side effects, such as cardiopulmonary complications and seizures, must be accomplished, and emergency equipment/medications must be immediately available. Specific anesthetics used for trauma patients in the emergency department are listed in Table 11-8.

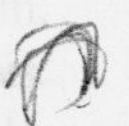

SPECIAL CONSIDERATIONS

Infants Younger Than 6 Months of Age

Dosing guidelines for young infants begin at a lower starting dose than for older infants and children. Morphine tends to have a longer half-life and a lower clearance rate in this population (Lynn & Slattery, 1987; Purcell-Jones, Norman, & Sumner, 1987). The duration is highly variable. In this age group the recommended starting dose for morphine is 0.03 mg/kg. Continuous opiate infusions should start with a conservative dose and be titrated to clinical effect while minimizing the risk of respiratory depression and apnea.

Assessment for infants includes continuous oximetry and continuous cardiorespiratory monitoring. Naloxone and emergency airway should be immediately available.

Nurses need to advocate for the administration of opiates in this population and provide other measures for comfort. Sucrose nipples (nipples dipped in table sugar/water) have been demonstrated to be effective for infant pain relief (Anand and the International Evidence-Based Group for Neonatal Pain, 2001).

Pain Management in the Child With a Head Injury

Pain assessment and management of the child with a head injury creates a special challenge. For the child with an altered level of consciousness, pain assessment is often restricted to physiologic responses, such as increased heart rate, blood pressure, and ICP. However, if the patient can perceive pain, appropriate analgesics are required to prevent further increases in ICP and to assist with patient comfort.

The main concerns with pharmacologic management of pain are blunting effects on neurologic assessment and potential decrease in mean arterial pressure and thus cerebral perfusion pressure. Pain is especially detrimental in the child with intracranial hypertension because it can further increase ICP and oxygen consumption.

Protocols for the child with a head injury must address pain management. After initial assessment and stabilization in the emergency department, analgesia should be optimized. Local anesthetics should be used for laceration repair and invasive procedures (see Table 11-8). Short-acting opioids, such as fentanyl, can be titrated intravenously to maximize analgesic and beneficial physiologic effects. Midazolam, or another short-acting benzodiazepine, may be given with an opioid to provide amnesia and synergistic effects on the provision of pain relief. The goal is to provide adequate analgesia, sedation, and ICP management while minimizing interference with clinical assessment.

Pain Management in the Child With Burns

The hospitalized child with burns experiences pain from the burn injury itself and during burn dressing changes. Optimal pain control is necessary because undertreatment can escalate anxiety. An opioid can be administered alone or with a benzodiazepine. The initial pain regimen may include a continuous opiate infusion with additional opiate and benzodiazepine boluses. Dosages are increased as needed to titrate to previous procedure response (if positive). For extensive debridement, deep sedation or general anesthesia may be required.

A variety of nonpharmacologic strategies to assist the child to cope with frequent dressing changes have been reported in the literature. These strategies include distraction, imagery, relaxation, and hypnosis (Elliott & Olson, 1983). Children have also been demonstrated to cope more effectively if they can participate and have some control over the environment, such as with scheduling of dressing changes and taking off old dressings (Kavanaugh, 1983). Care should be taken to keep the child's room "safe"; therefore dressing changes should be done in the treatment room.

NONPHARMACOLOGIC STRATEGIES

For pain relief, nonpharmacologic, noninvasive strategies should be used in addition to medication. Comfort

TABLE 11-8 Local Anesthetic Used in Emergency Departments

Drug	Indications	Application	Concentration	Maximum Dose	Comments
EMLA	Venipuncture, lumbar puncture, intravenous start	Apply dollop of cream and occlusive dressing 60 min (minimum) before procedure			Risk for developing methemoglobinemia
TAC	Dermal lesions	1-3 ml gel or liquid directly to wound for 15 min	1 ml liquid = 10 mg tetracaine Epinephrine 0.25 mg Cocaine 40 mg 1 ml gel = 5.0 mg tetracaine Epinephrine 0.125 mg Cocaine 12 mg	Tetracaine 1.5 mg/kg Cocaine 6 mg/kg	Blanching after 10 min correlates with blockade
LET	Dermal lesions	1-3 ml gel or liquid applied directly to wound for 20-30 min	Lidocaine in stock liquid is 4 mg/ml Tetracaine 0.5 mg/ml Epinephrine 1 mg/ml	Lidocaine with epinephrine: 7 mg/kg	Contraindicated for end arteries Wound blanching may or may not be associated with effective blockade
Lidocaine	Peripheral blockade	Subcutaneously	0.5%-1%	Without epinephrine: 5 mg/kg With epinephrine: 7 mg/kg	May cause seizures if given intravascularly

LET, Lidocaine/epinephrine/tetracaine; *TAC,* tetracaine/adrenalin/cocaine.

measures are complementary to analgesics/opiates, but they should not be the mainstay for pain management in the pediatric trauma patient.

Hospitalized children experience pain and anxiety from many sources, including treatment and procedures; separation from family and friends; loss of control, autonomy, and competence; and uncertainties regarding their diagnosis, prognosis, and length of hospitalization (Smith & Martin, 2001). The goal in using comfort strategies is to enhance effectiveness in decreasing anxiety and promoting children's comfort. This is the same in teaching comfort strategies to patients and families.

General Guidelines

The following guidelines are helpful when using comfort strategies:

- Involve the child and his or her parents in individualizing coping strategies. Allow parents to be present during a procedure.
- Educate them about the procedure and their supportive role.
- Do not have the parents restrain the child.
- Keep the child's bed and room "safe." Use a (different) treatment room for painful procedures. Ask a child older than 6 years of age where he or she prefers to have the procedure.
- Before a procedure, have the room set up.
- Reduce waiting time.
- Avoid deceptive statements.
- Establish a trusting alliance with the child.
- Speak calmly and quietly to the parents and child.
- Provide developmentally appropriate explanations of why the procedure is necessary.
- Use child life specialists, if available, to assist the patient and family with developing and implementing a plan of care regarding strategies and pain reduction techniques.
- Address environmental modifications, positioning and handling techniques, distraction techniques, cognitive-behavioral techniques, and family involvement in caregiving.

Developmentally Appropriate Comfort Strategies

The pediatric trauma patient requires diverse strategies that take into account the severity of illness and the child's neurologic status and developmental level. The critically ill patient with a head injury requires a calm, quiet environment; strategies are aimed at decreasing stimulation and ICP. On the other hand, a 6-year-old who has been in the hospital for 7 days, confined by traction in the bed, can use multiple nonpharmacologic strategies, such as distraction with music, video games, and art play. These strategies can be individualized to decrease boredom and provide comfort. For infants and very young children, interventions are aimed at decreasing distress and behavioral disorganization with calming measures, such as swaddling and rhythmic rocking.

Developmentally appropriate comfort strategies are outlined in Table 11-9. The goal is to have the patient, family, nurse, and child life specialist design, implement, and evaluate an individualized plan of care for pain management.

TABLE 11-9 Developmental Approaches to Complementary Nonpharmacologic Strategies

Developmental Age (yr)	Environmental Modification	Distraction Techniques	Cognitive-Behavioral Techniques	Touch/Physical Modalities	Spiritual Strategies
"Infants" (0-1)	• Decrease noise/light • Maintain calm demeanor • Use therapeutic positioning and containment • Speak calmly and reassuringly • Consider physical environment • Be aware of sleep/wake patterns • Consider anxiety level of child/parent(s)/practitioners	• Audio: music (transitions, Tibetan bells); soothing talk, soft/novel voice • Visual: mobiles, books for older children • Oral-meter stimulation: pacifiers, nonnutritive sucking	• Explanations: caregiver teaching	• Swaddling/ containment • Kangaroo care • Positioning • Developmental care • Massage • Therapeutic touch • PT/OT	• Passive dance • Music therapy
Young children (1-2)	As above	As above; consider variety below	As above	• Rocking, positioning, PT/OT, massage therapeutic touch	As above
Toddlers/ preschoolers (2-6)	As above	• Auditory: music, sing-alongs, ABCs • Visual: pop-up books, puppets, kaleidoscopes, videos, counting tiles, flashlights • Tactile: holding a Spinoza bear/favorite toy, squeezing a Koosh ball and release • Engaging: bubbles/party blowers/pinwheels; use of humor	• Explanations: child and caregiver teaching, therapeutic play • Imagery: magic circle/magic game, stories, use of images familiar to child, storytelling • Relaxation: "Go limp as a rag doll," yawn, "You are blowing your hurt away," "Pretend like you are blowing out your birthday candles," "Choo-choo like a train"	TENS • Heat/cold application • Massage • Therapeutic touch • Healing touch • Accupressure/ acupuncture • PT/OT	• Clown therapy • Dance therapy • Pet therapy • Music therapy
School-age children (7-11)	As above	• Auditory: Sony Walkman music	• Explanation: child, teen, and caregiver teaching	TENS • Heat/cold application	• Clown therapy • Dance therapy
Teenagers (12+)		• Visual: videos, books • Tactile: holding a Spinoza bear/favorite toy, squeezing a Koosh ball and release • Engaging: use of humor	• Imagery/hypnosis • Storytelling • Relaxation/progressive muscle relaxation • Biofeedback training • Modeling • Counseling	• Massage • Therapeutic touch • Healing touch • Accupressure/ acupuncture • PT/OT	• Pet therapy • Art therapy • Music therapy

OT, Occupational therapy; *PT*, physical therapy; *TENS*, transcutaneous nerve stimulation.

PATIENT AND FAMILY EDUCATION

Before a plan of care is developed, children and families require more information regarding pain, pain assessment (including how to use appropriate tools), and pain management. Children and their parents will be able to create an individualized pain management plan (Boxes 11-5 and 11-6). They can help plan an around-the-clock schedule for constant pain and a PRN approach for intermittent pain. If patient-controlled analgesia (PCA) is the treatment of choice, nurses must ensure that the child knows how to use this method. Nonpharmacologic strategies can be used on a trial basis until a plan is individualized for the patient.

For the pediatric trauma patient who has a prolonged hospitalization, creative strategies may need to be changed as the pain management plan must be modified. Self-care strategies should be taught.

NURSING RESPONSIBILITY FOR EFFECTIVE PAIN RELIEF: TEAM APPROACH

The American Pain Society (1999) and AHCPR (1992) have mandated that a team approach be used for pain management driven by "the rights of all children in any institution to receive the best level of pain relief that can be provided safely" (see Box 11-7 for the "Children's Pain Bill of Rights").

BOX 11-5 Family Education

Helping Your Child Cope With Pain

Pain is frightening for children and adults. As a parent, it can be frustrating not knowing if your child is experiencing pain and, if he or she is, what the nature of that pain experience may be. Because each child is unique, many factors, such as the child's age and personality, need to be taken into account.

Helping Your Child Express Feelings

As a parent, you can help your child express what he or she is feeling. Children often need a parent's permission to express what they are feeling. Children will usually respond after the door has been opened for them. Permission can be as simple as asking about their feelings and listening, regardless of the content. It is easier for children to talk about a doll's (or other fictitious character's) hurt than it is to talk about their own. Professionals use tools such as the Eland color scale to solicit pain information. Toys, such as dolls or crayons, and stories can be used to help your child express pain. For example, you can ask your child to show you where the doll is hurting and what makes that hurt go away. You could tell a story about how a child (or animal) goes to the doctor, gets medication (and/or other treatment), and is treated. Allow your creativity to help you facilitate your child's expression of pain.

Reassure and Comfort Your Child

Simple, uncomplicated language is best. Let your child know that you will be there and that everything is being done to help him or her. Never lie to your child. Speaking in an honest and caring way will help ensure that your child will trust and depend on you. Children can become protective of their parents, not wanting their parents to be burdened by their pain. You can redirect your child's need to protect you by having him or her play out this situation in caring for a doll.

Be Consistent

Routine and consistency are very important for children, especially during a time of illness when things can feel out of control. On the other hand, flexibility is essential.

Don't Forget the Siblings!

It is too easy to feel overwhelmed by the child who is in pain, leaving little time for other children. Siblings often feel that they are not getting enough attention and can harbor feelings of resentment and guilt. Make time for your other children so that they feel that their emotional needs are being met. As with your child who is experiencing pain, talk openly and honestly.

- Touch, massage, and rub your child's skin or hold your child's hand.
- Stay with your child or have someone else stay with him or her when you must be away.
- Record your voice or favorite music for your child to hear when he or she must be left alone.
- Approach your child in a calm, comforting way.
- Stimulate other senses (e.g., watch television, blow bubbles).
- Be honest with your child about what is going to happen.

Can My Child Become Addicted to Pain Medicine?

Some parents worry about their child becoming addicted to pain medicine. It is important for you to know the facts about addiction so that your concerns will not result in needless suffering for your child. Drug addiction means that a person is taking a drug to get a mental "high" instead of relief from real pain. Children take pain medicine so that they can function. When children are in pain, they need relief from their pain. Once the pain is gone, the medicine is no longer needed and it is gradually stopped. The truth is that addiction is extremely rare when medicine is taken for pain control.
Note: Feel free at any time to ask questions or share concerns about your child's pain care. Your child's health and well-being is the primary concern.

From James Whitecomb, Riley Hospital for Children, Indiana University Medical Center, Indiana University Medical Center Nursing Services.

BOX 11-6 Pain Management Recipe Care for Pediatric Procedures

Name: ______________________________
Date Developed: ______________________________

Preprocedure

___ 1. Use medical play. ______________________________
___ 2. Tell me what's going to happen. ______________________________
___ 3. Medication(s) that worked best in past; apply EMLA cream. ______________________________
___ 4. Please give me choices (e.g., books, songs, bubbles). ______________________________
___ 5. Parent input: ______________________________

During the Procedure

___ 1. I want this person with me: ______________________________
___ 2. For comfort/distraction/relaxation, I want (e.g., book, song, bubbles, puppet): ______________________________
___ 3. Important points on timing and positioning: ______________________________
___ 4. I don't like this: ______________________________
___ 5. I act like this during a procedure: ______________________________
___ 6. At critical moments, I need this: ______________________________
___ 7. Parent input: ______________________________

Postprocedure

___ 1. Information for parent, guardian, comforter: To comfort me, please (e.g., give me praise, spend time with me, validate my feelings): ______________________________
___ 2. How did it go this time (score on pain intensity scale): ______________________________
___ 3. Things I need after the procedure: ______________________________
___ 4. Gather information from me and my parent(s) on what worked/did not work and make changes on my plan. Thanks.
___ 5. Parent input: ______________________________

Comprehensive Pain Management

Inpatient Unit:

Analgesia Regimen:
Oral ___ PCA ___ Continuous
Infusion ___ Intermittent bolus ___

Pain Scale:

Nonpharmacologic Regimen:

PCA, Patient-controlled analgesia.

Nurses play a crucial role in pain assessment and management through direct patient care and coordination of institutional processes. Clinical nurse specialists and expert pain nurses should participate with other health care team members to research the standard of care; provide individual patient consultation; educate staff, patients, and families; and direct performance improvement efforts.

Ideally, a dedicated multidisciplinary pain management team that includes nurses, physicians, pharmacists, child life specialists, therapists, and social workers should direct the overall program and evaluate institutional standards, in addition to providing patient consultation services. A formal process should be developed in institutions to assess pain management practices and to obtain feedback from children and their parents regarding adequacy of pain management.

Performance improvement procedures should be used routinely to ensure that the following pain management practices are followed: Children and their parents are informed that effective pain relief is an important part of the treatment, communication of unrelieved pain is essential, nurses (and other team members) will respond quickly, and total absence of pain may not always be a realistic goal. Clear

BOX 11-7 Children's Pain Bill of Rights

As a parent, you have a right to do the following:

- Act on behalf of your child
- Have your child's pain prevented or controlled adequately
- Discuss your child's pain history and pain behavior
- Tell what special name for hurt your child uses (such as "boo-boo," "owie," or other)
- Do what comforts your child when he or she is in pain
- Know what kind of pain can be expected and for how long
- Know how pain will be controlled before, during, and after a medical procedure
- Know the risks, benefits, and side effects of pain medications
- Sign a statement of informed consent about a pain plan
- Be with your child before, during, and after a medical procedure
- Be with your child up to and immediately after surgery
- Have a commitment from doctors and nurses to assess your child's pain on a regular basis
- Know who is accountable for your child's pain relief
- Have doctors and nurses use topical and/or local anesthetic before any injections, needlesticks, or invasive procedures
- Have postoperative pain managed aggressively
- Request painless methods of administering medications (oral or intravenous line, instead of injection) (Avoid rectal administration in children older than age 2 years when possible.)
- Have doctors and nurses listen to your assessment of how much pain your child is experiencing
- Remind those who care for your child that pain management is an important part of any diagnostic, medical, or surgical procedure
- Request a second opinion if you feel your child's pain is being poorly managed or if doctors and nurses do not share your concerns about preventing and controlling your child's pain
- Act as an aggressive advocate for your child

Reminders

- You can never assume that your child's pain will be taken care of automatically. You should always ask about pain control.
- Do not assume that if your child has received medication for pain, the pain has been adequately or appropriately treated. Assessment should continue.

From Cowles, J. (1993). *Pain relief: How to say "no" to acute, chronic and cancer pain.* New York: Mastermedia Limited.

documentation exists that pain assessment and management are provided. Pain flow sheets "lead" staff through systematic, developmentally appropriate assessment and evaluation of strategies. There are institution-defined levels for pain intensity and relief, based on the Joint Commission on Accreditation of Healthcare Organizations (JCAHO) and other standards of care. When not followed, a sentinel event review is initiated for pain management team review. Periodically, as defined by their review plan, clinical units should assess a randomly selected sample of children receiving pain management. The assessment process should ensure a review of their current pain intensity, the worst pain intensity in the first 24 hours postoperatively (if applicable), the degree of pain relief obtained from pain management interventions, satisfaction with relief, and children's and parents' satisfaction with the staff's responsiveness (AHCPR, 1992).

Resources must be available to all health care providers caring for children in pain. Standardized references, such as the AHCPR guidelines (AHCPR, 1992), American Pain Society guidelines (1999), and current pediatric medication formulary, should be available for all staff to use.

Nurses are in a pivotal position to coordinate pain management team efforts. It is the responsibility of all health care team members to provide the best, current, individualized pain management for all children in the institution.

SUMMARY

Pediatric trauma patients deserve expert pain management. Nurses need to assess and treat pain early in the admission of a child who has sustained trauma. Nurses require knowledge about research in pediatric pain, such as advances in strategies, new medications and delivery systems, and applicability to children in their practice. The pain management team format is necessary, with recommendations communicated to the trauma team.

The diagnosis of trauma implies that tissue injury has occurred and that pain is part of the child's experience. Pain and anxiety must be addressed throughout the entire continuum of care, admission through discharge, to provide optimal care for the pediatric trauma patient.

BIBLIOGRAPHY

Agency for Health Care Policy and Research. (1992). *Acute pain management in infants, children and adolescents. Quick reference guide for clinicians* (AHCPR Publication No. 92-0020). Rockville, MD: U.S. Department of Health and Human Services.

American Academy of Pediatrics, Committee on Drugs. (1992). Guidelines for monitoring and management of pediatric patients during & after sedation for diagnostic & therapeutic procedures. *Pediatrics, 89*(6 Pt. 1), 1110-1115.

American Pain Society. (1999). Principles of analgesic use in the treatment of acute pain & cancer pain. Glenview, IL: American Pain Society.

Anand, K. J. S. (1996). Developmental neurobiology of pain in neonatal and pediatric I.C.U. patients. In D. Tibboel & E. van der Voort (Eds.), *Intensive care in childhood: A challenge to the Future* (pp. 507-516). Berlin: Springer-Verlag.

Anand, K. J. S., & Carr, D. B. (1989). The neuro anatomy, neuro physiology and neuro chemistry of pain, stress, and analgesia in newborns and children. *Pediatric Clinics of North America, 36*(4), 795-821.

Anand, K. J. S., & Hickey, P. R. (1987) Pain and its effects in the human neonate and fetus. *New England Journal of Medicine, 317,* 1321-1329.

Anand, K. J. S., & Shapiro, B. S. (1993). Pharmacotherapy with systemic analgesics. In K. J. S. Anand & P. S. McGrath (Eds.), *Pain in neonates* (pp. 157-200). London: Elsevier Science.

Anand, K. J. S., & the International Evidence-Based Group for Neonatal Pain. (2001). Consensus statement for the prevention and management of pain in the newborn. *Archives of Pediatric and Adolescent Medicine, 155,* 173-180.

Berde, C. B., Lehn, B. M., Yee, J. D., Sethna, N. F., & Russo, D. (1991). Patient-controlled analgesia in children and adolescents: A randomized prospective comparison with intramuscular administration of morphine for postoperative analgesia. *Journal of Pediatrics, 118,* 460-466.

Beyer, J. (1984). *The Oucher: A user's manual and technical report.* Evanston, IL: The Hospital Play.

Blanchard, N. (1998). *Children's Hospital and Regional Medical Center's formulary of medications* (4th ed.). Hudson, OH: Lexi-Comp. Inc.

Curley, M. A. Q., McDermott, B., Berry, P., Hurley, J., Mackey, C., McAleer, D., & Alsip, C. (1992). Nurses' decision making regarding the use of sedatives and analgesics in pediatric ICU. *Heart and Lung, 21*(3), 296.

Eland, J. (1983). Children's pain: Developmentally appropriate efforts to improve identification of source, intensity, and relevant intervening variables. In G. Feldon & M. Alberts (Eds.), *Nursing research: A monograph for non-nurse researchers.* Iowa City: University of Iowa.

Eland, J., & Anderson, J. E. (1977). The experience of pain in children. *Pain: A sourcebook for nurses and other health professionals.* Boston: Little, Brown

Elliott, C. H., & Olson, R. A. (1983). The management of children's distress in response to painful medical treatment for burn injuries. *Behavioral Research and Therapy, 21,* 675-683.

Finnegan, L. P., Connaughton, J. F., Jr., Kron, R. E., & Emich, J. P. (1975). Neonatal abstinence syndrome: Assessment and management. *Addiction Diseases, 2*(2-1), 141-158.

Foster, R. L. (1996). Pain management. *Journal of the Society of Pediatric Nursing, 1*(2), 93-94.

Gaffney, A., & Dunne, E. A. (1987). Children's understanding of the causality of pain. *Pain, 29,* 91-104.

Hester, N. O. (1979). The preoperational child's reaction to immunization. *Nursing Research, 28,* 250-254.

Hurley, A., & Whalen, E. G. (1988). Cognitive development and children's perception of pain. *Pediatric Nursing, 14*(1), 21-24.

Kavanaugh, C. (1983). A new approach to dressing change in the severely burned child and its effects on burn-related psychopathology. *Heart and Lung, 12,* 612-619.

Lynn, A. M., & Slattery, J. T. (1987). Morphine pharmacokinetics in early infancy. *Anesthesiology, 66,* 136-139.

McCaffery, M., & Beebe, A (1989). *Pain: Clinical manual for nursing practice.* St. Louis: Mosby.

McGrath, P. A. (1990). *Pain in children: Assessment and treatment.* New York: Guilford.

Melzack, R., & Wall, P. (1965). Pain mechanisms: A new theory. *Science, 150,* 971-979.

Oakes, L. L. (2001). Caring practices: Providing comfort. In M. A. Q. Curley & P. A. Moloney-Harmon (Eds.), *Critical care nursing of infants and children* (2nd ed., pp. 547-576). Philadelphia: WB Saunders.

O'Hara, D. A., Fragen, R. J., Kinzer, M., & Pemberton, D. (1987). Ketorolac tromethamine as compared with morphine sulfate for treatment of postoperative pain. *Clinical Pharmacology and Therapeutics, 41*(5), 556-561.

Purcell-Jones, G., Norman, F., & Sumner, E. (1987). The use of opioids in neonates. A retrospective study of 933 cases. *Anesthesia, 42,* 1316-1320.

Sanedra, M. C., Tesler, M. D., Holzema, W. L., & Ward, J. A. (1992). *Adolescent pediatric pain tool (APPT).* San Francisco: University of California, San Francisco.

Schechter, N. L. (1989). The under treatment of pain in children: An overview. *Pediatric Clinics of North America, 36*(4), 781-794.

Schechter, N. L., Allen, D. A., & Hanson, K. (1986). Status of pediatric pain control: a comparison of hospital analgesic usage in children and adults. *Pediatrics, 77*(1), 11-15.

Smith, J. B., & Martin, S. A. (2001). Caring practice: Providing developmentally supportive care. In M. A. Q. Curley & P. A. Moloney-Harmon (Eds.), *Critical care nursing of infants & children* (2nd ed., pp. 17-46). Philadelphia: WB Saunders.

Wong, D. L., & Hess, C. S. (2000). *Wong and Whaley's clinical manual of pediatric nursing* (5th ed.). St. Louis: Mosby.

World Health Organization Expert Committee. (1990). *Cancer pain relief and palliative care.* Geneva, Switzerland: World Health Organization.

Yaster, M., Krane, E. J., Kaplan, R. F., Cote, C. J., & Lappe, D. G. (1997). *Pediatric pain management and sedation handbook.* St. Louis: Mosby.

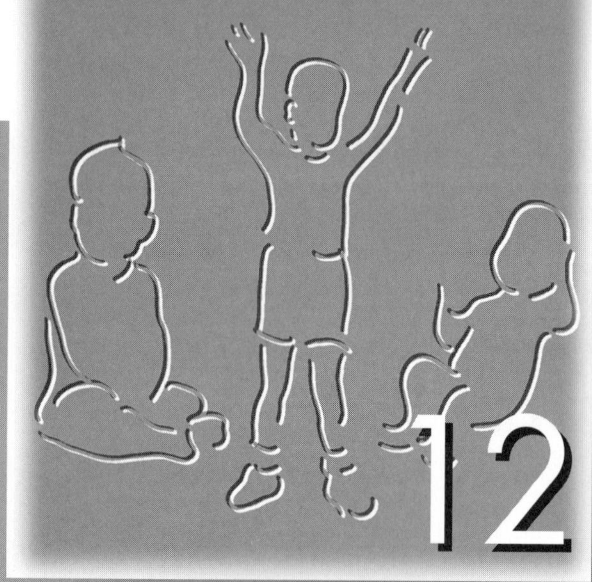

12 Nutritional Support of the Pediatric Trauma Patient

Jennifer Thorpe • Rosemary Eikov

Nutritional support is a key component in the care of the pediatric trauma patient. The small size, rapid growth, low calorie reserve, and varied fluid requirements of children can make the provision of nutritional support seem like an unruly task. However, research has clearly shown multiple benefits of aggressive nutritional support for children of all ages who have sustained a traumatic injury. It is well documented in nursing and medical literature that traumatic injury sets in motion a metabolic response that leads the patient to a hypermetabolic and hypercatabolic state. Without appropriate nutritional support, patients in this state may suffer from malnutrition, delayed wound healing, immune deficiency, prolonged recovery, multisystem organ failure, and increased morbidity and mortality (Pollack Wiley, Kanter, & Holbrook, 1982; Wesley & Coran, 1995).

In this era of advanced technology, it is hard to believe that any patient could suffer the effects of poor nutrition, yet a variety of studies done in pediatric tertiary care centers show that malnutrition is a reality in critical care settings (Pollack et al., 1982). Young children are at increased risk for developing iatrogenic malnutrition because of their higher metabolic rates, which can lead to more rapid utilization and depletion of energy substrates (Ford, 1996).

This chapter assists the nurse in identifying and preventing nutritional problems in pediatric trauma patients. Nurses will gain the knowledge to improve assessment and management of the nutritional needs of the pediatric patients who are most affected by trauma: teenagers, young children, and toddlers.

METABOLIC RESPONSE TO INJURY

Injury and stress impose great metabolic demands on the body. A sequence of hormonal responses after injury causes dramatic changes in protein and carbohydrate metabolism as the body instinctively tries to limit further injury, heal wounds, prevent infection, and restore hemodynamic stability (Buckley & Kudsk, 1994).

Phases of the Metabolic Response to Injury

Two distinct postinjury phases—the "ebb" phase and the "flow" phase—were first described by biochemist David Cuthbertson nearly 70 years ago (Hill & Hill, 1998). The ebb phase, or the immediate, postinjury phase, is characterized by an initial hypometabolic response. Catecholamine, glucocorticoid, antidiuretic hormone, and mineralocorticoid levels rise; cardiac output drops; tissue perfusion and core body temperature decrease; and water is retained (Hill & Hill, 1998; Wesley & Coran, 1995). After resuscitation and hemodynamic stabilization, the patient enters the flow phase, which is characterized by a hypermetabolic state. Cardiac output and core body temperature increase, insulin levels rise, protein catabolism occurs at a tremendous rate, and tissue perfusion begins to return to normal (Hill & Hill, 1998).

Scientists since Cuthbertson's time have attempted to further define this cascade of events, subdividing the flow phase into a catabolic phase and an anabolic phase (Rogers & Lobe, 1995). The anabolic phase is marked by protein synthesis and a gradual return to positive nitrogen balance (Wesley & Coran, 1995). Regardless of the terminology used to classify phases of the metabolic response to injury, the cascade of events is the same, and the extent of the response depends on the severity of the injury (Buckley & Kudsk, 1994; Wesley & Coran, 1995).

The patient's preexisting nutritional status may affect the metabolic response (Rogers & Lobe, 1995). Because young children and rapidly growing adolescents have less fatty tissue than adults, they have proportionately fewer fat stores (Wesley & Coran, 1995). This causes a greater degree of protein catabolism to occur in children to meet increased energy demands after trauma (Rogers & Lobe, 1995). Lipolysis occurs throughout the metabolic response to injury, and in the face of inadequate nutritional support, stored body fat can become a major fuel source in a trauma patient (Hill & Hill, 1998; Rogers & Lobe, 1995). Restoration of fat stores occurs later in the anabolic recovery phase (Rogers & Lobe, 1995).

DETERMINING REQUIREMENTS

Trauma victims are rarely able to eat or drink enough to meet the increased energy demands of the flow phase. The injured body quickly uses up any available glucose, including that from glycogen stores, while supporting itself immediately after sustaining an injury (Wesley & Coran, 1995). Once all available glucose and glycogen stores are used up, generally after approximately 24 hours, the body will begin to break down stores of fat and protein to preserve lean body mass (Buckley & Kudsk, 1994). This breakdown will ultimately have a direct effect on the immune system and muscle function (Wesley & Coran, 1995). Although a previously healthy child can theoretically withstand a deficit in calorie intake for 3 to 7 days, initiation of nutritional support should not be delayed (Wesley & Coran, 1995). The negative effects of limited protein and calorie intake on an injured body in a hypermetabolic state can readily be seen. Signs and symptoms include increased muscle weakness, impaired immune function, poor wound healing, unstable cardiac output, and problematic respiratory function or difficulty weaning from the ventilator (Pollack et al., 1982). To ensure positive outcomes for pediatric trauma patients, nurses must be vigilant in preventing malnutrition. Their input into both planning and monitoring the effectiveness of nutrition interventions is essential.

FLUID REQUIREMENTS

WATER

Infants and small children have a higher proportion of body mass as water (70% to 75% of body weight) than do adults (60% to 65% of body weight); therefore they have greater fluid requirements (Wesley & Coran, 1995). Increased energy expenditure due to stress, the hypermetabolic state, and fever also increase fluid needs (Ford, 1996).

LOSSES

Fluid losses must be considered. In a healthy state approximately 50% of water is excreted via the kidney, 3% to 10% is lost via the gastrointestinal tract, and the remaining proportion (40% to 50%) is lost insensibly (Wesley & Coran, 1995). Table 12-1 lists equations for calculating a child's fluid needs.

TABLE 12-1 Fluid Requirements

Weight (kg)	Fluid Requirements
1-10	100 ml/kg
10-20	1000 ml + 50 ml/kg over 10 kg
>20	1500 ml + 20 ml/kg over 20 kg

ENERGY REQUIREMENTS

DETERMINING CALORIE NEEDS

Once the child's fluid needs have been determined, calorie goals may be established to meet the child's needs for healing and for the maintenance of body functions. It is important to remember that children have higher energy demands than adults because of their periods of rapid growth or extreme physical activity (Wesley & Coran, 1995). However, during stress the calories normally required for growth may be shifted to support the metabolic response, and growth will not occur until the child is recovering (Ford, 1996). Calorie goals should be reevaluated periodically as the child progresses through the phases of the metabolic response to injury from a catabolic state to an anabolic recovery to prevent underfeeding or overfeeding (Trocki, 1993).

A variety of methods are used to calculate the caloric needs of infants and children. They all provide an estimate of calorie needs to use in developing a nutrition care plan, but they should not be viewed as absolute requirements. Ongoing monitoring of the child's weight and overall nutritional status is necessary so that goals can be adjusted on the basis of clinical outcomes.

METHODS FOR ESTIMATING ENERGY REQUIREMENTS

Recommended Dietary Allowances. One method commonly used to determine a healthy child's energy and protein requirements is the recommended dietary allowances (RDA), which were established by the National Research Council in 1989 and differ for age and gender. Energy recommendations provided by the RDA are derived from longitudinal intake data and represent average energy intake for appropriate growth in healthy individuals.

Because the RDA recommendations are for healthy individuals rather than sick children, they may not present an accurate estimate of a child's posttrauma energy needs. Adjustments may be needed to maintain an appropriate rate of weight gain or growth in a sick child. Such adjustments should account for the patient's current nutritional state, activity level, and effect of traumatic injury. Use of the RDAs to determine energy needs may be more appropriate in the final stages of rehabilitation. Table 12-2 lists the RDAs for energy intake in children.

The World Health Organization Equations. The World Health Organization's (WHO) prediction equations provide an estimate of the child's resting energy expenditure (REE) or, more simply stated, what the healthy body needs at rest. For children older than 1 year, the WHO recommendations have proven to be reliable determinants of energy needs for healthy, nonobese children. Table 12-3 lists the WHO equations for calculating REE.

Once the REE has been calculated, total calorie needs can be estimated by multiplying the REE by additional factors that represent additional stresses affecting the child's total energy expenditure. These factors include fever, injury, activity, growth, nursing care activities, and some medications. Box 12-1 lists commonly used activity and stress factors.

Schofield Height/Weight Method. For obese children the Schofield height/weight prediction equations may predict REE more accurately. These equations take into account the greater proportion of the body mass as fat, which is not metabolically active. Table 12-4 specifies the Schofield method for estimating REE in obese children.

Indirect Calorimetry. Indirect calorimetry offers a significant advantage over the use of prediction equations to estimate energy needs in a trauma patient. An indirect calorimeter, commonly referred to as a *metabolic cart,* directly measures a patient's oxygen consumption and carbon dioxide production. From this information the REE can be calculated and expressed in terms of kilocalories per day.

In a trauma patient whose metabolic demands are changing rapidly, indirect calorimetry eliminates the guesswork in trying to determine energy needs. However, this measurement is best obtained in a standardized setting, with a patient who is awake and resting, who has undergone an 8- to 12-hour fast, who has not done any physical activity, and who has not received any medications known to change the heart rate (Stallings, 1998). Accuracy of the measurement may be affected because the trauma setting and circumstances may not be optimal for obtaining a measurement. In addition, performing a metabolic cart study on a trauma patient who receives mechanical ventilation may pose even more of a challenge because of abnormal ventilatory patterns, elevated oxygen concentrations, humidification, and air leaks (Weissman & Kemper, 1995). Interpretation of these measurements in trauma patients should include critical comparison to the clinical condition of the patient and recent nutrient intake (Weissman & Kemper, 1995).

TABLE 12-2 **Recommended Dietary Allowances for Energy and Protein Intake in Children**

Gender	Age	kcal/kg	Grams Protein/kg
Male and female	0-6 mo	108	2.2
	6-12 mo	98	1.6
	1-3 yr	102	1.2
	4-6 yr	90	1.1
	7-10 yr	70	1.0
Male	11-14 yr	55	1.0
	15-18 yr	45	0.9
Female	11-14 yr	47	1.0
	15-18 yr	40	0.8

Modified from National Research Council. (1989). *Recommended dietary allowances* (10th ed.). Washington, DC: National Academy Press.

Protein Requirements

Protein Metabolism

In normal protein metabolism, the ongoing excretion of nitrogen is matched by protein intake (Wesley & Coran, 1995). Protein synthesis and breakdown occur simultaneously; this protein flux is measured as nitrogen balance. During trauma or any stressed state, the rate of protein catabolism increases while intake is drastically reduced (Wesley & Coran, 1995). Once glucose and glycogen stores have been exhausted, the body in effect "cannibalizes" itself by breaking down skeletal muscle to provide the fuels necessary to survive (Buckley & Kudsk, 1994). This leads to negative nitrogen balance.

When a patient is in negative nitrogen balance, protein synthesis does not stop. In fact, the synthesis of antibodies, new cells, coagulation factors, and other biologic proteins occurs at an accelerated-rate. The negative balance simply arises from an inability to match destruction with synthesis (Rogers & Lobe, 1995). A critical goal of early nutritional support of a trauma patient is to provide a balanced and sufficient energy source to minimize catabolism of lean body mass (Wesley & Coran, 1995).

The specific amino acid content of proteins given to infants and children is important. Essential amino acids are those that cannot be produced by the body and therefore must be supplied daily to the patient. There are eight essential amino acids for infants and children: threonine, leucine, isoleucine, valine, lysine, methionine, phenylalanine, tryptophan, and histidine (essential in infancy). The amino acids tyrosine and cysteine are regarded as conditionally essential amino acids in premature infants (Wesley & Coran, 1995). All essential amino acids must be present simultaneously if new tissue is to be formed.

TABLE 12-3 **World Health Organization Method for Estimating Resting Energy Expenditure (kcal/day) in Children**

	Age (yr)			
	0-3	3-10	10-18	18-30
Male	60.9 W – 54	22.7 W + 495	17.5 W + 651	15.3 W + 679
Female	61.0 W – 51	22.5 W + 499	12.2 W + 746	14.7 W + 496

Modified from World Health Organization. (1985). Energy and protein requirements: Report of a Joint FAO/WHO/UNU Expert Consultation (WHO Technical Report Series No. 724). Geneva: Author.

W, Weight in kilograms.

The absence of any essential amino acid can lead to negative nitrogen balance (Wesley & Coran, 1995).

Protein provides the body with approximately 4.0 kcal/g and 4.5 kcal/L of oxygen consumed; this gives it a respiratory quotient (RQ) of 0.8 (Wesley & Coran, 1995). The RQ is the ratio of carbon dioxide produced to oxygen consumed. It is particularly important to consider RQ when planning nutritional support for patients with respiratory problems.

Methods for Determining Protein Needs

Recommended Dietary Allowances. The RDA for protein is determined to be the minimum amount needed to maintain nitrogen balance in all growing, healthy individuals. It also accounts for varying protein requirements, adding a degree of safety for those with special dietary needs. Adjustments may need to be made when determining optimal protein intake for traumatized children; increased protein may be needed to account for exogenous protein losses, and conversely, protein restrictions may be needed if renal or hepatic function is impaired. See Table 12-2 for the RDAs for protein intake in children.

Nitrogen Balance Studies. Nitrogen balance studies are the most accurate method for determining the adequacy of protein intake (Skipper, 1989). Nitrogen balance can be calculated as follows:

$$N_2 \text{ balance} = N_2 \text{ intake} - N_2 \text{ excretion}$$

where N_2 *intake* equals protein intake (in grams)/6.25 and N_2 *excretion* equals 24-hour urine urea nitrogen (UUN) + 4 (4 estimates N_2 losses in unmeasured fluids).

Most daily nitrogen is lost in the urine as UUN; however, under normal circumstances a small amount is also lost through the skin and feces (Skipper, 1989). Additional losses may occur in the trauma patient who has open wounds, draining chest tubes or fistulas, or diarrhea. For practical purposes in a clinical setting, typically only urinary nitrogen loss is measured (Trocki, 1993).

Accuracy of a nitrogen balance study depends on accurate urine collection, which may be difficult in a young child in diapers (Skipper, 1989). Although appropriate for children with various types of traumatic injury, a nitrogen balance study is not a reliable or practical tool in children with burns because of the difficulty of determining nitrogen losses in burn wound exudates (Trocki, 1993).

Carbohydrate Requirements

Carbohydrates are the most important energy source in the metabolically stressed patient but often the source in shortest supply (Wesley & Coran, 1995). Carbohydrate supplies approximately 4.0 kcal/g. Because a child's liver and skeletal muscle mass are proportionally smaller than those of an adult, carbohydrate reserves (primarily glycogen) are significantly smaller in children (Wesley & Coran, 1995). Glycogen is converted to glucose in the liver and is then metabolized aerobically or anaerobically throughout the body. Aerobic metabolism, which produces carbon monoxide and water, requires 1 L of oxygen for each 5 kcal produced to give off equal amounts of carbon dioxide, yielding an RQ of 1.0 (Wesley & Coran, 1995). A nutritional support regimen that is high in carbohydrate will yield a higher RQ, which may greatly affect a patient's ability to be weaned from respiratory support.

In the altered hormonal state of the metabolic response to injury, neuroendocrine mediators are released, which have an antiinsulin effect, increasing gluconeogenesis and glycogenolysis and in turn creating hyperglycemia. Peripheral cell uptake of glucose is unchanged, but insulin resistance increases (Rogers & Lobe, 1995; Skipper, 1989). Trauma patients then may exhibit higher blood glucose levels, even while they are receiving relatively low concentrations of intravenous glucose.

Fat Requirements

Infants and young children have higher needs for fat than adults to support their rapid growth and development and the need for nerve sheath myelinization (Wesley & Coran, 1995). In infants and young children, 35% to 50% of total calories should come from fat. The need for fat decreases with age.

BOX 12-1 Activity/Stress Adjustment Factors

REE × 1.3

For a well-nourished child at bed rest with mild to moderate stress (minor surgery)

REE × 1.5

For a normally active child with mild to moderate stress, an inactive child with severe stress (e.g., trauma, sepsis, cancer, extensive surgery), or a child with minimal activity and malnutrition requiring catch-up growth

REE × 1.7

For an active child requiring catch-up growth or an active child with severe stress

REE, Resting energy expenditure.

TABLE 12-4 Schofield Equations for Predicting Resting Energy Expenditure in Obese Children

Gender	Age (yr)	ccal/day
Male	0-3	0.1673 W + 1517.4 H – 617.6
	3-10	19.598 W + 130.3 H + 414.9
	10-18	16.252 W + 137.2 H – 515.5
	>18	15.057 W – 10.04 H + 705.8
Female	0-3	16.252 W + 1023.2 H – 413.5
	3-10	16.969 W + 161.8 H + 371.2
	10-18	08.365 W + 465.6 H + 200.0
	>18	13.623 W + 283.0 H + 98.2

Modified from Schofield, W. N. (1985). Predicting basal metabolic rate, new standards and review of previous work. *Human Nutrition 39C*(Suppl. 1), 5-42.

H, Height in meters; *W,* weight in kilograms.

Fat provides a substantial source of calories. It provides 9 kcal/g and 4.7 kcal/L of oxygen consumed, yielding an RQ of 0.7, the lowest of the three energy sources (Wesley & Coran, 1995). Because of its low RQ, fat can be an especially important nutrient for patients with impending respiratory failure or those who are having difficulty being weaned from a ventilator.

Essential fatty acids are those that cannot be produced by the body and therefore must be supplied daily to the patient. To prevent essential fatty acid deficiency, it is recommended that 2% to 4% of total daily calories be provided as the essential fatty acid linoleic acid. Essential fatty acid deficiency is characterized by hair loss; mental status changes; and a dry, flaky, erythematous skin rash (Wesley & Coran, 1995).

Electrolyte, Vitamin, Mineral, and Trace Element Requirements

Micronutrients play an important role in a well-balanced nutrition regimen. Vitamins, minerals, and trace elements are the cofactors that help achieve anabolism. An adequate supply of electrolytes is vital; in particular, potassium, calcium, magnesium, and phosphorus are utilized in increased amounts during tissue anabolism (Wesley & Coran, 1995). One important difference between pediatric and adult trauma patients is that infants and young children have a more significant negative calcium and phosphorus balance because of their rapidly growing skeleton (Wesley & Coran, 1995). For this reason, providing adequate amounts of these nutrients is crucial to the growing infant.

Because of their small size yet high metabolic demands, infants and young children require more vitamins per kilogram of body weight than do adults (Trocki, 1993; Wesley & Coran, 1995). Hypermetabolic patients catabolize vitamins more rapidly than do normal healthy children (Wesley & Coran, 1995). A stressed or injured child may develop deficiencies of the fat-soluble vitamins A, D, E, and K and the water-soluble vitamins B, C, and folic acid if sufficient amounts are not provided in the nutritional support regimen.

Trace elements are important components of a balanced nutritional support regimen. Trace elements with known metabolic functions include zinc, copper, fluoride, chromium, manganese, and selenium (Ford, 1996; Wesley & Coran, 1995).

Guidelines for vitamin, mineral, and trace element supplementation have been established for children who have sustained burns but not for other types of trauma (Trocki, 1993). The RDAs provide guidance in determining appropriate vitamin, mineral, and trace element intakes.

NUTRITION ASSESSMENT OF THE PEDIATRIC TRAUMA PATIENT

Thorough assessment of the child's nutritional status and identification of risk factors for malnutrition are critical to the development of an appropriate nutritional support regimen. Nutrition assessment includes many elements and should begin immediately after resuscitation and stabilization of the patient.

Physical Assessment

Every child who has sustained a traumatic injury should have his or her growth parameters plotted on a growth chart upon admission to the hospital. An accurately plotted growth chart can serve as a valuable baseline assessment tool that is helpful in setting short- and long-term nutritional support goals; it also serves as a reference against which to gauge progress made in meeting nutrition goals during recovery (Trocki, 1993).

Weight

Baseline weights of trauma patients are often estimated in the field for medical purposes before the child's arrival to the hospital; therefore they may be unreliable measures of the child's usual, preinjury weight. An actual measure of the child's weight should be obtained upon admission to the intensive care unit (ICU) so that medications can be appropriately dosed and to serve as a baseline for monitoring fluid shifts and edema. Because of the critical and intense nature of the child's first few hours in the ICU, the baseline weight measurement is apt to be overlooked. When possible, bed scales should be zeroed before the child's arrival to the ICU to facilitate future weight measurements. The child's usual, preinjury weight should be documented for reference.

Length/Height

A measurement of the child's standing height (or recumbent length, for infants younger than 36 months) should be included in the baseline nutrition assessment, with close attention paid so that the appropriate growth chart is used. National Center for Health Statistics (NCHS) growth charts for children from birth through age 36 months use recumbent length. NCHS growth charts for children aged 2 to 18 years use standing height. Height measurements are apt to be overlooked or cannot be measured upon admission to the ICU, depending on the nature and extent of the child's injury.

When a height measurement cannot be obtained, alternative measurements, such as upper arm and lower leg lengths, may lend insight into the child's linear growth; however, such measurements require that the child be stable enough to be manipulated for proper positioning. The pediatric registered dietitian is trained to obtain and interpret such alternative height measurements. Contacting the child's primary pediatrician for a copy of the child's growth chart may provide information about the child's pretrauma growth and overall nutrition status.

Weight for Height

Comparison of the child's preinjury weight for height serves as a useful measure of the degree of preexisting malnutrition or obesity. It can be plotted on the reverse of the NCHS growth chart using measured or reported weight and height measurements.

Head Circumference

Head circumference should be measured and plotted on the growth chart for all children younger than 36 months unless the injury or presence of head wound dressings precludes accurate measurement. A valuable indicator of brain growth, head circumference measurements are also useful in monitoring for hydrocephalus.

Arm Anthropometry

Arm anthropometric measurements, such as triceps skinfold and midarm circumference, may reveal the adequacy of the child's pretrauma fat and muscle reserves, respectively, and may be helpful assessment tools to determine trends in changes in body composition throughout the course of recovery. These measurements, which can also be obtained by a pediatric registered dietitian, require the child to be able to sit upright for proper positioning, which often is difficult for a critically ill child. Such measurements are subject to alterations in the presence of total body edema and therefore may not be the most sensitive nutritional markers in the immediate, postinjury phase.

Laboratory Assessment

Serum protein levels can be used to lend insight into the trauma victim's nutritional status after injury and throughout recovery. Low levels may indicate inadequate provision of protein or total calories.

Albumin

Albumin functions as a carrier protein for multiple elements and is needed to maintain serum oncotic pressure. Serum albumin levels correlate to the degree of malnutrition present, but its half-life is approximately 20 days, which makes it a relatively insensitive indicator of acute changes in nutritional status and a more appropriate indicator of long-term nutritional status. Low serum albumin levels can be seen in a variety of conditions, including metabolic stress and infection.

Transferrin

Transferrin acts as a carrier protein for iron. It may be more sensitive to acute changes in nutritional status than albumin. In addition, it has a shorter half-life (8 to 10 days) than albumin; however, like albumin, decreased transferrin levels may be seen in acute catabolic states.

Thyroxine-Binding Prealbumin

More commonly referred to simply as *prealbumin,* thyroxine-binding prealbumin is a more sensitive indicator of acute changes in nutritional status because of its short half-life of 2 to 3 days. Although its name suggests it is related to albumin, prealbumin is not directly related to albumin. Instead, prealbumin functions as a carrier protein for retinol-binding protein and as a transport protein for thyroxine. Decreased levels can be expected in acute catabolic states, after surgery, and with infection. Falsely elevated levels are seen with renal dysfunction or failure.

Retinol-Binding Protein

Retinol-binding protein (RBP) acts to transport retinol, the alcohol of vitamin A. RBP has a short half-life of approximately 12 hours; however, low levels can be expected in acute catabolic states and after surgery. As with prealbumin, falsely elevated RBP levels are seen with renal dysfunction or failure.

Visual Assessment

Visual assessment of the child is another important component of the nutrition assessment because signs of preexisting malnutrition may be detected. A thorough review of the child's skin, hair, nails, teeth, and gums may signal the presence of preexisting vitamin and mineral deficiencies that will require special attention to replete. The child who is a victim of abuse and neglect may manifest such preexisting nutritional deficits. Table 12-5 lists the visible signs and symptoms of micronutrient deficiencies.

Ongoing visual reassessment for micronutrient deficiencies during recovery should not be overlooked. Suspicion of micronutrient deficiencies may, in some cases, be confirmed with a serum micronutrient level. Recovery from trauma marks a time of increased energy, protein, and micronutrient demands to promote tissue repair, wound healing, and the restoration of blood volume and organ function. The child with multiple trauma or burns who appears, upon baseline nutritional assessment, to have been previously well nourished is not exempt from developing such deficiencies in the hospital. Inadequate nutrition repletion, increased micronutrient needs during recovery, and type of injury sustained predispose the child to further risk of vitamin and mineral deficiencies. For example, the child who has sustained burns has increased requirements for supplemental vitamins A and C and zinc, in addition to daily multivitamin supplementation (Gottschlich, 1993; Trocki, 1993). The child with extensive abdominal trauma who requires resection and removal of portions of the small bowel may be at risk for fluid and electrolyte imbalances, steatorrhea, and malabsorption of a variety of vitamins and minerals, depending on the location and extent of the bowel resection (Jeejeebhoy, 1994).

Diet History

A thorough diet history should be obtained from the parent or caregiver. The presence of food allergies; special dietary practices, such as vegetarianism; or religious affiliations associated with special dietary practices, such as kosher in the Jewish faith or pork restrictions in the Muslim faith, will remain special considerations throughout the child's recovery. Such factors may directly affect the type of formula or supplement chosen to augment the child's oral intake. Notation of the child's food preferences, likes, and dislikes may be of great assistance in boosting oral intake when it becomes appropriate to transition back to oral feeds. Quantification of usual intake, methods of food or formula preparation, use of nutritional or herbal supplements, and unusual dietary

TABLE 12-5 Visible Signs of Nutrient Deficiencies

	Clinical Findings	Deficiency
Hair	Alopecia, dry, easily pluckable, brittle, sparse; dyspigmentation; flag sign	Protein-energy malnutrition (PEM); biotin, PEM; protein
Skin	Xerosis, follicular hyperkeratosis; perifollicular petechiae; dermatitis; nasolabial seborrhea	Vitamin A, essential fatty acids; vitamin C; vitamin K; niacin; riboflavin; vitamin B_6
Eyes	Xerophthalmia, Bitot spots, night blindness; angular palpebritis	Vitamin A; riboflavin
Lips	Cheilosis; angular stomatitis	Niacin, riboflavin, vitamin B_6, iron
Gums	Bleeding, spongy	Vitamin C
Tongue	Magenta tongue; atrophic papillae; glossitis	Riboflavin; iron, niacin, folate, vitamin B_{12}, vitamin B_6
Nails	Koilonychia	Iron
Subcutaneous tissue	Edema	PEM, thiamine
Musculoskeletal system	Muscle wasting; bowlegs; beading of ribs	PEM; vitamin D, calcium

Data from Hopkins, B. (1993). Assessment of nutritional status. In M. Gottschlich, L. Matarese, & E. Shronts (Eds.), *Nutrition support dietetics core curriculum* (2nd ed.). Silver Spring: American Society for Parenteral and Enteral Nutrition.

BOX 12-2 Diet-Related Questionnaire

Sample Questions for Nurses to Ask About a Child's Diet History

1. Does the child have any food allergies or intolerances?
   - If so, what type of reaction does he or she exhibit for each food?
2. Does the child follow any special dietary restrictions or practices at home? Please describe what foods the child may or may not have.
3. Does the child take any nutritional, herbal, or multivitamin supplements at home? Please describe.
4. Has the child recently gained or lost weight?
   - If so, how much weight was gained or lost and over what time period?
5. Does your child require assistance with oral feeding? Please describe what type of assistance is needed.
6. Does your child drink from a bottle or a cup? (for infants and toddlers)
7. Does your child have difficulty chewing or swallowing?
8. Please describe your child's usual meal pattern. (Note volume and formula concentrations for infants.) Examples: 3 meals/day; 1 snack/day; 8-oz bottle every 4 hours; 3 meals/day plus tube feedings over 10 hr at night.
9. Tell me a few of your child's
   - Favorite foods
   - Least favorite foods

practices at home can lend insight into the child's preinjury nutritional status, appropriateness of diet, and developmental level. Particularly in cases where abuse or neglect is suspected, inconsistencies between the child's physical appearance (e.g., malnutrition, overnutrition, visible signs of nutrient deficiencies) and the caregiver's report of the child's diet history warrant further investigation. Box 12-2 lists some sample questions that nurses should ask about the child's diet upon the child's admission to the ICU.

PARENTERAL NUTRITION

Although the enteral route is the preferred route for feeding trauma patients, parenteral nutrition should be considered for the nutritional support of pediatric trauma patients when the child's injuries and/or the severity of the child's condition preclude the ability to provide full enteral support (Cox & Cooning, 1993). Advances in technology and research have helped improve the safety of nutritional support via the parenteral route.

Intravenous Access

Peripheral Lines

Parenteral nutrition can be administered through either a peripherally placed catheter or a centrally placed catheter. Use of a peripheral catheter to infuse parenteral nutrition limits the concentration of dextrose that can be provided because the risk of venous thrombosis increases with the higher osmolalities that are associated with dextrose concentrations greater than 10% (Ford, 1996). Lower dextrose concentrations, in turn, limit the ability to meet the increased energy and protein demands of the trauma patient, which is further exacerbated by fluid restrictions (Cox & Cooning, 1993).

Central Lines

Use of a centrally placed catheter for administration of parenteral nutrition allows for infusion of solutions of greater concentration, which results in an improved ability to meet increased energy and protein needs. Administration of parenteral nutrition through a central catheter, however, carries the increased risk of line sepsis, an important consideration in the trauma patient whose immune function is already compromised. Peripherally inserted central catheters (PICCs) offer a substantial alternative for parenteral nutrition administration. PICCs can be inserted at the bedside of most trauma patients, much like a peripheral catheter. The

PICC line can be threaded into a larger vessel so that the tip ends at the superior vena cava for safe delivery of concentrated parenteral nutrition solutions (Goodwin & Carlson, 1993). A PICC line reduces the risk of venous thrombosis associated with peripherally administered parenteral nutrition. PICC lines can remain in place for longer durations than peripheral catheters but do not have the surgical risk associated with traditional, surgically placed central catheters.

Composition of Solutions

Parenteral nutrition solutions are composed of carbohydrate, protein, fat, fluid, electrolytes, vitamins, minerals, and trace elements.

Carbohydrate

Carbohydrate in parenteral nutrition solutions is provided in the form of dextrose monohydrate, which provides 3.4 kcal/g (Cox & Cooning, 1993). A desirable macronutrient balance is achieved when 50% to 60% of the total calories are provided by carbohydrates.

In general, carbohydrate in parenteral nutrition is started with a 10% dextrose concentration and gradually increased as tolerated to goal concentration. Patients who receive parenteral nutrition through a peripheral line should not receive greater than 10% to 12.5% dextrose concentrations because of increased risk of venous thrombosis with higher osmolality solutions.

Attention must be paid to the patient's glucose tolerance, particularly in stressed patients who are at increased risk for hyperglycemia. Calculation of the glucose infusion rate (GIR), which expresses carbohydrate administration in terms of milligrams per kilogram body weight per minute (mg/kg/min), is useful in monitoring tolerance (Skipper, 1989). A normal GIR for an adult is 4 to 6 mg/kg/min. Young children often require and can tolerate a GIR as high as 12 to 14 mg/kg/min (Lee & Werlin, 1997). Symptoms of hyperglycemia during infusion of parenteral nutrition include glucosuria, elevated blood glucose levels, and excessive urination. Abrupt cessation of concentrated parenteral nutrition solutions can result in rebound hypoglycemia; therefore it is advised to gradually taper parenteral nutrition solutions with a concentration greater than 10% or simply continue a dextrose-containing stock intravenous fluid.

Protein

Protein in parenteral nutrition solutions is provided in the form of crystalline amino acid solutions and provides 4.0 kcal/g. Standard amino acid solutions provide sufficient quantities of essential amino acids to allow for normal protein synthesis. TrophAmine is a standard amino acid solution formulated for infants younger than 6 months. It contains tyrosine and histidine, which are conditionally essential amino acids in infancy, as well as taurine, which may be conditionally essential in premature infants. Novamine and Aminosyn are formulated for infants and children older than 6 months and contain appropriate essential and nonessential amino acids necessary for normal growth in children (Mascarenhas & McCoy, 1998).

Specialized amino acid solutions are available for adult patients with chronic renal failure and hepatic failure, conditions associated with preferential amino acid requirements. The effectiveness of these solutions in young children has not been well studied, however. Specialized amino acid formulations are also available for patients with inborn errors of metabolism. Protein is recommended to comprise 10% to 15% of the total calories provided by the parenteral nutrition solution. Renal and hepatic function should be monitored carefully in the stressed patient who receives parenteral nutrition to ensure that adequate, not excessive, protein is provided.

Fat

Fat is provided in the form of lipid emulsions. Currently available for use are 10% lipid emulsions, which provide 1.1 calories/ml, and 20% lipid emulsions, which provide 2.0 calories/ml. The 20% lipid emulsion is preferred for use in pediatric patients because of its higher caloric density and more efficient clearance in the blood. It is generally recommended that fat comprise less than 30% of the total calories provided by parenteral nutrition; however, larger amounts may be tolerated, depending on the patient's age and condition (Cox & Cooning, 1993).

Electrolytes

Electrolytes are provided individually in the parenteral nutrition solution to aid in fluid and electrolyte homeostasis. Requirements vary depending on the child's age, medical condition, fluid balance, and losses.

Vitamins, Minerals, and Trace Elements

Vitamin, mineral, and trace elements are provided in parenteral nutrition solutions to complete the intravenous nutrition regimen. Requirements vary depending on the child's age, medical condition, and losses.

Other Additives

Heparin is commonly added to parenteral nutrition in small quantities to maintain line patency and prevent the formation of a fibrin sheath, which will clog the catheter (Wesley & Coran, 1995).

Iron may be added to parenteral nutrition solutions in the form of iron dextran; however, its use is routinely avoided in patients who receive large quantities of blood products. Regular monitoring of iron status is recommended to prevent iron overload.

Certain medications are considered compatible with parenteral nutrition and may be added directly to the solution, which may help simplify the child's medication routine. This may be particularly helpful in cases in which intravenous access is limited or if the central line has only a single lumen. A pharmacist should be consulted to assist in determining the compatibility of medications with parenteral nutrition.

Administration of Solutions

Parenteral nutrition solutions typically are provided as two solutions that are piggybacked together during infusion. A lipid emulsion is piggybacked to a solution that contains dextrose, amino acids, vitamins, minerals, trace elements, and electrolytes. Lipids have traditionally been separated from the other components to allow for easy visual inspection of additive precipitation, which usually appears as an opaque, chalky precipitate. Newer technology has allowed for the creation of total nutrient admixtures (TNA) or "three-in-one" solutions, which combine all ingredients into one solution. They require only one pump for administration. Such solutions are commonly used in patients who require long-term parenteral nutritional support at home.

Parenteral nutrition generally is initiated as 24-hour therapy in a critically ill child. This allows for more constant infusion of fluid, electrolytes, and glucose in a stressed patient and therefore reduces the risk of intolerance. Critically ill children often receive multiple other fluids and medications that may be incompatible with parenteral nutrition, thereby necessitating brief, but often numerous, interruptions in the delivery of parenteral nutrition. A nurse's heightened awareness of the potential for such interruptions is critical to the medical team's ability to provide adequate nutritional support to the stressed patient. When such interruptions are found to result in suboptimal delivery of energy and protein, medication routines can be altered or parenteral nutrition cycled over a shorter time frame to maximize parenteral nutrition delivery.

Monitoring for Complications

Laboratory Monitoring

Use of parenteral nutrition may be associated with metabolic or septic complications. Patients who receive parenteral nutrition require careful monitoring and excellent catheter care to minimize the risk of infection. Serum glucose levels should be monitored, especially in patients with trauma, stress, and sepsis because these patients are already at increased risk for abnormalities in glucose metabolism. Serum triglyceride levels should be checked with each increase in lipid dose and then weekly once the goal lipid dose is achieved. Elevated levels of circulating triglycerides are expected during sepsis, infection, and continuous lipid infusion; therefore it is prudent to monitor lipid tolerance more closely. Lipid administration in preterm infants has been associated with decreased pulmonary diffusion capacity, alteration in leukocyte function, lipid deposits in various tissues, displacement of bound bilirubin by free fatty acids, and changes in prostaglandin metabolism (Friedman, Marks, Maisels, Thorson, & Naeye, 1978; Heird, 1986; Levene, Wigglesworth, & Desai, 1980; Pereira, Fox, Wiley, Kaner, & Holbrook, 1980). However, given the risks of essential fatty acid deficiency and the inability to provide adequate calories or a regimen that is disproportionately high in carbohydrate, it is common practice to provide a reasonable, not excessive, dose of lipids with parenteral nutrition.

Serum electrolytes, calcium, phosphorus, and magnesium should be checked daily until the patient is stable on a goal regimen. Fluid and electrolyte shifts are expected as part of the normal stress response; however, many trauma patients also have increased uptake and exogenous losses of fluid and electrolytes, as well as the potential for medication interactions that directly affect fluid and electrolyte shifts. Hydration and fluid status should be monitored carefully when parenteral nutrition is given. Dehydration may indicate the need to liberalize fluid provided by the parenteral nutrition solution. Edema, regardless of the cause, may necessitate changes to the concentration of the parenteral nutrition solution and changes to the electrolyte balance to maintain the desired fluid and electrolyte balance. Replacement of gastrointestinal losses with parenteral nutrition solutions is generally not recommended.

Additional biochemical markers that should be monitored in patients who receive parenteral nutrition include albumin, total protein, total bilirubin, conjugated bilirubin, unconjugated bilirubin, alkaline phosphatase, alanine aminotransferase, aspartate aminotransferase, and gamma-glutamyltransferase. Each should be checked weekly to assess liver function.

Long-Term Complications

Complications that may occur with long-term use of parenteral nutrition include metabolic bone disease, hepatobiliary complications such as cholestasis, carnitine deficiency, and vitamin and trace element abnormalities.

Metabolic bone disease may occur in patients who require long-term parenteral nutrition and who have a history of severe illness, malnutrition, or skeletal abnormalities. The cause of metabolic bone disease remains unclear; however, it is speculated that its development may be related to disturbances in calcium or vitamin D balance as a result of the physiologic nature of parenteral nutrition.

The cause of hepatobiliary complications associated with prolonged use of parenteral nutrition remains unclear. Care must be taken to provide a reasonable total calorie level, protein intake, and macronutrient distribution. Additional laboratory monitoring of specific vitamin, mineral, and trace element levels may become necessary to ensure prevention of deficiency or toxicity in patients who require long-term parenteral nutrition.

ENTERAL NUTRITION

Benefits of Enteral Feeding

The benefits of early enteral feeding in critically ill patients who have sustained trauma and burns are well documented. Early enteral feeding has been shown to play a role in the preservation of gut integrity, thereby reducing the risk of bacterial translocation; the maintenance of intestinal barriers; and the reduction of infectious risk and septic complications (Cerra et al., 1997; McDonald, 1991; Minard & Kudsk, 1998; Mochizuki, Trocki, Dominioni, Brackett, Joffe, & Alexander, 1984). In adult and pediatric burn patients, early enteral feeding has been shown to have significant metabolic benefits and a reduced infectious risk compared with the use of parenteral nutrition. It has been proven to be a safe and effective means of nutritional support (Trocki, 1993).

Gastric function is often compromised in critically ill patients without specific abdominal trauma who demonstrate gastric ileus and absence of bowel sounds; however, feeding distal to the pylorus has been shown to be effective, as evidenced by the fact that small bowel function appears to be preserved (Bengmark & Gianotti, 1996; Cerra et al., 1997). Bedside transpyloric, nasoenteric tube placement has been shown to be a safe alternative to transporting an otherwise unstable, critically ill pediatric patient for fluoroscopic feeding tube placement (Chellis, Sanders, Dean, & Jackson, 1996). In those pediatric ICU patients who tolerated bedside transpyloric, nasoenteric feeding tube placement, early enteral feedings have been shown to be effective alternatives to parenteral nutrition (Chellis et al., 1996). Concurrent gastric decompression during small bowel feedings may also help improve tolerance to enteral feedings; however, unavailability of pediatric tubing that allows for nasojejunal feeding with gastric decompression may hamper such efforts. Enteral feeding also provides a cost advantage over parenteral nutrition.

In pediatric patients who have sustained abdominal trauma, attempts to initiate enteral feeds may understandably be delayed until gastric function is stabilized. In such cases calories and protein should be provided via the parenteral route so as not to delay initiation of nutritional support. Feeding via the oral route is commonly delayed in pediatric trauma patients because the child's ability to resume oral feeds is largely dependent on the type of injury and level of hemodynamic support, ventilatory support, and sedation required.

Formula Selection

Many commercial formula preparations are available for the enteral nutritional support of infants and children. Important factors to consider when choosing the appropriate formula include age of the patient; gut function and ability to digest the formula; caloric density of the formula; nutrient source and distribution of carbohydrate, protein, and fat; osmolality; renal solute load; and route of delivery.

Infant and Pediatric Formulas

Maternal breast milk is the preferred source of nutrition for infants, but when the mother's milk is unavailable, infant formulas modeled after breast milk may be used instead (Groh-Wargo & Antonelli, 1993). "Standard" formulas that contain intact protein are preferred for infants and children with normal gastrointestinal function. Unlike pediatric and adult enteral formulations, infant formulas contain approximately 45% to 50% of their calories from fat, which reflects the increased need for fat during infancy for growth and development. Easier to digest, more elemental formulas are available for infants and children with altered gastrointestinal function. Formulas that are available as a powder or concentrated liquid base may be concentrated to achieve appropriate calorie levels in less volume for fluid-restricted patients. Table 12-6 gives a categorized listing of enteral products designed for infants and children and their specific attributes.

Infant and pediatric enteral formulas contain vitamins and minerals that meet the RDA for age as long as adequate calories are consumed. Therefore consumption of dilute formulas or inadequate volumes may contribute to inadequate micronutrient intake over time. Such circumstances may occur in pediatric trauma patients who have impaired gastrointestinal function or who are fluid restricted. Provision of an age-appropriate daily multivitamin and mineral preparation may help to cover such deficiencies until enteral feeds can be advanced to achieve the intake goal.

Use of Adult Formulas

Although disease-specific and immune-enhancing enteral formulations have been developed for use in adults, such products have yet to be developed for use in infants and children. Pediatric enteral formulas generally are designed to meet the RDAs for vitamins and minerals in children aged 1 to 10 years; therefore the use of adult enteral products is common in adolescent trauma patients. Routine use of adult enteral formulas in infants and young children is not recommended because of the higher protein and electrolyte content, higher osmolality, and macronutrient distribution of the adult formulas that are ill designed to meet the needs of a growing child (Lingard, 1993). In circumstances that may necessitate use of an adult enteral formula in a pediatric patient, renal function, fluid and electrolyte balance, and gastrointestinal tolerance should be monitored closely until the child is able to be transitioned back to an age-appropriate product. Table 12-6 gives a categorized listing of adult enteral products and their attributes.

Modular Components

Modular fat, carbohydrate, and protein components are available for addition to commercial formulas in the event that manipulation of the macronutrient balance of the formula or the addition of calories is required. Table 12-7 gives a categorized listing of available modular components.

Tolerance to Enteral Feeding

Monitoring Tolerance

Tolerance to enteral feedings must be monitored closely as tube feedings are advanced and once a goal regimen is achieved. Diarrhea and vomiting may be signs of intolerance to the feeding regimen as a result of mechanical dysfunction of the gut (e.g., obstruction, ileus); intercurrent illness or infection (e.g., viral gastroenteritis, *Clostridium difficile*, rotavirus); or intolerance to formula volume, osmolality, or ingredients. However, there may be other nonrelated causes as well (Trocki, 1993). Constipation may be caused by poor gastrointestinal motility, inadequate fluid intake, and too much or too little fiber. Dehydration may occur if adequate free fluid is not provided, particularly when a calorically dense or hypertonic formula is being given.

TABLE 12-6 Commercially Available Enteral Products

Product Category	Characteristics	Product Examples
Infant Formulas	**For use in the first year of life; standard concentration is 20 kcal/oz**	
Milk based	Intact protein derived from cow's milk; contain lactose	Similac (Ross) Enfamil (Mead Johnson) Carnation Good Start (Carnation)
	Lower electrolyte content	Similac PM 60/40 (Ross)
	Do not contain lactose	Lactofree (Mead Johnson) Similac Lactose Free (Ross)
Soy based	Intact protein derived from soy; do not contain lactose	Isomil (Ross) ProSobee (Mead Johnson)
Predigested	Partially hydrolyzed protein only	Nutramigen (Mead Johnson)
	Partially hydrolyzed protein; modified carbohydrate; added MCT	Alimentum (Ross) Pregestimil (Mead Johnson)
	Free amino acids as protein source; hypoallergenic	Neocate (Scientific Hospital Supplies)
Premature	Standard 24 kcal/oz concentration; high protein; added MCT	Similac Special Care (Ross) Enfamil Premature (Mead Johnson)
Premature transitional	Standard 22 kcal/oz; concentration to bridge transition from premature to term infant formulas	Similac NeoSure (Ross) Enfamil 22 (Mead Johnson)
Special modifications	86% of fat from MCT	Portagen (Mead Johnson)
	Carbohydrate free; modular carbohydrate source must be added to make a complete formula	RCF (Ross) 3232A (Mead Johnson)
Pediatric Formulas	**Designed to meet RDAs for vitamins and minerals in children aged 1-10 yr; standard concentration is 1.0 kcal/ml**	
Standard formulas	Intact protein derived from cow's milk; lactose free; appropriate for tube feeding or oral supplementation; may be flavored	Pediasure (Ross) Nutren Jr. (Mead Johnson) Resource Just for Kids (Novartis)
	Contain fiber	Kindercal (Mead Johnson)
Predigested	Hydrolyzed whey protein	Peptamen Jr. (Nestle)
	Free amino acids as protein source	Neocate One Plus (Scientific Hospital Supplies) EleCare (Ross) Vivonex Pediatric (Novartis)
Adult Formulas	**Designed for use in adults; use in children must be monitored closely**	
Standard formulas	Intact protein; some with added MCT; 1.0-2.0 kcal/ml density; unflavored for use in tube feedings	Nutren (Nestle) Isocal (Mead Johnson) Deliver 2.0 (Mead Johnson) Osmolite (Ross)
	Flavored for use as oral supplement or tube feeding; osmolality tends to be higher	Sustacal (Mead Johnson) Resource (Novartis) Ensure (Ross)
	Have added fiber; unflavored for use in tube feedings	Nutren 1.0 with fiber (Nestle) Fiber Source (Novartis) Jevity (Ross)
	Have added fiber; flavored for use as oral supplement	Sustacal with fiber (Mead Johnson) Ensure with fiber (Ross)
Elemental	Hydrolyzed protein; added MCT; 1.0-1.5 kcal/ml	Peptamen (Nestle) SandoSource Peptide (Novartis)
	Free amino acids as protein source; some with added MCT; 1.0 kcal/ml	Tolerex (Novartis) Vivonex TEN (Novartis) Vivonex Plus (Novartis)

TABLE 12-6 **Commercially Available Enteral Products—cont'd**

Product Category	Characteristics	Product Examples
Condition specific: Critical care, healing support	1.0-1.5 kcal/ml; higher levels of intact and hydrolyzed proteins; may contain MCT and/or structured lipid blend; may have increased vitamin and mineral content for healing support	Crucial Diet (Nestle) Impact (Novartis) Perative (Ross) Replete (Nestle) TraumaCal (Mead Johnson) Promote (Ross)
Condition specific: Hepatic failure	1.2-1.5 kcal/ml; high branched-chain amino acid content	NutriHep Diet (Nestle) Hepatic-Aid II (McGaw)
Condition specific: Pulmonary	1.5 kcal/ml; high-fat/low-carbohydrate formulations designed to minimize CO_2 production; may contain specialized fat blends	Nutrivent Diet (Nestle) Respalor (Mead Johnson) Pulmocare (Ross) Oxepa (Ross)
Condition specific: Renal	2.0 kcal/ml for fluid-restricted renal patients; varying protein and electrolyte contents for use before and during dialysis	Renalcal Diet (Nestle) Nepro (Ross) Suplena (Ross) Magnacal Renal (Mead Johnson)

MCT, Medium-chain triglyceride.

TABLE 12-7 **Modular Components**

Macronutrient	Product Characteristics	Nutrient Density	Examples
Carbohydrate	Glucose polymers available in liquid or powder form; may increase osmolality of formula	2 kcal/ml; 23 kcal/Tbsp	Polycose (Ross)
Fat	Long-chain fat; liquid miscible form will not separate from formula	4.5 kcal/ml	Microlipid (Mead Johnson)
	Medium-chain triglycerides for patients with altered fat absorption	7.7 kcal/ml	MCT oil
	Long-chain fats; add to solid foods only	Approximately 45 kcal/tsp	Butter, margarine
	Long-chain fats; can add to liquids or foods; will separate out from liquids	Approximately 9 kcal/ml	Vegetable oil
Protein	Intact protein	4.4 g protein/Tbsp	Casec (Mead Johnson)
	Intact protein	5 g protein/Tbsp	ProMod (Ross)
Blends	Powdered calorie booster made from fat and carbohydrate; add to liquids and solids	35 kcal/Tbsp	Scandical (Scandipharm)
	Powdered calorie booster made from fat and carbohydrate; add to liquids and solids	64 kcal/Tbsp	Duocal (Scientific Hospital Supplies)

MCT, Medium-chain triglyceride.

Transitioning to Oral Diets

Oral Supplements

As the pediatric trauma patient gradually recovers, it is appropriate to transition the child back to an oral diet as tolerated. Tube feedings may be scaled back gradually to stimulate appetite and promote oral intake. Oral intake should be monitored closely for adequacy through documentation of calorie counts (Lingard, 1993). The child who has difficulty consuming enough to meet increased energy and protein needs for recovery may benefit from the use of high-calorie, high-protein oral supplements and between-meal snacks to boost their intake and allow for the complete withdrawal of tube feedings. A variety of appealing supplements rich in calories, protein, vitamins, and minerals are available for supplementation of the oral diet. Box 12-3 lists such products.

Adequacy of Oral Intake

It is important to remember the effect that a hospital setting can have on a child's appetite. Foods may be prepared differently than at home; menu choices may be limited, particularly if the child's family observes special diet restrictions; and favorite foods may not be readily available. In addition, the social environment of mealtime is missing with the rest of the family not present, availability of between-meal snacks may be limited, and food temperatures can be easily affected if the child is not present or able to eat when the

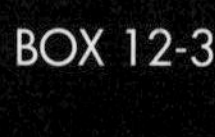

BOX 12-3 Product Characteristics and Names of High-Calorie, High-Protein Oral Supplements

Clear Liquid Supplements

Enlive (Ross)
Resource Fruit Beverage (Novartis)
Resource Nutritious Juice Drink (Novartis)
Citrotein (Novartis)
NuBasics Juice Drink (Nestle)

Broths and Soups

NuBasics Complete Nutrition Soup (Nestle)
Resource High Protein Broth (Novartis)

Bars

DuoBar (Scientific Hospital Supplies)
NuBasics Complete Nutrition Bar (Nestle)
Boost Nutritional Energy Bar (Mead Johnson)
Ensure Bar (Ross)

Puddings/Gelatin

Ensure Pudding (Ross)
Boost Pudding (Mead Johnson)
Resource Frozen Nutritious Pudding (Novartis)

Shakes

Boost (Mead Johnson)
Carnation Instant Breakfast (Nestle)
Forta Shake (Ross)
NuBasics Drink (Nestle)
NutraShake (NutraBalance)
Resource Health Shake (Novartis)
Resource Shake (Novartis)
Resource Yogurt Beverage (Novartis)
Scandishake (Scandipharm, Inc.)

meal is delivered. Special attention should be paid to the recovering trauma patient who is consuming an oral diet to ensure adequate food variety and adequate intake, as well as to ensure that special preferences are met. Depending on the institution's guidelines, parents may be encouraged to bring in favorite foods on occasion and to dine with their recovering child when possible.

SUMMARY

Pediatric patients who sustain trauma or burns have rapidly changing needs throughout the continuum of their recovery and rehabilitation. Timely assessment of nutrition risk and appropriate nutritional intervention can have a positive influence on clinical outcomes.

As primary caretakers, nurses are uniquely qualified to continually reassess and monitor the nutrition status of pediatric trauma patients. Nurses need to be equipped with the skills necessary to identify patients at risk for malnutrition and intervene appropriately.

BIBLIOGRAPHY

Bengmark, S., & Gianotti, L. (1996). Nutritional support to prevent and treat multiple organ failure. *World Journal of Surgery, 20*(4), 474-481.

Buckley, S., & Kudsk, K. (1994). Metabolic response to critical illness and injury. *AACN Clin Iss Crit Care Nurs, 5*(4), 443-449.

Cerra, F. B., Benitez, M. R., Blackburn, G. L., Irwin. R. S., Jeejeebhoy, K., Katz, D. P., Pingleton, S. K., Pomposelli, J., Rombeau, J. L., Shronts, E., Wolfe, R. R., & Zaloga, G. P. (1997). Applied nutrition in ICU patients: A consensus statement of the American College of Chest Physicians. *Chest, 111*(3), 769-778.

Chellis, M. J., Sanders, S. V., Dean, J. M., & Jackson, D. (1996). Bedside transpyloric tube placement in the pediatric intensive care unit. *Journal of Parenteral and Enteral Nutrition, 20*(1), 88-90.

Chellis, M. J., Sanders, S. V., Webster, H., Dean, J. M., & Jackson, D. (1996). Early enteral feeding in the pediatric intensive care unit. *Journal of Parenteral and Enteral Nutrition, 20*(1), 71-73.

Chiarelli, A., Enzi, G., Casadei, A., Baggio, B., Valerio, A., & Mazzoleni, F. (1990). Very early nutrition supplementation in burned patients. *American Journal of Clinical Nutrition, 51*(6), 1035-1039.

Cox, J. H., & Cooning, S. W. (1993). Parenteral nutrition. In P. Queen & C. Lang (Eds.), *Handbook of pediatric nutrition* (pp. 279-314). Gaithersburg, MD: Aspen Publishers.

Ford, E. (1996). Nutrition support of pediatric patients. *Nutrition in Clinical Practice, 11*(5), 183-191.

Friedman, Z., Marks, K. H., Maisels, J., Thorson, R., & Naeye, R. (1978). Effect of parenteral fat emulsion on the pulmonary and reticuloendothelial systems in the newborn infant. *Pediatrics, 61*(5), 694-698.

Gartner, J. (1994). Pediatric nutrition and gastroenterology. In B. Zitelli, H. Davis, & F. Oski (Eds.), *Atlas of pediatric physician diagnosis* (2nd ed., p. 10.6). St. Louis: Mosby.

Goodwin, M., & Carlson, I. (1993). The peripherally inserted central catheter. *Journal of Intravenous Nursing, 16*(2), 92-103.

Gottschlich, M. (1993). Nutrition in the burned pediatric patient. In P. Queen & C. Lang (Eds.), *Handbook of pediatric nutrition* (pp. 536-559). Gaithersburg, MD: Aspen Publishers, Inc.

Groh-Wargo, S., & Antonelli, K. (1993). Normal nutrition during infancy. In P. Queen & C. Lang (Eds.), *Handbook of pediatric nutrition* (pp. 107-144). Gaithersburg, MD: Aspen Publishers, Inc.

Heird, W. (1986). Lipid metabolism in parenteral nutrition. In S. Fomon & W. Heird (Eds.), *Energy and protein needs during infancy* (pp. 215-229). San Diego: Academic Press.

Hill, A. G., & Hill, G. L. (1998). Metabolic response to severe injury. *British Journal of Surgery, 85*(7):884-890.

Hopkins, B. (1993). Assessment of nutritional status. In M. Gottschlich, L. Matarese, & E. Shronts (Eds.), *Nutrition support dietetics core curriculum* (2nd ed., p. 42). Silver Spring, MD: American Society for Parenteral and Enteral Nutrition.

Jeejeebhoy, K. (1994). Intestinal disorders: Short bowel disease. In M. Shils, J. Olson, & M. Shike (Eds.), *Modern nutrition in health and disease* (8th ed., pp. 1036-1042). Philadelphia: Lea & Febiger.

Kaplan, A. S., Zemel, B. S., Neiswender, K. M., & Stallings, V. A. (1995). Resting energy expenditure in clinical pediatrics: Measured versus prediction equations. *Journal of Pediatrics, 127*(2), 200-205.

Lee, P., & Werlin, S. (1997). Carbohydrates. In R. Baker, S. Baker, & A. Davis (Eds.), *Pediatric parenteral nutrition* (p. 100). New York: Chapman & Hall.

Levene, M., Wigglesworth, J., & Desai, R. (1980). Pulmonary fat accumulation after intralipid infusion in the preterm infant. *Lancet, 2*(8199), 815-818.

Lingard, C. D. (1993). Enteral nutrition. In P. Queen & C. Lang (Eds.), *Handbook of pediatric nutrition* (pp. 249-278). Gaithersburg, MD: Aspen Publishers.

Mascarenhas, M., & McCoy, B. (1998). Nutrition support services appendix: Parenteral nutrition. In R. Jew (Ed.), *The Children's Hospital of Philadelphia pharmacy handbook and formulary* (p. 395). Hudson, OH: Lexi-Comp.

McDonald, W. S. (1991). Immediate enteral feeding in burn patients is safe and effective. *Annals of Surgery, 213*(2), 177-183.

Minard, G., & Kudsk, K. (1998). Nutritional support and infection: Does the route matter? *World Journal of Surgery, 22*(2), 213-219.

Mochizuki, H., Trocki, O., Dominioni, L., Brackett, K. A., Joffe, S. N., & Alexander, J. W. (1984). Mechanism of prevention of postburn hypermetabolism and catabolism by early enteral feeding. *Annals of Surgery, 200*(3), 297-310.

National Research Council. (1989). *Recommended dietary allowances* (10th ed.). Washington, DC: National Academy Press.

Pereira, G. R., Fox, W. W., Stanley, C. A., Baker, L., & Schwartz, J. G. (1980). Decreased oxygenation and hyperlipemia during intravenous fat infusions in premature infants. *Pediatrics, 66*(1), 26-30.

Pollack, M. M., Ruttimann, U. E., & Wiley, J. S. (1985). Nutritional depletions in critically ill children: Associations with physiologic instability and increased quantity of care. *Journal of Parenteral and Enteral Nutrition, 9*(3), 309-313.

Pollack, M. M., Wiley, J. S., Kanter, R., & Holbrook, P. R. (1982). Malnutrition in critically ill infants and children. *Journal of Parenteral and Enteral Nutrition, 6*(1), 20-23.

Rogers, D., & Lobe, T. (1995). Metabolic response to major injury and shock. In W. L. Buntain (Ed.), *Management of pediatric trauma* (pp. 106-119). Philadelphia: WB Saunders.

Schofield, W. N. (1985). Predicting basal metabolic rate: new standards and review of previous work. *Human Nutrition, 39C*(Suppl. 1), 5-42.

Skipper, A. (1989). *Dietitian's handbook of enteral and parenteral nutrition* (pp. 12-13, 152-154, 329-330). Rockville, MD: Aspen Publishers.

Stallings, V. A. (1998). Resting energy expenditure. In S. Altschuler & C. Liacouris (Eds.), *Clinical pediatric gastroenterology* (pp. 607-611). Philadelphia: Churchill Livingstone.

Trocki, O. (1993). Nutritional management of children with burns and trauma. In M. Eichelberger (Ed.), *Pediatric trauma: Prevention, acute care, rehabilitation* (pp. 591-605). St. Louis: Mosby.

Weissman, C., & Kemper, M. (1995). Metabolic measurements in the critically ill. *Critical Care Clinics, 11*(1):169-197.

Wesley, J. R., & Coran, A. G. (1995). Nutritional management in pediatric trauma. In W. L. Buntain (Ed.), *Management of pediatric trauma* (pp. 663-689). Philadelphia: WB Saunders.

World Health Organization. (1985). Energy and protein requirements: Report of a Joint FAO/WHO/UNU Expert Consultation (WHO Technical Report Series No. 724). Geneva:

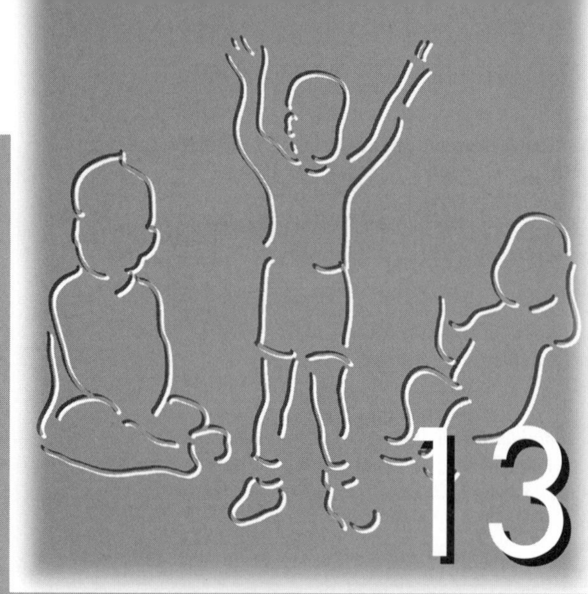

INTENTIONAL INJURIES

Sandra J. Czerwinski

• *Patricia A. Moloney-Harmon*

Violence, with its associated consequences of emotional trauma, injury, and death, is a fact of life for millions of American children. It has emerged as the single most significant and persistent threat to the health of American children. Violent behavior affects children of all ages, and it occurs in every geographic area, on all socioeconomic levels, and in all ethnic groups. Unfortunately, violence has become such a common part of our lives that it is often viewed as a normal, rather than an abnormal, event. This chapter discusses two major issues related to violence in children: firearm injury and child maltreatment.

FIREARM INJURY

Death resulting from firearm injuries is an increasingly important public health problem. Approximately 38,000 people die from firearm injuries each year, and many more are wounded (National Center for Injury Prevention and Control, Centers for Disease Control and Prevention, 1996). In 1997, 32,436 firearm-related deaths (12.12/100,000) occurred in the United States, of which 4223 of the victims were children and adolescents younger than 20 years old (National Center for Injury Prevention and Control, Centers for Disease Control and Prevention, 2000). Unintentional shootings are responsible for nearly 20% of all fatalities related to firearms in children 14 years and younger (National Safe Kids Campaign, 1999).

The cost per firearm fatality is higher than for nearly all of the other common causes of death (Max & Rice, 1993). In 1990 firearm injuries cost more than $20.4 billion in both direct costs for hospital and other medical care and indirect costs for long-term disability and premature death (Max & Rice, 1993). One study specifically focusing on firearm injuries from 1994 to 1995 estimates that the average per person lifetime cost per nonfatal hospitalized gunshot injury is $35,367 (Cook, Lawrence, Ludwig, & Miller, 1999). At least 80% of the economic costs for treating injuries resulting from firearms are paid for by taxpayer dollars (Max & Rice, 1993).

Firearm injuries to children are a serious medical and public health problem. Violent injury and death disproportionately affect children, adolescents, and young adults in the United States. Overall, mortality rates for children and youths in the United States have dropped sharply over the last decade. Even death rates from motor vehicle accident injuries have declined steadily during this period (Centers for Disease Control and Prevention, 1996). Firearm fatalities peaked in 1993 and have declined slightly since then. Despite this trend, the rate of victimization and involvement in violent crimes for children and adolescents has increased dramatically over the past decade (Centers for Disease Control and Prevention, 1997; Fox, 1996; Rachuba, Stanton, & Howard, 1995). The adolescent victimization rate is almost twice the rate for adults aged 25 to 34 years (Hennes, 1998). The Centers for Disease Control and Prevention predicts that firearms will replace motor vehicles as the leading cause of injury death in the United States by the year 2003 (Cherry, Annest, Mercy, Kresnow, & Pollock, 1998). This change has already occurred in 10 states and the District of Columbia according to mortality data from the National Vital Statistics System (Centers for Disease Control and Prevention, 1996). Increased homicide rates in 15- to 19-year-olds are largely responsible for this trend (Max & Rice, 1993).

Every day in the United States, 15 firearms kill children aged 19 and younger. Regardless of the type of shooting, most children are shot in a familiar location by someone close to their own age or by an adult family member (Laraque, Barlow, & Durkin, 1995). Beaver, Moore, Peclet, and Haller (1990) conducted a study that examined the incidence of fatal gunshot injuries in an eastern state from 1979 to 1987. During that time, 132 children between the ages of 0 and 16 years were shot and killed. Ninety-nine (75%) of the fatal injuries occurred in a home environment; seventy-nine (60%) occurred in the victim's home. The person committing the shooting was a member of the immediate family in 24 cases (18%), a relative in 3 (2%), a friend in 28 (21%), and an acquaintance in 10 (7%). Strangers committed the shooting in 26 cases (20%). The remaining deaths were children shot as bystanders (2 cases [2%]) or self-inflicted (39 [30%]) (Beaver et al., 1990). Other studies and information sources developed since then have generated data supporting these findings (Feero, Hedges, & Simmons, 1995; Laraque et al., 1995; National Safe Kids Campaign, 1999).

Several surveys and studies have shown that guns are easily accessible (Callahan & Rivara, 1992; L.H. Research, Inc., 1993; Rand Health, 2001; Sheley, McGee, & Wright, 1992). Young people are reportedly carrying firearms and other weapons at high rates. In 1995 1 in 12 students reported carrying a firearm for fighting or self-defense (Kann, Warren, & Harris, 1995). The rate was higher among male high school students and still higher among minority males. In 1996 researchers found that 40% of juvenile males reported possessing a firearm at some time, and 38% believed that it was acceptable to shoot someone who may inflict harm (Snyder, Sickmund, & Poe-Yamagata, 1996).

Handguns account for the majority of firearm deaths and injuries in the United States (Christoffel & Naureckas, 1994). Sheley and Wright (1993) reported on a survey that described how and why firearms were chosen by about 1600 teenage boys. Handguns were by far the weapons of choice for this group (Senturia, Christoffel, & Donovan, 1996; Sickmund, Snyder, & Poe-Yamagata, 1997). Use of small-caliber weapons has decreased while use of large-caliber semiautomatic handgun use has increased (Hartgarten, Karlson, O'Brien, Hancock, & Quebbeman, 1996). However, children have also been injured and killed by nonpowder weapons, such as BB, pellet, and air guns. Of people treated for BB and pellet wounds, 81% are children and teenagers 19 or younger (Centers for Disease Control and Prevention, 1995). Long guns are less prevalent and seen predominantly in rural areas (Christoffel & Naureckas, 1994; National Safe Kids Campaign, 1999).

Firearm deaths occur across the life span, beginning in infancy, increasing in frequency through childhood, and accelerating into late adolescence. Table 13-1 provides an overview of firearm death rates based on age and gender. Most unintentional injuries occur in children and adolescents younger than age 15 years, whereas the majority of homicides are seen in youths aged 15 to 19 years (Dahlberg, 1998; Fingerhut, Jones, & Makuc, 1994). Mortality rates for young males are twice as high as those for young females (Dahlberg, 1998; Fingerhut et al., 1994; Sheley et al., 1992). Violence affecting female adolescents is more frequently expressed as rape, sexual assault, and physical beating (Cohall, Cohall, & Bannister, 1998). African American males and females have a homicide rate more than twice the rate of their Hispanic counterparts and almost 14 times the rate

TABLE 13-1 **Death Rates for Firearm-Related Injuries According to Age and Gender: United States, Selected Years 1990-1999**

	1990	1995	1996	1997	1998	1999
Male						
1-4 yr	0.7	0.8	0.5	0.5	0.6	0.5
5-14 yr	2.9	2.9	2.4	2.1	1.9	1.5
15-24 yr	44.7	47.6	42.2	38.9	34.7	31.3
Female						
1-4 yr	0.8	0.8	0.7	0.6	0.7	0.5
5-14 yr	1.0	0.9	0.8	0.7	0.8	0.6
15-24 yr	6.0	6.0	5.1	4.8	4.5	4.0

From Centers for Disease Control and Prevention/National Centers for Health Statistics. (2001). Firearm deaths, death rates, and age-adjusted death rates. *National Vital Statistics Report, 49*(8), 72.

of the white non-Hispanic group (Anderson, Kochanek, & Murphy, 1997).

Mortality statistics alone do not reveal the full impact that violence has on children. The psychologic injuries that result from violence are often more extensive than the physical wounds (Berton & Stabb, 1996; Schwartz, 1996). A study of high school students reveals that exposure to physical violence has a positive and significant association with depression, anger, anxiety, and posttraumatic stress (Singer, Menden, Song, & Lunghofer, 1995). Development of these feelings has been linked to school failure and suicide (Berman & Jobes, 1991).

Homicide is the extreme outcome of violence against children. It is the second leading cause of death among children and the leading cause of death among African American males between the ages of 15 and 34 years in the United States (Singh, Kochanek, & MacDorman, 1996). In each year since 1988, more than 80% of homicide victims aged 15 to 19 years were killed with a firearm. In 1994 the rate rose to more than 90% (Hennes, 1998). Homicides vary by geographic area. New England states have lower rates, and the south Atlantic states have the highest rates (Hennes, 1998). Numerous studies indicate that homicide rates are higher in urban centers than rural areas (Centers for Disease Control and Prevention, 1997). International comparisons between the United States and 25 industrialized countries indicate that children between the ages of 5 and 14 years who are living in the United States are 5.8 times more likely to become a victim of homicide than children in any other industrialized country. The rate was 8.6 times higher for firearm homicide and 4.3 times greater for children aged 0 to 4 years (Centers for Disease Control and Prevention, 1997).

The relationship between victim and murderer, the means of death, and the circumstances surrounding child homicide vary with the age of the victim. Homicide in children younger than 1 year of age is usually the result of a beating inflicted by a parent. As children get older, they are more often victims of acquaintances and strangers; however, family members are still responsible for many of the fatalities. Older children are more likely to be victims of injuries caused by lethal weapons. Firearms and knives are used in the majority of these homicides. The proportion of homicides inflicted with firearms increases with age, regardless of sex or race (Hennes, 1998).

Firearms are now used in the majority of all completed teenage suicides, and handguns are the weapons of choice. In 1993 Fingerhut (1993) documented 1446 firearms-related suicides in children and adolescents 0 to 19 years of age. Suicide nearly ties homicide as the second leading cause of death among adolescents in the United States. There has been a dramatic rise in the rates among children aged 10 to 14 years (National Center for Injury Prevention and Control, Centers for Disease Control and Prevention, 2000). It is more prevalent among white teens than among black teens; however, suicide rates increased most rapidly among young black men. Female teenagers are more likely to attempt suicide than are males, and many will use a firearm (National Center for Injury Prevention and Control, Centers for Disease Control and Prevention, 2000). According to a case-controlled study by Brent, Perpur, and Moritz (1993), the presence of a gun in the home raises the suicide rate fourfold. Unfortunately, the availability of firearms increases the likelihood that a suicide attempt will be fatal because of the lethal nature of the weapon.

Contributing Factors

Many complex issues contribute to the unacceptably high rate of violence among children. Subcultural issues, poverty, urbanization, family disruption, and erosion of basic law and order are just a few. Box 13-1 provides an outline of the key risk factors.

Cappel and Heiner (1990) report that children with disruptive behavior disorders often grow into violent criminals as adults. Other physical conditions, such as head trauma; neuromotor deficits; seizures; and prenatal exposure to opiates, cocaine, and alcohol, may lead to aggressive tendencies (Reiss & Roth, 1993). Violence has numerous precursors and is a learned behavior that is part of a long developmental process that begins in early childhood. One of the strongest predictors of later aggression and criminal activity is a history of early aggression (Farrington, 1991). Children who grow up in families where there is child abuse and maltreatment, spousal abuse, and a history of violent behavior learn early to act out physically when they are frustrated and upset. Research provides evidence that there is a greater risk for aggressive behavior and antisocial behavior in children who experience rejection, neglect, or parental indifference (McCord, 1983; Tolan, 1988). These children are also at high risk for suicide. It has been shown that children who have low parental attachment have higher risk of delinquency (Huizinga, Loeber, & Thornberry, 1994). Aggression and other behavior problems are increased in homes where a parent has a history of criminal behavior or drug or alcohol abuse or has an antisocial personality. Poor parenting practices, such as poor communication, ineffective problem-solving skills, poor negotiation skills, and lack of supervision, increase aggressive behaviors.

BOX 13-1 Key Risk Factors for Aggression, Violence, and Delinquency

Individual Factors

History of early aggression
Beliefs supportive of violence
Attributional biases
Social cognitive deficits

Family Factors

Problem parental behavior
Low emotional attachment to parents/caregivers
Poor monitoring and supervision of children
Exposure to violence
Poor family functioning

Peer/School Factors

Negative peer influences
Low commitment to school
Academic failure
Certain school environments/practices

Environmental/Neighborhood Factors

High concentrations of poor residents
High levels of transiency
High levels of family disruption
Low community participation
Diminished economic opportunity
Access to firearms

From Dahlberg, L. (1998). Youth violence in the United States: Major trends, risk factors, and prevention approaches. *American Journal of Preventive Medicine, 14,* 261.

Problems in school also increase the likelihood that children will turn to violence out of frustration and inability to learn. Research shows that academic failure and low commitment to school are associated with an increased risk for violent behavior (Farrington, 1991). Poverty, violent subculture, unemployment, and substance abuse often exacerbate the situation. Children raised in neighborhoods where they are continuously exposed to the sights and sounds of sirens, gunshots, and blood-spattered sidewalks begin to see these conditions as normal and grow up thinking of violence as an acceptable way to solve problems. Crime and violence are high in poverty areas, where at least 20% of the residents are poor (Lamison-White, 1996). These communities are characterized by large numbers of people living in poverty, high levels of transience, family disruption, crowded housing, low community participation and organization, and the presence of firearms and drug distribution networks. These neighborhoods have high rates of school dropouts, substance abuse, unemployment, and teenage pregnancy. They generally lack neighborhood cohesion and are without common values and norms. Individuals who live in these environments experience a sense of social isolationalism and do not form community attachments. Over time, children who grow up in these neighborhoods are more likely to adopt lifestyles and behaviors that put them at greater risk for violence.

Adolescents are especially vulnerable to firearm death and injury because of certain basic developmental characteristics in their age group. Teenage males often see gun ownership as an initiation into manhood. Studies support the belief that males are much more likely than females to engage in serious violence (Elliott, 1994; Loeber & Stouthamer-Loeber, 1998), possibly because they are socialized into roles that encourage higher levels of physical aggression (Oliver, 1989; Spivak, Hausman, & Prothrow-Stith, 1989). Adolescents believe they are invincible and often behave recklessly with weapons. Teenagers are increasingly independent and autonomous, which allows them more unsupervised time and contributes to their desire to challenge adult rules. They distance themselves from parental authority, struggle to establish an individual identity and self-worth, and try to develop mature behaviors. Curiosity about firearms and peer pressure may prompt teenagers to use firearms in ways they might otherwise resist. Although peer groups are generally positive, they can be negative if they pressure individuals to engage in risky behaviors. Numerous researchers have shown that delinquency is a group phenomenon (Elliott, Huizinga, & Ageton, 1985; Thornberry, Huizinga, & Loeber, 1995). Immaturity and impulsiveness can often result in dangerous experimentation and potentially lethal situations. Commonly, a shooting is precipitated by an argument that is generally impulsive and unplanned. Adolescents are much more likely to participate in negative activities if their friends encourage those behaviors.

No place in American society today is untouched by violence. It intrudes into all aspects of life and touches everyone in homes, schools, workplaces, highways, churches, recreational areas, and shopping malls. In this heightened atmosphere of violence, normal rules of behavior do not apply. Traditional social supports, such as home, school, church, and community, have disappeared, and new role models have taken their place. All too often children receive their direction from peers on the street, local drug dealers, and a variety of criminals. Prison is rapidly becoming the dominant institution that shapes the culture of our children, replacing church and school.

Increased gang activity and readily available firearms are largely responsible for high rates of homicide and violent crimes. Studies in several cities indicate that gangs may be responsible for 60% to 89% of all serious violent adolescent offenses (Thornberry, 1998). The formation of gangs has been a social and criminal problem in the United States for several decades. However, the number of young people involved in gangs and the violence produced by the gangs have proliferated dramatically. Gangs no longer are limited to big cities; they are active in 94% of all U.S. cities with populations greater than 100,000 (Klein, 1995). Today's gangs are also larger, more violent, and more inclined toward criminal activities (Kyriacou, Hutson, Anglin, Peek-Asa, & Kraus, 1999).

Children join gangs for various reasons, such as for protection, fun, and acceptance, as well as to gain a sense of family. Some young people join gangs for economic reasons, whereas others join for a sense of excitement. Various studies have associated gang formation with poverty, unemployment, delinquency, lack of family structure, lack of education, and racism (Castiglia, 1993; Clark, 1992; Klein, 1995). Interviews with gang members reveal that they often have a fascination with firearms. They see firepower as a means of empowerment. Often, these young people have already given up on the idea of conventional success and long-term survival. They seize the opportunities that are readily available. These gangs are well-equipped armies whose members embrace no socially accepted value system and have little conscience about using their weapons.

Children receive false ideas about violence from the media, where violence is glorified and sensationalized. Heroes are portrayed as invulnerable supermen who commonly use violence to solve their problems (Yokota & Thompson, 2000). The scientific literature strongly suggests that long-term exposure of children to television is an important cause of violent behavior in later years (Centerwall, 1992). By the end of their teenage years, the average adolescent has witnessed more than 200,000 violent acts on television, including 40,000 murders (Huston, Donnerstein, & Fairchild, 1992). Young children are unable to differentiate fact from fantasy, which increases their vulnerability to media-produced violence. Unfortunately, much of what children know about violence and its role in society is learned from the media. In addition to information obtained from the media, realistic toy guns and nonpowder firearms are frequently purchased for children. It is not surprising, then, that they feel comfortable with guns and develop a gun habit.

Another factor that contributes to the increase in childhood violence is the revolving-door justice system for juveniles. This system allows youthful offenders to repeatedly commit crimes and escape significant punishment or appropriate rehabilitation. Over the past decade, however, there has been a growing trend toward more severe punishment and incarceration for juvenile offenders. This practice has resulted in significant overcrowding within facilities and more blending of juvenile offenders with hardened adult criminals. Unfortunately, this places juveniles at greater risk for physical abuse and exposes them to individuals and influences that may interfere with future attempts at rehabilitation and redirection (Sickmund et al., 1997).

Mechanism of Injury

Penetrating forces occur from firearms, knives, and other objects. The mechanism of penetrating injuries in children is the same as it is for adults. However, when one understands how a knife or bullet can produce such devastating injuries and transfers that understanding to the smaller body of a child, the potential for significant damage becomes clear.

The severity of a wound caused by a knife or other sharp object is related to the anatomic site of the wound, the length of the projectile, and the angle of penetration (Creel, 1988). An exit wound may or may not be present, and the object may remain in place.

The characteristics and severity of a gunshot wound depend on the design of the weapon, the size or caliber of the bullet, the bullet's velocity or speed, the trajectory of the bullet, and the distance of the victim from the weapon. A bullet can take multiple routes once it is within the body, causing injury to multiple organs, and it may lodge in the body or exit through a separate wound. Injury may also be caused by fragments of bone that is struck by the bullet, creating secondary paths. Bullets that penetrate blood vessels can enter the cardiovascular system and embolize to the pulmonary, cerebral, or peripheral circulation, causing infarcts in these areas (White, 1989). Bullet embolization can occur hours after the actual shooting when the patient's position changes, causing movement of the bullets that have entered the cardiovascular system (White, 1989).

The nature of the wound is determined by the missile characteristics, such as the mass, shape, and construction of the bullet, as well as by the type of weapon. Characteristics of the tissue, such as elasticity, anatomic relationships, and density, also affect the wound. When a bullet strikes the victim, two major wounding mechanisms occur: (1) crushing of tissues in the bullet's path (permanent cavity) and (2) creation of a cavity by the transfer of kinetic energy from the bullet to the tissue (temporary cavity) (Hollerman, Fackler, & Coldwell, 1990).

Crushing of Tissues

A missile injures the victim initially by crushing the tissues it strikes, thereby creating a permanent cavity (Figure 13-1). Tissue destruction occurs because of a number of factors. *Yaw* is the deviation of a bullet from a straight path. If the bullet strikes the body at an angle, the angle of yaw is increased and more damage occurs as a result of a slowing of the bullet and increased energy lost to the tissues. *Tumbling* is the somersault action of a bullet that can create significant damage. Because both yaw and tumbling increase the area of the bullet as it strikes its target, the wound becomes more severe.

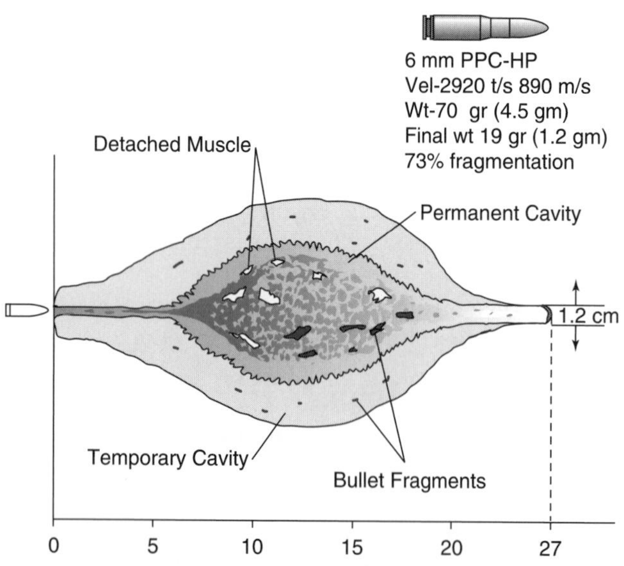

FIGURE 13-1 Permanent and temporary cavities. (From Fackler, M. L., & Malinowski, J. A. [1985]. The wound profile: A visual method for quantifying gunshot wound components. *Journal of Trauma, 25*, 525.)

Other factors that increase the degree of tissue destruction are bullet deformation and fragmentation. Soft-point and hollow-point bullets mushroom on impact, increasing surface area and wound severity (Berlin, Janzon, & Liden, 1988). Bullets that fragment increase the surface area and the volume of tissue crushed. Bullets can also cause secondary missiles, such as bone fragments, which increase the severity of the wound.

Temporary Cavitation

The energy lost by the missile as it enters the body is directly transferred to the tissues. As the bullet penetrates, kinetic energy is transmitted to the surrounding tissues, causing stretching, tearing, and displacement of tissues. The creation of this temporary cavity is called *cavitation.* The maximum size of the cavity, which can be many times the size of the bullet, is reached milliseconds after penetration. The pressure exerted against the cavity walls can approach 100 times that of atmospheric pressure (White, 1989). The negative pressure created behind the missile can draw outside contaminants into the cavity and along the entire wound tract. Structures not in the bullet path can be injured from the effects of cavitation.

Bullet velocity defines the extent of cavitation and tissue deformation. Low-velocity bullets travel at speeds of less than 1000 feet/sec, and injury is confined to a small area around the center of the tract. These bullets cause little cavitation. High-velocity bullets lose large amounts of energy to the tissue and produce large degrees of cavitation. These missiles travel at speeds of greater than 3000 feet/sec and can cause cavities with diameters 30 to 40 times greater than the diameter of the bullet (Weigelt & Klein, 1993). The potential for wounding is great, depending on the characteristics of the body tissue. Dense, less elastic tissue, such as bone, brain, liver, and spleen, and fluid-filled organs (e.g., the heart or the gastrointestinal tract), can be damaged severely by the formation of a temporary cavity because of the greater amount of energy imparted (Hollerman et al., 1990). Lower-density elastic tissues (e.g., the lung) are less affected by cavitation because less energy is transferred to the tissue (Creel, 1988).

The extent of injury can be extremely severe because of the mechanisms associated with high-velocity missiles, such as cavitation, yawing, and tumbling. Mortality rates are high.

Severe injury with penetrating trauma can occur as the result of *muzzle blast,* which refers to the combustion of gas and powder whenever the gun is held close to or in contact with the victim. The gas and powder enter the cavity and cause an internal explosion, which creates a burn (Hollerman et al., 1990). Cavitation is produced from the effects of combustion and is commonly seen with shotgun wounds.

Assessment and Management of Pediatric Gunshot Wounds

Despite advances in emergency medical and hospital care, many victims of gunshot injuries die before medical care personnel arrive (Meislin, Conroy, Conn, & Parks, 1999). The most effective means for decreasing morbidity and mortality associated with pediatric gunshot wounds are rapid transport, effective resuscitation, and immediate surgical intervention. The basic principles for pediatric trauma care are the foundation for management, with airway, breathing, and circulation having top priority. Little attention is given to the wound during the primary survey unless there is extensive bleeding, in which case direct pressure should be applied. The child is observed for the presence of a patent airway. If one does not exist, as evidenced by the presence of nasal flaring, grunting, stridor, or other signs of airway obstruction, immediate intervention takes place. This may include ventilation with 100% oxygen via a bag and mask and intubation. The need to establish an airway at the scene has been shown to be a poor prognostic indicator (Kountakis, Rafie, Ghorayeb, & Stiernberg, 1996).

It is important to clearly and concisely describe the wound. This will help reconstruct the events and injuries of the trauma. The location of the center of the wound and position in relation to anatomic landmarks, as well as the size and shape of the wound, are important pieces of information. Injury tattooing, strippling powder, or abrasions around the wounds should be described in detail. Evidence of gunshot residue on the clothing or skin should be documented (Nayduch, 1999). This description is especially important in the emergency center because wounds change with healing and make accurate reconstruction of events more difficult.

Penetrating injury has the potential to produce significant bleeding in the child. Because of the child's small blood volume (80 ml/kg), a small amount of blood loss can quickly produce hypovolemic shock. The child compensates effectively for blood loss and may not show a decrease in systolic blood pressure until 25% of the blood volume has been lost. Early signs of hypovolemic shock in the child include tachycardia, capillary refill greater than 2 seconds, cool and mottled extremities, pallor, and narrowed pulse pressure. Later signs include decreased urine output, decreased level of consciousness, and hypotension. Immediate intervention is restoration of the circulating blood volume by establishment of intravascular access and administration of fluids at 20 ml/kg.

During the primary survey a quick examination of the child's neurologic status takes place. In addition, the child is exposed and closely examined, especially for entrance and exit wounds and hidden injuries. Entrance and exit wounds are meticulously examined once the child has been stabilized and the appearance of the wounds is carefully documented.

Specific treatment of gunshot wounds depends on their location. A thorough discussion of these injuries and specific treatment regimens are presented in each system-specific chapter. Skull and cranial cavity wounds are often the result of firearm injury. Unfortunately, morbidity and mortality from these injuries are extremely high (Beaver et al., 1990). For gunshot wounds to the head, the child is stabilized and computed tomography scan is obtained if time permits. Surgical debridement will be necessary if the bullet has entered the intracranial compartment.

When neck injuries occur, the presence of neurovascular, neuromuscular, and aerodigestive structures creates complex management problems (Kountakis et al., 1996). Gunshot wounds to the neck can produce severe airway compromise as a result of an expanding hematoma or direct injury to the larynx. Close assessment for respiratory distress is necessary. If the child needs airway assistance, endotracheal intubation is the treatment of choice. If this is not possible, a cricothyroidotomy is performed.

Penetrating thoracic injuries are uncommon in children. Rib fractures indicate severe chest trauma and injury to underlying organs; however, serious injury may be present in the absence of obvious chest wall injury (Webster, Grant, Slota, & Kilian, 1998). The child is initially assessed for airway patency and the presence of respiratory compromise. If a pneumothorax or hemothorax is present, an appropriate-sized chest tube is inserted. Indications for a thoracotomy are massive or persistent bleeding, esophageal injury, or cardiac tamponade. Penetrating cardiac injuries always require surgical repair, but they are associated with a high mortality rate.

Gunshot wounds to the abdomen cause significant injury and in most cases require surgical intervention. Stab wounds may not require surgery if they are believed to be superficial. The high kinetic energy released by the projectile often results in unpredictable organ injury. The most common injuries are to the hollow viscera. Major vascular injuries are common, and the onset of peritonitis may be immediate (Martin & Derengowski, 1998). Individual organ injuries are treated specifically.

Injured major vessels often require debridement and anastomosis. Because significant bleeding usually results from these injuries, mortality is high. Wounds that are close to major vessels require careful observation for hematoma formation and frequent neurovascular checks, especially in the area of the neck where a hematoma can cause airway compromise. Gunshot wounds that result in injury to the bones are treated as compound fractures with exploration and debridement.

Collaborative Management

After surgical intervention, the general principles of postoperative care and wound management apply. The wound is assessed for epithelial resurfacing, closure, exudate, hematoma, and the presence of delayed bleeding (Bates-Jensen, 1999). Tables 13-2 and 13-3 list the positive and negative outcome measures for surgical wound healing, respectively. The child with a penetrating head injury is assessed for the presence of increased intracranial pressure and the development of seizures. Neck wounds require close observation for airway compromise. Pneumonia is a

TABLE 13-2 **Positive Outcome Measures for Incisional Wound Healing**

Outcome Measure	Days 1-4: Inflammation	Days 5-9: Proliferative	Days 10-14: Proliferative	Day 15-years 1-2: Proliferative Remodeling
Incision color	Red, edges approximated	Red, progressing to bright pink	Bright pink	Pale pink, progressing to white or silver in light-skinned patients; pale pink, progressing to darker than-normal skin color in dark skinned patients
Surrounding tissue inflammation	Edema, erythema, or skin discoloration; warmth, pain	None present	None present	None present
Exudate type	Bloody or sanguineous, progressing to serosanguineous and serous	None present	None present	None present
Exudate amount	Moderate to minimal	None present	None present	None present
Closure materials	Present, may be sutures or staples	Beginning to remove external sutures/staples	Sutures/staples removed; Steri-Strips or tape strips may be present	None present
Epithelial resurfacing	Present by day 4 along entire incision	Present along entire incision	Present	Present
Collagen deposition (healing ridge)	None present	Present by day 9 along entire incision	Present along entire incision	Present

From Bates-Jensen, B., & Wethe, J. (1998). Acute surgical wound management. In C. Sussman & B. Bates-Jensen (Eds.), *Wound care: A collaborative practice manual for physical therapists and nurses* (p. 229). New York: Aspen Publishers.

common complication after thoracic injury. Pulmonary toilet and pain management are necessary to decrease the incidence of pulmonary infections. Abdominal abscesses may develop after treatment of an abdominal gunshot wound; therefore the child is closely assessed for this complication. Repair of penetrating injury to the bone demands assessment for neurovascular deficits and the development of osteomyelitis.

Treatment with antibiotics in the postoperative period is often indicated only if the child develops signs of an infection. For children with complicated or infected wounds, nutritional support is critical to promote wound healing. Age-related factors, such as large obligate energy needs and low macronutrient stores, make the child more prone to nutritional depletion when adequate nutritional support is not provided. Pain management is essential, especially when considering the severity of gunshot wounds. Standard analgesic therapy is initiated immediately. A combination of opioids with benzodiazepines, such as midazolam or lorazepam, can maximize the child's pain relief. Attention to maintenance of mobility and skin integrity and prevention of further complications are essential components of nursing care. Chapter 11 presents a discussion of pain management issues in children.

An important consideration in the care of the pediatric gunshot wound victim is addressing the psychosocial needs. Regardless of the circumstances of the shooting, the child may have symptoms of posttraumatic stress disorder (PTSD). Symptoms include nightmares, flashbacks, sleeping disorders, anxiety, fear, and extreme stress when the child is exposed to situations similar to the traumatic event. The child and family should receive treatment and may require referral to a psychiatric liaison nurse, mental health practitioner, social worker, and/or psychiatrist. Treatment is initiated as soon as possible because PTSD may become chronic and persist for years. Chapter 23 discusses with the psychologic effects of trauma.

Prevention

The approach to violence prevention must be multifaceted; one method will not work for all situations. Innovative prevention approaches must focus on all forces that affect delinquency and violence. Strategies that address issues such as violent media messages, poverty, unemployment, family and school dysfunction, poorly developed coping skills, and the influence of drugs and alcohol must be developed.

The first step is to recognize violence as a public health problem. Prevention of violence must become a national priority if we want to stop losing our children to senseless acts of aggression. The advantage to the public health approach is that it is a proven method for reducing the encumbrance of illness, suffering, and early deaths among a population. The public health approach consists of health-event surveillance, epidemiologic examination, intervention design, and prevention of a particular illness or injury (Rosenberg, O'Carroll, & Powell, 1992). This approach has

TABLE 13-3 Negative Outcome Measures for Incisional Wound Healing

Outcome Measure	Days 1-4: Inflammation	Days 5-9: Proliferative	Days 10-14: Proliferative	Day 15-Years 1-2: Proliferative Remodeling
Incision	Red, edges approximated but tension evident on incision line	Red, edges may not be well approximated; tension on incision line evident	May remain red, progressing to bright pink	Prolonged epithelial resurfacing, keloid or hypertrophic scar formation
Surrounding tissue inflammation	*No* signs of inflammation present: *no* edema, *no* erythema or skin discoloration, *no* warmth, and minimal pain at incision site; hematoma formation	Edema, erythema, or skin discoloration; warmth, pain at incision site; hematoma formation	Prolonged inflammatory response with edema, erythema, or skin discoloration; warmth and pain; hematoma formation	If healing by secondary intention, may be stalled at a plateau (chronic inflammation or proliferation), with no evidence of healing and continued signs of inflammation
Exudate type	Bloody or sanguineous, progressing to serosanguineous and serous	Serosanguineous and serous to seropurulent	Any type of exudate present	Any type of exudate present
Exudate amount	Moderate to minimal	Moderate to minimal	Any amount present	Any amount present
Closure materials	Present, may be sutures or staples	No removal of any external sutures/staples	Sutures/staples still present	For healing by secondary intention, failure of wound contraction or edges not approximated
Epithelial resurfacing	Present by day 4 along entire incision	Not present along entire incision	Not present along entire incision, dehiscence evident	Not present or abnormal epithelialization, such as keloid or hyper trophic scarring
Collagen deposition (healing ridge)	None present	Not present along entire incision	Not present along entire incision; dehiscence evident	Abscess formation with wound left open to heal by secondary intention

From Bates-Jensen, B., & Wethe, J. (1998). Acute surgical wound management. In C. Sussman & B. Bates-Jensen (Eds.), *Wound care: A collaborative practice manual for physical therapists and nurses* (p. 230). New York: Aspen Publishers.

been proven successful in reducing the numbers of deaths attributed to infectious diseases, heart disease, and motor vehicle accidents. Former U.S. Surgeon Generals Antonia Novello, M.D., and C. Everett Koop, M.D., advocated for interventions based on a health care approach rather than a criminal justice approach (Weber, 1996). They and many others believe that punitive measures should be considered and reserved for incorrigible chronic offenders.

Many propose enhancing the criminal justice system as a means to prevent violence. High-visibility policing patrols directed at confiscating weapons and aggressive gun-oriented policing have been linked to decreased firearm violence (Fagan, Zimring, & Kim, 1998; Sherman, Shaw, & Rogan, 1995). Comprehensive firearm tracing systems have made it easier to identify illegal suppliers and weapons. Although this is an important approach to violence prevention, itself it is not enough by itself. The incidence of injuries and deaths from violence remains high despite ever-greater resources being directed toward the criminal justice system. Efforts should be directed at separating low-level juvenile offenders from chronic or violent offenders. The majority of time and resources should be directed toward rehabilitation of juveniles who show the most promise and who will benefit the most. Alternatives to incarceration, such as residential programs, day treatment, or community-restitution projects for low-risk offenders, may be better options. Programs that emphasize education, hard work, and social bonding, combined with effective after-care options, have been shown to facilitate the individual's return to the community and to decrease recidivism (Coordinating Council on Juvenile Justice and Delinquency Prevention, 1996). Even though the criminal justice system is critical in enforcing already existing laws and providing harsh penalties for crimes committed with firearms, criminal justice is dealing with the episode of violence after the fact. Comprehensive evaluations and development of treatment plans that focus on vocational, educational, psychologic, and familial risk factors may reduce recidivism. Prevention initiatives are necessary to avoid the episode in the first place.

The American Academy of Pediatrics recommends eliminating handguns from the environment of children and adolescents and changing society's attitude toward guns so that it becomes socially unacceptable for children and youths to have access to deadly weapons. They have issued several policy statements, which recognize that the solution to preventing firearm injuries and death must be multifaceted. There is no controversy about the fact that children and adolescents should not have unsupervised access to deadly weapons. However, not enough is being done to prevent children and adolescents from having this access. Child access prevention laws, which create criminal liability for owners of firearms used by children to cause death or injury, may be useful if the penalties are adequate and the offenses are not just misdemeanors (Wintemute, 1999).

The reduction of the number of injuries resulting from firearms may come from legislative and regulatory measures. Unfortunately, enforcement of existing laws will probably have a limited effect on the incidence of injuries, and additional regulations under existing legislation are highly dependent on the political climate (Christoffel & Naureckas, 1994). There have been a variety of attempts at legislation to reduce access to firearms. One of the most well-known laws is the Brady Handgun Violence Prevention Act, enacted in 1994. This law requires a background check for prospective handgun owners.

In February 1995, the 1-year anniversary survey of the effectiveness of the Brady Handgun Violence Prevention Act was released. The Bureau of Alcohol, Tobacco and Firearms (ATF) surveyed 30 law enforcement authorities from a cross section of the law enforcement population from around the country. The data collected included the number of applications to purchase handguns submitted to law enforcement officials since the Brady law went into effect, the number of applications denied, and the grounds for denial. This report revealed that from March 1994 to January 1995, the applications of more than 15,500 persons in the 30 surveyed jurisdictions (3.5% of those who applied for a handgun) were denied. The ATF confirmed through discussions with the firearms industry that the overall volume of handgun sales remained relatively constant during the survey period. The Brady law and associated state statutes prevent the purchase of firearms by 70,000 to 80,000 felons and other prohibited persons each year (Manson & Gilliard, 1999).

Other legislative measures have been proposed. Increased taxation on firearms and ammunition may be effective at reducing discretionary purchases of firearms. Banning certain kinds of ammunition, handguns, assault weapons, and deadly air guns may reduce the severity of associated injuries, but not the frequency of injury. New design standards for firearms have been proposed, such as locks on guns that can be unlocked only by those who know the code. This approach would prevent children from accidentally shooting a gun and may be helpful in preventing suicides.

Some states have implemented a one-gun-a-month law. This law makes the purchase of more than one gun in a 30-day period illegal. The law is limited to handguns and does not regulate rifles and shotguns. Limiting the number of guns that can be purchased takes the profit out of interstate gunrunning and will put many gun traffickers out of business.

Implementation of a national firearm fatality and injury reporting system has been suggested. This would provide information about the type of weapon that was used and the circumstances under which the injury or death occurred. It would also allow public health providers to determine the effect of the injuries and assess the associated factors (Cherry et al., 1998). A model for this already exists in the fatal accident reporting system, which communicates information on all motor vehicle–related fatalities (Teret, Wintemute, & Beilenson, 1992).

There are a large number of suggested legislative and regulatory approaches. The language is often complex, but health care providers should become familiar with the content of the legislation so that they can make informed decisions about support.

Often, health care providers find that families keep guns in their homes. One study examined gun storage by families owning at least one firearm and the factors associated with keeping the gun loaded. The majority of the 1682 families who owned guns were white (95%), lived in single-family dwellings (94%) in suburban neighborhoods (63%), and had one or more children younger than 5 years (69%). It was reported that 1033 families (63%) had at least one unlocked gun in the house, and 253 (15%) had at least one loaded gun in the house. In addition, 144 (7%) admitted to keeping at least one gun loaded and unlocked in the house. Factors associated with keeping a loaded weapon in the house were gun ownership for self-protection, job-related gun ownership, owning a handgun, keeping a gun in the bedroom, not having any men in the house, and having an unlocked gun (Senturia et al., 1996). Even though a common reason for having a gun in the house is self-protection, several studies report a correlation between guns in the home and homicide risk. The *New England Journal of Medicine* reports that guns kept in the home for self-protection are 43 more times likely to kill a family member, friend, or acquaintance than to kill an intruder. A later study found that the presence of a gun in the home led to a tripling of the risk of homicide in the home (Kellermann & Reay, 1986; Kellermann, Rivara, & Rushforth, 1993).

If guns are kept in the home, pediatric health care providers must encourage families to create a gun-safe home environment. This should include asking about the presence of guns, counseling on the dangers of having a gun, advising about the removal of guns, and emphasizing gun safety rules. This is particularly important when dealing with families that include alcohol- or drug-addicted individuals.

Better education of health care providers on how to define family issues, including violence, is a priority. More information is needed about the child who is exposed to violence in the home because of the possible development of response patterns that lead to violence in later life (Schwartz, 1996). Unfortunately, children exposed to violence do not receive adequate psychosocial assessment or treatment. Parents should be encouraged to talk to their children about violence and discuss alternative ways of dealing with anger and conflict. They should actively discourage aggression and sensitize children to the harmful effects of violence on others. All prevention programs should encourage strong parental participation.

Attempts must be made to identify children at highest risk for violence and to provide appropriate services. High-risk youths include those with a history of family or peer violence, substance abuse, depression, previous suicide attempt, the carrying of weapons, poor school performance, and delinquency (Schwartz, 1996). Active interventions should include psychosocial assessment, family counseling, and referral for support services. The most important prevention efforts concentrate on eliminating risk factors, and these programs must start very early. Efforts targeted at improving social interaction and problem-solving skills among aggressive and defiant children can possibly decrease behavior problems in adolescence (Kipke, Simon, Montgomery, Unger, & Iverson, 1997). Increasing efforts to diagnose and treat symptoms of hyperactivity when they first emerge may also prevent the development of more serious problems as the child matures. Interventions directed at improving academic achievements have been shown to be successful in reducing aggressive behavior (Ellickson & McGuigan, 2000; Hawkins, Catalano, & Kosterman, 1999). Waiting until the teenage years is often too late.

Certain behaviors and situations can signal a problem and be warning signs of more serious violence to come. Angry outbursts, cruelty toward animals, fascination with weapons, threats of causing harm, destruction of property, negative attention-seeking behaviors, and feelings of being victimized all can be signs of a growing problem. Immediate evaluation is required if these behaviors increase in frequency and intensity (Steger, 2000).

Development of community-based coalitions of professionals, parents, schools, police, and other groups is another strategy to address the issue of violence. These groups can deal with the issues of public education about violence and play a significant role in promoting protective interventions and societal action necessary to reduce firearm injury and death. Numerous curricula have been developed to deal with violence in the community. The curricula focus on increasing knowledge about issues related to violence or on building skills in young people (Schwartz, 1996; Tucker, Barone, Stewart, Hogan, Sarnelle, & Blackwood, 1999). The STAR (Straight Talk about Risks), which was developed by the Center to Prevent Handgun Violence, is a curriculum that has been implemented by several school boards and large city school districts. This program, which targets children in grades kindergarten to 12, provides education about firearms (Schwartz, 1996). The Harlem Hospital Injury Prevention Program has developed youth programs that address violence prevention in collaboration with groups such as Juvenile Justice, the Tactical Narcotic Task Force, the District Attorney's community outreach program, schools, and community-based organizations (Laraque et al., 1995). Over a 9-year period, the percentage of injuries, homicides, and other violence in the community has declined by nearly 50% (Durkin, Kuhn, Davidson, Laraque, & Barlow, 1996). Health care organizations across the country, in collaboration with community groups, have developed violence prevention programs that range from providing health care services in the community to lobbying for antiviolence legislation to participating in statewide community development initiatives. Schools are providing classes aimed at preventing violence. Many of these programs deal with conflict resolution, coping skills, and risk awareness. Studies suggest that these programs should be introduced in elementary school to positively influence the early onset of violence (DuRant, Krowchuk, Kreiter, Sinal, & Woods, 1999).

Often, these programs offer role modeling opportunities and the chance for children to learn other ways to resolve disputes and vent anger nonviolently. Children have an opportunity to get to know members of their community personally, and barriers are often removed. Community partnerships with businesses can be developed to offer structured work experiences. Peer mentoring has been shown to play a role in violence prevention and can be a valuable part of community-based violence prevention programs (Sheehan, DiCara, LeBailly, & Christoffel, 1999).

Gang prevention is a priority for pediatric health care providers. Prevention strategies that can be implemented include the following: identifying children at high risk for gang membership, involving parents, working on gang prevention programs, supporting firearm legislation, and encouraging responsible publicity by the news media and advertisers (Rollins, 1993). Reducing exposure to antisocial peers and strengthening bonds to family, school, and community groups can counteract negative peer influences (Resnick, Bearman, & Blum, 1997). Effective parenting is also a highly effective tool against antisocial peer influences.

Efforts to reduce the glorification of gun use in the media must be attempted. Because a correlation between television and violence has been demonstrated, parents must be encouraged to screen their children's viewing choices and limit the amount of time their children watch television. Parents should encourage children to discuss what they are watching and explain the consequences of violence. It is also helpful for parents to point out the positive behaviors and explain that violence is not the most effective solution to problems. Consumer groups must target media violence and lobby for changes. Support should be provided to the media for developing public service announcements that discourage violence. The media should be encouraged to offer a more balanced portrayal of violence and the consequences. Toy guns should meet certain safety standards and look like toys, not like real guns.

Obviously, there are no easy solutions when developing prevention strategies to reduce childhood firearm injuries. As mentioned earlier, a number of approaches will be necessary. Some suggested approaches with pros and cons are listed in Table 13-4. Research on the causes and contributing factors of firearm injuries is critical, as are studies dealing with interventions and prevention strategies. All health care providers need to use their knowledge in creative ways, demonstrate a willingness to allocate necessary resources, and take on the difficult issues required to turn the tide of violence.

CHILD MALTREATMENT

Child maltreatment or *abuse* refers to any adult behavior that is destructive to the normal growth, development, and well-being of the child. It includes both action and inaction that results in physical, sexual, emotional, or neglectful abuse of infants, children, and adolescents.

Different forms of abuse have been accepted for centuries in different societies. In the past, children who were considered undesirable for religious or economic reasons or because they were defective or female were often killed; this was usually culturally sanctioned. During the fourteenth century, unwanted children were thrown into the Thames River in England. During the Industrial Revolution, young children were forced to work long hours in dangerous settings in unhealthy conditions (Moloney-Harmon & Adams, 2001).

EPIDEMIOLOGY

In 1999 there were an estimated 826,000 victims of maltreatment nationwide (U.S. Department of Health and Human Services, 2001). Approximately 58.4% of the victims suffered neglect, 21.3% experienced physical abuse, and 11.3% were sexually abused. More than 35.9% of all victims were reported to have experienced other or additional forms of maltreatment. The highest rate for maltreatment was for the 0- to 3-year-old age group. This age group experienced 13 maltreatments per 1000 children in this population (U.S. Department of Health and Human Services, 2001). Children who were victims of maltreatment prior to 1999 were almost three times more likely to experience a recurrence during the 6 months after the first incident in 1999 than children without a history of maltreatment.

Approximately 1100 children died as a result of abuse and neglect (1.62 deaths per 100,000 children in the general population) (U.S. Department of Health and Human Services, 2001). Children younger than 1 year accounted for 42.6% of the deaths; 86.1% of the victims were younger than 6 years of age. Deaths were most often the result of neglect (38.2%) compared with other forms of maltreatment.

A study published in 2000 by DiScala, Sege, Li, and Reece examined children who were victims of abuse over a

TABLE 13-4 Possible Regulatory and Legislative Approaches to Reduce Firearm Injuries Affecting Children and Adolescents

Approaches	Pros	Cons
1. Enforce existing laws	• No new laws needed	• Private use limits effectiveness of laws addressing use (rather than ownership)
2. Owner liability for child use	• Clear social expectations set by new legislation • Gun promoters may support	• Requires repetitive owner actions that have been shown to be less successful with a variety of prevention initiatives • Entire burden on owner (none on manufacture or retailer)
3. Firearm registration and licensure	• Other potentially deadly products are so treated (e.g., motor vehicles)	• Current registration and licensure systems have had little effect • Effective tracking system could be extremely costly and difficult to enforce
4. Background checks	• Reduce impulse purchases • Reduce purchases by ineligible individuals • A survey of compliance with the Brady law has suggested that the criminal element's access to handguns is decreased with little inconvenience to law-abiding citizens	• Many shootings do not involve new purchases, felons, or deranged individuals • Impossible to identify all mentally ill individuals • Would not affect private sales
5. Ammunition modification	• Consumable, so changes will enter market quickly • Likely to reduce injury severity • Current civilian bullets pack needlessly high power	• Does not reduce gun accessibility, so it would not affect frequency of injuries
6. Assault weapon ban	• Rapid deadliness of these guns • Popular support for ban • Increasing use predicts increasing death and injury	• A minority of deaths and injuries are due to these weapons
7. Handgun bans where there are children	• Focus on children • Avoids adult choice and privacy issues • Wide popular support likely	• Unenforceable • Entire burden on owner (none on manufacturer or retailer) • Would not protect against loss of parents and other adult loved ones

10-year period. Children injured by child abuse compared with nonintentional injury were more likely to be younger and have a preinjury medical history. They were more likely to be injured by battering and shaking and to sustain intracranial injury. They were more likely to be admitted to intensive care and have a longer length of stay.

The majority (87.3%) of all victims were abused by at least one parent (U.S. Department of Health and Human Services, 2001). Female parents were identified as the perpetrators of neglect and physical abuse in the highest percentage of children. Male parents were identified as the perpetrators of sexual abuse in the highest percentage of children. Children who were abused by persons other than their parents were more likely to be maltreated by a male than by a female (Sedlak and Broadhurst, 1996).

Definitions of Child Maltreatment

Child maltreatment, also known as *abuse and neglect,* affects children from across all age groups, races, and socioeconomic groups. *Child abuse and neglect* has been defined by the Child Abuse Prevention and Measurement Act as any act or failure to act on the part of a parent or caretaker that results in death, serious physical or emotional harm, or sexual abuse or exploitation, or an act or failure to act that presents a risk of serious harm (National Clearinghouse on Child Abuse and Neglect, 2001). Various forms of child maltreatment exist, including physical abuse and neglect, sexual abuse, and emotional abuse and neglect.

Physical Abuse

Physical abuse involves the intentional injury of a child, especially an injury that requires medical treatment. When an assessment of physical injury is made, two elements are essential to consider. First is whether the explanation given is plausible as a means of causing the injury, and second is whether the developmental level of the child is consistent with the history (Theodore & Runyan, 1999). Physical injuries labeled by the parents as self-inflicted accidents require certain motor skills on the part of the child. This requires the nurse to determine the child's developmental level.

TABLE 13-4 Possible Regulatory and Legislative Approaches to Reduce Firearm Injuries Affecting Children and Adolescents—cont'd

Approaches	Pros	Cons
8. Handgun bans	• Addresses cause of most deaths • Has been enacted in some locales and upheld in federal courts • Avoids most of the limitations of other approaches • Appears to have growing popular support • Work toward this goal will provide many opportunities for public education	• Wide popular support must be built • It will take a long time because there are so many handguns in homes now • Not now politically feasible in many places
9. Regulate toy gun construction	• Some toy gun injuries occur • Criminals can use realistic toy guns • Adults and children sometimes mistake real guns for toys and vice versa • Children may learn to be comfortable with guns	• Few injuries involve toy guns • Possibility of toy-colored real guns could undermine effectiveness • Best approaches not clear
10. Omnibus child firearm safety legislation	• Cover all approaches for greatest effect • Would be a useful means of public education	• Long complicated bills are inevitable • Results will differ greatly in different locales, maintaining an ineffective patchwork of pertinent laws
11. Required gun safety education	• Easy to implement • Not opposed by gun promoters	• Safety message may be lost in fantasy • Developmental characteristics of children may make them incapable of learning to consistently avoid handling guns • May decrease adult vigilance and increase risk
12. Increased taxation	• Taxes exist and are accepted • Would affect discretionary purchases	• Would not affect private sales • May not be effective for less expensive guns
13. New design standards for firearms (device that would indicate when the gun is loaded, locks that can be opened only by those who know the code)	• May prevent accidental shootings • May prevent homicides and suicides	• Would not prevent gun owner from using the weapon in the commission of a crime or suicide • Would take a very long time, if ever, to replace all guns currently in private ownership

Modified from Christoffel, K.K. (1991). Toward reducing pediatric injuries from firearms: Charting a legislative and regulatory course. *Pediatrics* 88, 294.

BOX 13-2 Examples of Neglect

Delay or failure to provide physical or mental health care
Inadequate supervision
Lack of protection from household/environmental hazards
Poor personal hygiene
Poor nutrition
Inappropriate substitute child care

From Moloney-Harmon, P. A., & Adams, P. (2001). Trauma. In M. A. Q. Curley & P. A. Moloney-Harmon (Eds.), *Critical care nursing of infants and children* (2nd ed., pp. 947-979). Philadelphia: WB Saunders.

Physical Neglect

Physical neglect is the failure to provide the necessities of life, such as medical care, nourishment, housing, and supervision. This form of maltreatment may be fatal as a result of inadequate physical protection, failure to provide the essentials of life, and inadequate health care. It is often described as an act of omission rather than commission and may or may not be intentional. Although neglect can result in obvious physical signs, such as malnutrition, other forms, such as emotional neglect, can have a negative affect on the child's future development. Box 13-2 provides examples of physical neglect.

Sexual Abuse

Sexual abuse is any sexual activity between an adult and child and includes assaultive or nonassaultive abuse. *Assaultive abuse* results in physical injury and often severe emotional trauma. *Nonassaultive abuse* often results in little or no physical injury, yet the child who is chronically sexually misused often suffers severe emotional trauma and disruption in the development of sexuality. Sexual abuse is the least reported form of child abuse, particularly nonassaultive chronic abuse (Moloney-Harmon & Adams, 2001).

Emotional Abuse and Neglect

Emotional abuse and neglect are the failure of parents or caregivers to provide an environment in which the child can thrive and develop. This form of abuse can be extremely difficult to identify.

Munchausen Syndrome by Proxy

Munchausen syndrome by proxy (MSBP) is a form of child abuse that occurs when a child's parent or guardian falsifies a medical history or actually causes an illness or injury to the child (Moloney-Harmon & Adams, 2001). Additional elements of MSBP include the denial of responsibility for the illness and the resolution of symptoms when the child is separated from the perpetrator. Generally, clinicians regard MSBP as different from other forms of child abuse for three reasons: (1) MSBP may be symptomatic of a psychiatric disturbance in the perpetrator; (2) mortality and morbidity rates are higher; and (3) MSBP seems to be premeditated rather than motivated by acute frustration and impulsive behavior (Donald & Jureidine, 1996). MSBP is a complicated interaction among the parent, child, and the medical establishment. The priority is to ensure the child's safety and prevent further harm (Moloney-Harmon & Adams, 2001).

Risk Factors

There are certain risk factors that may be present in families and environments. When considering the risk factors shown in Table 13-5, keep in mind that the spectrum of child maltreatment covers all people in all socioeconomic groups.

Maltreatment is most likely to occur when there is a combination of negative forces affecting the family because these forces interact and reinforce each other. Such combinations can be overwhelming, especially for a family that is not as well equipped to cope with problems as are other families.

Common Indicators of Child Maltreatment

Nurses, physicians, and other members of the health care team must be suspicious for child abuse to make an accurate diagnosis. The mechanism of injury, the extent of the injury, and the timing are factors that lead to consideration of child abuse (Leventhal, 1999). Other presentations suggestive of child abuse include denial of the existence of injuries or how they occurred, an explanation inconsistent with the physical findings, and a marked delay in seeking medical attention (Moloney-Harmon & Adams, 2001). A history of prior trauma and review of the medical record may reveal a pattern indicative of prior abuse. All details of the elected history are evaluated carefully in the context of their consistency or discrepancy with the physical findings. Box 13-3 provides indicators of child maltreatment.

Collaborative Interventions

The priority for the abused child is to assess and stabilize airway, breathing, and circulation (the ABCs). The child is treated as any trauma patient, and system-specific injuries are managed.

Diagnostics tests are invaluable in supporting the diagnosis of child abuse. Table 13-6 lists diagnostics tests associated with child maltreatment.

The child is protected from further immediate injury. Abused and neglected children are often too young and too frightened to seek help themselves. In the case of suspected abuse, a decision is made as to whether it is safe to return the child to the home. If hospitalization is required because of a medical condition, the matter is temporarily solved. If hospitalization is not medically warranted, the practitioner, in collaboration with a social worker or protective services worker, makes the decision. The custody and possible placement of children during the investigative process are often controver-

TABLE 13-5 Risk Factors for Child Maltreatment

Parental Characteristics	Child Characteristics	Social/Cultural Issues	Family/Situational Stressors	Triggering Events
Young/inexperienced parents with limited resources	Prematurity	Younger parents	Loss of job	Difficulties in normal child rearing
History of violence as a child	Congenital anomalies, especially visible anomalies such as cleft lip	Single-parent families	Death of partner	Arguments or family conflict
Substance abuse	Developmental delays	Poverty and lower educational level (as reported by some studies; however, these factors do not mean that poverty or less education can be used to conclude that a particular child has been abused)	Financial problems	Acute alcohol or drug abuse
Poor parenting role models	Temperament: Child perceived as different or difficult, hyperactive, or fussy	Values and norms about discipline and punishment*	Marital conflict	
Social isolation		Life changes		
Unrealistic expectations of child's capabilities		Crowded living conditions		
Domestic violence		Violence common in family interactions		

Data from Ludwig, S. (1999). Child abuse. In G. Fleisher & S. Ludwig (Eds.), *Textbook of pediatric emergency medicine* (4th ed.). Baltimore: Williams & Wilkins.
*Need to differentiate between abuse and cultural health care treatments such as cupping and coin rubbing, which produce bruises that may look like child abuse.

sial. These decisions entail careful scrutiny of a number of factors, such as the child's age, nature of the injury, past treatment of injuries, and family characteristics (Moloney-Harmon & Adams, 2001). Such a decision is not made lightly because it could result in additional harm to the child or even a potentially fatal injury. Severity of abuse is not always the contributing factor to removal; instead, perceived future risk is of greater significance (Crosson-Tower, 1999).

All 50 states have laws requiring practitioners to report child maltreatment. Professionals who are mandated to report child maltreatment include physicians, nurses, other medical professionals, counselors, social workers, and school personnel (Crosson-Tower, 1999). These state laws have a number of provisions designed to remove legal impediments to reporting. These provisions include immunity from civil and criminal liability for reporting, abolition of doctor-patient privilege in situations of suspected maltreatment, and penalties that vary from nominal fines to imprisonment for failure to report (Zellman & Faller, 1996).

DOCUMENTATION

Inadequate documentation of pediatric injuries often makes the diagnosis of child abuse difficult. When injuries are documented, the information should be objective. Only what is seen, heard, smelled, tasted, and touched is documented (Salassi-Scotter, Jardine, & Lawson, 1994).

The history of the injury should be well documented. The date, time, and place of occurrence; the entire sequence of events with associated times; time lapses between injury occurrence and arrival for medical care; and both the child's and caretaker's accounts of the incident in their exact words (i.e., use quotation marks) should be recorded (Salassi-Scotter, Jardine, & Lawson, 1994).

The actual behaviors of the child and family in response to injury, to each other, and to hospital setting and staff should be described. In addition, behaviors that demonstrate the child's current developmental level should be noted.

Physical findings should be described in qualitative and quantitative detail. The number and location of injuries; the measured size, shape, and symmetry; color; distinguishing

BOX 13-3 Common Indicators of Child Maltreatment

Family Behaviors

Inappropriate parent-child interaction
Extremes of reactions to hospital staff (e.g., hostile or unconcerned)
Unrealistic expectations of the child
Parental denial of any knowledge of how injury occurred
Attribution of blame to sibling for injury
Inappropriate response to severity of injury by parent, such as underreacting or overreacting to child's condition

Child Behaviors

Extremes of behaviors (e.g., withdrawn or acting out)
Lack of opposition to painful procedures
Developmental delays
Inappropriate sexual behavior
Somatic complaints (e.g., chronic headaches, sleep disorders, enuresis)
Suicidal behavior and threats
Drug or alcohol abuse

Historical Findings

Story inconsistent with physical findings or developmental level
Delays in seeking medical treatment
Direct disclosure
Repeat visits to the emergency department

Physical Findings

Multiple injuries in various stages of healing
Injury type and location inconsistent with child's developmental level
Characteristic pattern reflective of object used to cause injury (e.g., belt marks)
Signs of poor overall care
Genital bleeding or discharge in prepubescent children

Radiographic Findings

Multiple fractures
Cortical metaphyseal fragmentation
Traumatic involucrum*
Skull fractures†
Suture separation*

Data from Salassi-Scotter, M., Jardine, J. M., & Lawson, L. (1994). Child maltreatment. In D. Henderson & D. Brownstein (Eds.), *Pediatric emergency manual* (pp. 293-322). New York: Springer.
*Not visible radiographically until 7 to 18 days after trauma.
†Evident immediately after trauma.

characteristics (especially those that give clues to injury cause); and evidence of previous injuries should be recorded. Pictures, body diagrams, or photographs should be used as necessary to clarify narrative descriptions (Salassi-Scotter, Jardine, & Lawson, 1994).

The abused child's hospital record is part of the substantive evidence that is used in court; thus detailed descriptions are critical. Failure to recognize and document, in accurate detail, the presence of injuries and the pattern of illnesses that are possibly related to child abuse may lead to recurrent trauma or death (Boyce, Melhorn, & Vargo, 1996).

Managing Staff Reactions

Caring for the victims of child maltreatment is extremely difficult for any health care provider. Especially difficult is offering support to the family. Salassi-Scotter, Jardine, and Lawson (1994) offer excellent suggestions for nurses caring for the child and family. They suggest that nurses recognize that families may be seeking help for themselves and for the child. A wide range of emotional responses may be seen in families confronted with suspected child abuse. Anticipation of these emotions will assist the nurse in supporting the family. A nonjudgmental attitude is essential, and extremes of reactions in responses (direct confrontation or completely ignoring) must be avoided. All discussions should be kept nonaccusatory and focused on the child. Emotional reactions can be deescalated by focusing on the health care team's and family's mutual concern for the child. Competition with the family for the child's attention or affection is avoided.

Staff often have strong feelings about the situation and require support themselves. Staff should acknowledge their personal feelings and recognize their potential effect on the care of abuse victims and families. The family should be viewed as the patient and the child as the victim, with the focus of care on assessment and treatment rather than punishment. Blame is not placed on the family. The health care team's responsibility is not to prove that abuse occurred or to identify the perpetrator but to file a report of suspicion. It is useful to have a written protocol for child abuse management to focus attention on safe care of child and family. Staff often discuss feelings of frustration and powerlessness. Learning more about child abuse and becoming involved in local prevention efforts may help combat these feelings.

SUMMARY

The continued high rates of violence-related deaths in the last few years demand that violence be recognized as a public health emergency. Even though mortality rates in children have decreased overall and deaths from injuries have also decreased, the rate of violence-related mortality has remained unacceptably high. Violence does not know the limits of cities, age, sex, or race; everyone, everywhere is

TABLE 13-6 Diagnostic Tests Associated With Suspected Child Maltreatment

Laboratory Studies	Comments/Rationale
Complete blood count	
Hematocrit, hemoglobin	Rules out shock, anemia Rules out organic cause of bruising or bleeding
Coagulation Studies	
Prothrombin time, partial thromboplastin time, platelets	Elevated levels may be the first indicator of abdominal injury Elevated levels are indicative of extensive soft tissue and muscle injury
Serum	
Amylase Creatine phosphokinase Syphilis serology Human chorionic gonadotropin Toxicology screen	Rules out sexually transmitted disease; all ages; suspected sexual abuse Rules out pregnancy; all postmenarche girls with history suggesting sexual abuse Rules out forced or voluntary ingestions and chemical abuse Rules out renal trauma, dehydration, ingestions, sexual abuse
Urine	
Red blood cells, specific gravity, toxicology screen, culture, pregnancy test, sperm	Culture for gonorrhea, *Chlamydia,* and other sexually transmitted diseases is especially important with suspected sexual abuse Microscopic examination for sperm; may be omitted if >72 hr since abuse incident or if child has bathed
Cultures	
Wounds, throat, vaginal, rectal	
Vaginal secretions	*Trichomonas,* yeast, or *Gardnerella* infections
Vaginal wet preparation	
Saline and potassium hydroxide with whiff test	
Radiologic studies	
Skeletal x-ray film; skull, ribs, extremities Bone scans Ultrasound, computed tomography scan, magnetic resonance imaging	Rules out fractures; common findings are multiple fractures of varying ages Detects remote injuries and extremely recent injuries Important in detecting subtle intracranial and internal abdominal injuries

From D. Henderson & D. Brownstein (Eds.). (1994). *Pediatric emergency textbook manual.* New York: Springer Publishing.

affected. Recognition of violence as a leading cause of mortality and morbidity in children must become a national priority. By making a commitment to tackle the problem of violence, nurses and other health care professionals can make a significant contribution to society at large.

BIBLIOGRAPHY

Anderson, R., Kochanek, K., & Murphy, S. (1997). Report of final mortality statistics, 1995. *Monthly Vital Statistics Report, 45,* 11.

Baker, S. P. (1976). 28,000 gun deaths a year: What is our role? *Journal of Trauma, 16,* 510-511.

Bates-Jensen, B. (1999). Chronic wound assessment. *The Nursing Clinics of North America, 34,* 799-846.

Beaver, B., Moore, V., Peclet, M., & Haller, J. (1990). Characteristics of pediatric firearm fatalities. *Journal of Pediatric Surgery, 25, 97-102.*

Berlin, R., Janzon, B., & Liden, E. (1988). Terminal behavior of deforming bullets. *Journal of Trauma, 28*(Suppl), S58.

Berman, A., & Jobes, D. (1991). Adolescent suicide assessment and intervention. Paper presented at the annual meeting of the American Psychological Association, Washington, DC.

Berton, M., & Stabb, S. (1996). Exposure to violence and post-traumatic stress disorder in urban adolescents. *Adolescence, 31,* 489-498.

Boyce, M. C., Melhorn, K. J., & Vargo, G. (1996). Pediatric trauma documentation: Adequacy for assessment of child abuse. *Archives of Pediatrics and Adolescent Medicine, 150*(7), 730-732.

Brent, D., Perpu, J., & Moritz, G. (1993). Firearms and adolescent suicide: A community case-controlled study. *American Journal Disease Children, 147,* 1066-1068.

Bureau of Justice Statistics. (1998). *Criminal victimization in the United States, 1986: A national crime survey report,* Washington, DC: U.S. Department of Justice.

Callahan, C., & Rivara. F. (1992) Urban high school youths and handguns: A school-based survey. *Journal of the American Medical Association, 267,* 3038-3042.

Cappel, C., & Heiner, R. (1990). The intergenerational transmission of family aggression. *Journal Family Violence, 52,* 135-140.

Castiglia, P. (1993). Gangs. *Journal Pediatric Health Care, 7,* 39-41.

Centers for Disease Control and Prevention. (1995). *BB and pellet gun-related injuries—United States.* Atlanta: Author.

Centers for Disease Control and Prevention. (1996). *Injury mortality: National summary of injury mortality data, 1987-1993.* Atlanta: U.S. Department of Health and Human Services, Public Health Service.

Centers for Disease Control and Prevention. (1997). Rates of homicide, suicide, and firearm-related death among children—26 industrialized countries. *MMWR Morbidity and Mortality Weekly Report, 46,* 101-105.

Centerwall, B. (1992). Television and violence: The scale of the problem and where to go from here. *Journal of the American Medical Association, 267,* 3059-3062.

Cherry, D., Annest, J., Mercy, J., Kresnow, M., & Pollock, D. (1998). Trends in nonfatal and fatal firearm-related injury rates in the United States, 1985-1995. *Annals of Emergency Medicine, 32,* 51-59.

Christoffel, K., & Naureckas, S. (1994). Firearm injuries in children and adolescents: Epidemiology and preventive approaches. *Current Opinion in Pediatrics, 6,* 519-522.

Clark, C. (1992). Deviant adolescent subcultures: Assessment strategies and clinical interventions. *Adolescence, 27,* 283-293.

Cohall, A., Cohall, R., & Bannister, H. (1998). Adolescents and violent crime. *Current Opinions in Pediatrics, 10,* 356-362.

Cook, P., Lawrence, B., Ludwig, J., & Miller, T. (1999). The medical costs of gunshot injuries in the United States. *Journal of the American Medical Association, 282,* 447-454.

Coordinating Council on Juvenile Justice and Delinquency Prevention. (1996). *The National Juvenile Justice Action Plan.* Combating violence and delinquency.

Creel, J. (1988). Mechanisms of injury due to motion. In J. Campbell (Ed.), *Basic trauma life support: Advanced prehospital care* (2nd ed.). Englewood Cliffs, NJ: Prentice Hall.

Crosson-Tower, C. (1999). *Understanding child abuse and neglect* (4th ed.). Boston: Allyn & Bacon.

Dahlberg, L. (1998). Youth violence in the United States: Major trends, risk factors and prevention approaches. *American Journal of Preventive Medicine, 14,* 259-272.

DiScala, C., Sege, R., Li, G., & Reece, R. M. (2000). Child abuse and unintentional injuries: A 10-year retrospective. *Archives of Pediatric and Adolescent Medicine, 154,* 16-22.

Donald, T., & Jureidine, J. (1996). Munchausen syndrome by proxy: Child abuse in the medical system. *Archives of Pediatrics and Adolescent Medicine, 159*(7), 753-758.

DuRant, R., Krowchuk, D., Kreiter, S., Sinal, S., & Woods, C. (1999). Weapon carrying on school property among middle school students. *Archives of Pediatric Adolescent Medicine, 153,* 21-26.

Durkin, M., Kuhn, L., Davidson, L., Laraque, D., & Barlow, B. (1996). Epidemiology and prevention of severe assault and gun inquiries in an urban community. *Journal of Trauma, 41,* 667-730.

Ellickson, P., & McGuigan, K. (2000). Early predictors of adolescent violence. *American Journal of Public Health, 90,* 566-72.

Elliott, D. (1994). Serious violent offenders: Onset, developmental course, and termination. *Criminology, 32,* 1-22.

Elliott, D., Huizinga, D., & Ageton, S. (1985). *Explaining delinquency and drug use.* Thousand Oaks, CA: Sage.

Fagan, J., Zimring, F., & Kim, J. (1998). Declining homicide in New York City: A tale of two trends. *Journal Criminal Law Criminology, 88,* 1277-1323.

Farrington, D. (1991). Childhood aggression and adult violence: Early precursors and later-life outcomes. In D. Pepler & K. Rubin (Eds.), *The development and treatment of childhood aggression.* Hillsdale, NJ: Lawrence Erlbaum.

Feero, S., Hedges, J., & Simmons, E. (1995). Intracity regional demographics of major trauma. *Annals of Emergency Medicine, 25,* 788-792.

Fingerhut, L., Jones, C., & Makuc, D. (1994). Firearm and motor vehicle injury mortality: Variations by state, race, and ethnicity—U.S., 1990-1991. *Advance Data From Vital and Health Statistics, 242,* 1-12.

Fingerhut, L. (1993). Firearm mortality among children, youth, and young adults 1-34 years of age-United States, 1985-1990. *Advance Data from Vital and Health Statistics, 231,* 1-17.

Fox, J. (1996). *Trends in children and adolescents violence: A report to the U. S. Attorney General on current and future rates of children and adolescent arrest.* Washington, DC: U.S. Department of Justice, Bureau of Justice Statistics.

Hartgarten, S., Karlson, T., O'Brien, M., Hancock, J., & Quebbeman, E. (1996). Characteristics of firearms involved in fatalities. *Journal of the American Medical Association, 275,* 42-45.

Hawkins, J., Catalano, R., & Kosterman, R. (1999). Preventing adolescent health-risk behavior by strengthening protection during childhood. *Archives of Pediatric Adolescent Medicine, 153,* 226-234.

Hennes, H. (1998). A review of violence statistics among children and adolescents in the United States. *Pediatric Clinics of North America, 45,* 269-280.

Hollerman, J., Fackler, J., & Coldwell, D. (1990). Gunshot wounds: Bullets, ballistics, and mechanisms of injury. *American Journal of Roentgenology, 155,* 685-692.

Huizinga, D., Loeber, R., & Thornberry, T. (1994). *Urban delinquency and substance abuse: Initial findings.* Washington, DC: U.S. Department of Justice.

Huston, A., Donnerstein, E., & Fairchild, H. (1992). *Big worlds, small screen: The role of television in American society.* Lincoln, NE: University of Nebraska Press.

Kann, L., Warren, C., & Harris, W. (1995). Youth risk behavior surveillance. *MMWR Morbidity and Mortality Weekly Report, 45,* 6, 7, 32, 35.

Kellermann, A., & Reay, D. (1986). Protection or peril? An analysis of firearm-related deaths in the home. *New England Journal of Medicine, 314,* 1557-1562.

Kellermann, A., Rivara, F., & Rushforth, N., Banton, J. G., Reay, D. T., Francisco, J. T., Locci, A. B., Prodzinski, J., Hackman, B. B., & Somers, G. (1993). Gun ownership as a risk factor for homicide in the home. *New England Journal of Medicine, 329,* 1084-1092.

Kipke, M., Simon, T., Montgomery, S., Unger, J., & Iverson, E. (1997). Homeless youth and their exposure to and involvement in violence while living on the streets. *Journal of Adolescence Health, 20,* 360-367.

Klein, M. (1995). *The American street gang.* New York: Oxford University Press.

Kountakis, S., Rafie, J., Ghorayeb, B., & Stiernberg, C. (1996). Pediatric gunshot wounds to the head and neck. *Otolaryngology-Head and Neck Surgery, 114,* 756-760.

Kyriacou, D., Hutson, R. Anglin, D., Peek-Asa, C., & Kraus, J. (1999). The relationship between socio-economic factors and gang violence in the City of Los Angeles. *Journal of Trauma, 46,* 334-339.

Lamison-White, L. (1996). *Poverty areas in the United States, 1995.* Washington, DC: U.S. Government Printing Office.

Laraque, D., Barlow, B., & Durkin, M. (1995). Children who are shot: A 30 year experience. *Journal of Pediatric Surgery, 30,* 1072-1075.

Leventhal, J. M. (1999). The challenges of recognizing child abuse: Seeing is believing. *Journal of the American Medical Association, 281*(7), 657-659.

L.H. Research, Inc. (1993). *A survey of experiences, perceptions, and apprehensions about guns among young people in America: Report to the Harvard School of Public Health.* Boston: Joyce Foundation Grant.

Loeber, R., & Stouthamer-Loeber, M. (1998). Development of juvenile aggression and violence: Some misconceptions and controversies. *American Journal of Psychology, 53,* 242-259.

Manson, D., & Gilliard, D. (1999). *Presale handgun checks, the Brady interim period, 1994-98.* Washington, DC: U.S. Bureau of Justice Statistics.

Martin, S., & Derengowski, S. (1998). Gastrointestinal system. In M. Slota (Ed.), *Core curriculum for pediatric critical care nursing.* Philadelphia: WB Saunders.

Max, W., & Rice, D. (1993). Shooting in the dark: Estimating the cost of firearm injuries. *Health Affairs, 12,* 171-185.

McCord, J. (1983). A forty year perspective on the effects of child abuse and neglect. *Child Abuse Neglect, 7,* 265-270.

Meislin, H., Conroy, C., Conn, K., & Parks, B. (1999). Fatal injury: Characteristics and prevention of deaths at the scene. *Journal of Trauma, 46,* 457-461.

Moloney-Harmon, P. A., & Adams, P. (2001). Trauma. In M. A. Q. Curley & P. A. Moloney-Harmon (Eds.), *Critical care nursing of infants and children* (2nd ed., pp. 947-979). Philadelphia: WB Saunders.

National Center for Injury Prevention and Control, Centers for Disease Control and Prevention. (1996). National summary of injury mortality data, 1987-1994. *Firearm Injuries and Fatalities Fact Sheet*, 1-4.

National Center for Injury Prevention and Control, Centers for Disease Control and Prevention. (2000). *Suicide in the United States.* Available at: http://www.cdc.gov/ncipc/factsheets/suifacts.htm.

National Clearinghouse for Child Abuse and Neglect. (2001). *In focus: The risk and prevention of maltreatment of children with disabilities.* Available at: http://www.calib.com/nccanch/prevmnth/risk.htm.

National Safe Kids Campaign. (1999). *Unintentional firearm injury.* Available at: http://www.safekids.org/fact99/firearm99.html.

Nayduch, D. (1999). Trauma wound management. *Nursing Clinics of North America, 34,* 895-906.

Oliver, W. (1989). Sexual conquest and patterns of black-on-black violence: A structural-cultural perspective. *Violence Victim, 4,* 257-273.

Rachuba, L., Stanton, B., & Howard, D. (1995). Violent crimes in the United States: An epidemiologic profile. *Archives of Pediatric and Adolescent Medicine, 149,* 953-960.

Rand Health. (2001). Guns in the family: Firearm storage patterns in U.S. homes with children. Available at: http://www.rand.org/publications/RB/RB4535/.

Reiss, A., & Roth, J. (1993). *Understanding and preventing violence: Panel on the Understanding and Control of Violent Behavior.* Washington, DC: National Academy Press.

Resnick, M., Bearman, P., & Blum, R. (1997). Protecting adolescents from harm: Findings from the National Longitudinal Study of Adolescent Health. *Journal of the American Medical Association, 278,* 823-831.

Rollins, J. (1993). Nurses as gangbusters: A response to gang violence in America. *Pediatric Nursing, 19,* 559-567.

Rosenberg, M., O'Carroll, P., & Powell, K. (1992). Let's be clear: Violence is a public health problem. *Journal of the American Medical Association, 267,* 3071-3078.

Salassi-Scotter, M., Jardine, J. M., & Lawson, L. (1994). Child maltreatment. In D. P. Henderson & D. Brownstein (Eds.), *Pediatric emergency nursing manual* (pp. 293-331). New York: Springer Publishing.

Schwartz, D. (1996). Violence. *Pediatrics in Review, 17,* 197-202.

Sedlak, A. J., & Broadhurst, D. D. (1996). *Executive summary of the third national incidence study of child abuse and neglect.* Washington, DC: National Clearinghouse on Child Abuse and Neglect.

Senturia, Y., Christoffel, K., & Donovan, M. (1996). Gun storage patterns in US homes with children: A pediatric practice-based survey. *Archives of Pediatric and Adolescent Medicine, 150,* 265-270.

Sheehan, K., DiCara, J., LeBailly, S., & Christoffel, K. (1999). Adopting the gang model: Peer mentoring for violence prevention. *Pediatrics, 104,* 50-54.

Sheley, J., McGee, Z., & Wright, J. (1992). Gun-related violence in and around inner-city schools. *American Journal Disease Children, 146,* 677-82.

Sheley, J., & Wright, J. (1993). *Gun acquisition and possession in selected juvenile samples.* Washington, DC: U.S. Department of Justice.

Sherman, L., Shaw, J., & Rogan, D. (1995). *The Kansas City gun experiment research in brief.* Washington, DC: National Institute of Justice.

Sickmund, M., Snyder, H., & Poe-Yamagata, E. (1997). *Juvenile offenders and victims: 1997 update on violence.* Washington, DC: Office of Justice Programs. Office of Juvenile Justice and Delinquency Prevention, U.S. Department of Justice.

Singer, M., Menden, A., Song, Y., & Lunghofer, L. (1995). Adolescents exposure to violence and associated symptoms of psychological trauma. *Journal of the American Medical Association, 273,* 477-482.

Singh, G., Kochanek, K., & MacDorman, M. (1996). Advance report of final mortality statistics, 1994. *Monthly Vital Statistics Report, 45.* Hyattsville, MD: National Center for Health Statistics.

Snyder, H., Sickmund, M., & Poe-Yamagata, E. (1996). *Juvenile offenders and victims: 1996 update on Violence.* Washington, DC: U.S. Department of Justice, Office of Juvenile Justice and Delinquency Prevention.

Spivak, H., Hausman, A., & Prothrow-Stith, D. (1989). Practitioners' forum: Public health and adolescent prevention of adolescent violence prevention project. *Violence Victim, 4,* 203-212.

Steger, S. (2000). Killed in school. *RN, 63,* 36-38.

Teret, S., Wintemute, G., & Beilenson, P. (1992). The firearm fatality reporting system: A proposal. *Journal of the American Medical Association, 267,* 3073-3078.

Theodore, A. D., & Runyan, D. K. (1999). A medical research agenda for child maltreatment: Negotiating the next steps. *Pediatrics, 104*(1S-II), 168-177.

Thornberry, T. (1998). Membership in youth gangs and involvement in serious and violent offending. In R Loeber & D. Farrington (Eds.), *Never too early, never too late: Risk factors and successful interventions for serious and violent offenders.* Thousand Oaks, CA; Sage.

Thornberry, T., Huizinga, D., & Loeber, R. (1995). The prevention of serious delinquency and violence: Implications from the program of research on the causes and correlates of delinquency. In: *Sourcebook on juvenile offenders.* Washington, DC: U.S. Department of Justice.

Tolan, P. (1988). Socioeconomic, family, and social stress correlates of adolescent, antisocial, and delinquent behavior. *Journal of Abnormal Child Psychology, 16,* 317-331.

Tucker, J., Barone, J., Stewart, J., Hogan, R., Sarnelle, J., & Blackwood, M. (1999). Violence prevention: Reaching adolescents with the message. *Pediatric Emergency Care, 15,* 436-439.

U.S. Department of Health and Human Services. (2001). *Child maltreatment 1999: Reports from the states to the national child abuse and neglect data system.* Washington, DC: U.S. Government Printing Office.

Weber, D. (1996). Healing a violent society. *Healthcare Forum Journal, 39,* 22-28.

Webster, H., Grant, M., Slota, M., & Kilian, K. (1998). Pulmonary system. In M. Slota (Ed.), *Core curriculum for pediatric critical care nursing.* Philadelphia: WB Saunders.

Weigelt, J., & Klein, J. (1993). Mechanism of injury. In V. Cardona (Ed.), *Trauma nursing: From resuscitation through rehabilitation* (2nd ed.). Philadelphia: WB Saunders.

White, K. (1989). Injuring mechanisms of gunshot wounds. *Critical Care Nurse, 1,* 97-104.

Wintemute, G. (1999). The future of fire-arm violence prevention. *Journal of the American Medical Association, 282,* 475-478.

Yokota, F., & Thompson, K. (2000). Violence in G-rated animated films. *Journal of the American Medical Association, 283,* 2716-2720.

Zellman, G. L., & Faller, K. C. (1996). In J. Briere, L. Berliner, J. A. Bulkley, C. Jenny, & T. Reid (Eds.), *APSAC handbook on child maltreatment* (pp. 359-381). Thousand Oaks, CA: Sage.

SECTION

SYSTEM INJURIES

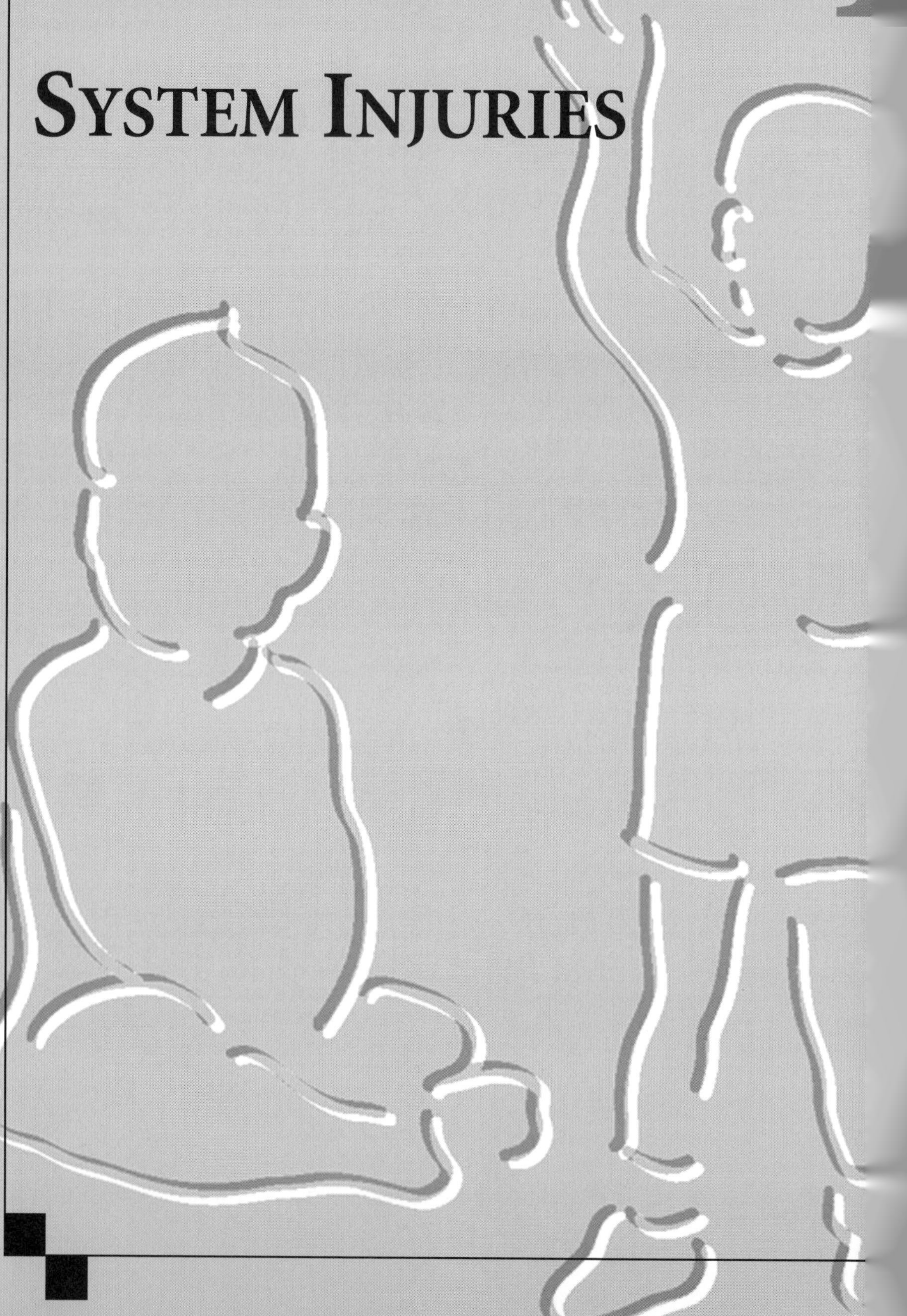

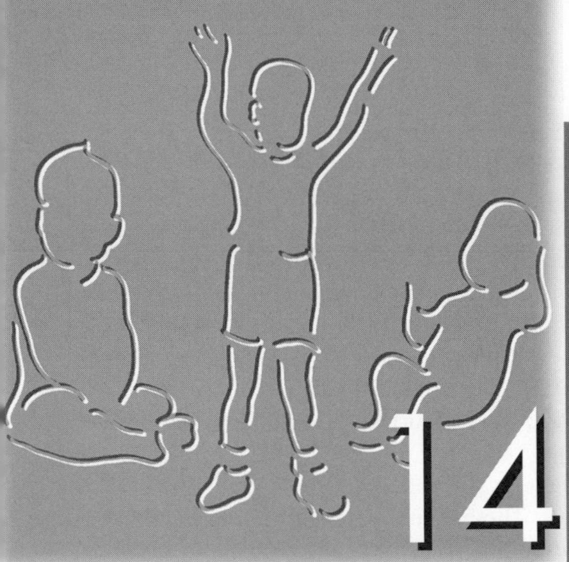

14 TRAUMATIC BRAIN INJURY IN CHILDREN

Paula Vernon-Levett

Accidental injury is the leading cause of death and disability among children. Although many organ systems may be injured in a child who has sustained a severe traumatic injury, it is injury to the central nervous system (CNS) that is responsible for most deaths and long-term disabilities (Sauaia et al., 1995; Tepas, Scala, Ramonofsky, & Barlow, 1990; Ward, 1995). In the past a universal term to describe accidental injury to the brain did not exist, making comparisons across groups and centers difficult. In recent years attempts have been made to search for a consistent term to describe acute neurologic injury. The most widely accepted term is *traumatic brain injury* (TBI). The National Head Injury Foundation (1986) defines a *TBI* as a CNS injury that occurs from an external source and is not of a degenerative or congenital nature. This definition attempts to decrease ambiguity by including only acute TBIs and by excluding extracranial injuries to the head and face.

Children with a TBI are particularly challenging to health care professionals because of different developmental aspects within this patient population. In children, organs develop and mature at different rates. The CNS is no exception. It has its own peculiarities of epidemiology, patterns of injury, pathophysiology, treatment, and outcome. Younger children have greater variability and unpredictability in their response to TBI compared with adults. This chapter presents a comprehensive overview of TBI in children and highlights developmental aspects of collaborative nursing care that are unique to the young child.

EPIDEMIOLOGY

The exact incidence of TBI in children is unknown, but it is estimated from epidemiologic studies of specific populations. Durkin, Olsen, Barlow, Virella, and Connolly (1998) reported the incidence of pediatric neurologic injuries resulting in hospitalization or death to be 155 incidents per 100,000 population per year. The mortality rate was 6 people per 100,000 population. TBIs vary among the pediatric population and depend in part on the characteristics of the community, age and sex of the child, and socioeconomic status of the child's family.

Children who live in large urban communities with high-rise living quarters are often victims of falls from windows, especially in warmer months and in warmer climates where windows are commonly left open. Injuries from violence and use of firearms are also more prevalent in urban settings. Suburban settings are associated with more sports-related injuries, and rural settings have the highest incidence of farm equipment–related injuries (Hall, 1994). Blunt trauma still predominates (approximately 80% to 90%) over penetrating trauma, but large urban centers have seen an increase in penetrating injuries in recent years. A decline in the incidence of TBI has been noted in communities that have high usage or mandatory helmet protection requirements (Kraus, Peek, McArthur, & Williams, 1994; Thompson, Rivara, & Thompson, 1989).

Mechanism of injury of TBI varies with age. In general, children in the 5- to 9-year age range have the greatest incidence of trauma. Infants and toddlers are often victims of falls and domestic violence. Injuries related to use of walkers and shopping carts also are unique to this age group. Older children have a higher incidence of pedestrian- and bicycle-related TBI. Assaults are most common in early adolescence (Durkin et al., 1998; Research and Training Center in Rehabilitation and Childhood Trauma, 1993). Individuals from all age groups are frequent victims of motor vehicle accidents. Males are involved in trauma more often than females at every age, and this predominance tends to increase with age (Durkin et al., 1998; Ward, 1994).

In an epidemiologic study, Durkin et al. (1998) reported an increase in risk for injury in low-income neighborhoods. Poverty is often associated with a family structure consisting of a young single parent with incomplete secondary education. These parental characteristics are markers for decreased use of automobile restraining devices and bicycle protective gear (Gotschall, 1993).

UNIQUE ANATOMIC AND PHYSIOLOGIC ASPECTS OF PEDIATRIC TRAUMATIC BRAIN INJURY

The CNS is in a continuous process of development that begins during the third week of gestation and proceeds at a rapid rate for the first 2 years postnatally. During this time the CNS grows quantitatively and qualitatively. Because of their unique anatomy and physiology, infants and young children have a predisposition for some types of neurologic injuries, but they are often protected from long-term neurologic sequelae. In adolescents anatomic and physiologic features of the CNS are more similar to those of adults; therefore their patterns of and responses to TBI tend to be similar.

Anatomic Features

Anatomic features of the young child that affect TBI include both skull and brain tissue components. The skull during infancy is very thin and pliable, with unfused suture lines and open fontanelles. The inner surface of the skull and orbital roofs and floors of the middle fossa are very smooth, and the subarachnoid space is smaller. The skull and subarachnoid space offer less resistance to brain shift and less protection for cerebral tissue (Rifkinson-Mann, 1993). A slowly expanding intracranial lesion is better compensated for in the infant than in any other age group. However, a rapidly expanding lesion is lethal in all age groups, especially in infants. Brain cell growth is incomplete at birth, and approximately five sixths of brain growth spurt is postnatal (Dobbing & Sands, 1973). Brain growth includes myelinization, glial cell population increase, dendritic arborization, and synaptic connection increase (Peacock, 1986). A significant injury during this growth period could presumably affect all of these processes. The total brain weight is 25% of adult weight at birth and increases to 70% of adult weight by age 4. Consequently, the center of gravity is higher in the young child who is "top heavy." If a young child is involved in a fall, the first part of the body to hit the ground is usually the head. Young children also have weaker neck muscles, which predispose them to cerebral damage from increased momentum as the result of deceleration forces.

Physiologic Features

The physiology of the immature brain has implications for TBI. Like the mature brain, the brain of the neonate and young child requires a constant supply of oxygen and nutrients. Cerebral blood flow (CBF) in the neonate and child is not well established. In the neonate CBF is believed to be low, corresponding to a low metabolic rate for oxygen (Altman, Powers, Perlman, Herscovitch, Volpe, & Volpe, 1988; Greisen, 1997). However, cross-brain oxygen extraction in the neonate is similar to that in adolescents and adults. This may provide a reserve capacity for low CBF states or when arterial blood has a low oxygen content (Greisen, 1997). The child's CBF is also closely coupled to cerebral metabolism. Reported values in normal children range from approximately 65 ml/100 g/min to 100 ml/100 g/min (Kennedy & Sokoloff, 1957; Settergren, Lindblad, & Persson, 1980). These values are significantly higher than CBF values in adults, which are approximately 50 ml/100 g/min. The ischemic threshold for infants and children is unknown.

Several physiologic mechanisms control CBF and are autoregulatory to maintain CBF within a constant range. Mean arterial pressure (MAP) and cerebral arteriolar vessel diameter are directly proportional to CBF, and vessel length and blood viscosity are inversely proportional to CBF. Pressure autoregulation represents the brain's intrinsic ability to maintain a constant CBF over a wide range of pressures. Vessel diameter increases with a decrease in MAP, and the opposite occurs when MAP increases (Figure 14-1). Cerebral tissue is no different than other organs when exposed to hypoxia. As PaO_2 decreases to levels of approximately 50 mm Hg, vessels compensate by dilating to increase CBF. $PaCO_2$ also affects cerebral vessel caliber; however, this response is not adaptive (i.e., autoregulatory) but rather primary. The relationship between $PaCO_2$ and vessel

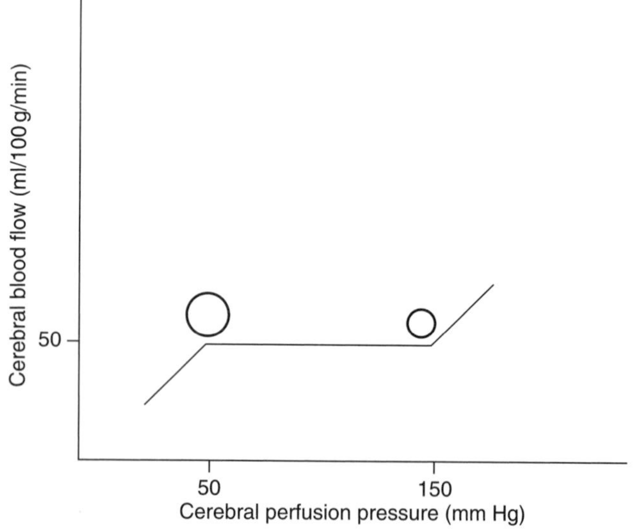

FIGURE 14-1 Autoregulation of cerebral blood flow. Blood flow remains constant at approximately 50 ml/100 g per minute over a range of cerebral perfusion pressures between 50 and 150 mm Hg. The circles represent cerebral blood vessels with different vascular resistance. The vessels constrict *(small circle)* or dilate *(large circle)* in response to cerebral perfusion pressure or decreases to maintain constant blood flow. (From Prociuk, J. L. [1995]. Management of cerebral oxygen supply-demand balance in blunt head injury. *Critical Care Nurse, 15,* 38-45.)

diameter is linear; an increase in Pa_{CO_2} causes an increase in vessel diameter and CBF. Figure 14-2 illustrates the linear relationships between CBF and Pa_{O_2}, Pa_{CO_2}, and blood pressure. Blood viscosity does not directly control vessel diameter, but a change in CBF velocity causes vessels to constrict or dilate.

In healthy newborn and term infants, pressure autoregulation is intact. However, unlike older children and adults, in whom pressure autoregulation is functional between a range of 50 and 150 mm Hg, the pressure range for the neonate is lower. Greisen (1997) suggests that the lower limit of arterial pressure autoregulation is below 30 mm Hg and the upper limit is above 60 mm Hg. His observations reinforce the idea that preterm infants have vascular sensitivity to oxygen and that Pa_{CO_2} vasoreactivity is intact.

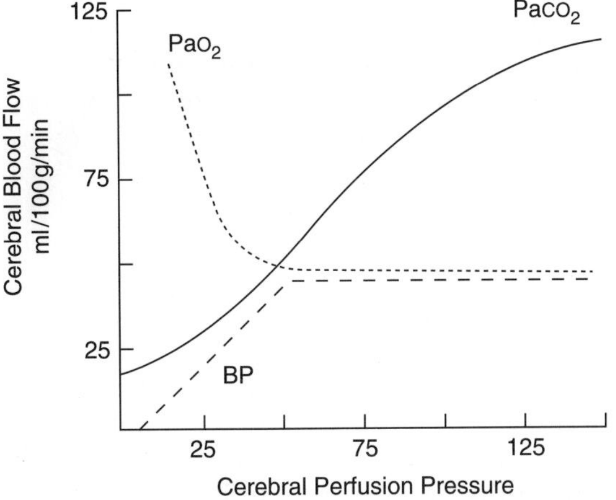

FIGURE 14-2 Cerebral blood flow alterations due to changes in Pa_{CO_2}, Pa_{O_2}, and blood pressure. (From Rogers, M. C., & Traystman, R. J. [1985]. An overview of the intracranial vault. Physiology and philosophy. *Critical Care Clinics, 1*[2], 195-204.)

PATHOPHYSIOLOGY OF TRAUMATIC BRAIN INJURY

There are two main pathophysiologic events that can occur intracranially after a severe TBI: cerebral hypertension and cerebral vascular ischemia. These secondary injuries may occur in tandem or, more frequently, simultaneously as a multidimensional process. If left untreated, both pathophysiologic events can result in further secondary injury to brain tissue in the form of endogenous biochemical cascades.

Cerebral hypertension develops from uncontrolled intracranial pressure (ICP). The rigid skull contains three different volume compartments: brain tissue (80% to 90%), cerebrospinal fluid (CSF; 5% to 10%), and blood (5% to 10%). According to the modified Monro-Kellie doctrine, an increase in one or more of the compartments requires a reciprocal decrease in volume in the other compartment(s). The relationship between ICP and volume is best described by the ICP-volume curve (Figure 14-3). The flat portion of the curve represents normal buffering (shifting of intracranial volumes) that takes place to avert abnormal increases in ICP; brain tissue has high compliance. The steep portion of the curve represents low compliance of brain tissue; the buffering capacity has been exhausted and abnormal increases in ICP are not controlled.

Normal ICP for children and adults is less than 10 mm Hg. In infants normal ICP is reported to be less than 3 mm Hg (Welch, 1980). Although there is no number that is universally accepted to define cerebral hypertension, most clinicians agree that an ICP of 20 mm Hg or more is pathologic and requires treatment. How an individual patient tolerates increases in ICP is variable and depends in part on where he or she is on the pressure-volume curve.

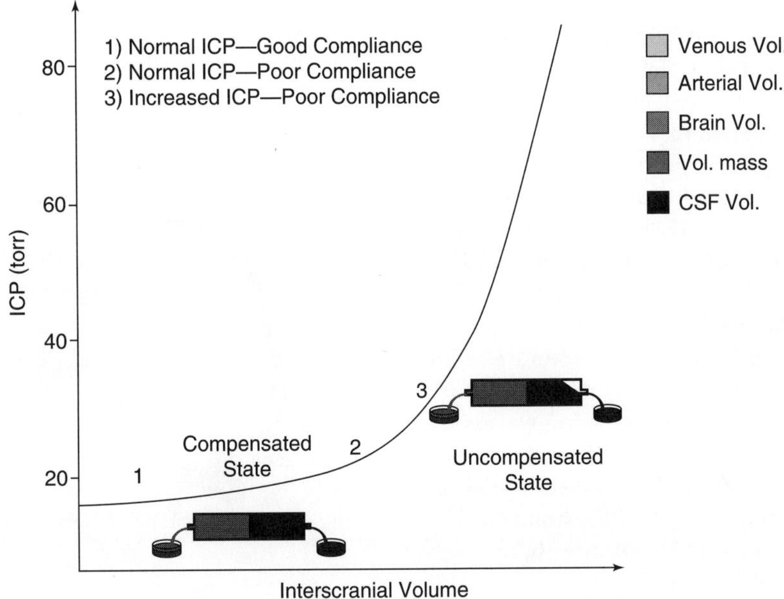

FIGURE 14-3 Pressure-volume curve of the intracranial vault. See text. (From Curley, M., & Moloney-Harmon, P. [2001]. *Critical care nursing of infants and children.* Philadelphia: WB Saunders.)

In patients with severe TBI, cerebral hypertension can evolve from a number of pathophysiologic processes. The most obvious cause is from a mass lesion (e.g., a hematoma) and a contusion. Less commonly, increased ICP results from excessive CSF accumulation. This can occur from obstruction of CSF pathways or from diminished reabsorption of CSF (e.g., blood in the subarachnoid space). The most common cause of cerebral hypertension in children is diffuse cerebral swelling.

Much of what is known about cerebral hypertension in children after a severe TBI was initially based on research and review articles from Bruce and associates (Bruce, Alavi, Bilaniuk, Dolinskas, Obrist, & Uzzell, 1981; Zimmerman & Bilaniuk, 1981; Zimmerman, Bilaniuk, Bruce, Dolinskas, Obrist, & Kuhl, et al., 1978). These researchers advanced the idea that children respond to TBI very differently than adults do. They reported general cerebral swelling was the most common finding on computed tomography (CT) scanning after acute head injury in children; this pattern was not seen in adults. This diffuse cerebral swelling was defined radiologically by CT scanning as an absence and compression of lateral and third ventricles and perimesencephalic cistern (Bruce et al., 1981; Zimmerman et al., 1978). Generalized cerebral swelling was believed to be caused by low cerebrovascular resistance resulting in increased CBF and increased cerebral blood volume but not true edema. Children were thought to have unique vasoreactivity that caused this malignant hyperemia. On the basis of these early reports, Bruce et al. (1981) advocated the use of hyperventilation and avoidance of mannitol (Osmitrol).

Recent studies have brought into question these earlier findings that describe cerebral swelling as a loss of cerebral vasomotor control leading to engorgement of cerebral vessels. In contrast to Bruce et al. (1981), Sharples, Stuart, Matthews, Aynsley-Green, and Eyre (1995) found cerebral swelling to be associated with low, rather than increased, CBF. A second study by Sharples, Matthews, and Eyre (1995) also showed that autoregulatory mechanisms and cerebrovascular resistance are preserved in most children after TBI. However, they also reported that there was a subpopulation of patients who died or had poor outcomes when their pressure autoregulation was disturbed. They further hypothesized that these patients may be more vulnerable to the development of cerebral ischemia. Aldrich et al. (1992), from the NIH Traumatic Coma Data Bank, reported that twice as many children developed diffuse cerebral swelling compared with adults, but this pathologic response was not unique to children. They also found that the highest incidence of lethal cerebral edema and hypertension was associated with early hypoxia and hypotension. Their conclusions support the concept that hypoxia and ischemia play an important role in the pathogenesis of diffuse brain swelling and edema and that this process is not directly or solely related to loss of cerebral vasomotor control.

Regardless of the pathogenic origin of diffuse cerebral swelling with increased ICP, the secondary insult to brain tissue has similar results. The most obvious consequence of cerebral hypertension is distortion, shifting, and herniation of brain tissue within the intracranium. A second detrimental effect is a significant reduction of blood supply to brain structures leading to focal or global ischemia. The consequences of ischemia are numerous and, in severe cases, lethal.

As previously discussed, it is becoming increasingly clear that children, as well as adults, experience early (the first few hours) ischemia after severe TBI (Adelson, Clyde, Kochanek, Yonas, & Marion, 1996; Muizelaar, Wei, Kontos, & Becker, 1983; Sharples, Stuart, Matthews, Aynsley-Green, & Eyre, 1995). In very simple terms, ischemia represents a mismatch between energy supply and demand with an excess of some substances (e.g., calcium and excitatory amino acid [EAA]) and a decrease in other substances (e.g., adenosine triphosphate, neurotropic factors). Figure 14-4 presents a schematic representation of the proposed pathologic events that can occur with TBI (Kochanek, 1993). Most notable are calcium ion disruption, increased EAAs, and inflammatory changes.

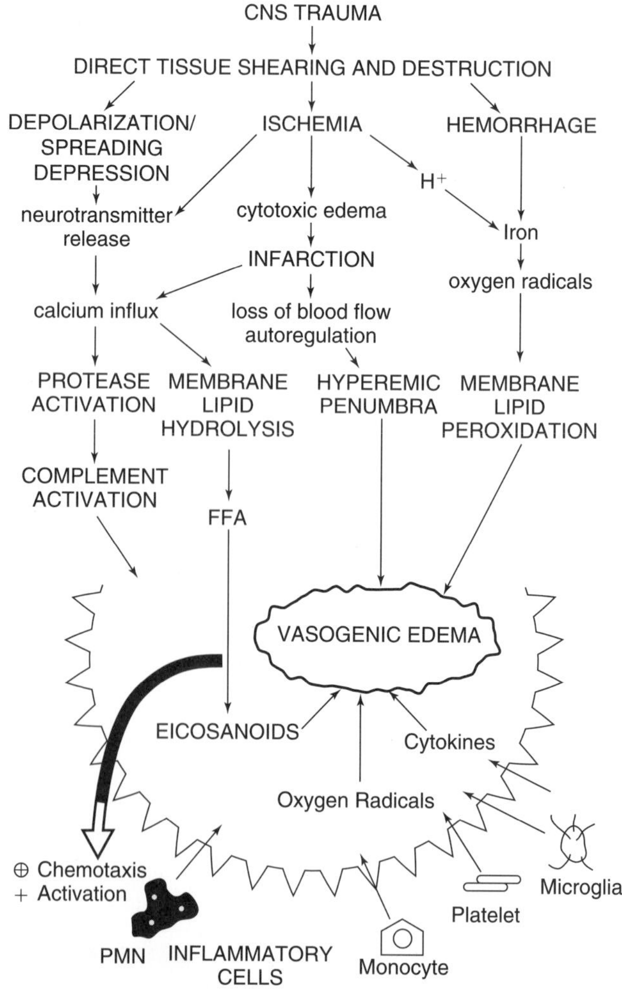

FIGURE 14-4 Schematic diagram of the proposed key events in the acute pathobiology of traumatic brain injury. (From Kochanek, P. M. [1993]. Ischemic and traumatic brain injury: Pathobiology and cellular mechanisms. *Critical Care Medicine, 21*[9, Suppl.], S333-S335.)

With ischemic injury, increased calcium is thought to play a major role in secondary injury after TBI. This event may initiate a number of biochemical cascades that eventually lead to cell lysis and death. EAAs (e.g., glutamate, aspartate) are known neurotoxic substances that accumulate after ischemic injury and, together with increased calcium, cause cell membrane dysfunction. There is evidence of a correlation between high levels of EAA and severity of brain damage (Choi, Barnes, Bullock, Germanson, Marmarou, & Young, 1994).

There is also a local inflammatory response initiated after TBI. Endogenous microglia are activated, and leukocytes increase. Both further the release of oxygen radicals, proteases, and local inflammatory mediators (Kochanek, 1993). The resulting vasogenic edema can lead to further ischemia and, in severe cases, cerebral hypertension.

Currently, the exact mechanism that causes cerebral edema remains unclear. Vasogenic edema may result from disruption of the blood-brain barrier. In contrast, cytotoxic edema may contribute to cerebral edema from secondary injury causing intracellular fluid fluxes. The blood-brain barrier can repair within 24 hours, and the commonly seen peak edema between 24 and 72 hours probably results from cytotoxic edema (Adelson & Kochanek, 1998). Most likely, a combination of toxic biochemical cascades and cerebrovascular vasomotor dysfunction plays a significant role in the development of uncontrollable increased ICP and brain damage.

TYPES OF TRAUMATIC BRAIN INJURY

TBIs are often classified into different groups: minor versus moderate-severe, closed versus penetrating, focal versus diffuse, and primary versus secondary. In all age categories, minor injuries prevail in incidence, and most cases go undetected. In children the majority of moderate to severe TBIs are diffuse closed head injuries (Levin et al., 1992). Primary injuries occur within seconds of the initial impact and include skull fractures, diffuse axonal injuries (DAIs), concussions, and penetrating injuries. Pathophysiologic responses that further tissue damage include endogenous biochemical cascades, which result in loss of autoregulation, disruption of the blood-brain barrier, and diffuse edema (cytotoxic and vasogenic). Clinical events that can contribute to secondary brain injury include systemic hypotension, infection, and hypoxemia (Adelson & Kochanek, 1998).

SKULL FRACTURES

Isolated skull fractures are usually minor injuries that require no further treatment; however, some are associated with intracerebral injuries that can be severe. Skull fractures in children are most often linear and occur along or perpendicular to a suture line. *Diastasis* refers to a fracture with a dural tear that continues to separate (grow) and is seen in infants and small children. Depressed fractures can be depressed bone fragments or an indentation of pliable bone without loss of bone integrity. Basal fractures can occur in different sinus locations of the skull: frontal, ethmoid, sphenoid, temporal, or occipital (Vernon-Levett, 1998).

Defining characteristics of skull fractures vary according to type and location. Patients with a simple isolated linear skull fracture are usually asymptomatic and are diagnosed with radiographs. Growing fractures are detected by radiographs or by palpation of an arterial pulse in the location of the fracture. Pathognomonic features of basilar skull fractures vary with location. Lee, Honrado, Har-El, and Goldsmith (1998) report a number of clinical signs associated with a temporal bone fracture: hearing loss (82%), hemotympanum (81%), loss of consciousness (63%), intracranial lesions (58%), and bloody otorrhea (58%). The raccoon or panda sign (periorbital blood collection) is seen with anterior basilar skull fractures, and rhinorrhea and anosmia are associated with middle fossa basilar skull fractures. Acute deterioration is associated with occipital basilar fractures because of the proximity and compression of vital centers in the brainstem.

Simple linear fractures usually heal without intervention. Growing fractures with dural tears require repair of the dura and cranioplasty. More extensive surgery is required with cysts or when brain tissue herniates through the bony defect. Most basilar fractures need only observation for 1 to 2 days. Meningitis, although rare, is a concern, but the use of intravenous antibiotics to treat CSF otorrhea is of questionable benefit (Lee et al., 1998). Most depressed skull fractures are uncomplicated and left untreated. Occasionally, they are surgically elevated when the depression is greater than the thickness of the skull.

CONCUSSION

A concussion is a diagnosis of exclusion and is based on patient history of loss of consciousness immediately after rapid deceleration of brain tissue. It represents a short-lasting disturbance of cerebral function without permanent morphologic changes. In most patients temporary or permanent retrograde amnesia is noted. Vomiting, headaches, and seizures may occur. In infants the presentation is less specific; loss of consciousness does not always occur. They have more generalized findings, such as lethargy, vomiting, pallor, and diaphoresis. No surgical treatment is required, and treatment is directed toward symptomatic relief.

DIFFUSE AXONAL INJURY

DAIs have been described more frequently in recent years because of better imaging technology. They are described as multiple focal lesions localized to the gray matter–white matter interface: the corpus callosum and dorsolateral aspect of the upper brainstem (Petitti & Williams, 1998). This injury is produced by rotational and shearing forces and is associated with sudden acceleration and deceleration injuries.

DAIs are characterized by loss of consciousness with a negative CT scan. Magnetic resonance imaging (MRI) can detect bleeding in the region of gray and white matter

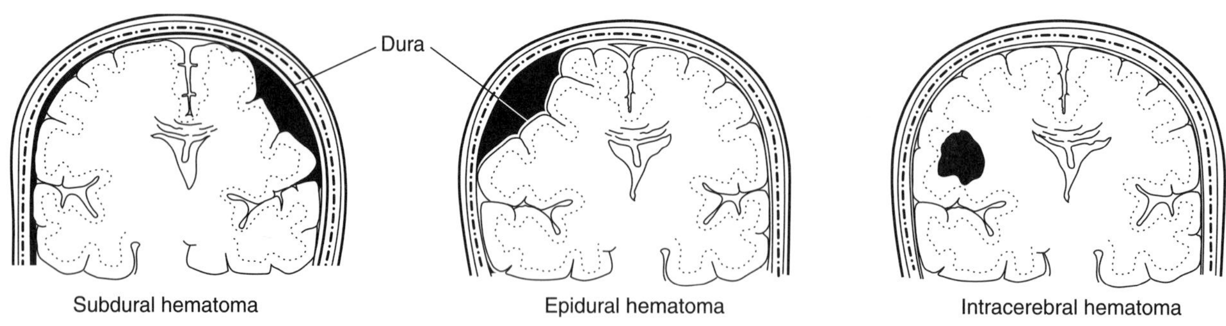

FIGURE 14-5 Types of hematomas. (From Luckmann, J., & Sorensen, K. C. [1993]. *Medical surgical nursing: A psychophysiologic approach* [4th ed., p. 753]. Philadelphia: WB Saunders.)

junction and in the brainstem (Magu, Mishra, & Gandhi, 1998). A DAI is a primary injury; no surgical intervention is required.

Intracranial Hemorrhage

Intracranial hematomas are classified into three types on the basis of anatomic location: epidural, subdural, and intracerebral (Figure 14-5). Epidural hematomas occur between the dura and the inner table of the skull. They have a characteristic biconvex, lenticular shape and rarely cross suture lines. In adolescents and adults bleeding usually occurs from the meningeal artery and is associated with a temporal bone fracture. In children, however, fractures are not always present, and bleeding most likely results from meningeal tears and dural vein tears (Bernardi, Zimmerman, & Bilaniuk, 1993).

Subdural hematomas occur between the inner table of the skull's dural surface and the thin meninges covering the brain. The most common source of bleeding is from stretching and tearing of the bilateral bridging veins between cortex and venous sinuses. Another source of bleeding is the tearing of dural sinuses, particularly the superior sagittal sinus. Large hematomas are commonly associated with contusion or laceration of underlying cerebral tissue (White & Likavec, 1992). Subdural hematomas are more common than epidural hematomas in children.

The last type of intracranial hemorrhage is an intracerebral hematoma or contusion. These injuries represent a heterogeneous area of hemorrhage and edema within brain tissue and can vary in size and location based on the mechanism of injury. They may occur directly opposite the point of impact (contrecoup injury) or at the site of impact (coup injury). Contusions and hemorrhages occur less frequently in infants and small children because they have a smoother inner table of the skull, which offers less resistance between bone and tissue with acceleration-deceleration forces. Also, demyelinized brain tissue has a softer consistency, which is believed to offer some protection against surface injuries (McLaurin & Towbin, 1986).

The defining characteristics of intracranial hemorrhage depend on the type, size, and location. Epidural hematomas from an arterial source represent a medical emergency because of rapid accumulation of blood that causes an increase in ICP. Children with epidural hematomas of venous origin may present with anisocoria, hemiparesis, or hemiplegia. Infants may present with a bulging fontanelle, separation of cranial sutures, and anemia (with significant bleeding). The clinical presentation of subdural hematomas is more nonspecific than that of epidural hematomas and may include lethargy or drowsiness, irritability, retinal hemorrhages, seizures, and bulging fontanelles (in infants). Contusions and intracranial hemorrhages of significant size produce classic symptoms of increased ICP: vomiting, headache, dizziness, blurred vision, dilated pupils, and respiratory arrest with central herniation.

Treatment depends on the type and size of intracranial hemorrhage. Epidural and large subdural hematomas are surgically evacuated. Small intracranial hemorrhages usually do not require surgical intervention. If they are large and continue to expand, producing significant increased ICP, they are surgically evacuated.

Generalized Cerebral Edema

Diffuse cerebral swelling (hyperemia) is the most common pathophysiologic feature occurring after TBI. However, it is differentiated from *true edema,* which is defined as an increase in brain volume resulting from an increase in water content. Cerebral edema may follow diffuse cerebral swelling, but the exact mechanism producing it is unclear and is probably multifactorial. Vasogenic edema represents disruption and increased permeability of endothelial cells allowing plasma filtrate to leak into the extravascular compartment. With cytotoxic edema, all brain cells (neurons, glia, and endothelial cells) undergo swelling. Severe endothelial swelling of the microcirculation can cause obstruction of the capillary lumens, producing a no-reflow phenomenon (Fishman, 1975).

The defining characteristics of cerebral edema are related to the severity and presence of significantly increased ICP. When increased ICP is present, symptoms include altered level of consciousness, vomiting, headache, and blurred vision. In severe cases the patient may present in coma with abnormal motor responses and unresponsive pupils. Increased ICP resulting from diffuse cerebral edema is not amenable to surgical intervention. An extensive discussion of the collaborative management is described later.

ASSESSMENT OF TRAUMATIC BRAIN INJURY

A complete assessment of neurologic function in the child with TBI encompasses four major areas. First and foremost is the clinical examination, followed by anatomic, physiologic, and electrophysiologic assessments. Without question, physical assessment of the patient begins at the time of initial contact. Depending on the patient's condition, the remaining assessment areas are conducted on an as-needed basis. In severely injured patients all areas of assessment are performed, some simultaneously.

CLINICAL ASSESSMENT

Clinical assessment of the CNS is unique from assessment of other organs: It cannot be inspected, percussed, palpated, or auscultated. Pediatric patients further complicate the assessment because of their different levels of CNS maturity. The examiner must adapt the examination to an age-appropriate level. In addition to the patient's condition, the degree of difficulty in obtaining the assessment may depend on the patient's degree of alertness, usual reaction to strangers, and communication skills. In the child with TBI, time is critical; an abbreviated and individualized neurologic examination is required to prevent delays in patient treatment.

HISTORY

How the neurologic examination progresses depends on the patient's level of consciousness and age. If the patient is young or has a diminished level of consciousness, the patient's history is obtained from significant others. Even in the alert, smiling, and cooperative child, it is almost always necessary to validate information with more reliable sources.

Important information obtained from the history that can give clues to the type and extent of TBI focuses on the mechanism of injury. Inquiries include how, when, and where the accident happened. Did the child lose consciousness, complain of headaches, or vomit? Pertinent information from the history includes perinatal course, developmental milestones, childhood illnesses, immunization status, allergies, significant or chronic illnesses, and current medications. If patient condition and time allows, a social history (e.g., school performance, play activities, substance abuse) is obtained to serve as a guide for planning rehabilitation and assessing outcome.

LEVEL OF CONSCIOUSNESS

The earliest and most sensitive indicator of neurologic function is level of consciousness. To accurately assess this function, the patient must be maximally aroused. If the child is not awake, the examiner should call him or her by name. If there is no response, a combination of verbal and tactile stimulation (e.g., shaking the shoulder) is used. In extreme cases when these measures are unsuccessful, painful stimuli (e.g., nail bed pressure, Achilles tendon compression) is necessary. When a stimulus does arouse the patient, it should be noted whether the patient stays alert when the stimulus is discontinued.

Altered states of consciousness are on a continuum ranging from lethargic to comatose. When communicating a state of consciousness, nonspecific terms (e.g., stupor, clouding) should be avoided; instead, the stimulus used and the behavior elicited should be objectively described. An example might be "opens both eyes when left index finger nail bed compressed."

Coma scales are often used to grade the degree of unresponsiveness in patients by standardizing assessments. The Glasgow Coma Scale (GCS) is the most commonly used coma scale (see Table 4-3, p. 36). The GCS was introduced by Teasdale and Jennet (1974) and later revised with one additional motor response category. It provides an objective measure of consciousness and therefore assesses the degree of central neurologic impairment. Three functional areas of behavior are assessed: eye opening assesses arousal state, verbal response assesses content of consciousness, and motor response assesses both arousal and content of consciousness. Each of the three components is given a score (verbal response, 1 to 5; eye opening, 1 to 4; motor response, 1 to 6) based on the best response elicited. The sum of numbers ranges from 3 (unresponsive) to 15 (normal). The GCS has been adapted by others to accommodate preverbal children.

MOTOR FUNCTION

Assessment of motor function requires an understanding of normal motor development in infants and toddlers. Motor development precedes cephalocaudal and proximodistal. Knowledge of previously acquired milestones (e.g., sitting, crawling, walking) is essential for comparison to postinjury function. A number of primitive reflexes are normally present in infants and toddlers and are included as part of the motor assessment. Assessment includes determining the presence or absence of a reflex and its symmetry. Responses are compared with the child's preinjury baseline. A complete discussion of normal primitive reflexes is given elsewhere (Vernon-Levett, 1998).

If the patient can follow commands, muscle groups are assessed for strength, tone, and symmetry. Deep tendon reflexes are assessed and provide information on the integrity of corticospinal tracts. However, not all deep tendon reflexes are present in infants because of incomplete development of corticospinal tracts. When present in the infant, inequalities in response are not uncommon.

In the comatose patient there are several abnormal motor responses. Decorticate posturing is described as flexion and adduction of the upper extremities and extension of the lower extremities with plantar flexion. This response represents dysfunction of the cerebral hemispheres or the upper portion of the brainstem. A second possible abnormal motor response is decerebrate posturing, characterized by extension, adduction, and hyperpronation of the upper and lower extremities and plantar flexion. It is indicative of pontomesencephalic level dysfunction. The most ominous of motor responses is no response at all, that is, flaccidity. In the absence of spinal cord injury or stroke, this represents dysfunction of the brainstem and its vital centers.

Pupillary Signs

Assessment of pupillary signs and eye movement provides indirect information regarding brainstem function via cranial nerves. Oculomotor cranial nerve III controls pupillary constriction, upper eyelid elevation, and most extraocular movements. Direct pupillary response is assessed for briskness and completeness of response. Pupils are noted for size and equality. Pupils normally are 2 to 6 mm in diameter, are equal, and constrict briskly to direct light. Early signs of cerebral hypertension include sluggishly reactive pupils or incomplete constriction. Dilated and unresponsive pupils may indicate brainstem dysfunction, severe ischemia, or herniation.

In the awake and cooperative patient, extraocular movements are assessed. In the comatose patient with an intact cervical spine, the oculocephalic reflex (doll's eye maneuver) is performed. This test is performed by moving the patient's head laterally from side to side while observing eye movement. A favorable response is seen when the eyes move in the opposite direction of head movement. A poor prognostic sign is observed when the eyes remain fixed in midposition. This usually indicates a lesion of the midbrain or pons.

Vital Signs

Vital signs are important parameters to assess, but they are not a reliable index of deteriorating neurologic function; however, they can be used to validate other clinical signs of neurologic deterioration. Abnormal vital sign parameters usually occur late in the clinical course. Specific respiratory patterns have been identified with neurologic dysfunction and may provide clues to the location of brainstem neuropathology (Plum & Posner, 1982). Cheyne-Stokes breathing is described as periodic breathing (i.e., phases of hyperpnea alternating with apnea). It represents neuropathology in the bilateral hemispheres or diencephalon. Central neurogenic hyperventilation is sustained, rapid, and deep hyperpnea from damage to the rostral brainstem. Prolonged inspiration with a pause at full inspiration is called *apneustic breathing* and may be seen with mid- or caudal-pontine level damage. Ataxic breathing is an irregular pattern and results from medulla injury.

Pulse and blood pressure changes are seen later than respiratory changes and represent severe neurologic dysfunction. Cardiac arrhythmias are nonspecific signs of TBI and are not seen in all patients. More common is a widening of the pulse pressure (Cushing's reflex), which often accompanies increased ICP. Temperature changes are nonspecific, and traditional methods of temperature measurement are often inaccurate indicators of brain temperature. Henker, Brown, and Marion (1998) compared brain temperature with bladder and rectal temperatures in adults with severe TBI. They found that bladder and rectal temperatures differ significantly from brain temperature, particularly in hypothermic and hyperthermic states.

Anatomic Assessment

Computed Tomography

Anatomic assessment of intracranial contents usually includes a combination of radiologic studies. Because of its cost, speed, and availability, the CT scan remains the gold standard for diagnosing intracranial injury in the early phases of trauma care. It is based on computer-image reconstruction from a series of slices of the brain. The CT scan can differentiate densities of brain tissue relative to water. It is superior to MRI in detecting acute intracranial blood (e.g., subarachnoid hemorrhage) and in evaluating cortical bone structures. Contrast media can be used to enhance images. For example, large cerebrovascular structures and breakdown of the blood-brain barrier can be visualized with an enhanced CT scan.

Magnetic Resonance Imaging

Despite the speed and ease of performing a CT scan, image resolution of the CT scan is significantly inferior to that of MRI (Chestnut, 1994). When a precise anatomic picture is required and time is not critical, MRI is the procedure of choice. MRI differentiates tissues by their response to radiofrequency pulses in a magnetic field; lesions have a high or low signal. It has excellent spatial resolution and can follow metabolic processes and structural changes. MRI is preferred to CT scanning in detecting pathologic conditions in the posterior fossa because bone artifact obscures lesions on the CT scan.

The MRI is inferior to the CT scan in detecting acute intracranial blood; MRI is not sensitive to fresh blood until several hours after the hemorrhage. Other disadvantages of the MRI are primarily related to the ease of monitoring the patient during the study. The magnetic field used with MRI prevents the use of metallic devises that are commonly used to monitor the acute care patient. Furthermore, the scanner isolates the patient from the caregiver at a time when close monitoring is necessary.

Skull Radiographs

Skull radiographs demonstrate structural abnormalities of bone tissue. Radiation is absorbed to varying degrees by different tissues. In addition to visualizing bone, radiographs show air-fluid levels in sinuses, abnormal intracranial calcifications, and pineal gland location. It is also useful in identifying missile injuries and some depressed skull fractures. During initial resuscitation, cervical spine radiographs are taken in three standard views: anteroposterior, lateral, and open mouth. With the widespread availability of CT scans, the utility of routine radiographs has been questioned. A radiograph does not visualize the intracranial contents; therefore CT scanning with bone views is a superior anatomic study.

Physiologic Assessment

Intracranial Pressure Monitoring

ICP monitoring uses a fiberoptic or fluid-filled catheter placed in the intracranium to continuously measure ICP. It is used in the patient with TBI for ongoing evaluation of condition, evaluation of therapy, and prediction of patient outcome. Several catheter locations are used for ICP monitoring, including subarachnoid, subdural, epidural, intraparenchymal, and intraventricular catheters. Intraventricular catheters remain the gold standard for monitoring patients with TBI because of their accuracy and reliability, as well as their ability to provide a means of draining CSF. Unfortunately, placement of intraventricular catheters is often difficult or prohibitive with small or collapsed ventricles, a common problem resulting from existing increased ICP. Disadvantages of all catheters include infection and bleeding. An extensive discussion of nursing care related to ICP monitoring is described elsewhere (Curley & Vernon-Levett, 1996).

Cerebral Blood Flow Studies

CBF can be assessed in patients with TBI by using a radioisotope tracer. Tracers are injected intravenously or inhaled while CT scanning is performed. This technique allows calculation of transit time of blood from one cerebral region to another. Because of its relative safety, the inhaled method is preferred over the intravenous route. Usually, a xenon gas mixture is used to measure brain tissue buildup of this tracer. It is based on the principle that clearance of an inert gas is proportional to blood flow in the tissue. The brain is scanned before, during, and after the gas mixture is inhaled while end-tidal xenon concentration is measured. This technique can correlate anatomic lesions to CBF and identify global and focal areas of ischemia.

Transcranial Doppler (TCD) ultrasonography is another technique that can be used to supplement evaluation of cerebral perfusion pressure (CPP). It originally was used for detecting vasospasm in patients with subarachnoid hemorrhage, but recently, there has been interest in using the technique for monitoring CBF in patients with TBI. This noninvasive, real-time study is performed with a 2-MHz ultrasound probe held to thin bone areas of the skull (e.g., temporal bone). It does not measure CBF directly, but it calculates mean velocity and direction of blood flow in the cerebral arteries. A pulsatility index is calculated, which reflects CPP; the index increases with decreasing CPP. Practical applications in the patient with TBI include evaluation of regional blood flow velocity, autoregulation, and $Pa{CO_2}$ vasoreactivity.

Unfortunately, TCD has not been found to be a sensitive measure of ICP and CPP in patients with TBI. Chan Miller, Dearden, Andres, and Midgley (1992) compared jugular venous oxygen saturation and TCD pulsatility index. They reported the pulsatility index did not change until brain ischemia already occurred. Other researchers have also concluded that TCD provides only a qualitative measure of changes in CBF (Jorgensen, 1995; Sabatino, Quantulli, & Morgese, 1994).

Jugular Venous Oxygen Saturation

A technique that has increased in popularity in recent years is jugular bulb oximetry. This technique uses a 4-Fr fiberoptic catheter placed retrograde into the jugular bulb to supply continuous readings of venous saturation ($S_{jb}O_2$). The obvious value of $S_{jb}O_2$ monitoring is its ability to provide information on cerebral oxygen supply and demand. It also provides information on the effectiveness of therapies. Normal $S_{jb}O_2$ values range between 55% and 70%; values below 55% indicate oligemia, and values greater than 70% indicate hyperemia. Confirmation of oximetry values is determined by measuring venous saturation via a catheter blood sample.

Although application of $S_{jb}O_2$ in managing patients with TBI is desirable, it is associated with some disadvantages. Catheter limitations include artifactual desaturation and errors in measurement as a result of position of the catheter along the vessel wall and from fibrin formation on the catheter tip. Overestimation of oxygen values may result from contamination with extracerebral blood. It is also relatively insensitive to infratentorial blood flow; the brainstem and cerebellum contribute little to total venous outflow. Finally, a falsely high $S_{jb}O_2$ value may occur from a leftward shift of the oxyhemoglobin dissociation curve under alkaline conditions (Bohr effect) (Gopinath et al., 1994; Kerr, Lovasik, & Darby, 1995; Sikes & Segal, 1994). Despite these limitations, improvements in technology continue to evolve, and further study is needed, particularly in children.

Electrophysiologic Assessment

Electroencephalogram

An electroencephalogram (EEG) assesses spontaneous electrical activity across the surface of the brain. This noninvasive study can be performed at the bedside. Specific EEG changes associated with acute TBI are both focal and general abnormalities. Focal EEG abnormalities consist of various paroxysmal activities and without etiologic specificity. Generalized findings include diffuse voltage reduction and slowing. Again, these findings lack etiologic specificity. In addition, lack of an abnormal finding does not rule out a pathologic brain condition. Practical applications in the child with TBI are limited to determining depth of coma, detecting seizure activity, managing chemically induced coma, and predicting overall outcome.

Somatosensory Evoked Potentials

Evoked potentials are recordings that measure electrical activity produced by a specific response to stimulation of a sensory pathway. This measurement is called an *evoked response* (ER), and neurologic dysfunction is characterized by a delay in this response. Several neural pathways may be studied, including visual ER (VER), brainstem auditory ER (BAER), somatosensory ER (SSER), and multimodality ER (MMER). The usefulness of ER in patients with TBI lies in its ability to identify neurologic dysfunction in specific sensory pathways. Sequential studies often demonstrate signs of improvement before clinical signs are evident.

Evoked potentials can be performed in uncooperative or comatose patients. The study is unaffected by sedatives or anesthesia, agents commonly used in the critically ill patient (Mason, 1992). Limitations of the study are seen in patients with ocular, auditory, or peripheral nerve disease. For example, BAER study cannot be used in a patient with external trauma to the ear canal. Also, studies of evoked potentials do not evaluate function of the frontal lobes or cerebellum.

COLLABORATIVE MANAGEMENT

A primary TBI occurs at the moment of impact and, when left untreated, has the capacity to progress to secondary injury. Collaborative management efforts are directed at preventing secondary injuries. As described earlier, the two pathophysiologic processes causing secondary injury are uncontrolled ICP and ischemic CBF. The goal of emergent and intensive care management is control of intracranial volume components (i.e., blood, CSF, and brain tissue) and preservation of CBF, especially the microcirculation. A potpourri of management strategies is available for treating the patient with TBI, and there is considerable variation in the management of patients with severe TBI even within the United States (Ghajar, Hariri, Narayan, Iacono, Firlik, & Patterson, 1995). Research protocols are evolving, but consensus for a standard protocol does not exist. Patients have different types of and responses to injuries, thereby complicating the standardization of interventions. Collaborative management strategies are individualized to each patient.

EMERGENCY MANAGEMENT

Emergency management of the child with TBI requires simultaneous assessments and interventions. Like any emergent situation, airway, breathing, and circulation (the ABCs) take precedence in managing the child. The initial assessment systematically focuses on vital components of the ABCs, neurologic disability, and exposure for life-threatening injuries. The airway is the first area to be assessed. All patients are assumed to have a cervical spine injury until one is ruled out by clinical examination and radiograph confirmation. The cervical spine is stabilized, and jaw-thrust maneuvers are used to open the airway.

After the airway is opened, respiratory mechanics are assessed to determine the adequacy of ventilation. The child is evaluated for symmetry of chest movement, signs of increased work of breathing (e.g., retractions, nasal flaring, tachypnea, grunting), and signs of penetrating injuries. Indications for intubation of the airway include a GCS score of 8 or less, maxillofacial trauma, aspiration, or absent gag reflex.

Restoration of adequate tissue perfusion is vital to preventing secondary TBI. Preservation of cerebral microcirculation depends on an adequate MAP. The child is assessed for early signs of systemic hypoperfusion, such as decreased capillary refill, altered level of consciousness, mottled skin, and tachycardia. Intravenous access is secured with at least two large-bore catheters. Restoration of circulation is performed with rapid infusion of isotonic fluids, 20 ml/kg per bolus. During this phase of care, placing a Foley catheter, obtaining blood and urine specimens, and administering tetanus toxoid are additional interventions performed.

The initial assessment is completed with a rapid neurologic assessment. Components of this evaluation include assessing the patient's level of consciousness, motor function, pupillary response, and vital signs. The GCS or modified scales for infants are valuable tools to use during all phases of trauma care. Examination of pupils is part of the rapid assessment and includes evaluation of pupillary size, symmetry, and reaction to direct light. In the alert or cooperative patient, extraocular movements are assessed. In patients with suspected devastating injuries, doll's eye maneuver or cold calorics are performed to assess brainstem viability.

The secondary assessment includes a systematic detailed assessment of all body systems to identify injuries not previously recognized. An *AMPLE history* is taken, which consists of *a*llergies, *m*edications, *p*ast medical history, *l*ast meal, and *e*vents leading up to the injury. Radiographic assessment includes cervical spine evaluation and possibly a CT scan. There has been considerable controversy over which patients require radiographic testing, especially in children. Patients with obvious neurologic injury or suspected severe closed head injury are usual candidates for CT scanning. Although clinical examination is reliable in children and adolescents for determining when further neurodiagnostic testing is indicated, the same is not true in infants. Greenes and Schutzman (1998) report that the absence of clinical signs does not exclude intracranial injury in infants in the first year of life. They conclude that radiographic studies are reasonable strategies for screening infants.

INTENSIVE CARE MANAGEMENT

Beyond the emergent phase, the child with TBI is transported directly to surgery or to the intensive care unit. Surgery is indicated for removing expanding lesions, evacuating significant hematomas, controlling hemorrhage, inserting an ICP catheter, or performing decompressive craniectomy. More often, the child is transported to the intensive care unit for further resuscitation and stabilization. The goal of intensive care management is the same as emergency management: normalizing ICP and maintaining adequate CBF.

OPTIMIZE CEREBRAL OXYGEN DELIVERY

The first priority in managing neurologic injury is optimizing oxygen delivery. This allows for recovery of primarily damaged but potentially viable neurons and curtails secondary ischemic insults. Oxygen delivery to the brain is accomplished by maintaining adequate CBF and normalizing levels of arterial saturation and hemoglobin.

Normalize ICP. The obvious means for improving CBF is maintaining ICP in a normal range. This may be done by surgical interventions; however, most TBIs in children are nonoperative. More commonly, ICP is managed by reducing one or more of the three components of the intracranial compartment: blood, brain, or CSF.

An effective way to reduce brain tissue volume is to remove extravascular fluid. A number of diuretics have been used in the past; to date, however, mannitol (Osmitrol) is the only pharmacologic agent that has become established as routine therapy for ICP control. Mannitol has been shown to attenuate cerebral hypertension via two primary mechanisms. The most commonly understood mechanism is the osmotic gradient created between the intravascular and extravascular compartments. Mannitol increases the osmolality of the blood. When the gradient exceeds approximately 10 mOsm, there is a net movement of free water from the interstitium into the intravascular compartment. The second major benefit of mannitol is its rheologic effect. Mannitol decreases blood viscosity, which improves CBF. Decreasing blood viscosity can potentiate autoregulatory mechanisms in the intact brain and reduce cerebral blood volume and ICP (Muizelaar et al., 1983).

Mannitol can be given every 4 to 6 hours or as necessary to control ICP. Dosing guidelines vary, but smaller bolus doses (0.25 mg/kg) were found to have equivocal beneficial effects with fewer side effects compared with larger doses (Dean & Moss, 1992). The use of mannitol is limited by the serum osmolality. A serum osmolality level greater than 310 to 320 mOsm/L is associated with renal failure and possibly rebound cerebral swelling.

Furosemide (Lasix) is given alone or, more commonly, in combination with mannitol. When used in conjunction with mannitol, furosemide reduces the initial increase in intravascular volume that accompanies a mannitol bolus. Furosemide can be given alone in hypervolemic states; the benefit is total body fluid reduction and possibly decreased CSF production. Peak effectiveness of furosemide occurs approximately 30 to 60 minutes after administration, which limits its use in managing acute increases in ICP. Furosemide administration is monitored closely to prevent hypovolemia and electrolyte imbalance.

A second means of normalizing ICP is through reduction of CSF. Various medications have been used unsuccessfully to decrease CSF production (Fishman, 1995). Currently, the most effective way of eliminating CSF is by drainage via an intraventricular catheter connected to an external ventricular drainage bag. An external ventricular catheter is placed at a predetermined ICP level so that when ICP exceeds this level, drainage occurs. It can also be opened for drainage based on patient clinical findings (e.g., dilated pupils). The disadvantages of intraventricular catheters are increased risk of infection and occlusion of the catheter tip. Drainage is sometimes complicated with diffuse cerebral edema as a result of compression of the lateral ventricles.

A simple noninvasive intervention to promote CSF drainage is body positioning. Elevating the head of the bed approximately 30 degrees and maintaining head alignment in the midline allow for drainage of CSF from the intracranial compartment into the spinal subarachnoid space.

Reducing CSF and brain tissue volumes is less effective in lowering ICP in comparison to blood volume reduction. Consequently, many interventions used to treat TBIs are directed at reducing cerebral blood volume through manipulation of the cerebral vessel caliber. Cerebral arterioles are known to respond to $Paco_2$ when vasoreactivity is intact. This response is related to hydrogen ion concentration; vessels constrict with lower levels of $Paco_2$ and dilate with increasing levels of $Paco_2$. Spontaneous hyperventilation is frequently seen in patients with TBI and is most likely a reflex mechanism to combat neuronal acidosis (Gabriel & Borel, 1996a).

A traditional cornerstone for treatment of increased ICP has been prophylactic controlled hyperventilation to reduce $Paco_2$ levels to 28 to 30 mm Hg. In recent years, however, this therapy has become increasingly controversial. The effect of $Paco_2$ on cerebral arterioles begins to diminish after 4 to 6 hours and lasts approximately 20 hours (Adelson & Kochanek, 1998; Gabriel & Borel, 1996a). This limited therapeutic effect in conjunction with increasing concerns over inducing ischemic blood flow has dictated the use of more moderate hyperventilation (i.e., low normal levels, 35 mm Hg). There is less disagreement on using controlled hyperventilation in an acute situation (e.g., a patient in the field with unilateral pupil dilation). Like most interventions, controlled hyperventilation is used cautiously and is individualized to each patient.

Promoting venous drainage is another technique for reducing total cerebral blood volume. This is accomplished by keeping the patient's head in the midline in a neutral position. Elevating the head of the bed 15 to 30 degrees is usual practice; however, some researchers advocate no elevation of the head of the bed because of concerns regarding ischemic blood flow (Rosner & Daughton, 1990; Rosner, Rosner, & Johnson, 1995). Feldman et al. (1992) studied the effects of head position on ICP, CPP, and CBF in adults. They found that as the head of bed was elevated from 0 to 30 degrees, ICP and MAP decreased significantly while CPP and CBF remained unchanged. However, a negative effect on CBF was seen when the head of the bed was elevated 60 degrees. Comparable studies do not exist in children.

Normalize Oxygen Content. Normalizing oxygen content can optimize cerebral oxygen delivery. In addition to $Paco_2$, maintenance of normal Pao_2 levels is important for controlling cerebral blood volume. As Pao_2 levels decrease below 60 mm Hg, vasodilation of cerebral arterioles results. In an already-compromised patient, the excessive cerebral blood volume can cause ICP elevation and secondary injury to brain tissue. Maximizing oxygenation in the patient with severe TBI is best accomplished with elective intubation and artificial ventilation.

To facilitate ventilation and lower metabolic demand, sedation and paralysis are used. Sedatives and paralyzing agents reduce anxiety and diminish awareness of noxious stimuli. Kerr et al. (1998) report that neuromuscular blockers attenuate increases in ICP in adults that occur with suctioning. Analgesics are used in conjunction with sedatives and nondepolarizing muscle relaxants to blunt increases in ICP related to pain, discomfort, and agitation.

Limited information is available to guide in the selection of these medications. The most commonly used sedatives include midazolam (Versed), diazepam (Valium), lorazepam (Ativan), and propofol (Diprivan). Nondepolarizing agents include vecuronium (Norcuron) and pancuronium (Pavulon); analgesics include morphine (Morphine Sulfate) and fentanyl (Sublimaze). Mode of administration is also of concern. Continuous infusions offer more consistent blood levels. Albanese, Viviand, Potie, Rey, Alliez, and Martin (1999) compared continuous and bolus infusion of opioids in patients with head injuries. They found transient increases in ICP with bolus injections and no increase in ICP with continuous infusions. Despite the advantages of sedation and paralysis, a number of concerns must be considered when these agents are used. Paralysis prevents serial physical examination of neurologic function; therefore it is usually reserved for when situations in which sedation alone is inadequate (Gabriel & Borel, 1996b). Further concerns regarding these medications involve prolonged weakness, myopathy, and time of awakening after the drugs are discontinued. Propofol is used with caution because of its potential for causing hypotension.

Oxygen delivery not only requires adequate CBF but is also dependent on normal hemoglobin levels. Hematocrit is directly related to blood viscosity, which affects CBF. Hudak, Jones, Popel, Koehler, Traystman, and Zeger (1989) confirm that cerebral arteriolar constriction occurs with hemodilution down to approximately 70% of baseline hematocrit. Below this level, very little or no benefit in CBF is found. Hematocrit level is individualized to each patient, taking into consideration respiratory parameters, ICP, CPP, and jugular venous saturation.

Optimize Systemic Arterial Pressure. CBF requires significant inflow pressure (MAP) so that blood flow can traverse the entire intracranial compartment. Optimizing systemic arterial pressure is achieved with intravenous fluids and vasoactive agents (Scalea, Maltz, Yelon, Trooskin, Duncan, & Sclafani, 1994). Fluid resuscitation has always been controversial and continues to be debated. However, the goal of fluid resuscitation remains clear: maintenance of adequate CPP and prevention of cerebral swelling.

With increasing evidence that early postinjury hypotension is associated with poor patient outcome, early resuscitation to maintain normal or slightly elevated MAP is critical. Hypotension is treated aggressively with fluids and vasopressors. In patients with intact autoregulation, induced hypertension can be helpful in preventing ischemia (Adelson & Kochanek, 1998; Rosner & Daughton, 1990). Increasing CPP causes an initial increase in CBF that results in vasoconstriction, blood volume reduction, and lowering of ICP.

The choice of fluids may vary, but isotonic solutions are usually administered early in resuscitation. Plasma expanders and blood are used when laboratory and hemodynamic values provide an indication. Both hyperglycemia and hypoglycemia can complicate the patient's condition and must be considered when selecting fluids. Even though studies evaluating the effects of hyperglycemia on neurologic outcome are inconclusive, avoiding glucose-containing solutions in early resuscitation is prudent (Sieber & Traystman, 1992). Hypoglycemia can cause neurologic damage and is treated aggressively with glucose. In patients with refractory increased ICP, Suarez et al. (1998) found that intravenous bolus administration of 23.4% saline reduced ICP and augmented CPP. A similar study performed in children with TBI compared lactated Ringer solution with hypertonic saline (Simma et al., 1998). They reported similar findings: Hypertonic saline administration significantly correlated with lower ICP and higher CPP. Although more research is needed, treatment of cerebral hypertension with hypertonic saline is promising and may be used more frequently in the near future.

When fluids and CSF drainage are not successful in maintaining adequate CPP, inotropic agents are indicated. Systemic pressors are titrated to maintain an adequate CPP. Because of size variation in children, determining the MAP to maintain an effective CPP is complicated and is individualized for each patient. Phenylephrine (Neo-Synephrine) is a commonly used vasopressor to manage CPP. Its long-term toxic effects are well known; therefore low-dose (2.0 to 4.0 µg/kg/min) dopamine (Intropin) is always given concurrently (Rosner, et al., 1995).

Optimize Cerebral Oxygen Consumption

Cerebral oxygen consumption is optimized by reducing metabolic needs so that metabolic supply and demand is in balance. A number of pathologic conditions can cause an uncoupling of cerebral oxygen supply and demand; examples are seizures, hyperthermia, Valsalva's maneuvers, pain, and agitation. Interventions to maintain or reduce cerebral oxygen consumption include prevention or control of seizures, induction of therapeutic coma, and maintenance of normothermia.

Seizures. Early (less than 7 days) posttraumatic seizures are often seen in children after TBI (Temkin, Dikmen, Wilensky, Keihm, Chabal, & Winn, 1990). Some predisposing factors for the development of posttraumatic seizure include a GCS score of less than 8, penetrating injuries, depressed skull fracture, subdural hematoma, cerebral edema, or any injury causing parenchymal damage (Adelson & Kochanek, 1998; Ward, 1995). Seizure activity is of particular concern in the acute period because intracranial compliance is diminished. Even a small increase in cerebral metabolism from a seizure can increase cerebral blood volume and ICP.

Anticonvulsants are not routine prophylaxis for all patients with TBI. However, any risk factor warrants early use of an anticonvulsant. The choice of anticonvulsant depends on the patient's current clinical status. Phenytoin (Dilantin) is often used when preserving the neurologic examination is important because it has less depressive effects on neurologic function. Phenobarbital (Luminal) can be used when further neurologic depression is of no concern.

Chemically Induced Coma. Historically, therapeutically induced coma was used to treat refractory increased ICP; however, its use has always been controversial. Barbiturates, particularly pentobarbital (Nembutal), are known to be neuroprotective by reducing metabolic requirements of the brain. They produce a dose-dependent decrease in CBF, cerebral metabolic rate for oxygen ($CMRO_2$), and ICP. With large doses, there is burst suppression on EEG followed by electrical silence. The standard level of burst suppression is present when there is 10 to 20 seconds between cortical activity (Adelson & Kochanek, 1998).

A chemically induced coma is not without risk, and indications for its use are unclear. Even though barbiturates are known to lower $CMRO_2$, their use in TBI has not been shown to improve outcome (Trauner, 1986; Ward et al., 1985). Large doses are associated with myocardial depression, which limits its therapeutic benefits. Patients are monitored closely for hypotension, and dopamine administration is often necessary to balance the vasodilatory effects of barbiturates.

Temperature Control. Fever is known to increase cerebral metabolism and can result in increased ICP. Ideally, temperature is monitored continuously or at frequent intervals. However, rectal and bladder temperatures do not correlate well with brain temperature in hypothermic or hyperthermic states. In one study, average brain temperatures were higher than average rectal temperatures (Henker et al., 1998). Patients with TBI may need to be treated with antipyretics at a lower febrile threshold (e.g., 37.5° C versus the usual 38.5° C) when rectal or bladder temperature is monitored.

In the past, induced hypothermia to 30° C was attempted in patients with TBI and was effective in lowering $CMRO_2$ and ICP. Unfortunately, the therapy was associated with cardiac instability and coagulation abnormalities and therefore was abandoned. Two studies subsequently evaluated the effectiveness of induced mild (34° C) to moderate (32° C) hypothermia in patients with TBI (Marion et al., 1993; Shiozaki et al., 1993). Both studies reported significant improvement in ICP control and patient outcome at 3 months. Clinical trials are under way to test the efficacy of this form of therapy in children.

COMPLICATIONS OF TRAUMATIC BRAIN INJURY

Patients who have sustained a severe TBI are at risk for developing systemic complications. Most patients with TBI experience at least one systemic complication after the initial injury is sustained (Gabriel & Borel, 1996b). The list of potential complications is long and variable. Complications commonly seen in the intensive care setting include acute respiratory dysfunction, endocrine disturbances, and coagulopathies. Table 14-1 provides a comprehensive list of systemic complications associated with severe head injuries.

Respiratory Dysfunction

Respiratory complications are often seen with severe TBI from either extracranial (e.g., depressed level of consciousness, contusions) or intracranial (neurogenic pulmonary edema) origins. Bratton and Davis (1997) reviewed TBI cases from the Traumatic Coma Data Base (TCDB) and found that 20% of patients with an isolated TBI had acute lung injury. Patients are at risk for respiratory complications because of their depressed gag reflex, prolonged ventilation, and heavy sedation. These risk factors are associated with a high incidence of aspiration pneumonia and pulmonary infections, both of which cause reduced lung compliance and ventilation/perfusion mismatch. Neurogenic pulmonary edema is commonly associated with severe TBI and can cause significant hypoxia. The pathogenesis is not well understood, but it is thought to result from excessive hypothalamus-mediated α-adrenergic discharge secondary to increased ICP.

Treatment of respiratory complications starts with good pulmonary toilet to remove excessive secretions and prevent infection. With superimposed pulmonary infection, antibiotics are administered. Campbell, Hendrix, Schwalbe, Fattom, and Edelman (1999) report that nasal colonization with *Staphylococcus aureus* at the time of severe head injury increases the risk of acquiring pneumonia during hospitalization. They recommend culturing the anterior nares early in admission so that preventive antibiotics can be administered.

Long-term ventilation usually requires a tracheostomy to facilitate airway protection and effective pulmonary toilet. Early tracheostomy care may decrease the incidence of pulmonary infection (Gabriel & Borel, 1996b). Complications can occur with a tracheostomy, but limiting time to decannulation to less than 50 days may markedly reduce airway complications in the pediatric patient with TBI (Citta-Pietrolungo, Alexander, Cook, & Padman, 1993).

Controlling ICP, administering diuretics, and monitoring fluid balance are methods used to prevent pulmonary edema in patients with neurogenic pulmonary edema. Intubation and controlled ventilation with positive end-expiratory pressure (PEEP) are also used routinely to improve oxygenation. However, there has always been concern when administering PEEP in the patient with TBI because of the concern that PEEP increases ICP and CPP. McGuire, Crossley, Richards, and Wong (1997) studied the effects of different levels of PEEP (5, 10, and 15 cm H_2O) on ICP and CPP. They conclude that in patients with increased ICP, there is no significant increase of ICP and CPP at all three levels of PEEP.

Endocrine Dysfunction

Common endocrine problems complicating TBI include diabetes insipidus (DI) and the syndrome of inappropriate antidiuretic hormone secretion (SIADH). Less commonly, disturbances in adrenal and thyroid function and in glucose and catecholamine metabolism have been reported.

TABLE 14-1 Systemic Complications Associated With Severe Head Injuries

System/Disorder	Therapy
General	
Deep venous thrombosis	Prophylaxis: passive exercises, thigh-high elastic stockings, or sequential compression devices Treatment: vena cave filter Heparin use discouraged because it may extend the intracranial hemorrhage
Decubital ulcers	Prophylaxis: repositioning every 2 hr Treatment: positioning of patient to avoid weight bearing on ulcer; application of nonadherent, occlusive wound dressings
Infection	Prophylaxis (only for patients with ICP monitoring devices in place): vancomycin, plus changing the ventriculostomy catheter every 5-7 days Treatment: CSF, blood, sputum, and urine cultures; administration of broad-spectrum antibiotics until source is identified
Hypermetabolism	Treatment: nutritional support (10%-16% of total calories provided as protein; the remainder split evenly between carbohydrates and fat); maintenance of intravascular volume
Pulmonary	
Aspiration pneumonia	Prophylaxis: head elevation; avoidance of large gastric residua Treatment: mechanical ventilation; intravenous antibiotics (if a superimposed infection is present)
Acute respiratory distress syndrome	Treatment: mechanical ventilation; intravenous antibiotics (if a distress syndrome superimposed infection is present); avoidance of hypervolemia-induced pulmonary edema
Neurogenic pulmonary edema	Treatment: control of ICP; diuretics, PEEP
Retained secretions	Treatment: standard therapies (cough induction, deep tracheal suctioning, chest percussion, postural drainage) almost always increase ICP; thus they must be accompanied by either preadministration of lidocaine or thiopental Combination of hyperventilation, preoxygenation with 100% oxygen, and a maximum of two suction passes
Cardiovascular	
Arterial hypertension	Treatment: adrenergic blockers (only if CPP is elevated and ICP is well controlled) Vasodilator use discouraged because these drugs may increase ICP
Myocardial ischemia	Treatment: β-blockers; nitroglycerin and calcium channel blocker use must be individualized because these drugs may increase ICP
Endocrine	
Hyperglycemia	Treatment: slow correction of the glucose level with sliding scale insulin coverage or intravenous insulin infusion; frequent monitoring of serum glucose level
Diabetes insipidus	Treatment: volume repletion; vasopressin (preferably, administered in 1 L of water)
SIADH	Treatment: fluid restriction
Cerebral salt-wasting syndrome	Treatment: fluid replacement with isotonic or hypertonic solutions
Gastrointestinal	
Gastritis/ulcers	Treatment: H_2 blockers and/or antacids; sucralfate
Delayed gastric emptying	Treatment: regular checks for gastric residua; metoclopramide (migration past the duodenum is particularly important for patients with pancreatitis)
Coagulation	
Prolonged PT or aPTT	Treatment: fresh frozen plasma or platelet transfusions

From Gabriel, E. M. & Borel, C. O. (1996). Managing systemic complications in patients with severe head injury. *The Journal of Critical Illness, 11*(4), 212-222.
aPTT, Activated partial prothrombin time; *CPP,* cerebral perfusion pressure; *CSF,* cerebrospinal fluid; *ICP,* intracranial pressure; *PEEP,* positive end expiratory pressure; *PT,* prothrombin time; *SIADH,* syndrome of inappropriate antidiuretic hormone secretion.

Diabetes Insipidus

The presence of DI after a severe TBI is an ominous sign. It results from injury to ADH-producing cells in the hypothalamus or to the posterior pituitary. The injured pituitary fails to release ADH when stimulated. Without enough ADH, the distal tubules and collecting ducts of the kidneys become impermeable to water, with free water loss. DI is characterized by profound diuresis of dilute urine. In addition to polyuria, polydipsia and dehydration are hallmark signs. The urine specific gravity is usually 1.005 or less, and serum osmolality increases to above 300 mOsm/kg, with serum sodium levels greater than 145 mEq/L (Blevins & Wand, 1992; Davies, 1996).

Treatment of DI depends on the severity of fluid and electrolyte derangements. Initially, the patient is weighed and serum and urine osmolalities and sodiums obtained. When hypovolemic shock is present, resuscitation with isotonic fluids is required. Once the patient is hemodynamically stable, fluid volume deficits are replaced with hypotonic fluids for 48 hours. When fluid therapy alone is unsuccessful, ADH replacement therapy is used and titrated to keep urine specific gravity greater than 1.010. Throughout treatment, the patient is weighed daily, assessed for changes in level of consciousness, and monitored for hypernatremia and hyperosmolality.

Syndrome of Inappropriate Secretion of Antidiuretic Hormone

SIADH is a severe metabolic disorder that results in acute changes in fluid and electrolyte balance. It involves an excess in the production and/or release of ADH. Consequently, it has the opposite effect on the kidneys; water is retained with expansion and dilution of intravascular fluids. Clinical manifestations include decreased urine output with increased urine specific gravity, decreased serum sodium below 125 mEq/L, nausea and vomiting, mental status changes, and possibly seizures.

For treatment of SIADH, fluid is restricted, usually to replace insensible losses. Once serum sodium is greater than 135 mmol/L, fluids are increased to a maintenance rate. In severe cases in which serum sodium is less than 120 mmol/L and the patient is at risk for seizures, hypertonic saline (3%) 3 to 5 ml/kg is administered as a slow intravenous push. Like DI, ongoing monitoring involves daily weighings and close trending of fluids and electrolytes.

Coagulopathies

Coagulation abnormalities are common after severe TBI. The exact pathogenesis is unknown, but they are probably related to severe tissue damage and release of thromboplastin. There is no consistent pattern of coagulopathies. Prolonged prothrombin and activated partial thromboplastin times may be seen alone or in combination with other clotting derangements (e.g., thromboplastin time, fibrinogen level, fibrin split products). Treatment consists of close monitoring of clotting factors and platelet count. Blood products are used to maintain clotting factors and coagulation parameters in a normal range.

OUTCOME OF TRAUMATIC BRAIN INJURY

Mortality

According to the National Pediatric Trauma Registry (1999), overall mortality for multiple trauma is 3.4%. However, when a subset of patients with TBI is separated from the larger group with multiple trauma, the mortality rate increases to between 3% and 24% (Henry, Hauber, & Rice, 1992; Klauber, Marshall, Luerssen, Frankowski, Tabaddor, & Eisenberg, 1989; Ward, 1994). Children who arrive at the hospital comatose and remain in that condition for at least 6 hours have the highest mortality, reported at 40% (Mamelak, Pitts, & Damron, 1996). Many clinical factors have been shown to predict outcome in patients with a TBI, but they can be grouped into two categories: age and severity of injury.

Age

It is well documented that children have a better outcome from TBI compared with adults (Henry et al., 1992; Klauber et al., 1989; Luerssen, Klauber, & Marshall, 1988). Age by itself has been reported to be the strongest predictor of outcome. Mamelak et al. (1996) found a linear relationship between increasing age and diminishing survival. In their study, approximately 60% of patients 0 to 19 years survived, compared with less than 20% of patients older than 60.

Severity of Injury

Historically, the GCS has been used to predict severity of injury and outcome in patients with TBI. Its predictive value is variable in the first few hours of resuscitation, and most researchers find it most valid when performed after 6 hours (Kokoska, Smith, Pittman, & Weber, 1998). Nonetheless, the validity of the GCS in young children, intubated patients, sedated patients, and patients with facial trauma remains questionable. Of the three categories used in the GCS, motor response is the most predictive (Klauber et al., 1989; Mamelak et al., 1996). As one might expect, motor responses with the poorest outcome are flaccidity and decorticate and decerebrate posturing.

In addition to motor response, extraocular motility and pupillary reactivity have predictive value. Mamelak et al. (1996) found a well-defined trend between survival and improving motor score, pupillary reactivity score, and extraocular motility score when measured 24 hours after admission. Twenty-four hours was a key factor in this study. For example, less than 1% of survivors had no motor response at 24 hours, compared with 20% of survivors without a motor response on admission.

The effects of hypotension on neurologic outcome in patients with TBI is not a new concept. Several researchers found a strong relationship between hypotension and increased mortality (Klauber et al., 1989; Kokoska et al., 1998). Outcome is most likely affected by the number of hypotensive episodes and the clinicians' ability to intervene quickly and efficiently to prevent cerebral ischemia.

Morbidity

Much has been learned about the developing brain and its response to neurologic insult. Children who have sustained a mild head injury rarely show any neurologic deficits (Fay et al., 1993; Jaffe et al., 1993). However, the same is not true for children who have experienced moderate to severe injuries. The National Pediatric Trauma Registry (1999) reported that 41.6% of trauma patients experienced some impairment in functional status. Most of these impairments occurred in children between the ages of 5 and 8 years, and the greatest number of impairments (four or more) were found in children with TBI.

Children with the most severe TBIs have the greatest variability in outcome measures. As one might expect, this group also shows the greatest deficits in performance at initial testing. Less commonly known is that this same severely injured group shows the greatest recovery during the first year of follow-up (Jaffe et al., 1993).

Despite all that is known, clinicians continue to be frustrated in their attempts to predict long-term morbidity in children who have sustained significant TBI. Predicting outcome in young patients is particularly difficult because brain development is still evolving. Delays in cognitive and motor function may not be evident until time has elapsed and critical neurologic milestones are delayed or never expressed.

Investigations of recovery from severe TBIs in children have identified a wide range of alterations in cognitive and behavioral functioning (e.g., visual-motor, intelligence, attention and memory, language, school achievement, and behavior). This underscores the need for a broad-based assessment of abilities. Neuropsychologic assessment is an important element of trauma care; it maximizes functional capacity and academic adjustment.

PREVENTION OF TRAUMATIC BRAIN INJURY

As the scientific approach to injury causation continues to evolve, so does the development of prevention programs. TBI is an important subcategory of traumatic injuries and is responsible for the majority of injury-related morbidity and mortality. Prevention of TBI in children is the same as any general strategy to prevent accidental injuries in children (see Chapter 2). However, there are preventive measures and strategies specifically designed to prevent TBI. Recreational-related TBI, including injuries associated with bicycling, roller-blading, skateboarding, roller-skating, hockey sledding, and skiing, are prevented primarily with helmet use. Playground surfaces can be altered and equipment height can be lowered to cushion falls. Other fall-related TBIs can be reduced with window bars and gates for stairs. Baby walkers should continue to be banned, and grocery carts must have safety belts. Transportation-related TBIs are also reduced with helmet use, car restraints, air bags, and treatment and education for alcohol abuse.

BIBLIOGRAPHY

Adelson, P. D., & Kochanek, P. M. (1998). Head injury in children. *Journal of Child Neurology, 13*(1), 2-15.

Adelson, P. D., Clyde, B., Kochanek, P. M., Yonas, H., & Marion, D. W. (1996). Cerebral blood flow and CO_2 responsitivity following severe traumatic brain injury in children. *Journal of Neurosurgery, 84,* 357A.

Albanese, J., Viviand, X., Potie, F., Rey, M., Alliez, B., & Martin, C. (1999). Sufentanil, fentanyl, and alfentanil in head trauma patients: A study on cerebral hemodynamics. *Critical Care Medicine, 27*(2), 407-411.

Aldrich, E. F., Eisenberg, H. M., Saydjari, C., Luerssen, G. G., Foulkes, M. A., Jane, J. A., Marshall, L. F., Marmarou, A., & Young, H. F. (1992). Diffuse brain swelling in severely head-injured children. A report from the NIH Traumatic Coma Data Bank. *Journal of Neurosurgery, 76,* 450-454.

Altman, D. I., Powers, W. J., Perlman, J. M., Herscovitch, P., Volpe, S. L., & Volpe, J. J. (1988). Cerebral blood flow requirement for brain viability in newborn infants is lower than adults. *Annals of Neurology, 24,* 218-226.

Bernardi, B., Zimmerman, R. A., & Bilaniuk, L. T. (1993). Neuroradiologic evaluation of pediatric craniocerebral trauma. *Topics in Magnetic Resonance Imaging, 5,* 161-173.

Blevins, L. S., & Wand, G. S. (1992). Diabetes insipidus. *Critical Care Medicine, 20*(1), 69-79.

Bratton, S. L., & Davis, R. L. (1997). Acute lung injury in isolated traumatic brain injury. *Neurosurgery, 40*(4), 707-712.

Bruce, D. A., Alavi, A., Bilaniuk, L., Dolinskas, C., Obrist, W., & Uzzell, B. (1981). Diffuse cerebral swelling following head injuries in children: The syndrome of malignant brain edema. *Journal of Neurosurgery, 54,* 170-178.

Campbell, W., Hendrix, E., Schwalbe, R., Fattom, A., & Edelman, R. (1999). Head-injured patients who are nasal carriers of Staphylococcus aureus are at high risk for *Staphylococcus aureus* pneumonia. *Critical Care Medicine, 27*(4), 798-801.

Chan, K. H., Miller, J. D., Dearden, N. M., Andrews, P. J. D., & Midgley, S. (1992). The effect of changes in cerebral perfusion pressure upon middle cerebral artery blood flow velocity and jugular bulb venous oxygen saturation after severe brain injury. *Journal of Neurosurgery, 77,* 55-61.

Chestnut, R. M. (1994). Computed tomography of the brain: A guide to understanding and interpreting normal and abnormal images in the critically ill patient. *Critical Care Nursing Quarterly, 17*(1), 33-50.

Choi, S. C., Barnes, T. Y., Bullock, R., Germanson, T. A., Marmarou, A., & Young, H. F. (1994). Temporal profile of outcomes in severe head injury. *Journal of Neurosurgery, 81,* 169-173.

Citta-Pietrolungo, T. J., Alexander, M. A., Cook, S. P., & Padman, R. (1993). Complications of tracheostomy and decannulation in pediatric and young patients with traumatic brain injury. *Archives of Physical Medicine and Rehabilitation, 74,* 905-909.

Curley, M. A. Q., & Vernon-Levett, P. (1996). Intracranial dynamics. In M. A. Curley, J. B. Smith, & P. A. Moloney-Harmon (Eds.), *Critical care nursing of infants and children* (pp. 336-384). Philadelphia: WB Saunders.

Davies, P. (1996). Caring for patients with diabetes insipidus. *Nursing, 96*(5), 62-63.

Dean, J. M., & Moss, S. D. (1992). Intracranial hypertension. In B. P. Fuhrman & J. J. Zimmerman (Eds.), *Pediatric critical care* (pp. 577-587). St. Louis: Mosby.

Dobbing, J., & Sands, J. (1973). Quantitative growth and development of human growth. *Archives of Disease in Childhood, 48,* 757-767.

Durkin, M. S., Olsen, S., Barlow, B., Virella, A., & Connolly, E. S., Jr. (1998). The epidemiology of urban pediatric neurological trauma: Evaluation of, and implications for, injury prevention programs. *Neurosurgery, 42*(2), 30-310.

Fay, G. C., Jaffe, K. M., Polissar, N. L., Liao, S., Martin, K. M., Shurtleff, H. A., Rivara, J. B., & Winn, H. R. (1993). Mild pediatric traumatic brain injury: A cohort study. *Archives of Physical Medicine and Rehabilitation, 74,* 895-901.

Feldman, Z., Kanter, M. J., Robertson, C. S., Contant, C. F., Hayes, C., Sheinberg, M. A., Villareal, C. A., Narayan, R. K., & Grossman, R. G. (1992). Effect of head elevation on intracranial pressure, cerebral perfusion pressure, and cerebral blood flow in head-injured patients. *Journal of Neurosurgery, 76,* 207-211.

Fishman, R. A. (1975). Brain edema. *New England Journal of Medicine, 293*(14), 706-711.

Fishman, R. A. (1995). Brain edema and disorders of intracranial pressure. In L. P. Rowland (Ed.), *Merritt's textbook of neurology* (9th ed., pp. 302-310). Baltimore: Williams & Wilkins.

Gabriel, E. M., & Borel, C. O. (1996a). Managing severe head injury in the intensive care unit. *Journal of Critical Illness, 11*(3), 171-181.

Gabriel, E. M., & Borel, C. O. (1996b). Managing systemic complications in patients with severe head injury. *Journal of Critical Illness, 11*(4), 212-222.

Ghajar, J., Hariri, R. J., Narayan, R. K., Iacono, L. A., Firlik, K., & Patterson, R. H. (1995). Survey of critical care management of comatose, head-injured patients in the United States. *Critical Care Medicine, 23*(3), 560-567.

Gotschall, C. S. (1993). Epidemiology of childhood injury. In M. R. Eichelberger (Ed.), *Pediatric trauma: Prevention, acute care, rehabilitation* (p. 16). St. Louis: Mosby.

Gopinath, S. P., Robertson, C. S., Contant, C. F., Hayes, C., Feldman, Z., Narayan, R. K., & Grossman, R. G. (1994). Jugular venous desaturation and outcome after head injury. *Journal of Neurology, Neurosurgery, and Psychiatry, 57,* 717-723.

Greenes, D. S., & Schutzman, S. A. (1998). Asymptomatic infants with head trauma. *Annals of Emergency Medicine, 32,* 680-686.

Greisen, G. (1997). Cerebral blood flow and energy metabolism in the newborn. *Clinics in Perinatology, 24*(3), 531-546.

Hall, S. C. (1994). Pediatric trauma in the 90s: An overview. *International Anesthesiology Clinics, 32*(1), 1-9.

Henker, R., Brown, S., & Marion, D. (1998). Comparison of brain temperature with bladder and rectal temperatures in adults with severe head injury. *Neurosurgery, 42*(5), 1071-1075.

Henry, P. C., Hauber, R. P., & Rice, M. (1992). Factors associated with closed head injury in a pediatric population. *Journal of Neuroscience Nursing, 24*(6), 311-316.

Hudak, M. L., Jones, M. D., Popel, A. S., Koehler, R. C., Traystman, R. J., & Zeger, S. L. (1989). Hemodilution caused size dependent constriction of pial arterioles in the cat. *American Journal of Physiology, 257,* H912-H917.

Jaffe, K. M., Fay, G. C., Polissar, N. L., Martin, K. M., Shurtleff, H. A., Rivara, J. B., & Winn, H. R. (1993). Severity of pediatric traumatic brain injury and neurobehavioral recovery at one year: A cohort study. *Archives of Physical Medicine and Rehabilitation, 74,* 587-595.

Jorgensen, L. G. (1995). Transcranial Doppler ultrasound for cerebral perfusion. *Acta Physiologica Scandinavica, 154*(Suppl. 625)1-44.

Kennedy, C., & Sokoloff, L. (1957). An adaptation of the nitrous oxide method to the study of the cerebral circulation in children: Normal values for cerebral blood flow and cerebral metabolic rate in childhood. *Journal of Clinical Investigation, 36,* 1130-1137.

Kerr, M. E, Sereika, S. M., Orndoff, P., Weber, B., Rudy, E. B., Marion, D., Stone, K., & Turner, B. (1998). Effect of neuromuscular blockers and opiates on the cerebrovascular response to endotracheal suctioning in adults with severe head injuries. *American Journal of Critical Care, 7*(3), 205-217.

Kerr, M. E., Lovasik, D., & Darby, J. (1995). Evaluating cerebral oxygenation using jugular venous oximetry in head injuries. *AACN Clinical Issues, 6*(1), 11-20.

Klauber, M. R., Marshall, L. F., Luerssen, T. G., Frankowski, R., Tabaddor, K., & Eisenberg, M. (1989). Determinants of had injury mortality: Importance of the low risk patient. *Neurosurgery, 24*(1), 31-36.

Kochanek, P. M. (1993). Ischemic and traumatic brain injury: pathophysiology and cellular mechanisms. *Critical Care Medicine, 21*(9 Suppl.), S333-S335.

Kokoska, E. R., Smith, G. S. Pittman, T., & Weber, T. R. (1998). Early hypotension worsens neurological outcome in pediatric patients with moderately severe head trauma. *Journal of Pediatric Surgery, 33*(2), 333-338.

Kraus, J. F., Peek, C., McArthur, D. L., & Williams, A. (1994). The effect of the 1992 California motorcycle helmet use law on motorcycle crash fatalities and injuries. *Journal of the American Medical Association, 272*(19), 1506-1511.

Lee, D., Honrado, C., Har-El, G., & Goldsmith, A. (1998). Pediatric temporal bone fractures. *Laryngoscope, 108,* 816-821.

Levin, H. S., Aldrich, E. F., Saydjari, C., Eisenberg, H. M., Foulkes, M. A., Bellefleur, M., Luerssen, T. G., Jane, J. A., Marmarou, A., Marshall, L. F., & Young, H. F. (1992). Severe head injury in children: Experience of the Traumatic Coma Data Bank. *Neurosurgery, 31,* 435-444.

Luerssen, T. G., Klauber, M. R., & Marshall, L. F. (1988). Outcome from head injury related to patient's age. A longitudinal prospective study of adult and pediatric head injury. *Journal of Neurosurgery, 68,* 409-416.

Magu, S., Mishra, D. S., & Gandhi, S. B. (1998). Evaluation of computed tomograms in paediatric head trauma. *Journal of the Indian Medical Association, 96*(1), 13-15.

Mamelak, A. N., Pitts, L. H., & Damron, S. (1996). Predicting survival from head trauma 24 hours after injury: A practical method with therapeutic implications. *Journal of Trauma: Injury, Infection, and Critical Care, 41*(1), 91-99.

Marion, D. W., Obrist, W. D., Carlier, P. M., Penrod, L. E., & Darby, J. M. (1993). The use of moderate hypothermia for patients with severe head injuries: A preliminary report. *Journal of Neurosurgery, 79*(3), 354-362.

McGuire, G., Crossley, D., Richards, J., & Wong, D. (1997). Effects of varying levels of positive end-expiratory pressure on intracranial pressure and cerebral perfusion pressure. *Critical Care Medicine, 25*(6), 1059-1062.

McLaurin, R. L., & Towbin, R. (1986). Cerebral damage. In A. J. Raimondi, M. Choux, & C. DiRocco (Eds.), *Head injuries in the newborn and infant* (p. 183). New York: Springer-Verlag.

Muizelaar, J. P., Wei, E. P., Kontos, H. A., & Becker, D. P. (1983). Mannitol causes compensatory cerebral vasoconstriction and vasodilation in response to blood viscosity changes. *Journal of Neurosurgery, 59,* 822-828.

National Head Injury Foundation. (1986). *Definition of traumatic brain injury.* Southborough, MA: Author.

National Pediatric Trauma Registry. (1999). *Biannual report.* Boston: Tufts University School of Medicine, New England Medical Center.

Peacock, W. J. (1986). The postnatal development of the brain and its coverings. In A. J. Raimondi, M. Choux, & C. DiRocco (Eds.), *Head injuries in the newborn and infant* (pp. 53-66). New York: Springer-Verlag.

Petitti, N., & Williams, D. W. (1998). CT and MR imaging of nonaccidental pediatric head trauma. *Academic Radiology, 5,* 215-223.

Piper, P. (1994). Pediatric trauma. *Pediatric Surgical Nursing, 29*(4), 563-584.

Plum, R., & Posner, J. B. (1982). *The diagnosis of stupor and coma* (3rd ed.). Philadelphia: FA Davis.

Research and Training Center in Rehabilitation and Childhood Trauma. (1993). *Facts from The National Pediatric Trauma Registry.* Boston: New England Medial Center and Tufts University School of Medicine.

Rifkinson-Mann, S. (1993). Head injuries in infants and young children. *Contemporary Neurosurgery, 15*(11), 1-6.

Rivara, F. P. (1994). Epidemiology and prevention of pediatric traumatic brain injury. *Pediatric Annals, 23*(1), 12-17.

Rosner, M. J., & Daughton, S. (1990). Cerebral perfusion pressure management in head injury. *Journal of Trauma, 30*(6), 933-940.

Rosner, M. J., Rosner, S. D., & Johnson, A. H. (1995). Cerebral perfusion pressure: Management protocol and clinical results. *Journal of Neurosurgery, 83,* 949-962.

Sabatino, G., Quartulli, L. A., & Morgese, G. (1994). Cerebral Doppler velocimetry in newborn. *Journal of Perinatology Medicine, 22*(Suppl. 1)135-141.

Sauaia, A., Moore, F. A., Moore, E. E., Moser, K. S., Brennan, R., Read, R. A., & Pons, P. T. (1995). Epidemiology of trauma deaths: A reassessment. *Journal of Trauma, 38*(2), 185-193.

Scalea, T. M., Maltz, S., Yelon, J., Trooskin, S. Z., Duncan, A. O., & Sclafani, S. J. A. (1994). Resuscitation of multiple trauma and head injury: Role of crystalloid fluids and inotropes. *Critical Care Medicine, 22*(10), 1610-1615.

Settergren, G., Lindblad, B. S., & Persson, B. (1980). Cerebral blood flow and exchange of oxygen, glucose ketone bodies, lactate, pyruvate and amino acids in anesthetized children. *Acta Paediatrica Scandinavica, 69,* 457-465.

Sharples, P. M., Matthews, D. S. F., & Eyre, J. A. (1995). Cerebral blood flow and metabolism in children with severe head injury. Part 2: Cerebrovascular resistance and its determinants. *Journal of Neurology and Neurosurgery Psychiatry, 58,* 153-159.

Sharples, P. M., Stuart, A. G., Matthews, D. S. F., Aynsley-Green, A., & Eyre, J. A. (1995). Cerebral blood flow and metabolism in children with severe head injury. Part 1: Relation to age, Glasgow coma score, outcome, intracranial pressure, and time after injury. *Journal of Neurology and Neurosurgery Psychiatry, 58,* 145-152.

Shiozaki, T., Sugimoto, H., Taneda, M., Yoshida, H., Iwa, A., Yoshioka, T., Sugimoto, T. (1993). Effect of mild hypothermia on uncontrollable intracranial hypertension after severe head injury. *Journal of Neurosurgery, 79*(3), 363-368.

Sieber, F. E., & Traystman, R. J. (1992). Special issues: Glucose and the brain. *Critical Care Medicine, 20*(1), 104-114.

Sikes, P. J., & Segal, J. (1994). Jugular bulb oxygen saturation monitoring for evaluating cerebral ischemia. *Critical Care Nursing Quarterly, 17*(1), 9-20.

Simma, B., Burger, R., Falk, M., Sacher, P., & Fanconi, S. (1998). A prospective, randomized, and controlled study of fluid management in children with severe head injury: Lactated Ringer's solution versus hypertonic saline. *Critical Care Medicine, 26*(7), 265-270.

Suarez, J. L., Qureshi, A-I., Bhardwaj, A., Williams, M. A., Schnitzer, M. S., Mirski, M., et al. (1998). Treatment of refractory intracranial hypertension with 23.4% saline. *Critical Care Medicine, 26*(6), 118-122.

Teasdale, G., & Jennett, B. (1974). Glasgow coma scale. *Lancet, 2,* 81-83.

Temkin, N. R., Dikmen, S. S., Wilensky, A. J., Keihm, J., Chabal, S., & Winn, H. R. (1990). A randomized, double-blind study of phenytoin for the prevention of post-traumatic seizures. *New England Journal of Medicine, 323,* 497-502.

Tepas, J. J., III, Scala, D., Ramonofsky, C., & Barlow, M. L. (1990). Mortality in head injury: The pediatric perspective. *Journal of Pediatric Surgery, 25,* 92-96.

Thompson, R. S., Rivara, F. P., & Thompson, D. C. (1989). A case-control study of the effectiveness of bicycle safety helmets. *New England Journal of Medicine, 320,* 1361-1367.

Trauner, D. A. (1986). Barbiturate therapy in acute brain injury. *Journal of Pediatrics, 109*(5), 742-746.

Vernon-Levett, P. (1998). Neurologic system. In M. Slota (Ed.), *Core curriculum for pediatric critical care nursing* (pp. 274-359). Philadelphia: WB Saunders.

Ward, J. D. (1994). Pediatric head injury: A further experience. *Pediatric Neurosurgery, 20,* 183-185.

Ward, J. D. (1995). Pediatric issues in head trauma. *New Horizons, 3*(3), 539-545.

Ward, J. D., Becker, D. P., Miller, J. D., Choi, S. C., Marmarou, A., Wood, C., Newlon, P. G., & Keenan, R. (1985). Failure of prophylactic barbiturate coma in the treatment of severe head injury. *Journal of Neurosurgery, 62,* 383-388.

Welch, K. (1980). The intracranial pressure in infants. *Neurosurgery, 52,* 693-699.

White, R. J., & Likavec, M. J. (1992). The diagnosis and initial management of head injury. *New England Journal of Medicine, 327*(21), 1507-1511.

Zimmerman, R. A., & Bilaniuk, L. T. (1981). Computed tomography in pediatric head trauma. *Journal of Neuroradiology, 8,* 257-272.

Zimmerman, R. A., Bilaniuk, L. T., Bruce, D., Dolinskas, C., Obrist, W., & Kuhl, D. (1978). Computed tomography of pediatric head trauma: Acute general cerebral swelling. *Radiology, 126,* 403-408.

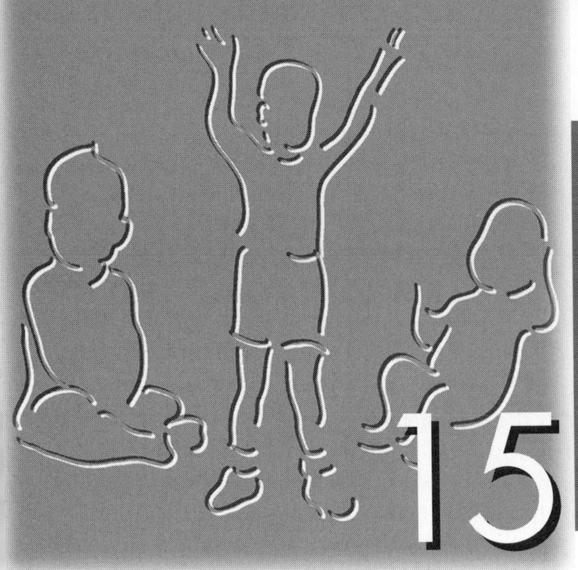

15

Spinal Cord Injury

Regina Muir • Deborah A. Town

Injury to the spine and spinal cord has devastating consequences in any patient, but the intensity is magnified when the patient is a child. Although spinal cord injury occurs less frequently than injury to other body systems, there is a lifelong impact on the child and the family. This chapter focuses on spinal cord injury in the pediatric patient, including anatomic differences in the pediatric spine, mechanism of injury, and specific spinal injuries. The chapter provides information on the assessment and care of the child who has sustained a spinal injury.

SCOPE OF THE PROBLEM

Although data related to the incidence of spinal cord injury have been collected, it is difficult to determine the exact number of cases. The National Spinal Cord Injury Association (NSCIA, 1998) estimates the incidence of spinal cord injury at 32 injuries per million population. This accounts for 7800 injuries in the United States each year. Population-based studies reveal that the greatest incidence of spinal cord injury occurs most frequently in persons between the ages of 16 and 30 years, with a male/female ratio of 2:1 (Gerhart, 1991; Go, DeVivo, & Richards, 1995). Children younger than 16 years account for a small percentage of the total number of patients with spinal cord injuries, estimated between 1% and 14% (Fesmire & Luten, 1989; Orenstein, Klein, Gotschall, Ochsenschlager, Klatzko, & Eichelberger, 1994).

In 1998 NSCIA estimated that approximately 250,000 to 400,000 people are living with a spinal cord injury or spinal dysfunction. Although the number of persons injured is relatively low, spinal cord injury has a significant effect on the medical and psychosocial well-being of the injured person and the patient's family. The financial impact of spinal injury cannot be minimized. NSCIA estimated that in 1992, a patient sustaining an injury that resulted in tetraplegia had an average hospital stay of 95 days and that on average one third to one half of all patients with spinal cord injuries were readmitted to the hospital annually. Torosian, Torosian, and Cogen (1995) estimated that after injury, approximately 20% of patients with tetraplegia will be employable. The remainder will require assistance from family members and governmental agencies. Although the occurrence of spinal injuries is low in the pediatric patient, there is considerable impact on the life of the child and family.

SPECIAL CONSIDERATION OF THE PEDIATRIC SPINE

The ability to correctly identify the pediatric patient with spinal injury can be challenging. The pediatric spine, like the rest of the body structures, is in a state of growth and development. The spine of the newborn is different from the spine of the adolescent. Knowledge of the development of the spine and the normal variations that occur will help the care provider identify the child with spinal injury.

Anatomic and Physiologic Considerations

Developmental Considerations

Development of the vertebral column begins within a few days of conception and continues throughout prenatal and postnatal life. Development of the spine occurs in a sequential manner with specific phases. Initially, there is membranous development. At approximately the sixth week after conception, chondrification centers appear. The first of three pairs fuses ventrally to the neural tube and forms the centrum of the vertebral body. The second pair forms dorsolaterally and fuses dorsally to the neural tube to become the posterior neural arch and spinous process. The third pair develops between the ventral and dorsal pairs and forms the transverse process. The anterior and posterior longitudinal ligaments, the intervertebral disc, and the vertebral cartilage also are formed during this phase (McLone & Dias, 1994).

Ossification of the spinal column begins in the second month after conception and continues after birth.

Ossification initiates in four primary ossification centers: two in the vertebral centrum and one in each side of the dorsal neural arch. The vertebral body becomes ossified from both the dorsal and ventral ossification centers, which fuse at about 20 weeks of gestation (McLone & Dias, 1994). The development of the craniovertebral junction is complex and requires more detailed discussion. Without knowledge of the location and sequential fusion of ossification centers, it is difficult to correctly interpret radiographs of the pediatric spine.

The first cervical vertebra, the *atlas,* is formed from three primary ossification centers: two neural arches and the body (Figure 15-1). The body of C1 is not ossified at birth, but one to two ossification centers will be visible on radiographs by 1 year of age. The neural arches of C1 appear at 7 weeks of gestation. The spinous process will fuse at approximately age 3 years, and the body of the vertebra will fuse by age 7. Before complete fusion, the chondrification centers may appear as fracture lines on radiographs (Bailey, 1952; Fesmire & Luten, 1989; Fielding, 1978; McLone & Dias, 1994).

The *axis,* the second cervical vertebra, has four ossification centers: odontoid, body, and two neural arches (Fesmire & Luten, 1989; Fielding, 1978) (Figure 15-2). The odontoid forms from two separate ossification centers that fuse in the midline by 7 months of gestation. Between the ages of 3 and 6 years, a secondary ossification center appears at the apex and fuses with the odontoid by age 12. The body of C2 develops from one to two ossification centers by 5 months of gestation. The body of C2 fuses with the odontoid by age 3 to 6 years. The fusion may remain visible on radiographs until adolescence. The neural arches fuse posteriorly by 3 years of age. By age 6, the neural arches have fused with the body/odontoid (Fesmire & Luten, 1989; Fielding, 1978).

The remainder of the cervical spine (C3 through C7) develops in a similar way. The body arises from a single ossification center by 5 months of gestation. The neural arches, which appear by the ninth fetal week, fuse posteriorly by age 3 years. Anterior fusion and the fusion of the neural arches and body occur by age 6 years. Secondary ossification centers appear at the tips of the vertebrae and at the superior and inferior aspects of the cervical bodies during puberty. They are commonly mistaken for fracture lines.

At birth the spine is elastic, and the ligamentous structures allow for up to 2 inches of distraction; however, the spinal cord can stretch only one fourth of an inch (Fielding, 1978; Leventhal, 1960). This may result in damage across spinal segments if a traction injury occurs. Other factors that influence the nature and location of spinal injuries in children are the presence of a large infantile head, the presence of lax ligaments and joint capsules, and nonsupportive musculature. In addition, the facets in the upper three cervical vertebrae have a horizontal orientation that permits increased motion (Bailey, 1952; Von Torklus & Gehle, 1972).

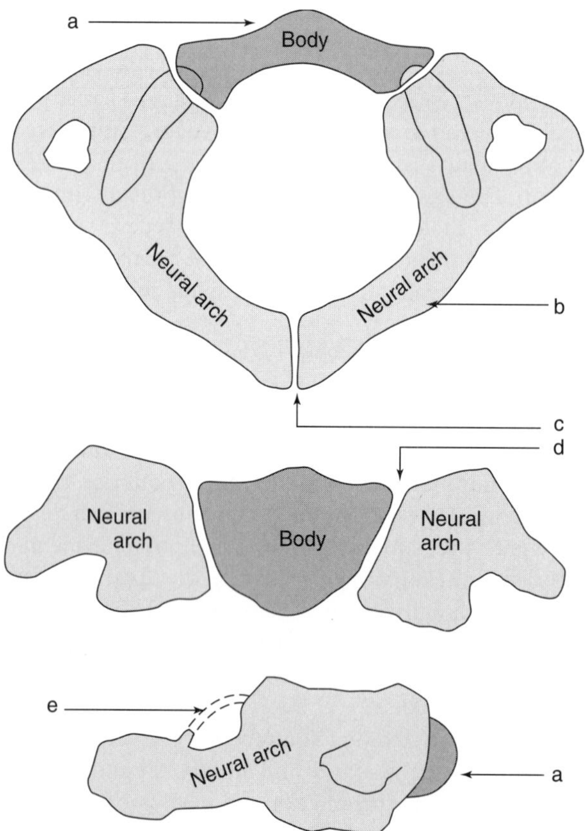

FIGURE 15-1 The first cervical vertebra (atlas). (From Fielding, J. W. [1983]. Cervical spine injuries in children. In Cervical Spine Research Society (Ed.), *The cervical spine* [pp. 268–281]. Philadelphia: JB Lippincott.)

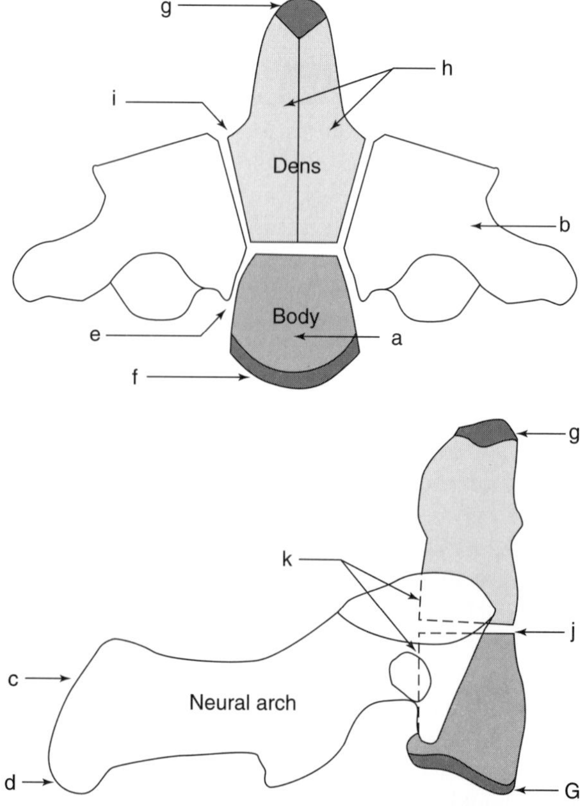

FIGURE 15-2 The second cervical vertebra (axis). (From Fielding, J. W. [1983]. Cervical spine injuries in children. In Cervical Spine Research Society (Ed.), *The cervical spine* [pp. 268–281]. Philadelphia: JB Lippincott.)

The combination of all of these factors accounts for the types of injuries that are often seen in the pediatric patient. The ability to identify injuries in the pediatric patient can be a difficult task.

Normal Radiologic Variants

Several normal anatomic variants have been noted in the spine of the pediatric patient compared with the spine of the adult patient. Normal variants can lead to confusion and misdiagnosis.

The first of the normal variants is the absence of lordosis in children younger than 16 years. When the neck is held in the neutral position, absence of lordosis of the lateral cervical spine is a common finding. Cattell and Filtzer (1965) reviewed lateral cervical spine radiographs of 160 children 1 to 16 years of age. They found that 14% of the children had absent lordosis on the x-ray film. This finding may be a sign of ligamentous injury in the adult patient.

A second normal variant found in the pediatric population is anterior wedging of the immature vertebral bodies of very young children. Anterior wedging can give the appearance of a compression fracture.

Pseudosubluxation is another normal variant found in the infant and young child. When the neck is mildly flexed, there may be an anterior pseudosubluxation, most marked at the level of C2 to C3. When Cattell and Filtzer (1965) performed flexion and extension x-ray examinations on 160 normal children, they found that 46% of the children younger than 8 years demonstrated anterior pseudosubluxation of C2 on C3. This pseudosubluxation occurs secondary to ligament laxity. Fielding (1978) believed that some of the excess mobility of the spine at the second and third cervical levels resulted from children having more horizontal facet surfaces, which allowed more forward displacement when the neck is flexed.

Another common variant in the pediatric spine is the presence of a widened predental space. A predental space, the distance between the odontoid process and the anterior arch of the atlas, less than 3.5 mm is considered normal in children younger than 8 years. A predental space greater than 2.5 to 3.0 mm in an adult is indicative of a ligamentous or subluxation injury (Cattell & Filtzer 1965).

An important radiographic finding in the adult patient with cervical spine injury is the presence of prevertebral soft tissue widening secondary to edema and hemorrhage. This indicator is not a reliable finding in the pediatric population. Small children may have marked increases in prevertebral soft tissue width when the neck is held in flexion or if the x-ray film is taken during expiration (Fesmire & Luten, 1989).

THE SPINAL CORD

Spinal Cord Anatomy and Physiology

Knowledge of the structure and function of the spinal cord is necessary to fully understand spinal injuries. The spinal cord is a cylindrical, pliable structure that extends from the brain. It starts at the foramen magnum and ends at the level of the first or second lumbar vertebra, where it terminates at the conus medullaris. The cord enlarges in the cervical and lumbar areas, corresponding with the large nerve supplies for the upper and lower extremities. The spinal cord consists of gray and white matter.

Gray Matter

The gray matter, or H-shaped center of the cord, contains groups of cell bodies. The gray matter is divided into columns: posterior, anterior, and lateral or horizontal.

- Posterior columns contain sensory cells that transmit information regarding sensation, proprioception, position sense, pressure sense, vibratory sense, movement, and stereognosis.
- Anterior columns contain motor cell bodies that transmit motor impulses from the brain to the skeletal muscle.
- Lateral or horizontal columns contain interconnecting neurons between the anterior and posterior columns. In the thoracic and lumbar regions these neurons give rise to the sympathetic nervous system.

White Matter

White matter in the spinal cord is composed of ascending and descending nerve fibers, which are myelinated. The fibers are organized into tracts, which act as transmission cables, sharing a common origin and destination (Figure 15-3). All tracts are bilateral for control of each side of the body. The major white matter tracts include posterior columns, spinothalamic tract, spinocerebellar tracts, and corticospinal tracts.

- The posterior columns contain sensory pathways for vibration, touch, and position sense.
- The spinothalamic tract originates in the spinal cord and ascends to the thalamus. The ventral spinothalamic tract transmits impulses of touch. The lateral spinothalamic tract transmits pain and temperature. The spinothalamic tract is unique in that the tracts cross in the ventral white commissure to ascend on the opposite side of the spinal cord.
- The spinocerebellar tract transmits information regarding position, sense, and body movement from the trunk and extremities to the cerebellum.
- The corticospinal tract originates in the motor cortex of the brain and crosses in the medulla to innervate the opposite side of the body. The corticospinal tract transmits impulses for voluntary motor movement.

Spinal Nerves

The spinal nerves provide pathways for involuntary movement in response to stimuli, controlled movement, and sensory input. The spinal nerves occur in pairs and correspond to the 31 segments of the spinal cord. Each nerve attaches to the cord by an anterior and posterior root. The nerve roots join in a common sleeve before exiting the cord to branch out to almost all parts of the body. Some spinal

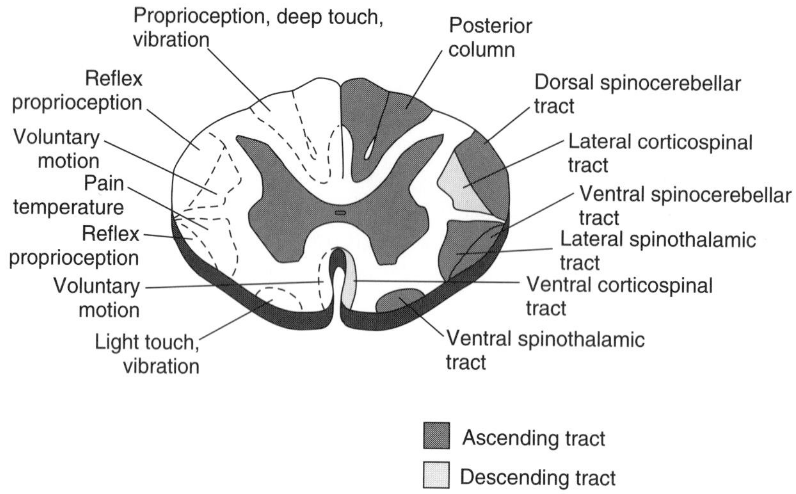

FIGURE 15-3 Cross section of the spinal cord. (From Zejdlik, C. [1992]. *Management of spinal cord injury* [2nd ed., p. 59]. Sudbury, MA: Jones and Bartlett.)

TABLE 15-1 Spinal Nerves

Spinal Nerve	Area Innervated
C4	Diaphragm
C5	Deltoids and biceps
C6	Wrist extensors
C7	Triceps
C8	Hands
T2-T7	Chest muscles
T9-T12	Abdominal muscles
L1-L5	Leg muscles
S2-S5	Bowel, bladder, sexual function

nerves join to form a plexus, complex nerve networks, which innervate certain areas. The brachial plexus controls most functions of the arm and hand. The lowest nerve roots, which fan out from the end of the spinal cord, are referred to as the *cauda equina* (horse tail) because of its appearance. Significant nerves and the areas they innervate are detailed in Table 15-1.

Nervous System Function

Autonomic Nervous System

The autonomic nervous system regulates the body's internal environment. It provides automatic control of all internal organ systems, including blood pressure, heart rate, thermoregulation, appetite, fluid balance, bowel and bladder control, sleep, and sexual functioning. The autonomic nervous system is activated by centers in the hypothalamus, brainstem, and spinal cord and, to a certain degree, by local reflex activity (Chipps, Clanin, & Campbell, 1992; Zejdlik, 1992). Neurons descend from the hypothalamus and end in one of three outflow tracts. The first group, *the cranial outflow tract,* is clustered in the brainstem. A second group of neurons is clustered between the first thoracic and first lumbar vertebrae and is referred to as the *thoracolumbar outflow.* The third group, *sacral outflow,* is centered between the second and fourth sacral cord segments. The sympathetic nervous system arises from the thoracolumbar outflow. The craniosacral outflow gives rise to the parasympathetic nervous system.

Sympathetic Nervous System. Stimulation of the sympathetic nervous system provides a generalized body response. This allows for maximum energy for stress defense, sometimes referred to as the *fight or flight response.* To prepare for a stressful situation, the sympathetic nervous system (1) shunts blood from less important areas to the cardiopulmonary system and increases heart rate and respiratory rate, (2) decreases gastrointestinal motility and urinary functions, (3) stimulates the adrenal gland to release epinephrine, and (4) releases red blood cells from storage in the spleen for additional energy.

Parasympathetic Nervous System. The parasympathetic division controls activities of nonstress everyday body functioning. The parasympathetic system initiates functions such as digestion and elimination and conserves body energy. Stimulation of the parasympathetic system results in a more specific response than stimulation of the sympathetic system, such as increased peristalsis. In normal stress-free situations, the parasympathetic and sympathetic systems work in harmony to maintain homeostasis within the body. When spinal cord injury interrupts intricate communications with the central nervous system, homeostasis is threatened. Generally, the higher the level of the spinal cord injury is, the more profound the effects are.

PATTERNS OF INJURY

Causes of Injury in the Pediatric Patient

The causes of spinal cord injury vary based on the child's age. Specific structural differences in the pediatric spine may influence the pattern of injuries seen. The fulcrum of cervical mobility becomes more caudal as the child ages. This accounts for the higher number of injuries in the area of the first through third cervical vertebrae. In children 8 to 12 years, the fulcrum changes to the third through fifth vertebrae, and in children older than 12 the fulcrum moves to the C5 to C6 region (Hall & Boydston, 1999). Although anatomic factors increase the likelihood of injury to the area of increased movement, it is not a guarantee that injury will not occur in other areas of the spine. In a study of 34 pediatric patients with spine injury, Givens, Polley, Smith, and Harden (1996) found that 50% of patients younger than 8 years had an injury below C4. Injuries to the thoracolumbar spine should be considered in all children with a significant mechanism of injury.

The most common causes of injury in the pediatric patient are motor vehicle accidents, motor-pedestrian collisions, and falls from a significant height. In addition, recreational activities play a role in injuries to children older than 8 years. The number of penetrating injuries to the spine has increased as a result of the increase in pediatric gunshot wounds (Torosian et al., 1995).

Spinal cord injury has been reported as a result of difficult cephalic or breech delivery with distraction and hyperextension of the head and neck. The infant spine has increased "stretchability" that is disproportionate to the ability of the spinal cord to stretch. Excessive traction and hyperextension placed during a difficult delivery may result in injury across spinal segments. Spinal injury may be an unrecognized cause of death in the newborn (Allen, Meyers, & Condon, 1969).

Mechanism of Injury

The mechanism of spinal injury is a result of the forces applied to the child. A direct relationship exists between the magnitude of the force applied and the extent of the injury. Most traumatic events result in multiple simultaneous forces. The most common mechanisms that cause injury to the spine are flexion injuries, flexion rotation, hyperextension, and compression. Any of these forces can produce an unstable spine injury if it results in disruption of the ligamentous structure, which provides support for the spine. Flexion injuries (Figure 15-4) are most often associated with motor vehicle accidents and occur when the head is thrown violently forward. Flexion injuries can also occur when a person falls backward and strikes the occipital area or when the spine is hyperflexed around a fixed axis, as with lap belt injuries. Forces that produce severe flexion may produce significant, unstable spinal injuries.

Flexion-rotation injury occurs when flexion forces combine with lateral force, which results in rotation. Flexion rotation (Figure 15-5) produces a shearing force of the upper vertebral body on the lower vertebral body. Injuries found in conjunction with flexion rotation include locking or dislocation of the facets (Torosian et al., 1995).

Hyperextension injuries (Figure 15-6) occur when the force is applied in such a way as to push the head backward. The force may occur secondary to a rear-end collision or from a fall in which the person lands on the chin, pushing the head back. Hyperextension injuries may also result from sport activity, such as football.

Compression forces or axial loading (Figure 15-7) occurs when the force is directed to the top of the head and is transmitted to the spine. This injury may occur during a fall when the child lands on the buttocks with the spine in a straight position. This injury occurs during falls and diving accidents, and when a child is ejected from a vehicle and hits another object.

SPINAL INJURIES

Vertebral Column Injuries

Fractures

The irregular shape of the vertebrae allows the bony structure to fracture easily. Fractures can occur in the vertebral body or arch in combination. Box 15-1 lists definitions of terms commonly used to describe vertebral fractures.

Stability

Vertebral injuries are classified as stable or unstable. An injury is considered *unstable* when the vertebral and ligamentous structures are unable to support or protect the injured area. The ability to distinguish a stable injury from an unstable injury requires radiologic diagnosis and clinical expertise. An injury is considered *stable* if the bony and ligamentous structures provide enough support to prevent further progression of neurologic deficit (Zejdlik, 1992).

Spinal Cord Injury

The diagnosis and classification of spinal cord injury can be confusing. Initial evaluation of a spinal cord injury should be geared to the determination of whether it is a complete or incomplete lesion. An injury is considered *complete* when there is a loss of all motor and sensory function below the level of the lesion, including the sacral segment. In the presence of spinal shock, it may be difficult to determine if a lesion is complete or incomplete. An injury is considered *incomplete* if there is partial preservation of sensory and/or motor function below the level of the injury, including the sacral segment. Incomplete injuries have been classified as spinal cord syndromes. The most common syndromes are as follows.

Anterior Spinal Cord Syndrome

Injury in anterior spinal cord syndrome involves the anterior two thirds of the spinal cord and is often associated with injury to the anterior spinal artery. The patient presents with loss of motor and sensory function below the level of the lesion. Deep sensation is preserved because this is mediated through the posterior columns (McGuire, 1998).

Central Spinal Cord Syndrome

In central spinal cord syndrome, injury involves the central portion of the spinal cord. Because the fibers that innervate the upper extremities lie more medial than the fibers that innervate the lower extremities, the child presents with motor and sensory deficit that is greater in the upper extremities than it is in the lower extremities (McGuire, 1998).

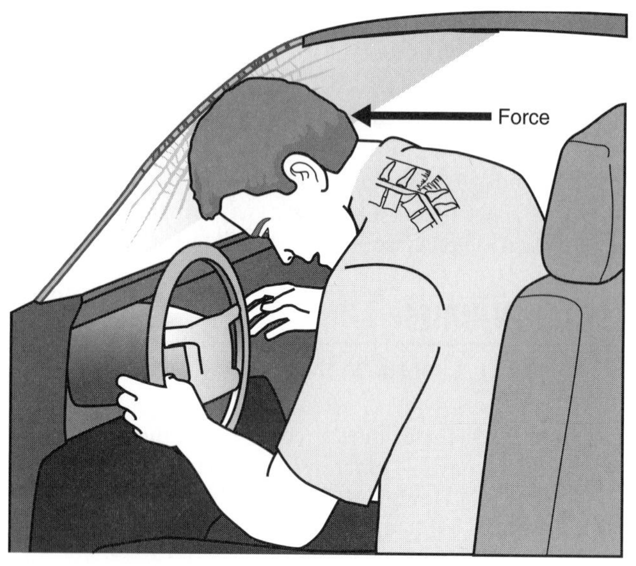

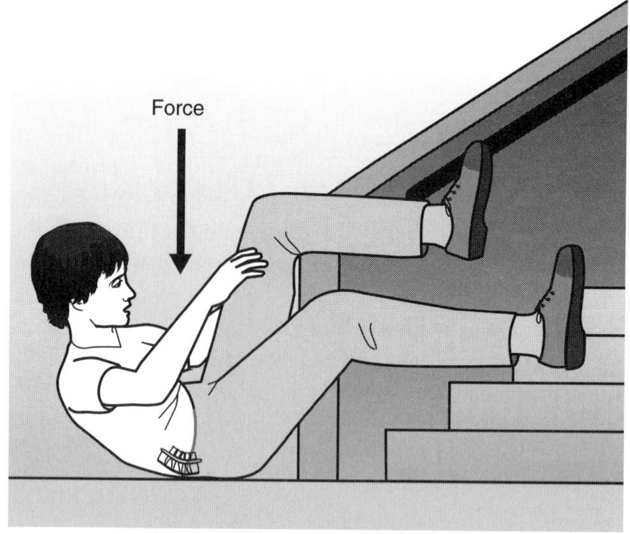

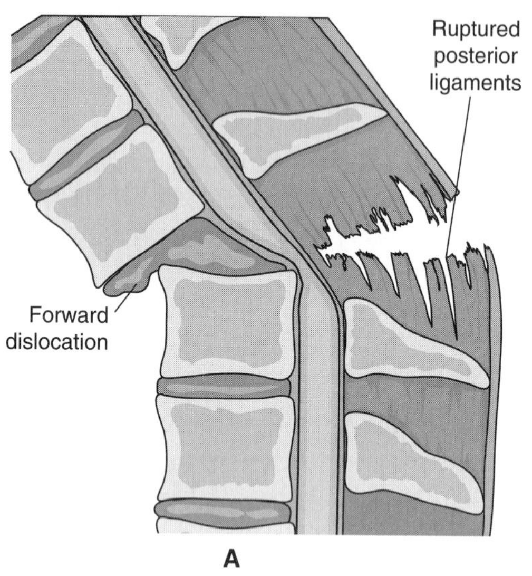

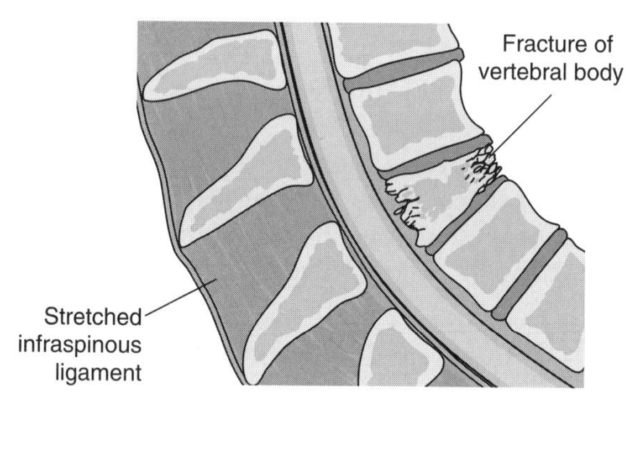

FIGURE 15-4 Forward-flexion injury can occur secondary to motor vehicle accidents or blunt force to the front or back of the head, as occurs when a person is struck with an object (**A**) or falls (**B**). (Redrawn from Zejdlik, C. [1992]. *Management of spinal cord injury* [pp. 63-65]. Sudbury, MA: Jones and Bartlett.)

Brown-Séquard Syndrome

Brown-Séquard syndrome is injury that results in a hemisection of the cord, leading to ipsilateral loss of motor function and contralateral loss of pain and temperature (McGuire, 1998).

Spinal Cord Injury Without Radiographic Abnormality

Pang and Pollack (1989) defined *SCIWORA (spinal cord injury without radiographic abnormality)* as the association of neurologic deficit in a trauma patient who has no evidence of skeletal injury or subluxation. This condition occurs almost exclusively in children, especially those younger than 8 years. Grabb and Pang (1994) believe that self-reducing, transient subluxation or distraction of the juvenile spine is responsible for the neurologic deficit. Signs and symptoms of SCIWORA include transient numbness, tingling, paralysis, paresthesia, generalized weakness, and pain radiating down the spine with neck movement. These sensorimotor complaints may progress in minutes to days (Marinier, Rodts, & Connolly, 1997).

Lap Belt Syndrome

The term *seat belt syndrome* or *lap belt syndrome* is used to describe a triad of injuries that may occur when there is a hyperflexion of the body around a fixed lap belt. The triad is made up of injuries to the abdominal wall, intraabdominal contents, and lumbar vertebrae (Shoemaker & Ose, 1997).

Autonomic Nervous System Dysfunction After Spinal Injury

After sustaining a spinal injury, hemorrhage, structural changes, cellular damage, and inflammatory responses cause secondary damage to the spinal cord. Complete transection

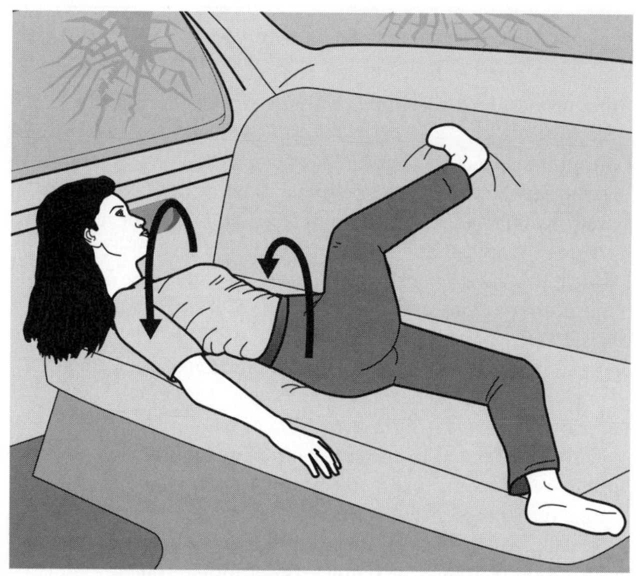

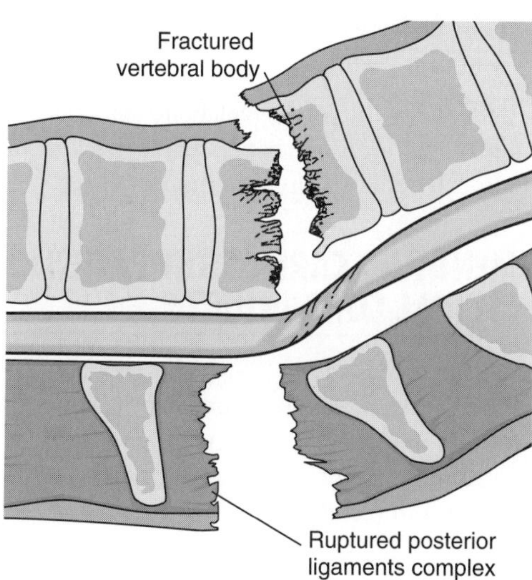

FIGURE 15-5 Flexion-rotation forces that occur concurrently are particularly potent and are associated with fracture dislocations. The posterior ligament is commonly ruptured and accompanied by a vertebral body fracture, making this a highly unstable injury. (Redrawn from Zejdlik, C. [1992]. *Management of spinal cord injury* [2nd ed., pp. 63–65]. Sudbury, MA: Jones and Bartlett.)

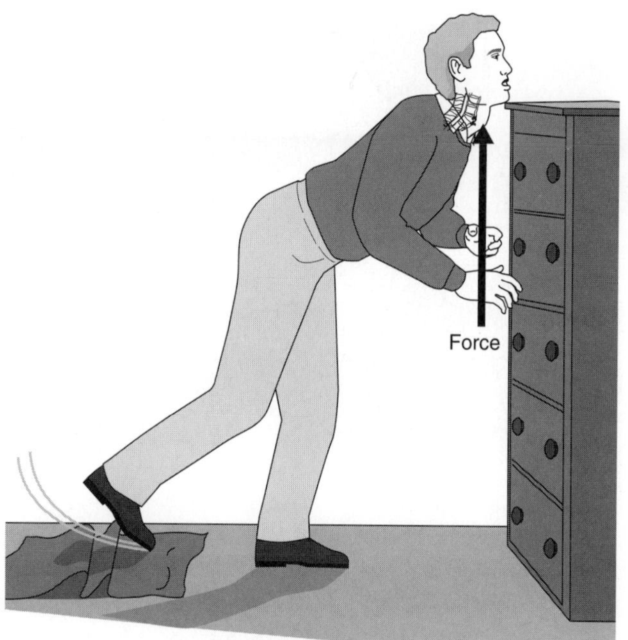

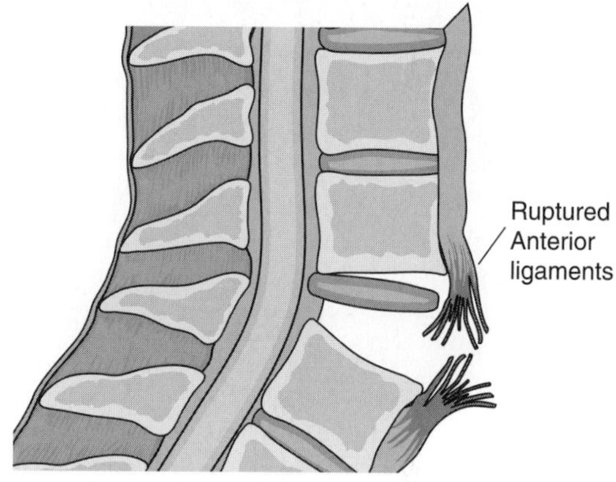

FIGURE 15-6 Hyperextension injury. Injuries are often related to falls in which the chin or face is struck, causing violent hyperextension of the neck. (Redrawn from Zejdlik, C. [1992]. *Management of spinal cord injury* [2nd ed., pp. 63–65]. Sudbury, MA: Jones and Bartlett.)

of the cord is rare. Usually, there is an injury to part of the cord, which results in hemorrhage and edema. Blood flow to the cord is impaired, leading to ischemia. Cell death results in an increased loss of spinal neurons, which do not regenerate, further impairing function (Emergency Nurses Association, 1995). The death of spinal neurons and loss of function usually lead to a "physiologic shock state." This shock state usually occurs immediately after injury, but it can occur up to several days later. The degree of intensity varies with the level of the lesion. Patients with injuries at the level of T6 or above are at greatest risk (Emergency Nurses Association, 1995). Spinal shock is often used to describe two different physiologic processes.

Spinal Shock. *Spinal shock* is the temporary loss of motor, sensory, and reflex activity below the level of the lesion. This is superimposed on either permanent or temporary neurologic loss. The patient presents with flaccid paralysis and bowel and bladder dysfunction. Spinal shock is considered resolved when there is a return of reflexes and a conversion to spastic paralysis.

Neurogenic Shock. Neurogenic shock refers to the body's reaction to the sudden loss of central nervous system control. A classic triad of symptoms exists in the patient with neurogenic shock. Loss of vasomotor tone and sympathetic innervation to the heart occurs as a result of parasympathetic predominance secondary to impairment of sympathetic pathways. The interruption of these pathways leads to passive vasodilation, which results in peripheral pooling of blood volume. Diminished venous return to the heart decreases stroke

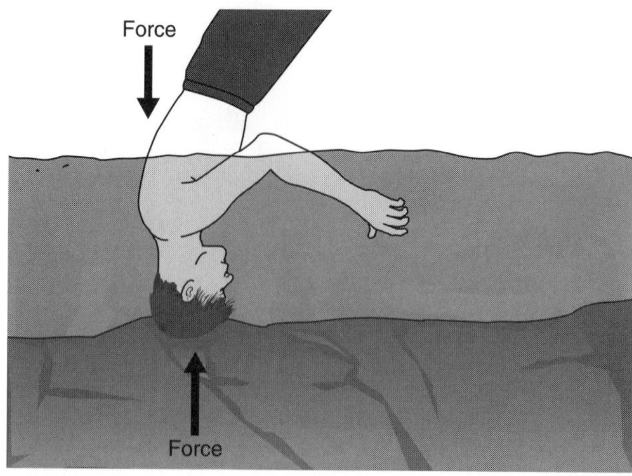

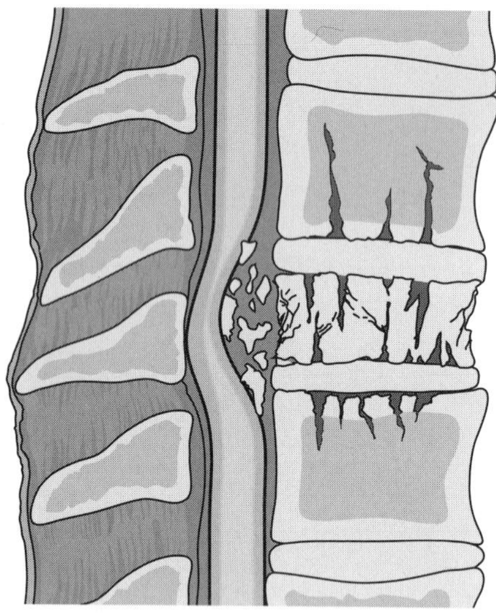

FIGURE 15-7 Compression injury. A high-velocity blow to the top of the head can cause a shattered vertebral body to burst into the spinal cord. Fractures frequently occur in the cervical or thoracolumbar area. (Redrawn from Zejdlik, C. [1992]. *Management of spinal cord injury* [2nd ed., pp. 63–65]. Sudbury, MA: Jones and Bartlett.)

volume, leading to decreased cardiac output. Loss of sympathetic pathways allows the parasympathetic nervous system to predominate. Unopposed effects of the vagus nerve lead to bradycardia. Abnormal vasovagal response, a dangerous phenomenon, may occur during this time. Sudden or noxious stimulation, such as endotracheal suctioning, chest physiotherapy, or sudden position changes, may result in severe bradycardia, possibly leading to asystole, hypotension, and loss of consciousness (Zejdlik, 1992). Infants and young children have very small stroke volumes and require higher heart rates to maintain cardiac output. Bradycardia is a life-threatening event in infants and young children. In addition, hypothermia occurs. Lack of vasomotor control results in dilation of the vascular bed, which allows for heat loss. The patient with a spinal cord injury who is experiencing neurogenic shock assumes the temperature of the environment, which is usually lower than body temperature. Hypothermia increases oxygen and glucose consumption, which compounds the physiologic stress the patient is undergoing. Increased metabolic demands, coupled with inability of the cardiovascular system to meet the increasing demands, may result in cardiopulmonary arrest.

BOX 15-1 Vertebral Injuries

Atlanto-occipital dislocation: Avulsion of the atlas from the occipital bone.

Comminuted fracture (burst): Shattering of the vertebral body. Bone may be driven into the spinal canal.

Compression (wedge) fracture: Vertebral body is compressed anteriorly. Spinal cord injury may or may not be present.

Dislocation: One vertebra overrides another and there is dislocation of one or both facets. This dislocation usually results in ligamentous injury.

Hangman's fracture: Fracture through the arch of C2. Patient often is asymptomatic.

Jefferson fracture: Bursting of the ring of C1 as a result of axial loading. Displaced fractures usually are fatal injuries.

Simple fracture: Fracture that generally involves the spinous or transverse process facets or pedicle. Alignment usually is intact. Spinal cord injury usually is not present.

Subluxation: Partial or incomplete dislocation of one vertebrae over another.

Teardrop fracture: Small fragment of the vertebrae becomes free and may lodge in the spinal canal.

ASSESSMENT AND CARE OF THE PATIENT WITH A SPINAL CORD INJURY

Initial Assessment

As with all trauma patients, assessment of the patient with a suspected spinal injury must be done in an orderly, systematic manner. Initial trauma assessment is divided into two phases: primary and secondary.

Primary Survey

Initial management of the injured child begins with evaluation of the airway for patency and the need to use adjunctive measures. At the same time, the patient's cervical spine must be protected. Spinal precautions are initiated for any patient who has sustained injury above the clavicles, complains of neck or back pain or neurologic signs after injury, or sustains an injury from severe forces (e.g., motor vehicle accidents, motor-pedestrian collisions, significant falls). The neck is maintained in a neutral position. Ideally, the patient should be secured to a spineboard, with tape and rigid rolls on each side of the head. Use of a standard spineboard in an infant or young toddler may force the neck into a degree of flexion because the head is disproportionately large.

Another technique is to lay the child so that the occiput is lower than the body, but using padding under the shoulders and trunk. A rigid cervical collar should be applied if a collar of proper size is available (Torosian et al., 1995). Standard cervical collars may not fit infants and young children (Figure 15-8). In this case the neck can be immobilized with towels or other padding. The patient with a spinal cord

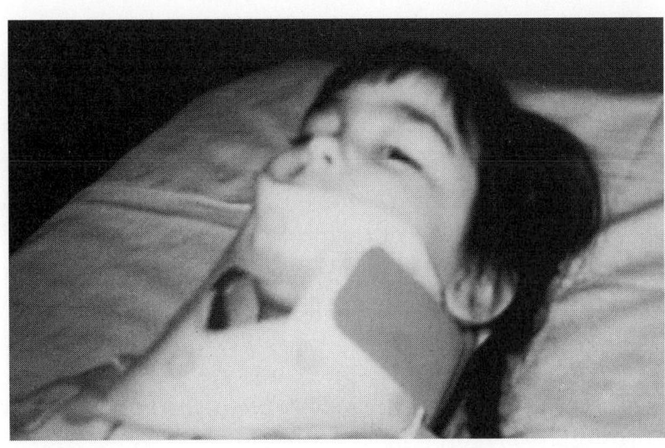

FIGURE 15-8 Example of a poorly fitting collar on a child. The collar occludes the patient's mouth and does not support the chin.

injury who requires an artificial airway must be treated with special consideration. Care must be taken not to manipulate the neck during the establishment of the airway. Initially, attempts to open the airway should be made using a jaw-thrust maneuver. Intubation can be done nasally or orally, with special attention paid to neck alignment.

Once patency of the airway is confirmed, breathing is evaluated. The patient is evaluated for the presence and quality of respirations. In patients with injuries to C1 through C4, phrenic nerve impairment results in the loss of diaphragmatic function and the inability to breathe spontaneously. In patients who have injury to the lower cervical and thoracic areas, paralysis of the intercostal and abdominal muscles may result in ineffective ventilation and the inability to cough and clear secretions effectively. The patient receives 100% supplemental oxygen via mask if ventilation is effective. Mechanical ventilation is initiated for patients with absent or ineffective ventilation.

Circulatory assessment is completed once airway and breathing are stabilized. The cardiovascular system remains unstable for the first several days after spinal cord injury. The patient is at high risk for the development of bradycardia, cardiac arrest, and hypotension. Identification of signs and symptoms of cardiovascular instability is essential.

Patients with spinal cord injury are also at risk for injuries to other organ systems. Detection of hypovolemic shock secondary to hemorrhage is difficult in the child with a spinal cord injury. The pediatric patient responds to hypovolemic shock by increasing the heart rate and vasoconstricting the peripheral blood vessels, resulting in the classic signs of tachycardia and poor perfusion. Unopposed parasympathetic innervation and the resultant bradycardia and vasodilation may mask the signs of hypovolemia and disable the normal methods of compensation that preserve blood flow to vital organs. Identification of internal bleeding may be further complicated by loss of sensation below the level of the injury. Pain and tenderness to palpation are symptoms of injury that are lost when the child has altered sensation. Initial treatment of the pediatric trauma patient with neurogenic shock is fluid resuscitation, but care is taken not to be too aggressive because the patient is at risk for the development of pulmonary edema. The patient who demonstrates persistent hypotension despite fluid resuscitation is thoroughly evaluated for areas of undetected bleeding. If no cause is found and neurogenic shock is suspected, vasopressor agents such as dopamine hydrochloride, epinephrine, or phenylephrine hydrochloride (Neo-Synephrine) can be initiated (Chameides & Hazinski, 1997; Torosian et al., 1995). Symptomatic bradycardia is treated with oxygenation and ventilation initially. Atropine or epinephrine can be administered if necessary (Chameides & Hazinski, 1997).

Once airway, breathing, and circulation (the ABCs) are stabilized, a brief assessment of the patient's neurologic status is performed. The patient is assessed for responsiveness to stimuli. The AVPU (*a*lert, responds to *v*erbal command, responds to *p*ain, *u*nresponsive). Method can be used to document the findings.

SECONDARY SURVEY

After the primary survey is completed, a more thorough examination is performed. This survey involves a head-to-toe examination, including a patient history and diagnostic tests. Discussion of the aspects of the secondary survey specific to the pediatric patient with spinal injury follows.

History. A patient history is obtained as soon as reasonably possible. In addition to details surrounding the injury, an assessment of conditions that place the patient at higher risk for spine injury is obtained. Patients with Down syndrome are at increased risk for cervical spine injury. Down syndrome is associated with multiple cervical anomalies. The most common anomaly is atlantoaxial instability (AAI), ligament laxity at the craniovertebral junction that leads to instability. It is believed that 10% to 20% of patients with Down syndrome have AAI (American Academy of Pediatrics, 1995; Citow, Munshi, Chang-Stroman, Sullivan, & Frim, 1998). AAI and other conditions, such as rheumatoid arthritis and osteogenesis imperfecta, increase the suspicion of spinal cord injury.

Exposure/Thermoregulation. Exposure of the patient is necessary to make an adequate assessment. The patient's clothing is removed while adequate measures are initiated to avoid heat loss, a particular problem for patients with spinal cord injury. The cervical collar is removed while the neck is stabilized manually. The neck is assessed anteriorly and posteriorly for the presence of pain, step-off, deformity, crepitus, bruising, and swelling. The patient is log-rolled while spine alignment is maintained.

With the child on his or her side, the physician assesses the entire spine for deformity, pain, step-off, bruising, and other signs of injury. Rectal sphincter tone may be assessed at this time.

Neurologic Examination. Performing a neurologic examination on a pediatric patient can be challenging.

Infants and young toddlers do not have the ability to cooperate with the examination. Older children may be frightened and may not cooperate. Attempts are made, within the child's developmental level, to perform a motor, sensory, and reflex examination.

The nurse begins by asking the child to follow simple commands, such as wiggling the toes or opening and closing the hands. Motor examinations include an assessment of all nerve roots and the muscles they innervate. Each extremity and the intercostal and abdominal muscles are assessed. Infants are observed for spontaneous movement and withdrawal from painful stimuli. Motor strength is scored on a 5-point scale (American Spinal Injury Association, 1992):

0 = Absent
1 = Palpable or visible contraction
2 = Active motion with gravity eliminated
3 = Motion against gravity
4 = Active motion against resistance
5 = Active motion against full resistance

Intercostal, abdominal, and perianal muscles are graded on a 2-point scale (Torosian et al., 1995):

0 = Absent
1 = Weak
2 = Strong contraction

If the child's cognitive condition allows, the nurse asks questions regarding the presence of pain or any altered sensation. Sensation is assessed in older children by testing the ability to distinguish between sharp and dull sensation to pinprick. The dermatome system (Figure 15-9) may be used to assess nerve root function. Using a pointed object, the examiner begins at the area where the patient has sensation, such as the side of the face, and proceeds, testing all dermatomes. The child can also be assessed for the ability to distinguish hot and cold. Proprioception can be tested by having the child tell which direction his or her finger or toe is facing when the examiner moves it. Sensory examination includes the assessment of sensation in the perianal area.

Radiologic Examinations. Once the patient is examined and stabilized, radiographic examination of the spine is performed, as indicated. Cervical spine radiographs are obtained on children considered to be at high risk for spine injury. Eight variables have been identified as indicators of cervical spine injury. These variables are neck pain and tenderness; abnormal strength, sensation, and reflexes; direct trauma to the neck; limitations in neck mobility; and altered mental status (Jaffe, Benns, Radkowski, Barthel, & Engelhand, 1987). Children who sustain minor trauma and have a normal neurologic examination, full range of neck movement, and no pain or tenderness are highly unlikely to have a spinal injury and may not require spine radiographs.

Once the decision is made to obtain radiographs, it is essential to obtain an adequate examination. The preferred initial cervical spine radiographs are lateral, anteroposterior, and odontoid views. The series must include a clear, unobstructed view of *all* seven cervical vertebrae and the first thoracic vertebra. Failure to obtain complete, clear radiographs may result in missed injury.

Flexion-extension views (Figure 15-10) may be ordered in patients whose radiographs are normal but who are suspected of having ligamentous injury. Flexion-extension views are performed with a physician present. The child should be alert and able to follow commands because he or she is instructed to actively flex and extend the neck and stop if there is pain or alterations in neurologic function. Passive flexion and extension are avoided because such actions may increase the risk of further damage to the cord (Hall & Boydston, 1999; Torosian et al., 1995).

Computed tomography (CT) scanning may be ordered if flexion-extension studies are contraindicated, the radiographs are suspicious, and injury is strongly suspected. CT scanning is not ordered routinely because it is not cost effective and sedation of the child may be required. For children experiencing neurologic symptoms who have normal radiographs, CT scans, and flexion-extension views, a magnetic resonance imaging (MRI) scan may be necessary. MRI may be able to detect contusion and edema of the cord, although the test is not ordered routinely because it is time consuming and expensive. MRI is difficult to obtain in the critically ill patient because it requires advanced preparation and specialized monitoring equipment.

Evaluation of the radiographs and scans is done by physicians familiar with the unique aspects of the pediatric spine. It is preferable to have the films officially read by a pediatric radiologist, neurosurgeon, or orthopedist. The child remains immobilized until the official reading of the films.

High-Dose Steroids

One of the goals of caring for the child with a spinal cord injury is to prevent secondary spinal cord injury. Bracken, Shepard, and Collins (1990) have advocated the use of methylprednisolone at high dosages. It is believed that the drug acts to decrease the formation of lipid peroxidases and hydrolases at the injury site and to decrease arachidonic acid metabolites, which decrease blood flow to the cord. A large, multicenter trial demonstrated that patients who received high dosages of methylprednisolone within 8 hours of injury and for 23 hours after the initial dose showed significant improvement in motor function and sensation 6 months after injury. One of the concerning factors related to the study is that it did not include children.

If methylprednisolone is given, it is administered at a dosage of 30 mg/kg intravenous bolus over 15 minutes. Forty-five minutes after completion of the bolus, a drip at 5.4 mg/kg body weight is infused each hour for 23 hours (Allen, Boyer, Cherney, & Fait, 1996).

Nursing Care of the Child With Spinal Cord Injury

Admission of the Patient to the Unit

Preadmission Preparation. Care of a child with a spinal cord injury begins at the scene of the injury and con-

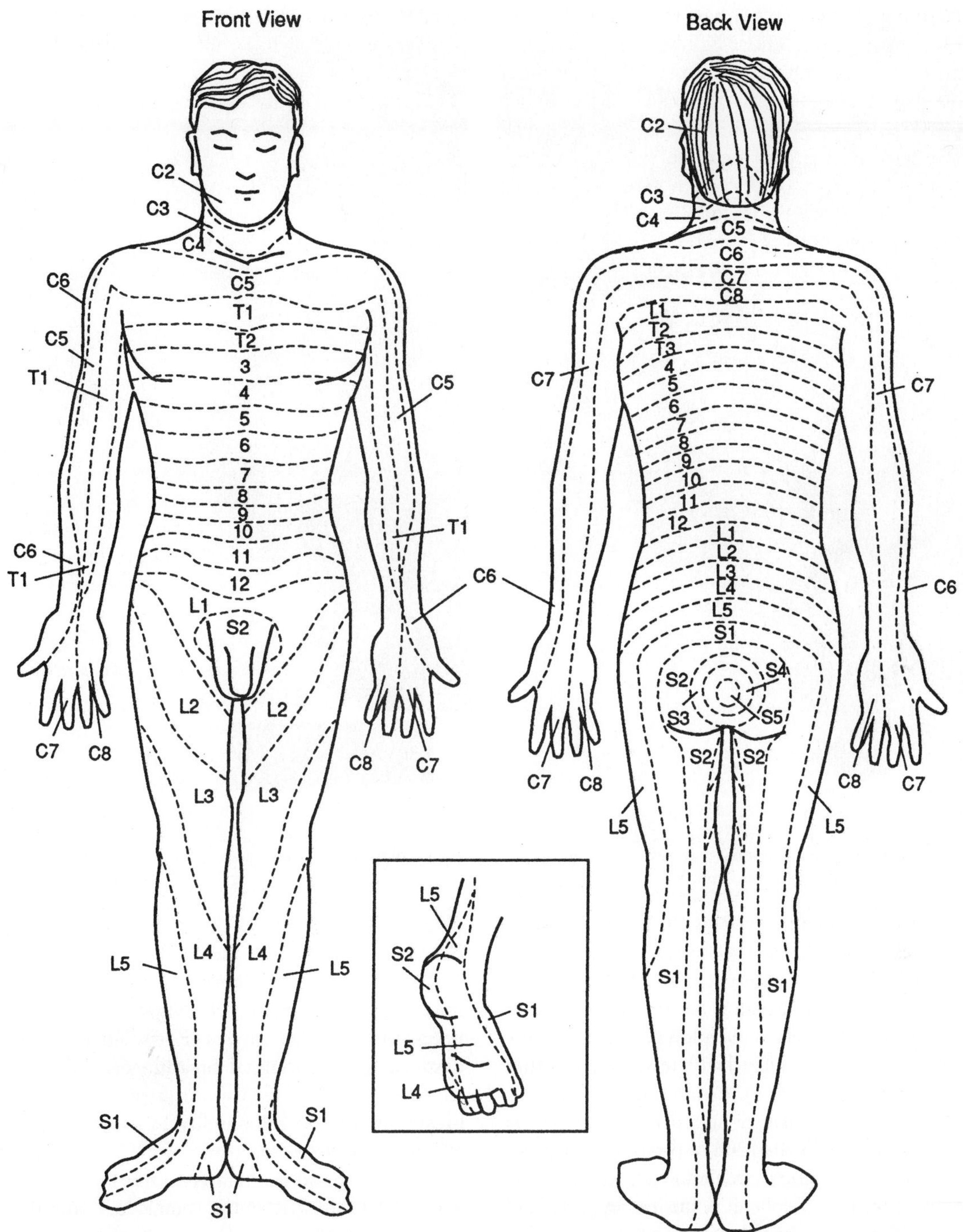

FIGURE 15-9 Dermatomes. (From McQuillan, K. A., Von Rueden, K. T., Hartsock, R. L., Flynn, M. B., & Whalen, E. [Eds]. [2002]. *Trauma nursing: From resuscitation through rehabilitation* [3rd ed.]. Philadelphia: WB Saunders.)

tinues throughout the rehabilitative phase. Before the patient's arrival in the unit, the admitting nurse obtains a detailed history, including preexisting conditions, mechanism of injury, events surrounding the injury, and therapeutic and preventive modalities initiated at the scene or the emergency center. The nursing report includes identified alterations in respiratory status, cardiovascular status, and neurologic deficits.

The nurse considers which methods of spinal immobilization will be used for the child and initiates measures to obtain the necessary equipment (e.g., rotating trauma bed, Stryker frame).

Initial Management. Upon the child's arrival to the unit, the priorities of care are to maintain adequate ventilation and hemodynamic stability while protecting the spine to prevent further injury. Assessment of the airway while maintaining spine alignment is the highest priority. If the patient has an artificial airway, the nurse assesses size, patency, and security. The patient is in the supine position, with the neck

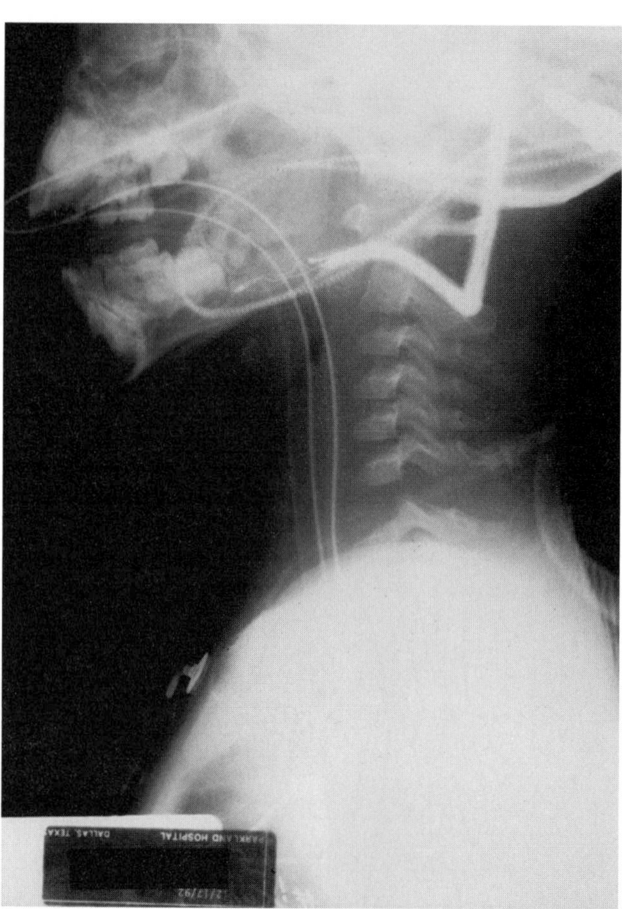

FIGURE 15-10 **A,** Example of a poor-quality cervical spine radiograph. A monitor cable obscures part of the view of the bones. **B,** Second radiograph without the obstruction reveals a significant injury.

in neutral alignment. A rigid cervical collar is applied if not previously done. Immobilizing the neck may be difficult because cervical collars may not fit young children. There are new pediatric spinal immobilization devices that take into account the anatomic differences in children. In certain situations the neck may be immobilized with towel rolls or other padding (Hall & Boydston, 1999). Breathing is assessed for rate and effectiveness. Ventilatory support is initiated for patients unable to maintain adequate respirations. After airway and breathing are stabilized, circulation is assessed. Heart rate, blood pressure, and peripheral perfusion are evaluated and appropriate therapies initiated. Once the ABCs are stabilized, rapid assessment of the patient's neurologic system, including motor sensory function, is completed.

Ongoing Care

Respiratory Assessment/Interventions. Alteration in respiratory function is a major problem for the patient with cervical and thoracic spine injury. Injury at or above C4 will disrupt the phrenic nerve, resulting in loss of diaphragmatic function. Spinal cord edema can cause alteration of function in areas above the true level of the lesion, resulting in ineffective breathing patterns. Injuries that paralyze the intercostal and abdominal muscles are problematic in infants and young children because they use these muscles for ventilation. In older children paralysis of the intercostal and abdominal muscles leads to ineffective cough and retained secretions.

The nurse assesses the respiratory status at least every hour until respiratory function is stable and then as deemed necessary. Any spontaneous efforts, altered chest excursion, dyspnea, and abdominal breathing are observed for. The character, rate, and rhythm of respirations; auscultation of breath sounds; and the ability to cough and deep breathe effectively are assessed.

Intubation and ventilatory support are used for patients with injuries that prevent spontaneous respirations. Patients with lower cervical injuries may be intubated prophylactically and mechanically ventilated to prevent respiratory muscle fatigue and maintain normal blood gas values.

Prevention of pulmonary complications is a goal for the patient with a spinal cord injury. Aspiration and pneumonia are two common complications in these patients. Patients are started on a regimen of chest physiotherapy, coughing, and suctioning at least every 4 hours. Positioning of the patient for postural drainage depends on the stability of the injury and the patient's condition. Unless contraindicated, the bed can be placed in the Trendelenburg position to facilitate postural drainage. Patients can be log-rolled from side to side for chest physiotherapy. Patients in a halo jacket can be turned onto their side and one side of the jacket opened for physiotherapy.

Assisted coughing can be used in patients with ineffective cough. When assisted coughing is performed, the caregiver places both hands on the chest wall, with the palms resting over the diaphragm area. After the patient takes a rapid succession of breaths, either spontaneous or assisted, the caregiver pushes downward and upward during the patient's exhalation. This process is repeated three to five times, until the secretions are cleared. The nurse or respiratory care practitioner provides gentle tracheal suctioning to clear secretions. Current practice includes administration of bronchodilators and mucolytic agents as needed to increase the diameter of the bronchioles. It is important to maintain adequate ventilation and monitor arterial blood gases frequently to prevent hypoxia, which may worsen the injury.

As the patient's condition stabilizes, the goals of treatment shift to long-term functioning. Patients with injuries below C5 generally can be weaned successfully from the ventilator. Weaning can be a long, tedious, and frightening process. Patients often become anxious and fearful as they are being weaned, fearing that they will not be able to breathe. The nurse can be instrumental in the success of weaning by allaying the patient's fears and offering encouragement. Respiratory therapists and physical therapists can assist by having the patient do breathing exercises, which will increase cardiopulmonary reserve.

Cardiovascular Assessment/Interventions. Cardiovascular assessment is performed every hour until the patient is stable and then as deemed necessary. Assessment includes monitoring of heart rate, blood pressure, skin color, temperature, strength and quality of peripheral pulses, capillary refill time, urine output, and level of consciousness. If the patient's condition warrants, arterial line and central venous pressure lines are placed.

The patient is assessed constantly for the presence of neurogenic shock. Hypotension in a patient with neurogenic shock is secondary to vasodilation and decreased venous return. Fluid resuscitation takes place with caution because the patient is at risk for development of pulmonary edema. Atropine can be used to treat bradycardia and vasopressors can be used for hypotension (Speer, 1999). Movement is minimized while the patient is in neurogenic shock because movement may exacerbate the vasovagal response. Application of antiembolism hose with or without sequential compression devices and/or wrapping of the lower extremities with elastic bandages from feet to groin may prevent venous pooling.

Patients with neurogenic shock are at high risk for hypothermia as a result of heat loss secondary to venous pooling. The patient with a spinal cord injury loses the ability to shiver and sweat, which impairs thermoregulation. Hypothermia can be treated with warm blankets, fluid warmers, and radiant warmers. Electrical warming devices and hot water bottles are never used in a patient with altered sensation. Fluid-filled warming blankets are used with caution.

Venous pooling secondary to peripheral vasodilation and immobility increase the risk for the development of deep venous thrombosis (DVT). The incidence of DVT is lower in children than in adults, but the risk is present. The patient with altered or absent sensation will not feel pain, a sign of DVT. The nurse assesses the patient for redness and swelling of the calves. Some practitioners advocate routine measurement of calf circumference to detect subtle changes.

DVT prophylaxis measures, such as antiembolism hose and sequential compression devices, can be used in older children and adolescents. The size of available equipment is a problem for infants and younger children. Modifications, such as wrapping the legs with elastic bandages (Ace wraps), can be made for the younger age groups. Use of prophylactic heparin in the pediatric age group is controversial, but it can be considered.

Patients with spinal cord injury at or above the level of T6 are at risk for autonomic dysreflexia. This condition usually occurs in the later course of the hospitalization or after the patient has been discharged. Noxious stimulation below the level of injury results in a massive sympathetic response and vasoconstriction of blood vessels, with resultant hypertension, pounding headache, and visual disturbances. The body responds by dilating vessels above the level of injury, causing flushing of skin, sweating, and goose bumps. Uncontrolled autonomic dysreflexia can lead to malignant hypertension and stroke. Treatment of autonomic dysreflexia involves removing the noxious stimuli, usually fecal impaction, bladder distention, or pressure ulcers. The patient is placed in an upright position, if possible, because this lowers blood pressure.

Stabilization of the Spine. Once the patient has been medically stabilized, the focus of care changes to the prevention of complications. The type of stabilization device depends on the type of injury and the stability of the spine. Initially, the patient is immobilized in a rigid cervical collar and a hard backboard. More definitive immobilization is initiated as soon as the patient is stable. Early immobilization of the unstable cervical spine injury is accomplished by applying skeletal traction. In the pediatric patient the most commonly used device is the halo ring (Figure 15-11). In young children a halo ring can be used with eight fixation

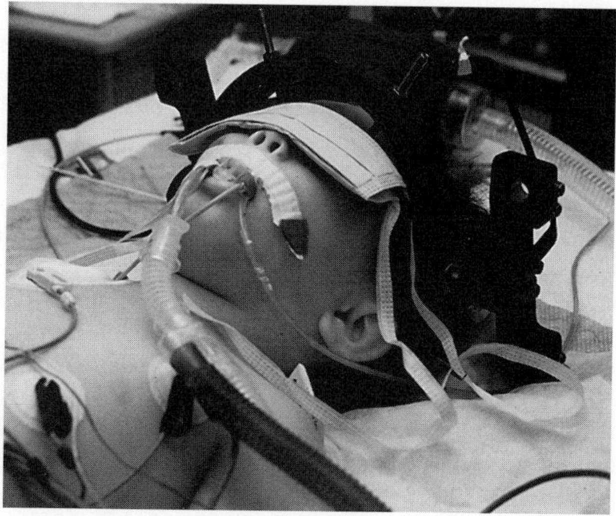

FIGURE 15-11 Patient in a halo ring without jacket.

pins. The pins allow for even distribution of forces at 2 psi of pressure. In the child younger than 2 years, finger tightening of the pins allows for pressures between 1 and 2 psi. Application of a halo jacket may be delayed in the young child because it may be necessary to order a specially sized jacket. Traction can be applied to the halo ring until the jacket is available. In the older child, traction can be applied via a standard halo ring and jacket. Once the halo jacket is in place, the child will be allowed more mobility. Because the jacket covers the chest wall, a contingency plan for removal of the jacket in the event of cardiopulmonary arrest is necessary. Many jackets now are made with bendable creases on the breast plate, which can be bent to allow access to the sternum for cardiopulmonary resuscitation (CPR). Older vests may not be equipped with this feature and require removal of the vest for CPR. As a safety measure, an Allen wrench and a torque wrench should be taped to the front of the halo vest of any patient wearing the vest. The staff caring for the patient should be competent in the removal of the vest. If the vest is removed, a rigid cervical collar is applied to the neck to maintain alignment. The nurse assures that the pins are secure in the skull and notifies the physician immediately if the pins loosen.

The nurse instructs all caregivers and family on the correct way to move and position the patient in a halo vest. The patient is never lifted by the stabilizing bars because this may pull the pins out of the skull. Skeletal tongs, such as Gardner-Wells tongs, may be used (Menezes & Osenbach, 1994). Stabilization devices are inspected for proper fit, alignment, stability of the pins in the skull, and correct amount of traction weight. Pin sites are assessed for redness, exudate, and any other signs of infection. Care of pin sites is institution dependent, but generally gauze soaked with povidone-iodine (Betadine) or topical antibiotic ointment is applied to the site for the first 24 to 48 hours. This is followed by a regimen of half-strength hydrogen peroxide or sterile normal saline every 6 to 8 hours.

Cervical traction is manipulated only by the physician. A thorough neurologic examination is completed before and after manipulation of stabilization devices to determine whether there has been a change. Cervical spine radiographs may be ordered after changes in cervical traction to assess alignment and reduction.

Thoracic and lumbar spine injuries are managed by immobilization in specialty beds or in specially fitted braces. These devices allow for movement to prevent complications associated with immobility while keeping the spine aligned (Yarkony, Formal, & Cawley, 1997).

In certain situations stabilization of the spine may be accomplished through surgical interventions. Spinal fusion may be done using an anterior or posterior approach. Postoperative care of the patient includes assessment of the cardiopulmonary system, neurologic evaluation, and specific regimens related to spinal immobilization.

Integumentary and Musculoskeletal Assessment/Interventions. All critically injured patients are at risk for complications secondary to immobility. The combination of altered tissue perfusion, immobility, and altered sensation magnifies this risk for the patient with spinal cord injury. The sacrum, occiput, and heels are the areas at greatest risk. Use of special beds and frames allows the spine to be immobilized while complications are prevented. Patients should be removed from the spineboard as soon as possible. Although the use of specialty beds may decrease the incidence of pressure ulcer formation, astute nursing assessment is mandatory. The most commonly used bed in the pediatric patient is the rotating trauma bed. The bed is a flat table with a series of pads that conform to the patient's body and allows the patient to be rotated from side to side (Figure 15-12). Some of the beds allow the patient to continuously rotate slowly in a 60- to 60-degree arc. The smaller rotating beds allow for manual turning of the patient. Continuous turning (16 to 20 hours per day) decreases the complications associated with immobility. The bed is equipped with a series of hatches and flaps, which permit access to the patient's back. When ordering a bed for the patient, the nurse should know the patient's height and weight to ensure that the bed is the proper size.

Skin is evaluated frequently for redness or breakdown because skin breakdown may occur in a short time. All areas of the skin are assessed, with special attention paid to high-risk areas such as the occiput, sacrum, and heels. The axilla and areas closest to the pads of the rotating bed are assessed carefully because they may break down secondary to friction and pressure.

Patients who require cervical immobilization with a cervical collar often experience pressure areas and skin breakdown. The chin, occiput, and ears are common sites of breakdown. At least every 8 hours the collar is removed, one section at a time, while the neck is manually stabilized and the skin of the neck inspected. It may be necessary to pad the collar or skin with a protective dressing such as DuoDERM. The key to maintaining healthy skin is prevention of break-

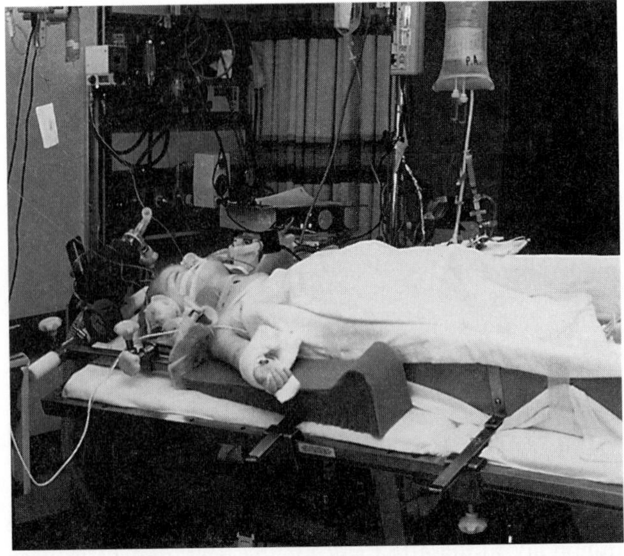

FIGURE 15-12 Child in a rotating trauma bed.

down by frequent repositioning and inspection. High-risk areas may be padded to prevent pressure areas. The use of gel pads, which conform to the patient, is acceptable. Donut-type devices are not used because they restrict circulation to the affected area.

Proper positioning of the patient is important for prevention of contractures and for facilitation into the rehabilitation phase. During the critical care phase the nurse can prevent contractures by performing passive range of motion several times a day. The extremities are extended and slightly abducted. The hands are kept in the anatomic position, which can be accomplished by placing a washcloth or small stuffed toy in the palms. Physical medicine and rehabilitation consultations are obtained soon after admission and physical and occupational therapy begun as soon as possible. Orthotic devices for the wrists and ankles may be necessary. Splinting regimens are initiated. Nursing care includes the removal of splints on a regular basis for passive range of motion and inspection of the skin. Once the patient is medically stable, more intensive therapies can be initiated, with the ultimate goal being transfer to a rehabilitation facility.

Gastrointestinal Assessment/Interventions. Paralytic ileus is a common occurrence in patients with spinal cord injuries. The goal of nursing care is to prevent abdominal distention, thereby reducing the risk of vomiting and aspiration. A nasogastric or orogastric tube is placed and attached to low intermittent suction. Oral and enteral feedings are restricted until peristalsis returns, as evidenced by the presence of bowel sounds and passing of flatus. Some form of nutrition is initiated within 72 hours because children have little reserve and develop protein catabolism in the initial hours after the injury. Antacids are administered as ordered to neutralize the pH of gastric secretions and to decrease the incidence of stress ulcers (Zejdlik, 1992).

As bowel function returns, a bowel regimen that is appropriate for the specific lesion is initiated. Upper motor neuron lesions result in a bowel that is reflexive, and the rectum empties every 2 to 3 days. These lesions can be managed on a set schedule with bowel training. In contrast, lower motor neuron lesions result in an areflexic bowel and require a bowel regimen that promotes daily emptying of the rectum to prevent incontinence.

Bowel training for children requires special consideration for age, developmental level, and cultural and psychosocial issues. Bowel training should occur at a specific time each day. The goal is to achieve complete emptying of the rectum on a set schedule, thereby decreasing the incidence of incontinence. Bowel training involves strict adherence to a daily schedule, digital manipulation, and administration of stool softeners and suppositories. This is combined with a well-balanced diet that includes fiber and adequate fluid intake (Edwards-Beckett & King, 1996). Caution is used when administering enemas because they may cause overdistention of the bowel, resulting in subsequent autonomic dysreflexia and/or fluid and electrolyte imbalances. Mineral oils are avoided to prevent the depletion of fat-soluble vitamins (Zejdlik, 1992). Adequate fluid intake and sufficient fiber in the diet are important to prevent impaction. Consumption of a warm liquid followed by digital stimulation approximately 1 hour after the chosen mealtime can be effective treatment in the bowel training program (Speer, 1999).

Genitourinary Assessment/Interventions. Preservation of renal function and urinary elimination is an important aspect in the nursing care of the child with spinal cord injury. The child will exhibit urinary retention and overflow incontinence as a result of an areflexic or flaccid bladder, secondary to spinal shock or lower motor neuron injury. In contrast, upper motor neuron injury results in a hyperreflexic bladder, which is not apparent during the spinal shock phase. The child will exhibit spasms of the bladder and internal sphincter and paralysis of the external sphincter, resulting in overdistention and incomplete emptying of the bladder. Overdistention can result in autonomic dysreflexia. Incomplete lesions can result in a combination of spasticity and flaccidity. The child may be able to detect fullness of the bladder yet may have limited or no control of voiding (Zejdlik, 1992).

During management of the acute phase, an indwelling urinary catheter is inserted and urine output monitored hourly. The urine should be clear yellow and free of blood or sediment. A minimal output of 1 to 2 ml/kg/hr should be maintained to preserve renal function. A urology consultation should be obtained early during treatment to assess renal function. Periodic urodynamic testing is an important part of ongoing therapy. Soon after spinal shock resolves, a bladder training regimen should be established that allows the child to achieve some control over elimination while providing complete emptying of the bladder. The ultimate goal is to preserve renal function, which is attributed to maintaining adequate bladder capacity (Pannek, Wolfgang, & Botel, 1997). Preventing associated complications, such as kidney and urinary tract infections, formation of renal calculi, and autonomic dysreflexia, is an ongoing challenge.

Progressive treatment after the acute phase involves intermittently clamping the urinary catheter, with gradual increases in time periods. This bladder training stimulates the micturition reflexes, promotes an improved level of bladder muscle tone and control, and decreases spasms associated with an overdistended or empty bladder (Speer, 1999).

Early in the subacute phase, the indwelling urinary catheter should be discontinued and intermittent catheterization or the Credé maneuver performed. Bladder capacity varies with the age of the child. Intermittent catheterization is done every 4 hours initially. Adjustments of time intervals are made in relation to the estimated amount of bladder capacity versus the amount of urine obtained. If the child voids spontaneously, the nurse assesses for residual amounts of urine by intermittent catheterization (Zejdlik, 1992).

Pharmacologic measures can be used to control some of the genitourinary symptoms associated with spinal cord injury. Antispasmodics or anticholinergics can be administered to decrease the bladder spasms associated with upper motor neuron injury.

Pain. Every person who sustains a spinal cord injury experiences pain. Acute pain syndromes often arise from nerve root or spinal cord damage that causes paresthetic pain. As the injury heals, most of the pain associated with the injury heals. However, for many people chronic pain syndromes develop. Usually, they develop months to years after the injury. Pain syndromes that occur after spinal cord injury can be classified into five types: mechanical, peripheral (nerve root in origin), visceral, central, or psychogenic. Chronic pain after spinal cord injury is a multifaceted problem that should be handled by an interdisciplinary team with a specialty in pediatric pain. Management of pain is multifactorial, and mechanical, neurologic, psychologic, and sociologic factors are considered. It is important for nurses to realize that pain is a real experience for patients with spinal cord injuries and is treated as such (Zejdlik, 1992). Chapter 11 provides information about pain management in critically injured children.

PSYCHOSOCIAL ASPECTS OF NURSING CARE FOR THE CHILD WITH SPINAL CORD INJURY

Sustaining a spinal cord injury is a devastating, life-altering experience. The nurse plays an important role in assisting the child and family to deal with the emotional stress associated with this catastrophic event. The nurse uses a holistic approach in the plan of care, one that incorporates the child's developmental level along with identified coping mechanisms, preferred methods of learning, and family dynamics. A multidisciplinary care team consisting of physicians, nurses, therapists, a social worker, a child life specialist, and a chaplain is assembled.

Early in the course of the injury, the family may be in denial or angry, both of which are normal coping behaviors. Information needs to be presented to them in a factual, honest manner. Frequent reinforcement of the information may be necessary. It is essential that all health care team members give the family the same information. Discrepancies in details related to injury, treatment plan, and prognosis will lead to confusion. Family members are encouraged to express their emotions related to their child's injury. They are also encouraged to participate in their child's care. As the child becomes more stable, the family receives information and resources to make informed decision regarding rehabilitation facilities.

The psychologic effect of the injury on even the youngest children cannot be minimized. These children are frightened, anxious, and often unable understand what has happened to them. The hospital environment is frightening, and their need for immobility affords them little in the way of comfort or entertainment. If it is necessary for the patient to lie supine for a length of time, measures are taken to make the environment more comforting. Posters can be hung on the ceiling or stuffed animals suspended from IV poles to make the environment more child-friendly. The child may feel vulnerable because he or she cannot see who is coming into the room. Staff members should announce to the child who they are and why they are there. Adjunctive devices, such as "prism glasses," allow the child to "see" who is entering the room and, when the glasses are worn, may allow the child to watch television or see pictures.

The nurse plays an instrumental role as child advocate by identifying himself or herself as someone who will stay with the child throughout the shift (Figure 15-13). The patient experiences the ultimate loss of control and is often afraid of being left alone. Patients with spinal cord injuries who are

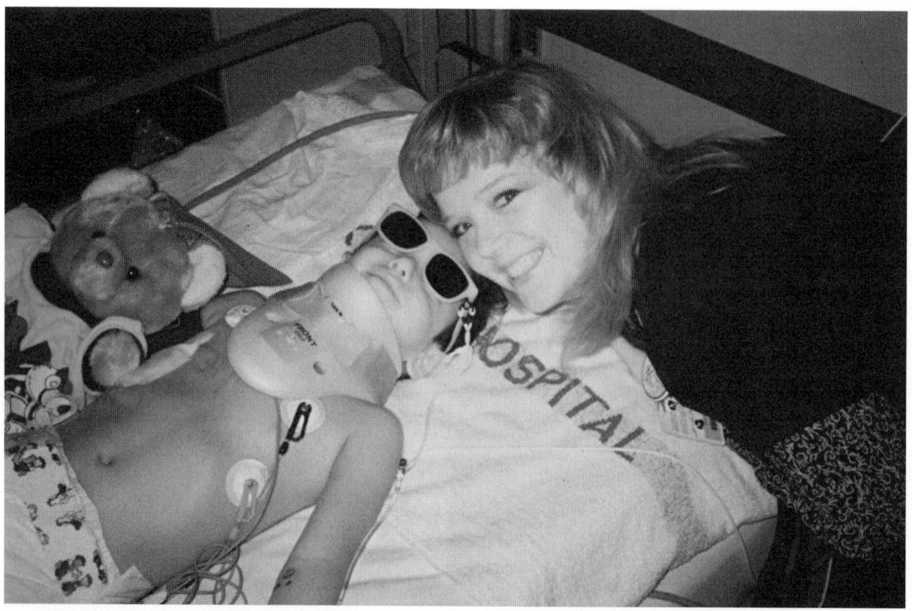

FIGURE 15-13 The nurse needs to remember that the patient is a child and allow for "playtime."

ventilatory dependent may fear not being able to breathe if the ventilator becomes disconnected and no one is in the room. The nurse provides constant reassurance. The nurse caring for a child with a spinal cord injury needs to be cognizant of making the patient feel secure while providing for some limit setting. The patient may make many requests to keep the nurse close to him or her. One technique that can be used with older children is to position a clock so that the child can see it. The nurse informs the child of a return time. It is imperative that the nurse return at that time to build a trusting relationship.

Child life specialists can be helpful in providing play therapy and distraction for the patient and the patient's siblings. They can also assist by setting up a daily routine for the patient. Within the routine the patient may be able to make choices, for example, which movie to watch or when to sit in the chair. When the child is stable and awaiting transfer to a rehabilitation facility, special consideration is given to activities such as trips to the playroom or walks outside. The child is encouraged to begin educational activities as soon as possible, with the goal of returning to school. Several studies have correlated educational achievement and employability in patients with spinal cord injuries (Alfred, Furher, & Rossi, 1987; DeVivo, Rutt, Stover, & Fine, 1987).

The child and family should be provided with a list of resources related to spinal cord injury. Box 15-2 lists some of the resources available to the child with spinal cord injury and the child's family.

BOX 15-2 Resources for Patients With Spinal Cord Injuries

Federation of Spine Associations
http://www.aaos.org

National Rehabilitation Information Center
http://www.cais.com/naric

National Spinal Cord Injury Association
8300 Colesville Road
Suite 551
Silver Spring, MD 20910
301-588-6959
http://www.spinalcord.org
Includes a program titled "In Touch with Kids," a free program for children 18 years and younger with spinal cord injury

National Statistical Center of the Model Spinal Cord Injury Care Systems
University of Alabama at Birmingham
http://www.spinalcord.uab.edu

Spinal Cord Injury Resources
http://www.eskimo.com/~jlubin/disabled/sci.htm

U.S. Department of Education, National Institute on Disability and Rehabilitation Research
http://www.ed.gov

CURRENT SPINAL CORD INJURY RESEARCH

Current research studies are focused on both acute and chronic spinal cord injury. For the acutely injured patient, the most strongly established treatment is the administration of methylprednisolone. An extended duration of treatment study is currently under way in the National Acute Spinal Cord Injury Study. Another medication that offers hope for the patient with acute spinal cord injury is ganglioside G_{M1}. Ganglioside G_{M1} is believed to work in several ways. It controls damage by reducing the toxicity of amino acids released after spinal cord injury. Another theory suggests that there may be a neurotropic effect that encourages the growth of injured neurons. Ganglioside G_{M1} is currently being used in a limited number of studies. A third medication, tirilazad mesylate, is believed to limit lipid peroxidation and acute spinal cord injury in animals (Yarkony et al., 1997).

Current research on chronic spinal cord injury includes functional electrical stimulation, omentum transposition, regeneration of severed axons, addition of new neurons, formation of new synapses, remyelination of axons, and supplementation of neurotransmitters. Future treatments may include any of these methods individually or in combination.

SUMMARY

Care of the child with spinal cord injury provides many challenges. The initial focus is on resuscitation and stabilization while protecting the spine. Ongoing care requires attention to supporting physiologic functions and meeting the psychologic needs of the child and family. Early involvement in a rehabilitation program is essential to integrating the child back into the community as soon as possible.

BIBLIOGRAPHY

Alfred, W. G., Fuhrer, M. J., & Rossi, C. D. (1987). Vocational development following severe spinal cord injury: A longitudinal study. *Archives of Physical Medicine and Rehabilitation, 68*(12), 854-857.

Allen, E. M., Boyer, R., Cherney, W. B., & Fait, V. F. (1996). Head and spinal cord injury. In M. C. Rogers (Ed.), *Textbook of pediatric intensive care* (3rd ed.). Baltimore: Williams & Wilkins.

Allen, J. P., Meyers, G. C., & Condon, V. R. (1969). Laceration of the spinal cord related to breech delivery. *Journal of the American Medical Association, 208,* 1019-1022.

American Academy of Pediatrics, Committee on Sports Medicine and Fitness. (1995). Atlantoaxial instability in Down syndrome: Subject review. *Pediatrics, 96*(1 Pt. 1), 151-154.

American Spinal Injury Association annual meeting, Toronto, Cananda, 8-10 May 1992. Abstracts. (1992). *Journal of the American Paraplegia Society, 15*(2), 73-152.

Bailey, D. K. (1952). The normal cervical spine in infants and children. *Radiology, 59,* 719.

Bracken, M. B., Shepard, M. J., & Collins, W. B. (1990). A randomized, controlled trial of methylprednisolone or naloxone in the treatment of acute spinal cord injury. *New England Journal of Medicine, 322,* 1405-1411.

Cattell, H. S., & Filtzer, D. L. (1965). Pseudosubluxation and other normal variants in the spine in children: A study of one hundred and sixty children. *Journal of Bone and Joint Surgery American Volume, 47,* 1295-1309.

Chameides, L., & Hazinski, M. F. (Eds.). (1997). *Textbook of pediatric advanced life support.* Dallas: American Heart Association.

Chipps, E., Clanin, N., & Campbell, V. (1992). Color atlas of neurologic structure and function. In E. Chipps, N. Clanin, & V. Campbell (Eds.), *Neurologic disorders* (pp. 2-17). St. Louis: Mosby.

Citow, J. S., Munshi, I., Chang-Stroman, T., Sullivan, C., & Frim, D. M. (1998). C2/3 instability in a child with Down's syndrome: Case report and discussion. *Pediatric Neurosurgery, 28*(3), 143-146.

DeVivo, M. J., Rutt, R. D., Stover, S. L., & Fine, P. R. (1987). Employment after spinal cord injury. *Archives of Physical Medicine and Rehabilitation, 68*(8), 494-498.

Edwards-Beckett, J., & King, H. (1996). The impact of spinal pathology on bowel control in children. *Rehabilitation Nursing, 21*(6), 292-297.

Emergency Nurses Association. (1995). *Trauma nursing core course provider manual* (pp. 195-224). Park Ridge, IL: Author.

Fesmire, F. M., & Luten, R. C. (1989). The pediatric cervical spine: Developmental anatomy and clinical aspects. *Journal of Emergency Medicine, 7,* 133-142.

Fielding, J. W. (1978). The cervical spine in the child. In M. S. O'Brien (Ed.), *Pediatric neurological surgery.* New York: Raven Press.

Gerhart, K. A. (1991). Spinal cord injury outcomes in a population based sample. *Journal of Trauma, 31,* 1529-1535.

Givens, T. G., Polley, K. A., Smith, G. F., & Hardin, W. D. (1996). Pediatric cervical spine injury: a three year experience. *Journal of Trauma Injury, Infection and Critical Care, 8,* 310-314.

Go, B. K., DeVivo, M. J., & Richards, S. (1995). The epidemiology of spinal cord injury. In S. L. Stover, J. A. De Lisa, & G. C. Whiteneck (Eds.), *Clinical outcomes from the model systems* (pp. 21-58). Gaithersburg, MD: Aspen.

Grabb, P. A., & Pang, D. (1994). Magnetic resonance imaging in the evaluation of spinal cord injury without radiographic abnormality in children. *Neurosurgery, 35*(3), 406-414.

Hall, D. E., & Boydston, W. (1999). Pediatric neck injuries. *Pediatrics in Review, 20*(1), 13-19.

Hjalmas, K. (1988). Urodynamics in normal infants and children. *Scandinavian Journal of Urology and Nephrology Supplement, 114,* 20-27.

Jaffe, D. M., Benns, H., Radkowski, M. A., Barthel, M. J., & Engelhand, H. H. (1987). Developing a clinical algorithm for early management of cervical spinal injury in child trauma victims. *Annals of Emergency Medicine, 16*(3), 270-276.

Leventhal, H. R. (1960). Birth injuries of the spinal cord. *Journal of Pediatrics, 56,* 447.

Marinier, M., Rodts, M. F., & Connolly, M. (1997). Spinal cord injury without radiologic abnormality. *Orthopedic Nursing, 16,* 57-63.

McGuire, R. A. (1998). Physical examination. In A. M. Levine, F. J. Eismont, S. R. Garfin, & J. E. Zigler (Eds.), *Spine trauma* (pp. 16-27). Philadelphia: WB Saunders.

McLone, D. G., & Dias, M. S. (1994). Normal and abnormal development of the spine. In W. R. Cheek (Ed.), *Pediatric neurosurgery: Surgery of the developing spine* (pp. 40-50). Philadelphia: WB Saunders.

Menezes, A. H., & Osenbach, R. K. (1994). Spinal cord injury. In W. R. Cheek (Ed.), *Pediatric neurosurgery: Surgery of the developing spine* (pp. 320-341). Philadelphia: WB Saunders.

National Spinal Cord Injury Association. (1998). Resource center web site. Available at: http://www.erols.com/nscia./resource/factshts/-fact02.html.

Orenstein, J. B., Klein, B. L., Gotschall, C. S., Ochsenschlager, D. W., Klatzko, M. D., & Eichelberger, M. R. (1994). Age and outcome in pediatric cervical spine injury: 11-year experience. *Pediatric Emergency Care, 10*(3), 132-137.

Pang, D., & Pollack, C. (1989). Spinal cord injury without radiologic abnormality in children. The SCIWORA syndrome. *Journal of Trauma, 29,* 651-664.

Pannek, J., Wolfgang, D., & Botel, U. (1997). Urodynamically controlled management of spinal cord injury in children. *Neurourology and Urodynamics, 16,* 285-292.

Ruge, J. R., Sinson, G. P., McLone, D. G., & Cerullo, L. J. (1988). Pediatric spinal injury in the very young. *Journal of Neurosurgery, 68,* 25.

Shoemaker, B. L., & Ose, M. (1997). Pediatric lap belt injuries: care and prevention. *Orthopedic Nursing, 16,* 15-23.

Speer, K. M. (1999). *Pediatric care planning.* Springhouse, PA: Springhouse Corporation.

Torosian, M. B., Torosian, C. M., & Cogen, P. H. (1995). Cervical spine injuries in children. In R. M. Arensman, M. B. Statten, D. J. Ledbetter, & T. Varsish (Eds.), *Pediatric trauma: Initial care of the injured child* (pp. 19-51). New York: Raven Press.

Vaccaro, A. R., & Pizzutillo, P. D. (1998). Management of pediatric spinal cord injury patients. In A. M. Levine, F. J. Eismont, S. R. Garfin, & J. E. Zigler (Eds.), *Spine trauma* (pp. 544-559). Philadelphia: WB Saunders.

Von Torklus, D., & Gehle, C. (1972). The upper cervical spine. Regional anatomy, pathology and traumatology. In G. T. Verlag (Ed.), *A systematic radiologic atlas and textbook* (pp. 2-91). New York: Grune & Stratton.

Yarkony, G. M., Formal, C. S., & Cawley, M. F. (1997). Spinal cord injury rehabilitation. 1. Assessment and management during acute care. *Archives of Physical Medicine and Rehabilitation, 78,* 48-52.

Yeung, C. K., Godley, M. L., Ho, C. K., Ransley, P. G., Duffy, P. G., Chen, C. N., & Li, A. K. (1995a). Some new insights into bladder function in infancy. *British Journal of Urology, 76*(2), 235-240.

Yeung, C. K., Godley, M. L., Duffy, P. G., & Ransley, P. G. (1995b). Natural filling cystometry in infants and children. *British Journal of Urology, 75*(4), 531-537.

Zejdlik, C. P. (1992). *Management of spinal cord injury.* Sudbury, MA: Jones and Bartlett.

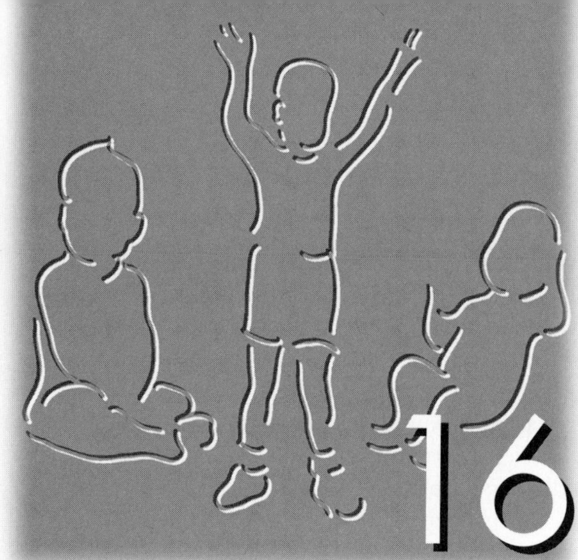

16

Thoracic Injury

Susan Nudelman Kamerling

Thoracic trauma in children results in significant morbidity and mortality. It ranges in severity from minor to immediately life threatening. The most serious thoracic injuries result in death immediately or while the child is in transit to an emergency department (ED). The likelihood for survival is in the favor of those children with thoracic injuries who do reach the hospital.

Thoracic trauma potentially compromises ventilation and perfusion. Therefore thoracic injuries complicate the treatment of patients with multiple trauma, especially those with associated neurologic injuries, and affect both morbidity and mortality. It is critical to have a high index of suspicion for severe multisystem injury for any child who presents with thoracic injury. In addition, the effect of the thoracic injury on other system injuries requires prompt recognition and treatment.

EPIDEMIOLOGY

The National Pediatric Trauma Registry (NPTR) reports the combined data of many U.S. pediatric trauma centers; therefore its representative data provide insight into pediatric trauma in the United States. As of April 1999, there were 85 participating pediatric trauma centers proceeding with Phase III of data entry. The total number of cases recorded in the data bank is 27,036. The 1999 distribution of injury diagnoses categorized by systems is depicted in Figure 16-1 (NPTR, April 1999). Traumatic brain injury leads the group in frequency, morbidity, and mortality. Following head injury, fractures, open wounds, and abrasions/contusions are the most common diagnoses in children sustaining trauma. Although these injuries may occur more frequently in children, the next significant group after central nervous system (CNS) injury in terms of mortality is injuries of the thorax/abdomen. Thoracic injury deaths in children exceed abdominal injury deaths, making thoracic trauma second only to head injury in lethal potential (Cooper, Barlow, DiScala, & String, 1994). This illustrates the absolute necessity for pediatric trauma nurses to be theoretically and technically equipped to care for young victims of thoracic trauma.

The NPTR (April 1999) has provided data specific to thoracic injuries in children by generating a report on patients admitted to participating level I pediatric trauma centers or their equivalents from April 2, 1994, to January 30, 1999. Of the 2058 patients with thoracic injuries included in the report, 60% were male and 75.8% were 5 years of age or older. Of the types of injuries reported, the mechanism was primarily blunt (91.4%) and the circumstances unintentional (87.4%).

Estimates of the true incidence of thoracic trauma in children differ in the literature. It is approximated that, in general, 15% to 20% of injured children will sustain serious chest injuries that require evaluation and treatment (Beaver & Laschinger, 1992). Another study, however, reports a lower incidence of thoracic trauma of less than 5% of pediatric trauma center admissions (Peclet, Newman, Eichelberger, Gotschall, Garcia, & Bowman, 1990).

There is strong consistent evidence that children with thoracic injuries tend to be more severely injured than those without and consequently have a high mortality rate. Because chest injuries are often multiple, the number and type of thoracic injuries obviously affect the mortality rate (Allshouse & Eichelberger, 1993). The overall mortality rate for children with thoracic injury is 26%. The mortality rate sharply increases for children with rib fracture (42%), lung laceration (43%), hemothorax (53%), and injury to the heart and great vessels (75%) (Peclet et al., 1990).

It has been suggested that the associated extrathoracic injury, rather than the chest injury itself, is the primary cause of high mortality. Black, Snyder, Miller, Mann, Copetas, and Ellis (1996) reported that the presence of any extrathoracic injury was associated with a higher mortality (29%) than chest injury alone (4.3%), with head and neck injuries resulting in the highest mortality (72%). Peterson, Tepas,

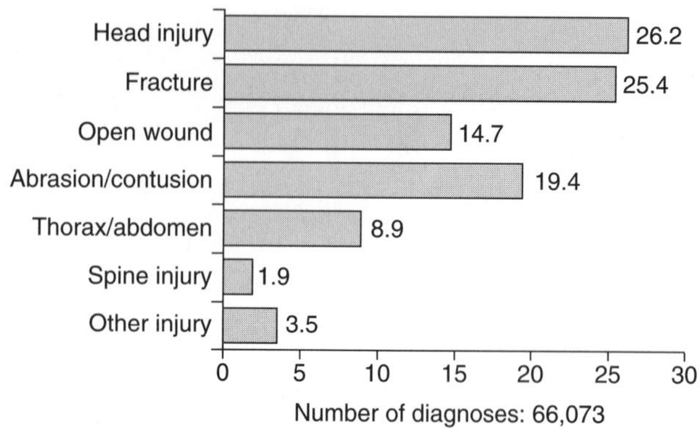

FIGURE 16-1 Injury diagnosis distribution (NTPR-3, April 1999).

Edwards, Kissoon, Pieper, and Ceithaml (1994a) found that 75% of the deaths from blunt thoracic trauma in their series were secondary to neurologic sequelae from CNS trauma. Statistics from the NPTR (May 1999) further support this finding; the primary cause of death in 67.2% of all children registered with thoracic trauma was CNS injury. Although neurologic injury may be the major determinant in predicting outcome, thoracic injuries affect ventilation and oxygenation and therefore greatly contribute to the morbidity of neurologic injuries.

MECHANISM OF INJURY

BLUNT

In children the overwhelming majority of all injuries, including thoracic, result from blunt trauma. Blunt chest trauma is primarily motor vehicle related. The number of children injured as occupants in motor vehicles, as pedestrians, or as bicyclists is overwhelming. In an analysis of adult and pediatric thoracic trauma data conducted by Peterson et al. (1994a), 81% of thoracic injuries in children were blunt trauma injuries. In a comparison of mechanisms of thoracic trauma between pediatric and adult populations, children were found to be more frequently injured as pedestrians (35% vs. 11%) and bicyclists (14% vs. 3%). Of the children injured while riding bicycles, 34% were involved in motor vehicle collisions. Geographic location greatly influences the mechanism of injury in children. For example, pedestrian injuries in children tend to predominate over other motor vehicle–related injuries when looking specifically at intercity areas.

Examination of NPTR data (May 1999) reveals specifics of motor vehicle–related thoracic trauma from a national data bank. In this report, 41.9% of children with thoracic injury were injured in motor vehicles and 19.9% were injured as pedestrians. Additional motor vehicle–related mechanisms in this report include injuries sustained as a result of bicycle (6.9%), all-terrain vehicle/recreational vehicle (2.4%), and motorcycle (1.8%) accidents. Of notable importance is that most of those injured in motor vehicle–related incidents failed to use protective devices. For example, only 33.8% of motor vehicle occupants were restrained, and only 9.2% of bicyclists wore a helmet. This points to the fact that increased emphasis needs to be placed on technological and educational aspects of child passenger safety, helmets, and pedestrian safety. Table 16-1 lists a complete breakdown of mechanism of injury of thoracic trauma in children as determined by the National Pediatric Trauma Registry.

Other reported mechanisms of chest trauma in children include falls and child abuse. Falls are a very common cause of injuries, especially in young children. Fortunately, they usually result in relatively minor injuries and are associated with low mortality and morbidity. This is in sharp contrast to child abuse, which often results in thoracic injury. The presence of thoracic injury in abused children greatly increases mortality (Peclet et al., 1990).

Management of chest injuries secondary to blunt forces is complicated by the reality that multisystem injuries are the rule rather than the exception in children. This is explained by the previously stated point that chest trauma is most commonly the result of high-energy trauma seen in motor vehicle–related accidents. Chest trauma is associated with multisystem injuries in approximately 80% of cases (Allshouse & Eichelberger, 1993). Because of the child's small size and the distribution of forces in blunt trauma, concomitant head, abdominal, and orthopedic injuries are common. Head injury is the most common associated injury, present in 57.7% of the children, followed by fracture or dislocation of the extremities (40.4%) and abdominal injuries (37.5%) (Peclet et al., 1990). Associated intraabdominal injury was similarly found to occur in 38% of children evaluated for thoracic injuries in a study by Rielly, Brandt, Mattox, and Pokorny (1993).

Motor vehicle–related accidents continue to be the primary culprit in pediatric trauma. To look specifically at the impact of motor vehicle–related trauma on thoracic injuries in children, Roux and Fisher (1992) analyzed 100 cases of blunt chest trauma from motor vehicle accidents. This classic study further attests to the extent of multiple injuries in

TABLE 16-1 Breakdown of Mechanism of Thoracic Injury in Children

Mechanism of Thoracic Injury	Incidence
Motor vehicle occupant	41.9%
Motorcycle	1.8%
Bicycle	6.9%
All-terrain/recreational vehicle	2.4%
Pedestrian	19.9%
Fall	5.3%
Beating	4.1%
Sports	3.2%
Gunshot wound	4.6%
Stab wound	3.4%
Other	6.5%

Data from National Pediatric Trauma Registry. (1999, May). *Children with thoracic injuries.* Boston: Tufts University School of Medicine, New England Medical Center.

children who sustain blunt thoracic trauma in motor vehicle–related incidents. Of the 100 children included in the study sample, all but three had serious extrathoracic injuries. Here, as in the studies previously cited, extrathoracic injuries were the major cause of mortality and morbidity and of increased length of hospitalization.

PENETRATING

Penetrating thoracic trauma is uncommon in children. However, when caring for the child with a penetrating thoracic wound to the chest, the trauma team must be prepared to rapidly assess and treat the resultant life-threatening injuries. In the analysis of mechanism of injury in pediatric thoracic trauma, it is important to consider young children and adolescents as separate entities. Although most thoracic injuries in children are the result of blunt trauma, a penetrating mechanism is more likely in the adolescent population. A study analyzing the impact of age on the presentation of thoracic trauma (Peterson et al., 1994a) found that 81% of thoracic injuries in children were blunt trauma in contrast to 42% in adolescents. The cause of the penetrating injury also differed between the two age groups. Whereas the vast majority of penetrating thoracic trauma in the adolescent age group were related to gunshot and stab wounds, younger children incurred penetrating injuries from mechanisms such as impalement, falls through plate glass, or accidents with farm equipment. When younger children sustain gunshot or stab wounds, the injuries are largely unintentional. In a study by Peterson, Tiwary, Kissoon, Tepas, Ceithaml, and Pieper (1994b), more that half of the penetrating thoracic injuries in the study sample were unintentional.

Nance, Sing, Reilly, Templeton, and Schwab (1996) looked specifically at thoracic gunshot wounds in children. Their data further supported the unintentional nature of gunshot wounds in younger children. In their study children younger than age 12 years were much more likely to be injured by unintentional crossfire (35.3%) or by a friend or relative (41.1%).

This is in sharp contrast to children older than 12 years, who most commonly were injured by assault. These statistics attest to the fact that the majority of penetrating thoracic injuries, especially in younger children, are preventable.

In sharp contrast to the multisystem nature of blunt trauma in children, penetrating trauma in children largely involves unisystem management and rarely involves injury to the CNS (Peterson et al., 1994b). In blunt trauma, death is most likely to occur secondary to associated brain injury, whereas death is the direct result of the chest injury in 97% of penetrating thoracic trauma victims (Cooper et al., 1994). This makes it possible to rapidly identify injuries and focus lifesaving resuscitative efforts early in the child's trauma resuscitation.

IATROGENIC

Iatrogenic thoracic trauma is a unique concern in children. Any instrumentation of the intrathoracic organs has the potential to cause injury. It is crucial that individuals treating children truly appreciate the anatomy of the infant or child and adjust assessment, diagnostic, and treatment techniques accordingly.

Properly sized equipment for airway management and appropriate volume/pressures for artificial ventilation prevent airway damage and barotrauma. The same concern of iatrogenic trauma lies with diagnostic tests such as bronchoscopy, esophagoscopy, and cardiac catheterization. Although these invasive tests provide valuable information on selected trauma and nontrauma cases, the possible risks associated with these procedures should be understood by staff and patients/families alike.

ANATOMIC AND PHYSIOLOGIC CONSIDERATIONS

PATHOPHYSIOLOGY

The mechanics of normal respiration are based on intrathoracic pressure changes resulting from coordinated actions of the muscles of respiration (Figure 16-2) (Campbell, 1996). During inspiration, respiratory muscles and diaphragmatic movement result in a decrease in intrapleural pressure, which normally is slightly lower than atmospheric pressure. The chest wall expands, and air enters the tracheobronchial tree into the lungs. The reverse occurs during expiration. The diaphragm and respiratory muscles relax, and air passively exits the lungs.

The primary goal of the respiratory system is ventilation. *Ventilation* is the process of gas exchange whereby oxygen moves from the air into the blood and carbon dioxide moves from the blood to the air (Zander & Hazinski, 1992). The alveolar-capillary bed of the lungs maintains a delicate balance as it allows for the diffusion of gases freely across the membranes. If this gas exchange is abnormal or disrupted in any way, the child becomes hypoxic and hypercarbic. Respiratory distress and respiratory failure will ensue.

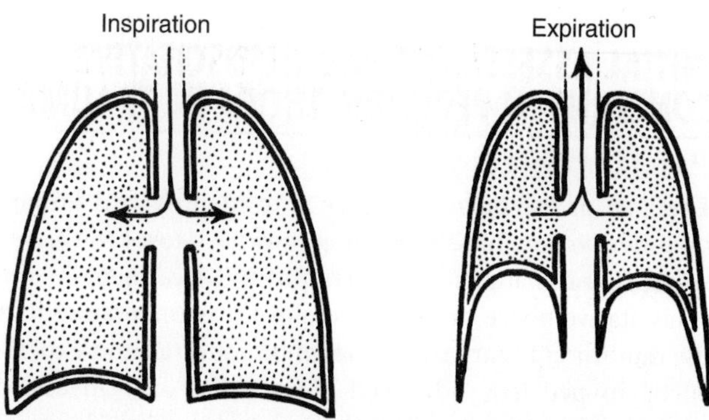

FIGURE 16-2 Normal respiration. (From Campbell, D. B. [1996]. Physiology and management of chest injuries. In J. A. Waldhausen, W. S. Pierce, & D. B. Campbell [Eds.], *Surgery of the chest* [6th ed.]. St. Louis: Mosby.)

The cardiovascular system supplies oxygenated blood to the tissues and carries the byproducts of respiration back to the lungs. Adequate blood volume is necessary to ensure the delivery of oxygen and nutrients to the tissues. Hypovolemia and hypoperfusion in the child result in tissue hypoxia and metabolic acidosis.

Thoracic trauma has a detrimental effect on both ventilation and perfusion. Any injury that affects the components of the respiratory system, including the airways, chest wall, muscles of respiration, and lungs, ultimately influences ventilation. The same holds true for components of the cardiovascular system. Impediments to circulation and perfusion directly interfere with oxygen and substrate delivery. Shock, hypoxia, hypercarbia, and acidosis require rapid identification and reversal during the primary and secondary surveys.

Pediatric Considerations

Children differ greatly from adults anatomically, physiologically, and emotionally. The distinct characteristics of children must be considered for successful management of pediatric thoracic trauma. The child's airway differs significantly from that of the adult. In adults, rib fractures provide a clue to underlying thoracic disease. The child, however, has a compliant chest wall, making rib fractures relatively uncommon. The absence of rib fractures does not preclude the absence of significant intrathoracic trauma. Significant intrathoracic injury may occur without any apparent external evidence of trauma. The child's cartilaginous ribs are unable to provide sufficient protection from blunt forces, and energy from a blunt force is readily transmitted to underlying intrathoracic and intraabdominal structures. On the other hand, if rib fractures are present, one must be suspicious of serious underlying injury.

Another major consideration in the pediatric chest is the mobility of the mediastinum as compared with that of the adult. An advantage of this mobility is that it may contribute to the low incidence of major vessel and airway injury in children. On the other hand, the child's mobile mediastinum may result in respiratory and circulatory collapse after a significant thoracic injury.

INITIAL ASSESSMENT AND RESUSCITATIVE CONCERNS IN PEDIATRIC THORACIC TRAUMA

Primary Survey

The goal of the primary survey is to identify and initiate treatment of any life-threatening injuries. Most life-threatening thoracic injuries requires prompt treatment in the resuscitative phase of care. Therefore it is imperative that the multidisciplinary trauma team be educated and experienced in pediatric advanced life support and advanced trauma life support protocols and techniques. Hypoxia, hypercarbia, and acidosis associated with inadequate ventilation and perfusion ultimately result in increased mortality and morbidity from both thoracic and associated injuries.

Airway

The first priority in the treatment of any trauma patient is the establishment of a stable airway and adequate ventilation. Because of their increased metabolic needs and associated increased oxygen demands, children rapidly decompensate from any compromise to the airway. Airway compromise in pediatric trauma can be caused by obstruction of the airway by edema, foreign material, blood, or vomitus or by depression of breathing resulting from central or mechanical reasons. Assessment of the pediatric trauma patient's airway is continuous and begins from the moment the child is examined. The child's respiratory efforts must be observed to assess the patency of the airway. The oropharynx should be inspected for potential causes of airway obstruction and auscultation performed to detect breath sounds in all lung fields to evaluate air movement.

Children understandably are often fearful of health care providers in the frightening and unfamiliar hospital environment. Therefore one should begin to gain as much clinical information while approaching the child. If the child is conscious, developmentally appropriate interactions help allay the child's fears and establish a rapport. Having a parent or family member at the bedside, if possible, provides further support to the injured child. Many resuscitations are unnecessarily noisy because a hemodynamically stable but terrified child is screaming for reassurance from a loved one. Assessments on a calm child are clearly more accurate and meaningful than those performed on an emotionally distraught one.

Endotracheal intubation of the pediatric airway requires a true appreciation and familiarity of the unique qualities of the child's airway. Immediate control of the airway while maintaining cervical spine immobilization is essential to prevent irreversible neurologic damage associated with hypoxemia. On the rare occasion when endotracheal intubation is unsuccessful, a needle cricothyroidotomy is performed.

Once an endotracheal tube is inserted, its position is evaluated clinically by observing chest excursion and listening for air movement bilaterally. Tube placement is ultimately confirmed by chest radiography. Pulse oximetry and end-tidal carbon dioxide monitoring provide vital continuous information regarding the effectiveness of ventilation, supplemented as needed by arterial blood gas determination.

Breathing

Once the airway is secured, adequate ventilation must be ensured. Supplemental 100% oxygen is always provided immediately upon the patient's arrival until proven unnecessary. The chest wall should be observed for symmetric movement the respiratory effort of the child evaluated, noting the respiratory rate and any signs of distress, such as intercostal or substernal retractions, nasal flaring, or stridor.

Young children are primarily diaphragmatic or abdominal breathers. In the presence of abdominal injury or in the presence of respiratory distress secondary to thoracic trauma, children will switch their breathing pattern and maximize the use of their intercostal muscles. Because these muscles are not well developed in the child, intercostal retractions demonstrate increased work of breathing. If left untreated, the child will fatigue quickly.

Breath sounds should be auscultated, noting the quality and equality of breath sounds in all lung fields. Because breath sounds easily radiate throughout the child's thoracic cavity, sequential respiratory assessments are essential. The position of the trachea is evaluated to provide clues of any mediastinal shifting. Tracheal deviation from excessive mediastinal shifting, as in the case of a tension pneumothorax, can result in rapid respiratory and circulatory collapse.

Aerophagia is a symptom unique to children that potentially compromises breathing. The child's natural response to trauma is crying, which results in swallowing of air or aerophagia. This subsequently results in a distended abdomen and compromises diaphragmatic excursion. Placement of a nasogastric or orogastric tube to decompress the stomach not only establishes the diagnosis but also provides the treatment.

Circulation

Appreciation of the child's ability to compensate in the presence of hypovolemia promotes a proactive approach to the resuscitation of the child. Circulation can be assessed easily by palpating pulses and noting the child's heart rate. The first sign of hypovolemic shock in the pediatric patient is tachycardia. The pediatric nurse needs to be familiar with normal heart rates for children of different ages. It is of equal importance to observe the trend of the heart rate to identify early signs of shock. Other reliable indicators of shock are physical signs, such as cool mottled skin, delayed capillary refill, and altered mental status (Moront & Eichelberger, 1994). It is imperative to identify the early signs of shock by closely monitoring heart rate and capillary refill. Urine output also provides an excellent measurement of the adequacy of tissue perfusion.

A decreased level of consciousness in the absence of head injury and decreased blood pressure demonstrates late signs of shock. A child who is hypotensive has already lost a considerable amount of blood volume and is exhibiting late signs of shock. This is viewed as a medical emergency and treated with aggressive fluid resuscitation.

If a patient is in shock, one of three possible thoracic etiologic factors must be considered: massive hemothorax, cardiac tamponade, or myocardial contusion (Beaver & Laschinger, 1992). Hypovolemia is the most likely cause of the shock and may result from intrathoracic or intraabdominal bleeding. The cardiovascular compromise associated with cardiac tamponade or myocardial contusion may also lead to cardiovascular collapse and therefore must be included in the differential diagnosis of shock for patients with thoracic trauma. If shock persists despite aggressive fluid resuscitation in the absence of an obvious source, cardiac tamponade is considered.

Two large-bore intravenous (IV) lines are inserted as part of the initial resuscitation. This allows rapid fluid resuscitation of crystalloids and colloids and administration of medication. If the infant or young child is in circulatory collapse and IV access is unobtainable, intraosseous line placement is a viable option.

Fluids infused for fluid resuscitation should be warmed in an attempt to keep the child normothermic. Injured infants and children readily lose heat to the environment, making them prone to hypothermia. Hypothermia is a major risk for infants and children and can be extremely detrimental to the resuscitative efforts of the trauma team. Nurses should be cognizant of the child's temperature and institute appropriate interventions to prevent the development of this serious complication.

Secondary Survey

The secondary survey provides a detailed head-to-toe assessment for further diagnosis of injuries while allowing constant reevaluation of the primary survey. When thoracic injuries specifically are looked at, previously undetected injuries are identified and diagnostic tests to support or refute specific injuries are initiated.

Assessment begins with as detailed a history as possible. The specifics of the mechanism of injury provide essential clues of where to place appropriate suspicions for injury. A history of a high-energy impact in cases of thoracic trauma is especially concerning for severe underlying injury.

Complete assessment of the thorax begins with a systematic physical examination of the chest by inspection, percussion, palpation, and auscultation. Complete exposure is necessary for complete visual inspection of the trunk, noting any clues of possible underlying injury, such as bruises, abrasions, lacerations, and penetrating wounds. Physical findings that are highly suggestive for thoracic injury include cyanosis, dyspnea, noisy breathing, tracheal deviation, hoarseness or stridor, subcutaneous emphysema, open or sucking chest wounds, reduced or absent breath sounds, venous engorgement, pulsus paradoxus, hypotension, and abnormal heart sounds (Wesson, 1998). Each of these signs is associated with specific injuries to the pulmonary or cardiovascular system and is regarded seriously.

If the initial resuscitation of a child with significant thoracic injuries is conducted in an adult trauma center that does not have pediatric trauma capabilities, arrangements for transfer to an appropriate facility should be made as soon as possible after the child arrives and is stabilized. Care should continue according to advanced trauma life support guidelines and as clinically indicated while awaiting transport. Ongoing communication, consultation, and collaboration with the receiving pediatric trauma center is indicated to prevent any unnecessary delays in treatment.

Diagnostic Tools

The physical examination is an essential step in the diagnosis of thoracic injuries in children. The clinical evaluation, however, must be supplemented by diagnostic tests. Selected diagnostic tests are routinely done as part of the initial trauma evaluation to support or further refine the diagnoses identified in the primary and secondary surveys (Box 16-1). The first-line diagnostic tests in the evaluation of thoracic

BOX 16-1 Thoracic Trauma Diagnostic Tools

First-Line Diagnostics
Clinical assessment
Chest radiography
Chest computed tomography
Electrocardiogram

Second-Line Diagnostics
Aortogram
Echocardiogram
Bronchoscopy
12-Lead electrocardiogram
Pericardiocentesis

trauma include the chest x-ray film, computed tomography (CT), and electrocardiogram.

Chest X-Ray Film

Because the thoracic cavity houses the primary organs of the pulmonary and cardiovascular systems, the chest x-ray film is considered one of the most important initial diagnostic tests completed on the pediatric trauma patient. A chest radiograph should always be done upon the patient's arrival to the trauma center, even if one was done at the referring hospital (Wesson, 1993).

The chest radiograph provides critical information regarding the patient's airway, breathing, and circulation—the focus of the primary survey. The x-ray film furthermore allows for rapid identification of life-threatening and potentially life-threatening injuries. Injuries are recognized through examination of the rib cage, lungs, cardiac silhouette, and mediastinum. In the evaluation of thoracic trauma, the chest radiograph demonstrates essential clues necessary for specific injury diagnosis. Some significant radiologic signs include hemothorax, pneumothorax, subcutaneous emphysema, rib or other fractures within the thoracic cavity, subcutaneous emphysema, pulmonary contusion, mediastinal shift or widening, and diaphragmatic rupture.

Not only does chest radiography identify potentially life-threatening injuries to the thoracic cavity, it also allows the evaluation of treatment modalities. Consider the child who requires needle decompression and chest thoracostomy as treatment for a pneumothorax. Chest radiography confirms evacuation of air and reexpansion of the affected lung.

Endotracheal tube placement for airway management should be confirmed with a chest radiograph regardless of whether the tube was placed in the field or in the resuscitation bay of the ED. For intubated children transferred from outside hospitals, the chest film is repeated upon the patient's arrival because the endotracheal tube can easily be displaced during transport. Central line and nasogastric tube placement are also readily confirmed by chest radiography.

The chest film as a gross screening tool serves as a springboard for determining supplementary diagnostic tests. For example, if the chest x-ray film is suspicious for widened mediastinum, further diagnostic testing, including chest CT and possibly aortogram, are indicated. Despite the reliance of the trauma team on the patient's chest film, it is important to balance the initial chest films done in the trauma room with the clinical presentation. This is especially true if the patient has a history of significant blunt trauma to the torso. These initial films are often of relatively poorer quality because they are portable films and may contain artifacts from the equipment involved in the resuscitation.

Chest Computed Tomography

If a child sustains a clinically significant blunt trauma to the torso, the supine chest film may be insufficient in revealing the extent of the injury. CT images of the head and abdomen are widely accepted diagnostic tools in the workup of the injured child. Peclet et al. (1990) further recommend the inclusion of several thoracic planes during the CT examination of the abdomen to improve the diagnosis of injury and contribute to the modification of treatment to enhance outcome. Work by Manson, Babyn, Palder, and Bergman (1993) further establishes that CT scanning can demonstrate the true extent of underlying injury in the presence of significant blunt thoracic trauma. In this study, parenchymal abnormalities of the lung were the most common abnormalities detected on CT examination, taking the form of either pulmonary contusions or lacerations. Concomitant abdominal injuries were also frequently seen in the presence of major pulmonary contusions. These injuries occur because the child's compliant rib cage is unable to provide adequate protection against blunt forces. The energy from these blunt forces is readily transmitted to the underlying thoracic organs. Here, CT increases diagnostic sensitivity and provides extremely valuable information upon which therapeutic decisions can be made more accurately.

Electrocardiogram

Continuous monitoring of the child's heart rate and rhythm allows for gross monitoring for arrhythmias that may be associated with thoracic trauma. Any child with chest trauma is at risk for myocardial injury.

One of the greatest concerns with myocardial injury is the development of arrhythmias. When there is considerable risk for potentially life-threatening arrhythmias, a more in-depth evaluation of the cardiac rhythm is warranted. A standard 12-lead electrocardiogram is specifically indicated in patients with anterior chest trauma, sternal fracture, or any arrhythmia, including unexplained tachycardia (Beaver & Laschinger, 1992).

Further diagnostic testing may be necessary to provide objective clinical data integral to proper injury management. Aortography and echocardiography are used to evaluate potential cardiac, aortic, and great vessel injuries. Bronchoscopy, 12-lead electrocardiography, and pericardiocentesis are additional diagnostic tools in the evaluation of specific thoracic injuries.

IMMEDIATELY LIFE-THREATENING THORACIC INJURIES

TENSION PNEUMOTHORAX

A tension pneumothorax occurs when there is a communication between the airways or lung parenchyma and the pleural space that causes air to accumulate in the pleural space. As the air continues to collect in the thoracic cavity, intrathoracic pressure increases, causing collapse of the affected lung, displacement of the mediastinum to the opposite side, and compression of the contralateral lung. Tension pneumothorax may result from a primary injury to the tracheobronchial tree or to the lungs themselves. Iatrogenic causes predominate, however, because tension pneumothorax is most commonly caused by the positive pressure of mechanical ventilation (Beaver & Laschinger, 1992).

Signs and symptoms include severe respiratory distress, decreased chest wall movement, diminished or absent breath sounds on the affected side, deviation of the trachea and mediastinum away from the defect, and distended neck veins. Because of the child's mobile mediastinum and subsequent angulation of the great vessels in the presence of a tension pneumothorax, profound and rapid circulatory compromise results. This is a direct consequence of increased impedance of venous return to the right side of the heart and the resultant decreased cardiac output. Tension pneumothorax should be suspected when an injured child, especially one receiving mechanical ventilation, suddenly deteriorates for no overt reason. If a tension pneumothorax is not treated instantly, death will rapidly ensue as a result of ventilatory and circulatory collapse.

Treatment of a tension pneumothorax necessitates immediate decompression of the pressure to allow for a shifting back of the mediastinum. Radiographic confirmation with x-ray film is not essential before treatment because of the detrimental effects of delaying decompression. A needle decompression in the second intercostal space in the midclavicular line is performed, followed by thoracostomy tube placement in the affected hemithorax.

OPEN PNEUMOTHORAX

A large defect to the chest wall with a direct opening into the thorax causes a sucking chest wound or open pneumothorax. This opening effectively eliminates the differences in intrathoracic and atmospheric pressure, making effective ventilation impossible. The ipsilateral lung collapses, and ventilation to the opposite lung is impaired. Air entering the thoracic cavity through the open chest wound causes shifting of the mediastinum toward the affected side on expiration and back toward the opposite side on inspiration (Figure 16-3). This mediastinal shift carries with it a potential associated disturbance in cardiovascular function.

A child who presents with an open pneumothorax will display signs of significant respiratory distress and mediastinal shift. Air may be heard through the open chest wound. Treatment of an open pneumothorax requires that the wound first be closed to reestablish the integrity of the chest wall. The wound is covered with a sterile occlusive dressing that is large enough to overlap the wound's edges, and the dressing is taped securely on three sides. Taping the occlusive dressing on three sides provides a one-way valve effect that prevents air from entering the thoracic cavity during inspiration while allows air to escape during exhalation (American College of Surgeons [ACS], 1997). Because the underlying pulmonary parenchyma may also be damaged, observation for a tension pneumothorax or simple pneumothorax is indicated. Definitive treatment involves chest tube placement and probable surgical closure of the defect.

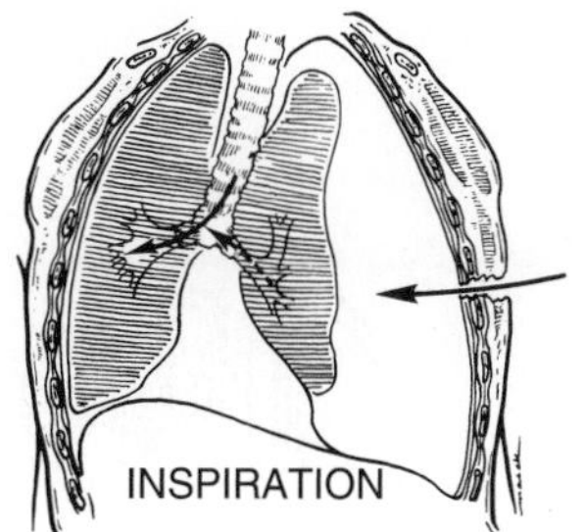

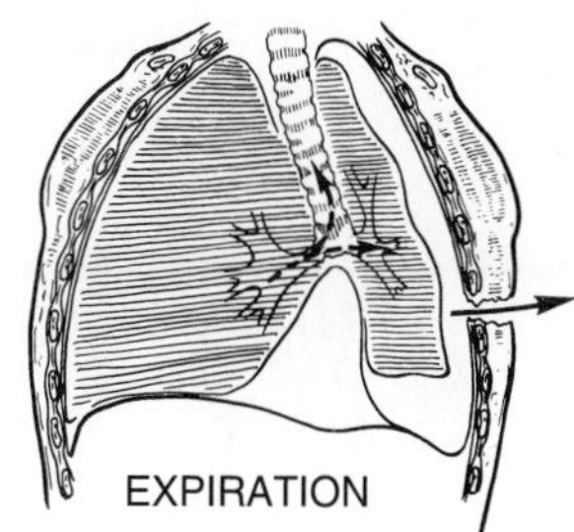

FIGURE 16-3 Open pneumothorax. (Redrawn from Jones, K. W. [1985]. Thoracic trauma. In T. A. Mayer [Ed.], *Emergency management of pediatric trauma.* Philadelphia: WB Saunders.)

FLAIL CHEST

Flail chest occurs when there is a free-floating segment of the rib cage caused by multiple fractures of adjacent ribs. It is rare in children and has been reported in less than 1% of children with thoracic trauma (Peclet et al., 1990). A tremendous amount of force is needed to cause a flail segment, so serious underlying parenchymal injury is to be expected.

A flail chest results in paradoxical respirations from the loss of the integrity of the rib cage, making it unable to support changes in intrathoracic pressure during normal respirations (Figure 16-4). On inspiration the flail segment will retract rather than expand, and on expiration the affected segment will protrude outward instead of retracting. The paradoxical movement decreases tidal volume by preventing full expansion of the lung, which results in ineffective ventilation. This, combined with associated pain, ineffective coughing, and chest wall splinting, obviously negatively affects ventilation, causing marked hypoxia and hypercarbia. The diagnosis may be evident on visualization of paradoxical chest wall movement during inspection accompanied by significant respiratory distress and is easily confirmed by chest x-ray film.

Children with flail chest and no other significant injuries are managed with supportive care consisting of supplemental oxygen, aggressive pain relief, and chest physiotherapy. If the flail chest precipitates significant impairment of gas exchange, intubation is necessary to allow for adequate healing and lung expansion. Ventilatory assistance is maintained until adequate stabilization of the flail segment occurs. Pulmonary contusion is frequently associated with flail

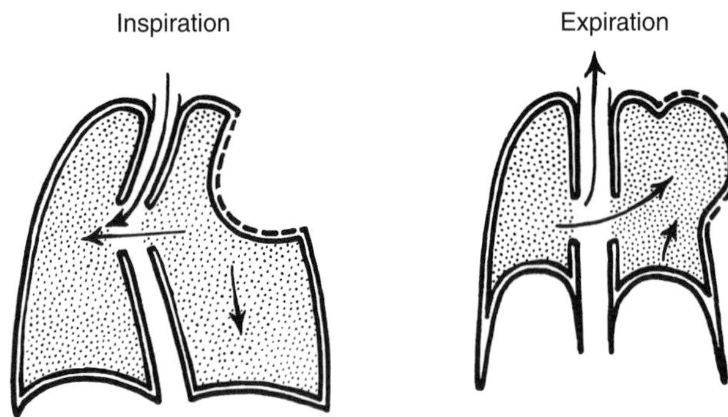

FIGURE 16-4 Paradoxical respirations in flail chest. (From Campbell, D. B. [1996]. Physiology and management of chest injuries. In J. A. Waldhausen, W. S. Pierce, & D. B. Campbell [Eds.], *Surgery of the chest* [6th ed., p. 17]. St. Louis: Mosby.)

chest, and its treatment must be taken into consideration for accurate management.

Massive Hemothorax

Massive hemothorax occurs when a large amount of blood accumulates between the lung parenchyma and the pleural space. A hemothorax of this degree usually signifies major intrathoracic vascular injury with a swift onset of hypovolemic shock. Possible causes of hemothorax include laceration of an intercostal or intermammary artery, the lung, or a mediastinal blood vessel (Wesson, 1993).

As blood accumulates in the thoracic cavity, it creates ventilatory insufficiency and a mediastinal shift, intensifying the cardiovascular compromise from hypovolemia. Breath sounds are decreased or absent on the affected hemithorax, and dullness to percussion is elicited. Compounding the clinical symptomatology is the strong likelihood of concomitant pneumothorax.

Chest tube placement is necessary to evacuate the hemothorax and to prevent a fibrothorax and restrictive lung disease from developing. However, caution is needed when evacuating a massive hemothorax because of the possibility of exsanguination from the chest tube as the tamponading effect of the hemothorax is relieved. Before chest tube placement, it is imperative that large-bore IV access be obtained and that ample warmed, crossmatched blood be readily available. Once circulating blood volume is restored, the hemothorax can be evacuated with a large-bore inferolateral chest tube. In cases of massive hemothorax, autotransfusion allows for safe return of the patient's own blood instead of exposing the patient to the various risks of multiple blood transfusions. In addition, autotransfusion is efficient and avoids depletion of the hospital's blood supply.

Thoracotomy may be indicated for patients who cannot be physiologically stabilized by thoracostomy tube and fluid replacement alone. This is evidenced if any of the following is present: initial drainage exceeds 20% of the estimated blood volume, continued bleeding exceeds 1 to 2 ml/kg/hr, bleeding increases rather than decreases, or the pleural space cannot be drained of blood and clots (Wesson, 1998). ED thoracotomy is reserved for extreme cases when the child cannot be stabilized before transfer to the operating room.

The operating room is alerted immediately upon ED presentation of a patient with hypovolemic shock. This expedites transfer of the patient from the ED to the operating room for definitive surgical treatment in a more controlled environment. The operating room is the most suitable environment for managing this immediately life-threatening injury.

Cardiac Tamponade

Cardiac tamponade occurs when blood accumulates in the pericardial sac and impinges on cardiac activity and function. Because a child has a small pericardial sac, a smaller volume of fluid is tolerated before the child decompensates. As pressure builds up in the pericardial sac, the constricting effect on the heart increases, making it increasingly difficult for the heart to pump. The consequence is decreased diastolic filling and pump failure.

The diagnosis of cardiac tamponade may be challenging because the typically reported diagnostic clinical findings may be absent in children with acute trauma. The signs and symptoms suggestive of cardiac tamponade include the classic findings of narrowed pulse pressure, muffled heart tones, and neck veins that are distended even in the presence of shock (Beaver & Laschinger, 1992). Assessment for distended neck veins, however, may be difficult in a small child who has a short fat neck, and muffled heart tones may be hard to ascertain during a trauma resuscitation. Another classic sign of cardiac tamponade is when pulsus paradoxus, the normal physiologic decrease in systolic blood pressure during inspiration, exceeds 10 mm Hg. This too may be extremely difficult to detect on a child in an emergency setting.

Tension pneumothorax may mimic cardiac tamponade and further confound the diagnosis. Just as in tension pneumothorax, cardiac tamponade may present as persistent hypotension despite maximal fluid resuscitation. However, cardiac tamponade can be distinguished from tension pneumothorax in that the trachea is not displaced and the chest is normal to percussion (Wesson, 1998). Cardiac tamponade must be ruled out in patients with pulseless electrical activity in the absence of hypovolemia and tension pneumothorax.

The definitive diagnosis and the initial resuscitative treatment are made by pericardiocentesis. Prompt evacuation of pericardial blood via pericardiocentesis is indicated for patients who do not respond to initial resuscitative efforts and have the potential for cardiac tamponade (ACS, 1997). Aspiration of this nonclotting blood from the pericardial sac results in prompt clinical improvement of the patient. Once the catheter is inserted, it remains in place in case repeated aspirations are needed before definitive surgical intervention. The ultimate treatment involves prompt operative management to inspect the heart, followed by repair of the causative pericardial, cardiac, or vascular injury.

POTENTIALLY LIFE-THREATENING THORACIC INJURIES

Pneumothorax

Pneumothorax is the result of air in the pleural space, which in turn causes collapse of the affected lung. A ventilation/perfusion mismatch occurs because perfusing blood cannot be oxygenated by the unventilated portion of the lung. The mechanism of injury is usually one of blunt trauma, but a pneumothorax may be the consequence of penetrating trauma to the chest as well. Air leakage within the thoracic cavity may be secondary to a laceration to the lung or may be caused by tears in the tracheobronchial tree, the esophagus, or the chest wall.

The child with a pneumothorax exhibits varying signs of respiratory distress depending on the size of the pneumothorax. On physical examination, breath sounds are decreased on the affected side and hyperresonance is noted on percussion (ACS, 1997). The diagnosis is confirmed with upright chest films. If left untreated, especially in a child receiving positive-pressure ventilation, a simple pneumothorax can progress into an immediately life-threatening tension pneumothorax.

Treatment of a simple pneumothorax usually necessitates placement of a chest tube in the fourth or fifth intercostal space, anterior to the midaxillary line. Only an asymptomatic child with a very small pneumothorax (less than 15%) can be managed conservatively without tube thoracostomy (Moloney-Harmon & Adams, 2001). When a chest tube is required, it is followed up with a chest film to document correct placement and reexpansion of the lung. Once the air leak resolves, the chest tube can be removed. A continued air leak is highly suggestive of a tracheobronchial injury.

Hemothorax

A hemothorax results from bleeding into the pleural space from a direct chest wall or parenchymal injury. What differentiates a small hemothorax from a massive hemothorax is that the bleeding involved is usually self-limiting (Beaver & Laschinger, 1992). This injury, which may be secondary to either blunt or penetrating trauma, causes collapse of the affected lung. On physical examination, this is clinically evidenced by respiratory distress, decreased breath sounds, and dullness to percussion over the affected area. An associated pneumothorax often is present.

The diagnosis is most likely made based on the chest film, and treatment involves tube thoracostomy drainage to evacuate the blood from the pleural cavity. Ongoing blood loss via the chest tube is monitored closely, along with the child's physiologic status, to evaluate the need for blood transfusion or possibly operative intervention. As in massive hemothorax, all blood is evacuated from the chest to prevent future development of a fibrothorax.

Tracheobronchial Injury

An injury to the tracheobronchial tree is a rare but very serious sequela of blunt thoracic trauma. This injury most commonly occurs secondary to high degrees of acceleration and deceleration associated with motor vehicle accidents (Gaebler, Mueller, Schramm, Eckersberger, & Vecsei, 1996). Otherwise, the mechanism of tracheobronchial injury can be divided into internal and external modalities (Vinograd & Udassin, 1993) (Figure 16-5). Internal injuries to the airway are usually iatrogenic in nature, whereby perforations result as a complication from bronchoscopy, intubation, or even application of vigorous suction via a catheter inserted too far into the endotracheal tube in a small infant. A tracheobronchial perforation also may occur from a previously unidentified long-standing foreign body in the airway, such as a disk battery or coin, which eventually erodes through the airway.

External causes of tracheobronchial injury include direct blunt trauma, as seen when a child rides a bike, motor bike, motorcycle, or snowmobile into an unseen wire or cable that strikes the neck. In rare cases, penetrating trauma to the tracheobronchial results from gunshot or stab wounds or even from impalement on a sharp object. Unintentional and intentional strangulation are also causative factors in young children who become entangled in their clothing and in child abuse, respectively.

Central airway ruptures are more common in children than in adults because the child's airways are susceptible to the excessive energy associated with blunt trauma to the chest. Injuries result from the compression, shear forces, traction, or crush forces between the chest and the vertebral column. Bronchial ruptures occur more frequently on the right versus the left, possibly because of the position of the right bronchus in front of the vertebral column; the shorter length of the right bronchus, which impedes energy dispersion; and the potential protection of the left bronchus by the aorta (Gaebler et al., 1996).

In cases of severe airway injuries, death from respiratory failure occurs before the patient reaches the hospital or soon thereafter. The initial symptoms of survivors of tracheobronchial rupture, may be relatively mild, such as persistent atelectasis, conceivably resulting in misdiagnosis or delay in diagnosis. This subsequently affects the timeliness of ultimate treatment of this serious injury. The diagnosis should be considered on the basis of an understanding of the kinematics of the mechanism of injury combined with clinical suspicion. Clinical symptoms, as described by Gaebler et al. (1996), include chest pain, hemoptysis, subcutaneous emphysema, pneumothorax, and pneumomediastinum. In addition to these symptoms, Barmada and Gibbons (1994) reported that dyspnea and cough were experienced almost universally in their series of patients with tracheobronchial injuries sustained from blunt and penetrating chest trauma. One should have an especially high index of suspicion for an tracheobronchial tree injury if chest tube placement does not lead to reexpansion of the lung and the child continues to have a very large air leak.

Subcutaneous emphysema occurs when air from the pleural space enters the tissues of the chest wall. In severe cases the air may extend beyond the chest wall upward into the neck and face and outward into the arms and hands

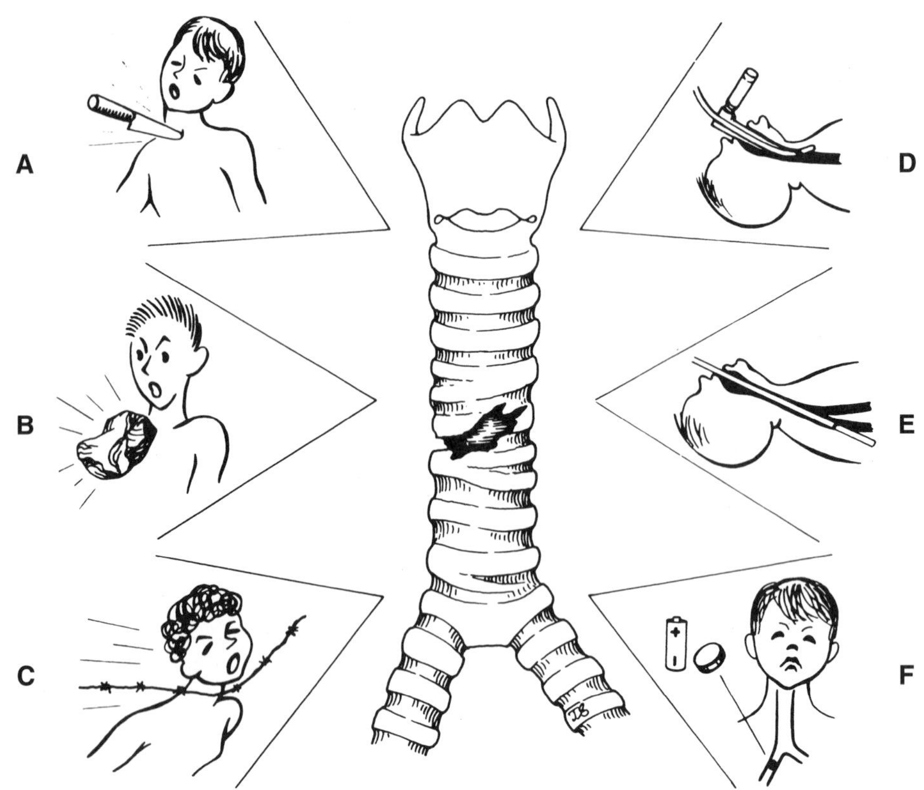

FIGURE 16-5 External (A-C) and internal (D-F) mechanisms of tracheobronchial injury. (From Vinograd, I., & Udassin, R. [1993]. Tracheobronchial injury. In M. R. Eichelberger [Ed.], *Pediatric trauma: prevention, acute care, rehabilitation* [p. 427]. St. Louis: Mosby.)

(Figure 16-6). In cases of tracheal injury, subcutaneous emphysema in the cervical region may be massive, making the child look unrecognizable. As the symptoms progress, stridor, dysphonia, and even aphonia may develop.

The key to successful management includes early diagnosis with plain radiographs of the chest and neck and CT of the chest. The child will likely display radiographic signs of thoracic trauma, including rib fractures, soft tissue air, pneumothorax, or pneumomediastinum. Although all of these signs are suggestive of underlying thoracic injury, they are not in themselves definitive for airway injury. A radiographic indication specific to a main bronchus transection is a dropped lung, where the affected collapsed lung actually drops down onto the diaphragm after loss of suspension from the upper tracheobronchial tree (Vinograd & Udassin, 1993). Bronchoscopy, preferably done in the operating room, confirms the diagnosis and determines the precise location and extent of the defect.

Early control of the airway, followed by prompt surgical management, optimizes recovery. Depending on the extent of anatomic distortion, tracheal intubation may not be possible, thus necessitating cricothyroidotomy or surgical tracheostomy placement for airway management. Flexible bronchoscopy is another option to facilitate endotracheal intubation distal to the injury.

Surgical intervention for bronchial injuries requires bronchial resection and anastomosis (Beaver & Laschinger, 1992). Tracheostomy may be indicated in cases of significant tracheobronchial injury until adequate healing takes place. The surgical approach may require lobectomy or even pneumectomy if massive lung parenchymal damage is present (Gaebler et al., 1996). Bronchoscopy and bronchial lavage are indicated during the early postoperative period to prevent complications such as obstruction and stenosis. Long-term follow-up includes further assessment for tracheal stenosis caused by scar formation.

Nonoperative management may be considered in select patients who have small lacerations in the membranous trachea or partial bronchial tears (Figure 16-7). These children are hemodynamically stable, reach full lung expansion with thoracostomy placement, and have only a transient air leak. These injuries may heal spontaneously with the supportive care involved in conservative treatment. Patients remain intubated and supported until the acute inflammation and edema are resolved. Close follow-up is necessary to detect any early complications or late stricture formation.

Children who are managed nonoperatively or who have small bronchial injuries that are not acutely diagnosed and heal spontaneously are at risk for complications. These children may present 1 to 2 months after sustaining their injury with recurrent pneumonia or atelectasis in the involved lung caused by a bronchial stricture (Wesson, 1993). Bronchial strictures can be mechanically dilated in some cases, but surgical repair is typically indicated.

Pulmonary Contusion

Pulmonary contusion is the most commonly seen pulmonary injury in children. It results from the direct applica-

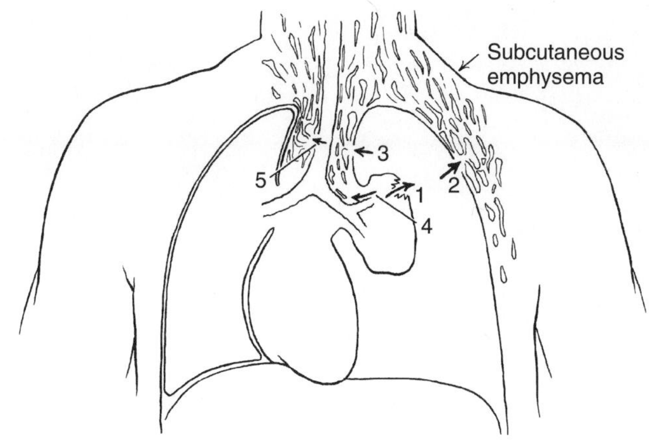

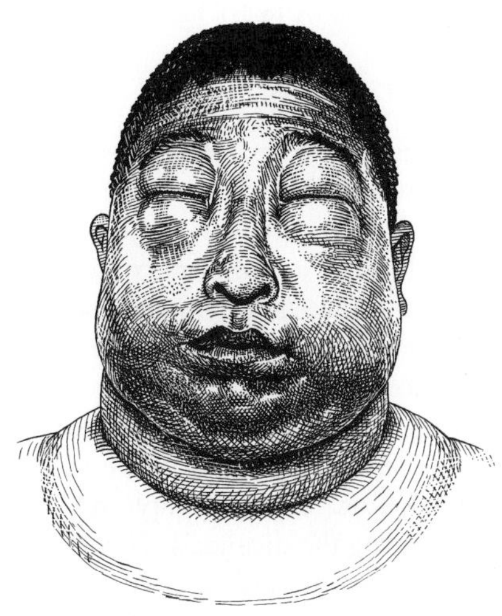

FIGURE 16-6 Subcutaneous emphysema. (From Campbell, D. B. [1996]. Physiology and management of chest injuries. In J. A. Waldhausen, W. S. Pierce, & D. B. Campbell [Eds.], *Surgery of the chest* [6th ed., p. 9]. St. Louis: Mosby.)

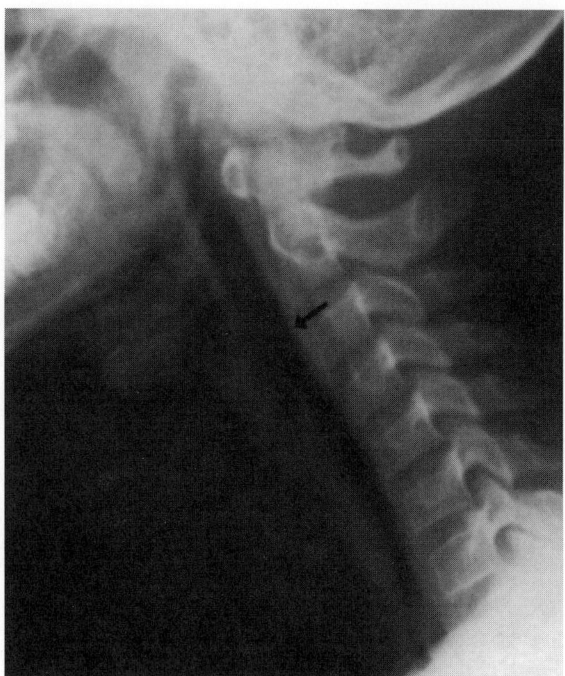

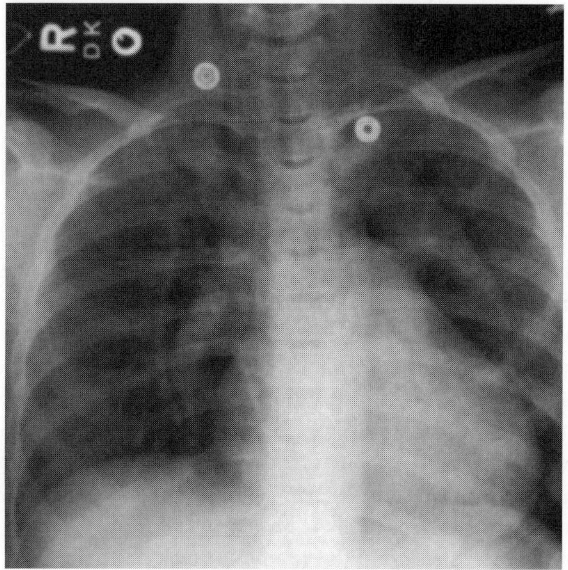

FIGURE 16-7 X-ray films depicting tracheal dissection and subcutaneous emphysema. (From Handler, S. D., & Meyer, C. M. [1998]. *Atlas of ear, nose, and throat disorders in children* [p. 144]. Philadelphia: BC Deeker.)

tion of force to the lung, which causes disruption of parenchyma, bleeding, and edema (Wesson, 1993). Because of the plasticity of the child's ribs, blunt forces are readily relayed to the underlying lung parenchyma, resulting in significant pulmonary contusion, often without any external signs of trauma. The hemorrhage and edema that result from the parenchymal injury disrupt alveolar-capillary integrity and therefore result in intrapulmonary shunting. This injury to the lung parenchyma negatively affects lung compliance, making ventilation increasingly difficult. Signs and symptoms vary depending on the extent of the injury, ranging from mild respiratory distress to tachypnea, dyspnea, hemoptysis, and fulminant respiratory failure.

Diagnosis of pulmonary contusion may be delayed if chest radiographs alone are relied on for diagnosis. Pulmonary contusion commonly occurs in the absence of rib fractures and may not be evident on initial radiographs of the chest (Moront & Eichelberger, 1994). This may result in underestimation of the severity of the underlying injury. As the contusion develops over time, fluffy infiltrates will be apparent on subsequent chest radiographs (Figure 16-8). Pulmonary contusion on chest x-ray film appears as air space consolidation that can be irregular and patchy, homogeneous, diffuse, or extensive (ACS, 1997).

CT scanning is much more sensitive in diagnosing pulmonary contusion (Figure 16-9). Parenchymal abnormalities of the lung were the most common abnormalities detected on CT examination in a study by Manson et al. (1993). CT scanning is very useful in evaluating the actual extent of the contusion, thereby providing valuable information for subsequent management of the injury.

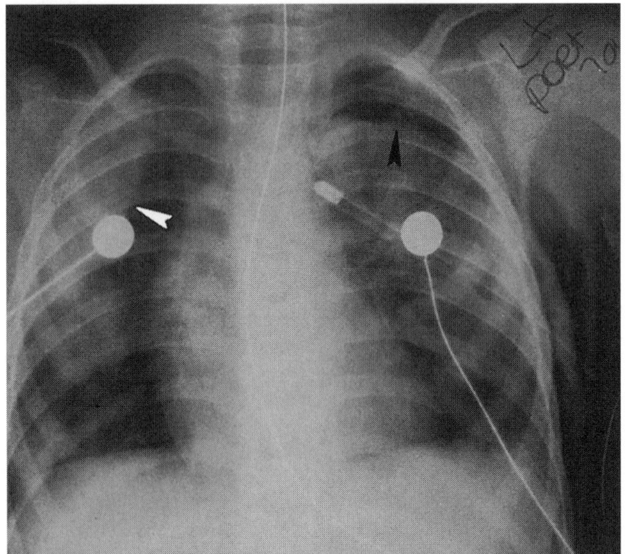

FIGURE 16-8 Progressing pulmonary contusion (*white arrow*) and pneumothorax persisting (*black arrow*) despite a chest tube. (From Othersen, H. B., Jr. [1990]. Cardiothoracic injuries. In R. J. Touloukian [Ed.], *Pediatric trauma.* St. Louis: Mosby.)

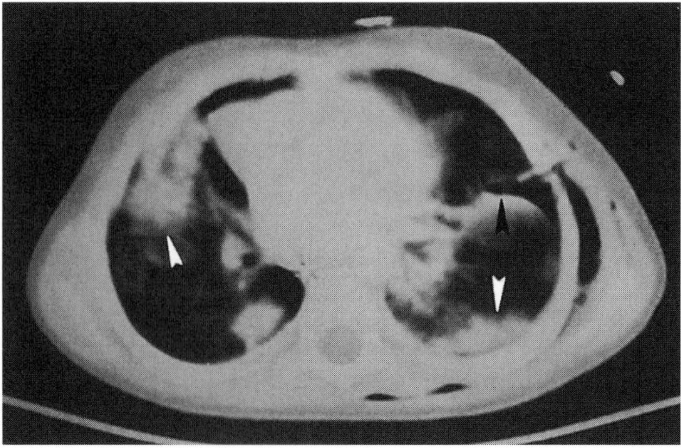

FIGURE 16-9 Computed tomographic view of the chest with contusion (*white arrows*) and pneumothorax (*black arrow*). (From Othersen, H. B., Jr. [1990]. Cardiothoracic injuries. In R. J. Touloukian [Ed.], *Pediatric trauma.* St. Louis: Mosby.)

Management of pulmonary contusion depends on the severity of the symptoms experienced by the child. Management can be complicated by associated thoracic injuries, such as rib fractures, hemothorax, pneumothorax, hemopneumothorax, and posttraumatic effusion, which rarely exist in the absence of pulmonary contusion (Roux & Fisher, 1992). Evaluation of oxygenation is essential and is accomplished by frequent respiratory assessments, pulse oximetry, and (if indicated) arterial blood gas determination. Treatment may be limited to supplemental oxygen and supportive care if the contusion is mild. In more severe cases, endotracheal intubation and mechanical ventilation with positive end-expiratory pressure (PEEP) are required. Close fluid management incorporating the judicial use of diuretics is important to combat pulmonary edema. Early mobilization, vigorous chest physiotherapy, and clearance of secretions are essential to expedite recovery and prevent, or at least minimize, respiratory complications.

Myocardial Contusion

Myocardial contusion is a cardiac muscle injury caused by forces significant to interrupt blood flow to areas of the heart and/or directly destroy myocardial cells. This injury is quite common in adolescent and adult drivers and results primarily from driver impact with the steering wheel during motor vehicle accidents. A study by Bromberg, Mazziotti, Canter, Spray, Strauss, and Foglia (1996) reports that nonpenetrating cardiac trauma in children is likely to be the consequence of a motor vehicle accident, although in this scenario the child is more likely to be a pedestrian or unrestrained passenger. Regardless of mechanism, any child with significant blunt trauma to the thorax is at risk for myocardial contusion. This is because the child's chest is capable of notable anteroposterior deformation during impact, which allows for compression of the heart between the sternum and spine (Allshouse & Eichelberger, 1993). Cardiac contusion is not uncommon in pediatric trauma patients, especially if the child has a pulmonary contusion or rib fracture(s). However, the clinical significance of this injury appears to be much less severe in children than in adults (Stafford & Harmon, 1993).

The child with a myocardial contusion may complain of chest pain, but because the pain may be easily attributed to associated thoracic injuries, this symptom does not necessarily aid in narrowing the diagnosis. There is no definitive, specific diagnostic test for cardiac contusion, although the tests proposed include electrocardiography, echocardiography, myocardial enzyme determinations, and radionuclide scans (Wesson, 1998). Because the most concerning consequence of a myocardial contusion is cardiac arrhythmias, the most logical initial diagnostic test for myocardial contusion is the electrocardiogram. The diagnosis is made by conduction abnormalities identified on electrocardiogram, such as tachycardia, premature ventricular contractions, or other arrhythmias. If the 12-lead electrocardiogram is normal, typically, no further testing is indicated. If an arrhythmia is present, creatine phosphokinase MB level is measured and may support the diagnosis if the level elevated. However, coexisting soft tissue and muscle trauma may result in elevated enzyme levels, making the specificity of this test somewhat unreliable.

Echocardiography is the most useful diagnostic tool in the identification of clinically significant cardiac contusion. It evaluates cardiac wall motion and intracardiac anatomy to identify any anatomic and physiologic abnormalities. Transthoracic echocardiography may not always be possible because of limited access to the chest in the patient with multiple traumas. Transesophageal echocardiography (TEE) provides a viable, although more technically complex, alternative; however, it frequently requires intubation and cannot be performed in patients with cervical spine or severe facial injuries (Prêtre & Chilcott, 1997).

A child with cardiac contusion requires close telemetric monitoring and cardiovascular assessment for clinical evaluation of cardiac output. Children typically tolerate myocardial contusion well, as evidenced by the series reported by Bromberg et al. (1996) in which all conduction abnormalities and arrhythmias resolved without medical intervention. Arrhythmias that compromise cardiac output must be treated promptly with antiarrhythmics and/or inotropic agents as needed. Serious sequelae of myocardial contusion are rare in children and are related to infarction, delayed rupture, rupture of papillary muscles or ventricular septum, and valvular dysfunction (Allshouse & Eichelberger, 1993).

Aorta and Great Vessel Injury

Injuries to the aorta and great vessels are usually the result of immense decelerating blunt forces, but they may result from penetrating trauma as well. Traumatic aorta rupture is a common cause of immediate death after a high-speed motor vehicle accident or fall from a great height. It occurs more frequently in adults, being responsible for approximately 10% of traumatic deaths, presumably because children cannot be injured by a steering wheel of a motor vehicle and because children's aortas are more resilient (Wesson, 1998). The most likely location for an aortic tear is at the site of the ligamentum arteriosum of the aorta. Patients quickly succumb from exsanguination if the aortic laceration represents a complete transection. Patients who survive aortic rupture are likely to have an incomplete laceration to the intimal lining. The adventitia of the aorta is believed to be much more resistant to rupture than the intima and media. The resistant adventitia contains the hematoma or pseudoaneurysm after traumatic aortic rupture. This in turn limits the amount of blood lost into the mediastinum and allows the 15% to 20% of patients who survive the injury to make it to the hospital (Trachiotis, Sell, Pearson, Martin, & Midgley, 1996). For patients who do not exsanguinate immediately, imminent rupture is unlikely to occur. This allows for a more controlled resuscitation, full diagnostic assessment, and prioritization of treatment to the aortic and concomitant injuries. It is of utmost importance not to mistakenly focus on a suspected aortic injury because hemorrhagic shock in a patient who reaches the ED is most often caused by bleeding from injuries to the abdomen, pelvis, or arms and legs, not aortic injuries (Prêtre & Chilcott, 1997).

A child with an aortic or great vessel injury may not display specific clinical signs and symptoms. The characteristics of acute coarctation syndrome (i.e., upper limb hypertension, pressure differences between upper and lower extremities, and loud murmur over the precordium or back) are uncommon in children (Wesson, 1993). The mechanism of injury and chest radiography provide the most pronounced clues to possible aortic injury. A history of massive decelerating, crush or compression forces to the chest, and radiographic signs on chest radiography or chest CT should clearly raise suspicion for a potential aortic injury.

The most notable radiographic signs of an aortic injury are a widened mediastinum and an abnormal aortic contour. A clearly abnormal chest film or a high clinical suspicion of an aortic injury requires a prompt aortogram (Stafford & Harmon, 1993). If the initial chest x-ray film is not definitive or is suggestive of an aortic injury and the child is hemodynamically stable, a chest CT scan can further delineate the presence of a mediastinal hematoma and subsequent need for aortogram. If any suggestion of an aortic injury is present on these initial radiographic studies, angiography has traditionally been considered the gold standard to make a definitive diagnosis. Angiography specifically identifies the precise location and extent of injuries to the aorta and the other great vessels of the chest and thereby provides direction for surgical repair of such injuries.

The diagnostic role of TEE in traumatic aortic rupture has been explored. Tobias, Rasmussen, and Yaster (1996) describe the potential benefits of TEE in their series of children with traumatic aortic rupture. Their experience suggests that the combination of chest CT and TEE versus aortography allows a more rapid diagnosis, thereby decreasing the time to definitive operative repair. Furthermore, TEE offers other advantages, including rapidity; avoidance of femoral artery puncture; lack of reliance on interventional radiology support; utilization of cardiologists with expertise in the evaluation of cardiac and great vessel anatomy; and the ability to be performed in the ED, intensive care unit, or operating room. Pearson, Karr, Trachiotis, Midgley, Eichelberger, and Martin (1997) also examined the role of TEE in aortic and cardiac trauma in children. Although the sample in their study was small, it too supports the use of TEE in the diagnosis of aortic trauma in children. Their results suggest that CT and TEE have similar diagnostic accuracy in identifying aortic trauma, especially with use of helical CT. However, TEE has the additional advantage of providing information on intracardiac structures and function and on blood flow patterns in the aortic lumen. As the role of TEE continues to expand, it ultimately may displace aortography in the diagnostic evaluation of potential aortic injuries.

A child will ultimately die from an untreated injury to the aorta, which will eventually rupture, causing exsanguination. Prompt operative management is necessary to restore distal perfusion to avoid lower extremity neurologic or vascular compromise and spinal myelopathy. Surgical intervention consists of either direct suture repair of the aorta or resection of the damaged area, followed by direct anastomosis or grafting.

Blunt and penetrating injuries to the chest can result in injuries to the other major vessels of the chest. These injuries are managed surgically via thoracotomy or median sternotomy. For aortic arch branch vessel injuries, contused arteries are explored closely because the outer arterial layers may appear to be nearly normal externally, despite clot and disruption present within (Roberts, Holder, & Ashcraft, 1995). Surgical repair of the majority of great vessel injuries involves resection and reanastomosis if possible.

Penetrating Cardiac Injury

Penetrating trauma to the thorax is rare in children, but as the frequency of penetrating trauma in children, especially adolescents, continues to increase, one can anticipate a concomitant increase in penetrating cardiac injuries. Any penetrating injury in the proximity of the mediastinum or that traverses the mediastinum carries with it the risk of injury to the heart. Stab wounds are limited to the tract of the instrument, making the differential diagnosis relatively simple. Gunshot wounds, on the other hand, have an unpredictable injury pattern, dissipate greater energy into the chest cavity, and are more likely to be multiple in number. This may explain differences in initial mortality between stab and gunshot wounds to the heart. The higher mortality of gunshot wounds within the first hour after wounding is attributed to the higher incidence of multiple and complex anatomic wounds of the heart, the greater incidence of associated potentially life-threatening injuries, the worse physiologic condition of patients with gunshot wounds on arrival, and the higher incidence of exsanguination and asystole (Buckman et al., 1993).

Because of the high mortality rate in the initial period of injury, it is imperative that patients with penetrating cardiac wounds expeditiously reach the nearest trauma center. Prehospital providers minimize scene time by practicing a traditional "scoop and run" technique to maximize survival. Attempts of stabilization at the scene are likely to be unsuccessful and are essentially detrimental because they prolong the critical time to definitive treatment.

Once the patient arrives in the ED, care is provided according to advanced cardiac life support guidelines. The diagnosis is made based on the clinical examination and chest radiography. Metallic markers placed on the wound(s) before radiography allow for identification of the trajectory of a gunshot wound to the torso.

The major concerns with penetrating cardiac injuries are cardiac tamponade and massive hemothorax with resultant exsanguination. The likelihood of survival is relative to the severity of cardiovascular derangement caused by blood loss or tamponade. Survival is much more likely for patients with cardiac wounds whose clinical deterioration is related to tamponade, a physiologically reversible event, as compared with patients whose demise is related to exsanguination (Nance et al., 1996). Tamponade is the primary cause of cardiovascular compromise in the vast majority of patients with stab wounds, whereas exsanguination is more likely among gunshot victims (Buckman et al., 1993).

Treatment is complicated, especially in gunshot wounds, by any associated injuries. Associated spinal cord, abdominal, pulmonary, tracheobronchial, vascular, or esophageal injuries may be present and must be searched for with vigilance. Finally, there is a risk of retained foreign bodies, such as bullets or pellets, in penetrating trauma and the secondary injury they may cause (Roberts et al., 1995). The potential hazards of removing such objects may far outweigh the benefits, making surgical intervention quite dangerous. Migration of the foreign bodies, infection, and other complications are obvious concerns.

In all cases of penetrating thoracic trauma, staff anticipate the potential need for massive infusion of warmed fluids and blood, tube thoracostomy, thoracotomy, pericardiocentesis, and rapid transport to the operating room. Prompt surgical repair of a penetrating injury to the heart is necessary for the ultimate survival of the child and requires the availability of bypass.

Diaphragmatic Injury

A diaphragmatic rupture occurs when there is a tear to the diaphragm and subsequent displacement of the abdominal contents into the thoracic cavity. This injury is most commonly caused by significant blunt forces to the lower chest or upper abdomen, as seen in motor vehicle accidents. The left side of the diaphragm is most likely to be affected after blunt trauma because the liver provides protection and support to the right hemidiaphragm. In high-energy incidents, herniation of the diaphragm can occur immediately. This is in contrast to penetrating injuries to the diaphragm, which may be small and initially unrecognized. These injuries often take time, even years, to develop into diaphragmatic hernias.

The child with a diaphragmatic disruption may be asymptomatic or present with a scaphoid abdomen and respiratory distress. The signs and symptoms are directly related to the amount of intraabdominal contents displaced into the thoracic cavity and the associated injuries. On physical examination, abdominal tenderness and decreased breath sounds on the same side of the defect will likely be noted. Bowel sounds may be auscultated in the chest on the affected side. Bowel sounds from the abdomen, however, normally may radiate through the child's thin chest wall, making this sign unreliable. Compromise of the lung may become bilateral and cardiorespiratory compromise severe if the mediastinum is deviated in response to displacement of the intraabdominal contents within the chest cavity (Reynolds, 1995). If the initial tear is small, symptoms may present gradually over time as the abdominal contents slowly enter the chest secondary to the negative intrathoracic pressure involved in normal inspiration.

A chest radiograph will establish the diagnosis if the herniation is significant. A nasogastric or orogastric tube should be placed before the radiograph is obtained so that displacement of the tube can be evaluated. Obviously, a nasogastric tube curled up in the lower chest or loops of bowel seen within the chest cavity confirm the diagnosis (Figure 16-10). In some cases the injury to the diaphragm may be missed if the chest x-ray film is misinterpreted as showing an "elevated left diaphragm," "acute gastric dilation," "a loculated pneumohemothorax," or a "subpulmonary hematoma" (Beaver & Laschinger, 1992). These radiographic abnormalities, at the very least, should arouse suspicion for diaphragmatic disruption. In these cases a gastrointestinal contrast study would establish the proper diagnosis. If the child is falsely believed to have a pneumothorax, placement of a chest tube could perforate the stomach or bowel and further complicate the management of the injury.

Treatment of a diaphragmatic tear involves definitive surgical management to reestablish the integrity of the diaphragm as soon as stabilization permits. Laparotomy

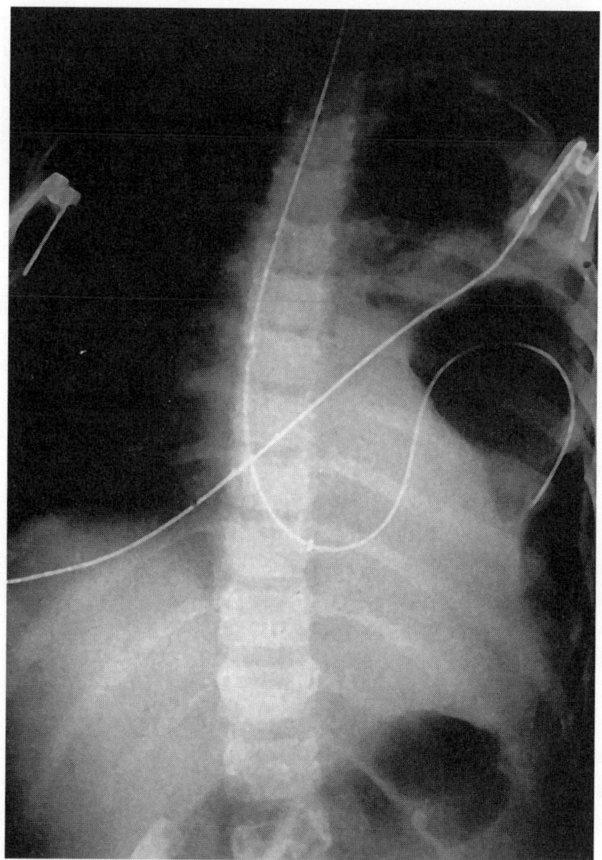

FIGURE 16-10 X-ray film demonstrating diaphragmatic hernia. (From Curley, M. A. Q., & Moloney-Harmon, P. A. [Eds.]. [2001]. *Critical care nursing of infants and children* [p. 963]. Philadelphia: WB Saunders.)

allows for repair of the diaphragm and complete evaluation for any abdominal organ injuries. In penetrating injury, close examination of the diaphragm is indicated to avoid missing even a small tear, which will enlarge over time and ultimately allow herniation of the abdominal contents into the chest.

Esophageal Injury

Injury to the esophagus is children is uncommon, primarily because the esophagus is relatively protected within the mediastinum. Esophageal injuries resulting from blunt trauma are usually the result of rapid deceleration from blunt forces to the upper abdomen. The forceful ejection of gastric contents into the esophagus produces a linear tear, usually in the lower esophagus, which is less supported. Penetrating injuries to the esophagus in children tend to be almost exclusively from iatrogenic causes rather than gunshot or stab wounds. Esophageal perforation may occur from passage of nasogastric tubes, suction catheters, or endoscopic instrumentation. Other causes of esophageal perforation include ingestion of foreign bodies and caustic agents, as well as anastomotic strictures secondary to the repair of congenital defects (Reynolds, 1995).

The signs and symptoms of esophageal perforation are directly related to the spillage of gastric contents and oral secretions into the mediastinum. The diagnosis of esophageal rupture is considered in a child who has a left pneumothorax or hemothorax without rib fracture, has a history of a severe blow to the lower sternum or epigastrium and is in pain or shock out of proportion to the overt injury, or has particulate matter in the chest tube after the blood begins to clear (ACS, 1997). Air leaking into the neck and mediastinum may be detected as subcutaneous emphysema on examination and/or be notable on chest radiography. Fever and dyspnea are additional clinical symptoms. The diagnosis is typically confirmed by contrast studies, which demonstrate extravasation of contrast material. Esophagoscopy is valuable to evaluate the injury in cases of caustic ingestion and may be worthwhile in other selected cases.

Management depends on the extent and location of the injury, the clinical presentation of the child, and the presence of associated injuries. Very small perforations in the neck and chest may be treated successfully through medical management involving the cessation of all oral intake, administration of broad-spectrum antibiotics, nasogastric suction, and possible chest tube insertion (Reynolds, 1995). Direct surgical repair of the injury and drainage of the pleural space and mediastinum are likely in most instances of esophageal injury. Efforts are made to perform a primary repair if possible. However, esophageal diversion with delayed surgical repair or even a colonic interposition may be necessary in more involved situations. In all cases of esophageal injury, fastidious attention must be paid to nutritional support and interventions to combat infection and sepsis.

CHEST WALL INJURIES

Rib Fractures

Rib fractures are relatively uncommon in children compared with adults because of the elasticity of the ribs in children. Still, the incidence of rib fractures in children with thoracic trauma is 32% (Peclet et al., 1990). Unlike in the adult, an extreme amount of force and chest deformation is required to fracture a child's ribs. Therefore the presence of rib fractures should alert staff to be highly suspicious of significant underlying thoracic and abdominal injuries.

Rib fractures result primarily from blunt trauma associated with motor vehicle–related injuries. Rib fractures in young children, especially if they are at various stages of healing, may signify intentional injury. It is crucial to examine whether the reported mechanism of injury explains the clinical presentation of the child. If the history is vague or seems relatively benign in the presence of rib fractures, child abuse is considered, followed by a complete medical workup and evaluation by social services. A radionuclide bone scan detects new and old fractures and is quite useful in cases of suspected child abuse.

The level of fracture may give insight to the underlying pathologic condition. First rib fractures demonstrate a high severity of trauma and were shown by Harris and Soper (1990) to be associated with a high incidence of thoracic, vascular, abdominal, and CNS injuries in children. Roughly two thirds of the children in this sample sustained an associated clavicle fracture, rib fracture, and/or pneumothorax. In addition, one third of the study population sustained a serious vascular injury. The patients diagnosed with proximal vascular injury exhibited distal signs of pulse deficit on the affected side and/or blood pressure discordance between upper extremities.

Injuries relative to the level of fracture are described further in the literature (Moloney-Harmon & Adams, 2001) and follow a logical pattern of injury according to the anatomic location of the fracture. The upper four ribs lie within the shoulder girdle, which provides a degree of protection. If any of these upper ribs are fractured, bronchial, tracheal, or great vessel injuries should be suspected. The middle ribs, ribs four through nine, commonly penetrate lung tissue and therefore put the child at risk for pneumothorax or hemothorax. Fracture to the bottom three ribs may result in liver, spleen, or kidney trauma.

In a classic study of rib fractures in children (Garcia, Gotschall, Eichelberger, & Bowman, 1990), rib fractures were found to be a marker of severity of injury as characterized by measures of physiologic derangement, anatomic injury, and mortality. The severity of injury and the probability of multisystem injury and mortality increase dramatically for patients with multiple rib fractures. The mortality rate for children in this series with both rib fractures and head injury was 71%. In contrast to the aforementioned citations, this study reported that it is the absolute number rather than the location or level of the fractured ribs that predicts severity of injury and mortality. Despite the fact that several children with fractures to the first or second ribs were included in the study, no significant thoracic vascular injuries were reported.

Regardless of the location of rib fractures, any child with a rib fracture is approached with a high index of suspicion for other significant associated injuries. The clinical presentation consists of some level of respiratory distress, depending on the severity of the thoracic injury, chest pain, and point tenderness or crepitus elicited on palpation. Aggressive pain management is necessary to optimize respiratory function and to minimize complications associated with immobility and poor respiratory effort. With adequate rest, analgesia, supplemental oxygen, and good pulmonary toilet, children recover well and have complete healing, usually within 6 weeks.

OTHER INJURIES TO THE CHEST

Traumatic Asphyxia

Traumatic asphyxia is an entity essentially unique to children because of the compliance of the child's chest wall and the absence of valves in the superior and inferior vena cavae. This injury is seen in cases of sudden severe compression to the chest and upper abdomen from a crushing force, for example, when a child is run over or pinned under a motor vehicle. In anticipation of the event, the child takes a deep breath, tenses the thoracoabdominal muscles, and closes the glottis. This increases the pressure in the thoracic cavity. Intrathoracic pressure increases exponentially when it is combined with severe compression to the chest, and this pressure is transmitted directly through the valveless superior and inferior vena cavae. Subsequently, the force is transmitted into the head and neck with ensuing disruption of superficial capillaries.

The physical presentation of the child is quite dramatic and consists of characteristic subconjunctival and petechial upper body cutaneous hemorrhages, cyanosis, and facial edema. The visible effects are limited to the areas above the impact; the skin below is normal. This is accompanied by variable degrees of pulmonary and CNS dysfunction.

Management of traumatic asphyxia involves the identification and subsequent treatment of associated injuries. Coexisting injuries may include great vessel injury, retinal hemorrhages, cardiac contusion, pneumothorax, rib fractures, pulmonary contusion, and brain injury. Close assessment for any respiratory insufficiency is mandatory to provide supplementary oxygen and mechanical ventilation if indicated.

If brain injury and increased intracranial pressure are present, they are treated accordingly. Fortunately, the skull is believed to provide some counterpressure, providing protection to the brain. Neurologic sequelae are believed to be related to the degree of hypoxemia rather than cerebral hemorrhage (Allshouse & Eichelberger, 1993). Although the child may be disoriented on initial presentation, neurologic outcome tends to be good.

MANAGEMENT OF THORACIC INJURIES

Although children differ greatly from adults anatomically and physiologically, the basic principles of thoracic trauma management are fundamentally the same for both groups. At least 85% of chest injuries can be definitively managed by pediatric advanced life support and advanced trauma life support techniques (Beaver & Laschinger, 1992). After the initial resuscitative phase of care, continued supportive and symptomatic care to ensure adequate oxygenation and treatment of affiliated injuries are key to successful management. Often, the only interventions required are supplemental oxygen, tube thoracostomy, analgesia, and good pulmonary toilet.

Because of the potential life-threatening nature of thoracic injuries and the child's superb ability to compensate for hypovolemia, the trauma team maintains an aggressive approach to the child with thoracic trauma. Vigilant clinical assessments are critical, and team members need to have an appropriate index of suspicion for a possible impending need for tube thoracostomy placement, thoracotomy, and operative management.

Tube Thoracostomy

The majority of life-threatening thoracic injuries require an appropriately placed chest tube or needle decompression to correct pleural space issues and thereby restore the integrity of the cardiothoracic system. Most children with thoracic injury require only tube thoracostomy and supportive cardiopulmonary care. In a series of children hospitalized for treatment of thoracic trauma, 78% were treated with observation or tube thoracostomy alone (Rielly et al., 1993).

Gunshot wounds to the thorax most commonly result in hemothorax, pneumothorax, and associated pulmonary injuries (Nance et al., 1996). The majority of hemothoraces and pneumothoraces can be managed by tube thoracostomy alone if the patient otherwise does not demonstrate clinical indications for urgent thoracotomy or laparotomy.

Placement of chest tubes depends on the clinical issue being addressed. In general, tubes placed to evacuate fluid are placed in a posterior and dependent location, and tubes placed to relieve a pneumothorax are inserted in an apical location (Campbell, 1996). The surgeon placing the chest tube needs to consider pediatric developmental and growth concerns to prevent future complications such as scoliosis and breast development problems. Once air and/or fluid is evacuated from the pleural space, the lung reexpands, which promotes return of pulmonary and cardiovascular stability in the patient. A chest tube is connected to underwater seal and may be discontinued once the air leak and/or bleeding resolves.

Thoracotomy

Thoracotomy is a heroic measure in thoracic trauma management. A resuscitative thoracotomy is performed to accomplish lifesaving therapeutic interventions. The surgical maneuvers consist of evacuation of pericardial blood in cases of cardiac tamponade, direct control of exsanguinating intrathoracic hemorrhage, open cardiac massage, and cross-clamping of the descending aorta to slow blood loss below the diaphragm and increase perfusion to the brain and heart (ACS, 1997).

Younger patients tend to undergo thoracic surgical procedures more frequently than older patients. Peterson et al. (1994a) found that there was no significant difference in the rate of thoracotomy among the blunt thoracic injuries in any of the age groups studied (i.e., child, adolescent, adult, elderly). However, when penetrating chest trauma was examined in isolation, the number of children undergoing thoracotomy was found to be significantly higher than in any of the other three age groups.

It is important to remember that the principles of ED thoracotomy do not differ between pediatric and adult populations. For patients who present to the ED in cardiac arrest after blunt trauma, the success of ED thoracotomy is negligible. Children whose injuries are severe enough to cause loss of vital signs after blunt trauma most likely have complex and irreparable injuries from which survival is not possible. Therefore it is recommended that ED thoracotomy not be performed on children with blunt trauma who sustain cardiopulmonary arrest at the scene of the injury and in whom cardiopulmonary resuscitation (CPR) does not result in return of cardiac function (Sheikh & Culbertson, 1993). The child should receive an aggressive resuscitation based on advanced trauma life support guidelines, but thoracotomy need not be performed.

With penetrating trauma, however, ED thoracotomy is performed in selected cases. It is generally believed that ED thoracotomy may offer a good outcome in the penetrating trauma patient who deteriorates while in the ED. Another case in point is if the patient's down time is reasonably low and adequate CPR and ventilation have been provided at the scene and on transport. If scene and transport times are short, the patient can receive definitive interventions more quickly, which improves the chances for survival. In these cases rapid treatment of hypovolemia is attempted along with open cardiac massage. Neurologic function in pediatric patients with penetrating thoracic trauma may be essentially normal unless the patient sustained hypoxic CNS damage after severe hemorrhagic shock.

Theoretically, ED thoracotomy in penetrating trauma is generally supported; however, reevaluation of this radical intervention is most likely indicated based on recent studies. Evidence supports that asystole and exsanguination caused by a cardiac gunshot wound carry such a low probability of survival that resuscitative thoracotomy should be withheld (Buckman et al., 1993). In another series studying thoracic gunshot wounds (Nance et al., 1996), all patients in whom ED thoracotomy was performed died as a result of their injuries. All patients in this subset presented pulseless and without detectable blood pressure, and all but one had evidence of cardiac electrical activity at initial presentation. More research clearly is indicated to evaluate the benefit of thoracotomy in patients who present to the ED without vital signs after they sustain a penetrating chest injury. Elimination of unnecessary ED thoracotomy clearly has financial ramifications but, more important, may have a long-lasting emotional impact on family members, who may be left to struggle with this extreme invasive intervention.

The decision to proceed with thoracotomy is made by the trauma chief in collaboration with surgical and emergency medical personnel, and the decision is based on objective facts rather than emotion. The ED staff should be familiar with individual team member responsibilities and equipment needs anticipated during an ED thoracotomy. A quick and coordinated team response is essential to optimize outcome and avoid unnecessary delays in treatment.

Operative Management

A patient who presents to the ED with cardiovascular instability after significant chest trauma may require expeditious operative management. ED thoracotomy may be indicated for imminently life-threatening injuries, but definitive surgical treatment ideally should take place in the operating room. Operative management of thoracic injuries is not limited to the chest cavity and often includes operative management of abdominal injuries. Immediate notification and close communication with the operating room personnel are critical to expedite the definitive treatment of the pediatric trauma patient in extremis. The operating room provides a more controlled environment in which to provide surgical interventions and maximizes the hospital's resources to optimize the patient's outcome.

Operative management may be required for children who sustain thoracic trauma regardless of the mechanism of injury. In a series studying blunt and penetrating thoracic trauma in children (Rielly et al., 1993), 22% required thoracotomy for resuscitation or repair of intrathoracic injuries and 32% of children admitted for treatment of thoracic trauma had injuries that required exploratory laparotomy secondary to associated abdominal injuries. Children with penetrating injuries to the thoracic cavity are even more likely to require operative intervention compared with adults, as evidenced by multiple studies. In a large series of both pediatric and adult thoracic trauma patients (Peterson et al., 1994a), 40% of children with penetrating thoracic trauma underwent a thoracic operation compared with 18% of adults in the same series. Peterson et al. (1994b) determined that more than half of the children with penetrating thoracic trauma in their study required operative intervention. Nance et al. (1996) reported similar findings; more than half of the children in this series required surgical interventions, which included sternotomy or thoracotomy, exploratory laparotomy, and orthopedic procedures.

The higher operative rate found in children who are victims of penetrating thoracic trauma probably reflects differences in mechanism of injury, chest wall anatomy, and intrathoracic size because the principles determining the need for surgical intervention are similar in all age groups. Vital organs in children occupy a proportionately larger space in the thorax, providing an easier target for the penetrating missile or weapon. Any patient with a penetrating injury below the nipple line and above the inguinal ligaments potentially has an injury to the thoracic and abdominal organs. A gunshot wound that penetrates the peritoneal cavity must be explored with laparotomy because of the unpredictable course of destruction.

Some specific injuries within the child's thoracic cavity require operative intervention independent of the patient's physiologic stability on initial presentation. These injuries include major airway lacerations, aortic injuries, structural cardiac and pericardial injuries, and esophageal perforations (Wesson, 1998). The key to proper management lies in accurate diagnosis and timely operative intervention.

COMPLICATIONS

Children are generally healthy before they sustain their trauma, making complications less common and less severe in children than in adults. The overwhelming majority of deaths from thoracic trauma in children occur early during hospitalization as a direct result of injury, not from complications. Most deaths result from associated head injury or hemorrhage rather than respiratory failure, sepsis, or multisystem organ failure as seen in adults (Wesson, 1993). Complications, however, are obviously a serious morbidity risk after thoracic trauma. Shock, sepsis, and impaired immune response can lead to serious pulmonary complications and development of acute respiratory distress syndrome or multisystem failure (Campbell, 1996). Proactive nursing interventions are aimed at prevention, early diagnosis, and prompt treatment of complications. Early mobilization, coughing, and deep breathing exercises combined with aggressive pain management, infection surveillance, and nutritional support promote healing and prevent respiratory complications during the recovery period. Astute nursing assessments are absolutely essential for early detection of complications and the evaluation of the various treatment modalities used.

PNEUMONIA

A child is at risk for developing pneumonia when he or she sustains a thoracic injury, especially when the injury renders the child immobile and mechanical ventilation is used. Clinical symptoms include fever, gastrointestinal symptoms, and respiratory symptoms (e.g., cough, tachypnea, or respiratory distress). Nursing assessments include monitoring for these signs as well as other signs of respiratory infection, such as an increased white blood cell count and changes in the quality and quantity of respiratory secretions. Sputum is sent for culture and Gram stain to isolate the causative pathogens. Chest x-ray film determines the location and extent of infection within the lung itself.

Antibiotics are necessary to effectively treat pneumonia. Broad-spectrum antibiotics are administered initially until specific sensitivities are determined. Treatment also involves close assessment and management of the child's hydration status. Fever and increased respiratory rate associated with pneumonia increase insensible water loss in the child, and the water must be replaced to prevent dehydration.

ASPIRATION PNEUMONIA

When a child is injured, all health care providers should consider the high likelihood that the victim has a full stomach. This, combined with the additional probability that the child has swallowed a lot of air, puts the child at great risk for aspiration. Children who sustain head or abdominal trauma have a high incidence of vomiting after they sustain their injuries. If the child requires an artificial airway and/or has a decreased level of consciousness, the child is rendered incapable of protecting his or her airway from secretions and vomitus. The threat of aspiration then increases substantially because vomitus can readily enter the lungs and cause a significant chemical pneumonitis.

Precautions are taken during the resuscitative phase of care in patients who have a decreased level of consciousness and/or are receiving positive-pressure ventilation. Placement of a nasogastric or orogastric tube during the resuscitative phase of care decompresses the stomach and thereby greatly minimizes the risk of aspiration. Cuffed endotracheal tubes should be used when appropriate and cricoid pressure applied if possible during intubation. If the child vomits during the resuscitation, the child is rolled on his or her side while cervical spine immobilization is maintained and the oropharynx is promptly suctioned.

Unfortunately, aspiration of vomitus and secretions may occur at the scene before any professional intervention. If a child presents with a history of vomiting at the scene and an inability to adequately protect his or her airway, one should have an especially high index of suspicion for subsequent development of aspiration pneumonia.

Signs and symptoms are basically indistinguishable from those of pneumonia, as addressed earlier. The most effective treatment for aspiration pneumonia is prevention through stomach decompression and close monitoring of feeding tolerance in patients receiving enteral nutrition. Once aspiration pneumonia has occurred, treatment consists of supportive care, which includes supplemental oxygen and ventilation as determined by the patient's ventilatory needs.

Atelectasis

Atelectasis is a common complication in patients with thoracic trauma and results from hypoventilation. Pain associated with thoracic injuries combined with decreased mobility makes it difficult for injured children to cough effectively. Furthermore, splinting of the chest and abdominal walls inhibits the child from taking deep breaths.

The child with atelectasis tends to take frequent shallow breaths and has decreased breath sounds over the involved hemithorax. Chest radiography provides objective confirmation of atelectasis. Again, prevention is the key to managing atelectasis after pediatric thoracic trauma. Nursing interventions are aimed at pain management and exceptional pulmonary toilet. Patients should be out of bed as soon as possible after their injuries unless associated injuries preclude their ability to do so. Frequent use of the incentive spirometer also aids in the prevention of atelectasis. If atelectasis occurs, aggressive pulmonary toilet is that much more important. Standard supportive respiratory therapy is used in treating the child with atelectasis. Use of mechanical ventilation with PEEP may be required in severe cases that significantly compromise oxygenation.

Acute Respiratory Distress Syndrome

Acute respiratory distress syndrome (ARDS) is an extremely serious respiratory complication that affects the alveolar-capillary unit, ultimately resulting in acute respiratory failure. Precipitating factors in the development of ARDS include systemic hypotension and/or severe direct lung injury. ARDS may also develop as a result of multisystem organ failure. The manifestations of ARDS include the clinical signs of tachypnea, dyspnea, and hypoxemia with radiographic evidence of diffuse alveolar infiltrates, decreased functional residual capacity, and increased extraparenchymal lung water in the setting of normal cardiovascular function (Tobias et al., 1996). The lung is noncompliant, and because the insult is at the level of the alveolar-capillary unit, a ventilation/perfusion mismatch becomes increasingly evident. If the arterial hypoxemia is not reversed, tissue perfusion will be grossly insufficient and death will ultimately occur.

Management of ARDS requires treatment of associated causative factors; supportive care; and a carefully calculated balance of supplemental oxygen, mechanical ventilation, and PEEP. PEEP is beneficial because it allows for reexpansion of collapsed alveoli and an increase in functional residual capacity. This delicate balance in turn maximizes oxygenation by using the lowest possible oxygen concentration in an effort to avoid oxygen toxicity and barotrauma.

SUMMARY

Thoracic trauma is the second leading cause of trauma death in children. Fortunately, the vast majority of thoracic injuries are fairly easy to diagnose and treat with conservative medical management. Even the most severe thoracic injuries can be managed successfully with a coordinated trauma team approach that includes astute nursing assessments and interventions. Quality management of thoracic injuries in children includes anticipation and careful scrutiny for multiorgan system injury.

A great deal of time and effort is involved in training emergency medical personnel, nurses, physicians, and other health care providers to care for injured children. The most effective training emphasizes the importance of injury prevention in children. The data of injuries in children repeatedly point to the fact that increased prevention efforts are needed. In looking specifically at pediatric thoracic injuries, continued coordinated efforts are especially needed to improve and enforce child passenger safety, pedestrian safety, and violence control. Only then will there be a substantial decrease in the incidence and severity of thoracic trauma in children.

BIBLIOGRAPHY

Allshouse, M. J., & Eichelberger, M. R. (1993). Patterns of thoracic injury. In M. R. Eichelberger (Ed.), *Pediatric trauma: prevention, acute care, rehabilitation* (pp. 437-448). St. Louis: Mosby.

American College of Surgeons. (1997). *Advanced trauma life support instructor manual.* Chicago: American College of Surgeons.

Barmada, H., & Gibbons, J. R. (1994). Tracheobronchial injury in blunt and penetrating chest trauma. *Chest, 106*, 74-78.

Beaver, B. L., & Laschinger, J. C. (1992). Pediatric thoracic trauma. *Seminars in Thoracic and Cardiovascular Surgery, 4*(3), 255-262.

Black, T. L., Snyder, C. L., Miller, J. P., Mann, C. M., Copetas, A. C., & Ellis, D. G. (1996). Significance of chest trauma in children. *Southern Medical Journal, 89*(5), 494-496.

Bromberg, B. I., Mazziotti, M. V., Canter, C. E., Spray, T. L., Strauss, A. W., & Foglia, R. P. (1996). Recognition and management of nonpenetrating cardiac trauma in children. *Journal of Pediatrics, 128*(4), 536-541.

Buckman, R. F., Badellino, M. M., Mauro, L. H., Asensio, J. A., Caputo, C., Gass, J., & Grosh, J. D. (1993). Penetrating cardiac wounds: Prospective study of factors influencing initial resuscitation. *Journal of Trauma, 34*(5), 717-727.

Campbell, D. B. (1996). Physiology and management of chest injuries. In J. A. Waldhausen, W. S. Pierce, & D. B. Campbell (Eds.), *Surgery of the chest* (6th ed., pp. 3-29). St. Louis: Mosby.

Cooper, A., Barlow, B., DiScala, C., & String, D. (1994). Mortality and truncal injury: The pediatric perspective. *Journal of Pediatric Surgery, 29*(1), 33-38.

Gaebler, C., Mueller, M., Schramm, W., Eckersberger, F., & Vecsei, V. (1996). Tracheobronchial ruptures in children. *American Journal of Emergency Medicine, 14*(3), 279-284.

Garcia, V. F., Gotschall, C. S., Eichelberger, M. R., & Bowman, L. M. (1990). Rib fractures in children: A marker of severe trauma. *Journal of Trauma, 30*(6), 695-700.

Harris, G. J., & Soper, R. T. (1990). Pediatric first rib fractures. *Journal of Trauma, 30*(3), 343-345.

Manson, D., Babyn, P. S., Palder, S., & Bergman, K. (1993). CT of blunt chest trauma in children. *Pediatric Radiology, 23*(1), 1-5.

Moloney-Harmon, P. A., & Adams, P. (2001). Trauma. In M. A. Q. Curley & P. A. Moloney-Harmon (Eds.), *Critical care nursing of infants and children* (2nd ed., pp. 947-980). Philadelphia: WB Saunders.

Moront, M. L., & Eichelberger, M. R. (1994). Advances in the treatment of pediatric trauma. *Current Opinion in General Surgery*, 41-49.

Nance, M. L., Sing, R. F., Reilly, P. M., Templeton, J. M., & Schwab, C. W. (1996). Thoracic gunshot wounds in children under 17 years of age. *Journal of Pediatric Surgery, 31*(7), 931-935.

National Pediatric Trauma Registry. (April 1999). *Biannual report.* Tufts University School of Medicine, New England Medical Center.

National Pediatric Trauma Registry. (1999, May). *Children with thoracic injuries.* Boston: Tufts University School of Medicine, New England Medical Center.

Pearson, G. D., Karr, S. S., Trachiotis, G. D., Midgley, F. M., Eichelberger, M. R., & Martin, G. R. (1997). A retrospective review of the role of transesophageal echocardiography in aortic and cardiac trauma in a level I pediatric trauma center. *Journal of the American Society of Echocardiography, 10*(9), 946-955.

Peclet, M. H., Newman, K. D., Eichelberger, M. R., Gotschall, C. S., Garcia, V. F., & Bowman, L. M. (1990). Thoracic trauma in children: an indicator of increased mortality. *Journal of Pediatric Surgery, 25*(9), 961-966.

Peterson, R. J., Tepas, J. J., Edwards, F. H., Kissoon, N., Pieper, P., & Ceithaml, E. L. (1994a). Pediatric and adult thoracic trauma: Age-related impact on presentation and outcome. *Annals of Thoracic Surgery, 58*(1), 14-18.

Peterson, R. J., Tiwary, A. D., Kissoon, N., Tepas, J. J., Ceithaml, E. L., & Pieper, P. (1994b). Pediatric penetrating thoracic trauma: A five-year experience. *Pediatric Emergency Care, 10*(3), 129-131.

Prêtre, R., & Chilcott, M. (1997). Blunt trauma to the heart and great vessels. *New England Journal of Medicine, 336*(9), 626-632.

Reynolds, M. (1995). Pulmonary, esophageal, and diaphragmatic injuries. In W. L. Buntain (Ed.), *Management of pediatric trauma* (pp. 238-247). Philadelphia: WB Saunders.

Rielly, J. P., Brandt, M. L., Mattox, K. L., & Pokorny, W. J. (1993). Thoracic trauma in children. *Journal of Trauma, 34*(3), 329-331.

Roberts, S. R., Holder, T. M., & Ashcraft, K. W. (1995). Cardiac and major thoracic vascular injuries. In W. L. Buntain (Ed.), *Management of pediatric trauma* (pp. 248-264). Philadelphia: WB Saunders.

Roux, P., & Fisher, R. M. (1992). Chest injuries in children: An analysis of 100 cases of blunt chest trauma from motor vehicle accidents. *Journal of Pediatric Surgery, 27*(5), 551-555.

Sheikh, A. A., & Culbertson, C. B. (1993). Emergency department thoracotomy in children: Rationale for selective application. *Journal of Trauma, 34*(3), 323-328.

Stafford, P. W., & Harmon, C. W. (1993). Thoracic trauma in children. *Current Opinion in Pediatrics, 5*(3), 325-332.

Tobias, J. D., Rasmussen, G. E., & Yaster, M. (1996). Multiple trauma in the pediatric patient. In M. C. Rogers & D. G. Nichols (Eds.), *Textbook of pediatric intensive care* (pp. 1467-1503). Baltimore: Williams & Wilkins.

Trachiotis, G. D., Sell, J. E., Pearson, G. D., Martin, G. R., & Midgley, F. M. (1996). Traumatic thoracic aortic rupture in the pediatric patient. *Annals of Thoracic Surgery, 62*, 724-732.

Vinograd, I., & Udassin, R. (1993). Tracheobronchial injury. In M. R. Eichelberger (Ed.), *Pediatric trauma: prevention, acute care, rehabilitation* (pp. 426-433). St. Louis: Mosby.

Wesson, D. E. (1993). Trauma of the chest in children. *Chest Surgery Clinics of North America, 3*(3), 423-441.

Wesson, D. E. (1998). Thoracic injuries. In J. A. O'Neill, Jr., M. I. Rowe, J. L. Grosfeld, E. W. Fonkalsrud, & A. G. Coran (Eds.), *Pediatric surgery* (5th ed., pp. 245-260). St. Louis: Mosby.

Zander, J., & Hazinski, M. F. (1992). Pulmonary disorders. In M. F. Hazinski (Ed.), *Nursing care of the critically ill child* (pp. 395-497). St. Louis: Mosby.

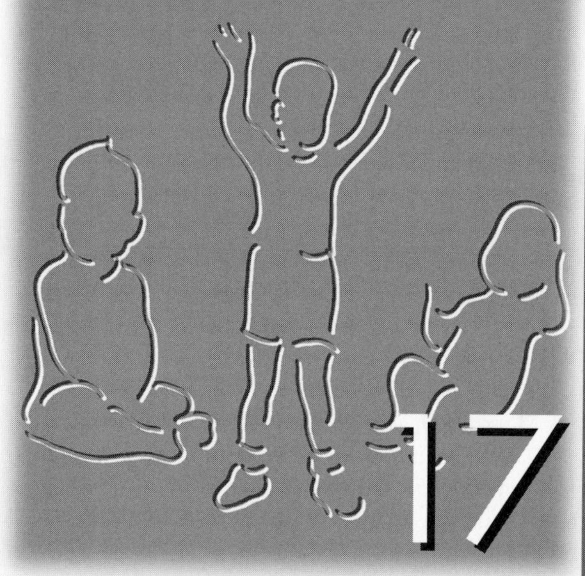

17 ABDOMINAL/ GENITOURINARY INJURY

Shari Simone

Trauma is the leading cause of morbidity and mortality in children. Most of these injuries result from blunt trauma rather than penetrating injuries, which occur more commonly in adults. Common mechanisms of injury from blunt trauma in children are motor vehicle accidents while the child is a passenger, pedestrian, or bicyclist; falls from windows or buildings; contact sports; and child abuse. These types of incidents often result in multisystem injuries. When a child sustains abdominal and head trauma, the mortality rate is markedly increased (Polhgeers & Ruddy, 1995; Rothrock, Green, & Morgan, 2000a). Although abdominal trauma is often not obvious, the health care team should maintain a high index of suspicion because of the potential morbidity of unrecognized injuries (Furnival, Woodward, & Shunck, 1996; Stylianos, 1998). Nurses play a critical role in the assessment and management of children with abdominal trauma.

This chapter describes in detail specific abdominal and genitourinary injuries in children. Particular emphasis is placed on assessment and management strategies of these injuries and the unique characteristics in children.

EPIDEMIOLOGY

Abdominal trauma is the third leading cause of traumatic death after head and thoracic injuries and the most common cause of unrecognized fatal injury in children (Cantor & Learning, 1998; Stylianos, 1998). Abdominal trauma in children results from blunt causes in 85% of cases, and penetrating trauma accounts for the remaining 15% (Cantor & Learning, 1998; Marx, 1994). Of children who present for other injuries, 9% die as a result of associated abdominal trauma (Cooper, Barlow, DiScala, & String, 1994; Gilbert & Bailey, 1998; Stylianos, 1998).

The mechanism of injury directs attention toward certain organ involvement and should raise the level of suspicion regarding certain injuries. Blunt trauma from motor vehicle accidents causes more than 50% of the abdominal injuries in children and is the most common fatal mechanism of injury (Pieper, 1994; Schafermeyer, 1993; Stylianos, 1998). Pedestrian–motor vehicle accidents commonly result in a phenomenon called *Waddell's triad* (Figure 17-1) (Haley, 1998). This phenomenon occurs in young children when they are struck as they dart into traffic. The crash results in a midshaft femur fracture, abdominal injury, and head injury. The injury occurs primarily to the left side of the body and often results in splenic injuries. However, there is some information that questions the occurrence of Waddell's triad (Orsborn, Haley, Hammond, & Falcone, 1999).

"Lap belt injury" occurs in approximately 10% of restrained children involved in motor vehicle accidents (Polhgeers & Ruddy, 1995). Trauma involving a shoulder-lap belt causes rib and lumbar spine injuries and duodenal and jejunal perforations, whereas injuries involving a lap belt alone produce contusion or perforation of the intestine or mesentery (Newman et al., 1990; Osberg & DiScala, 1992).

Head trauma is the predominant injury sustained in bicycle crashes; however, abdominal injury can occur if the child is hit by the handlebars or if the child falls to the ground. The effects of bicycle injuries may go unrecognized. In general, the mean elapsed time to onset of symptoms of abdominal trauma is almost 24 hours (Polhgeers & Ruddy, 1995; Rothrock et al., 2000a). Handlebar injuries represent a serious cause of hospitalization of children, with the mean length of stay exceeding 3 weeks (Polhgeers & Ruddy, 1995).

Sports-related injuries are another common cause of abdominal trauma. Sports-related injuries are primarily

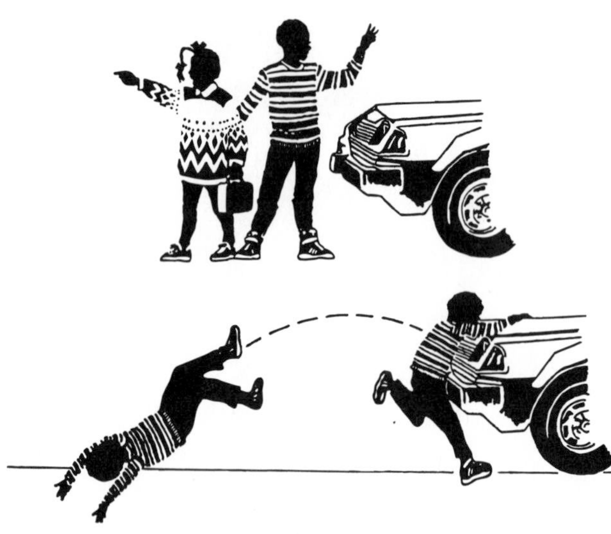

FIGURE 17-1 Injuries resulting from collision with a motor vehicle, referred to as the *Waddell triad.* (From Hazinski, M. F. [1992]. *Nursing care of the critically ill child.* St. Louis: Mosby.)

associated with isolated organ injury, such as a direct blow to the abdomen. Organs at particular risk include the spleen, liver, kidney, and intestinal tract.

Falls rarely cause isolated serious abdominal injuries unless there is a direct blow to the abdomen. Falls from higher than 15 feet usually cause injuries to other body systems, typically head injuries, long-bone fractures, and chest wall trauma (Colucciello, 1993; Haller, 1996).

Significant abdominal trauma occurs in only about 5% of child abuse cases, but it represents the second most common cause of death after head injury (Cantor & Learning, 1998; Gilbert & Bailey, 1998). Punching or kicking the abdomen commonly inflicts blunt abdominal trauma. The child may present with persistent bilious vomiting (indicating abdominal obstruction), abdominal pain, and hypovolemic shock. However, the diagnosis is often unrecognized because of delay in seeking treatment, lack of external signs of trauma, and the hidden nature of the visit. A high index of suspicion should be raised if the history does not coincide with the results of examination.

There are three types of blunt abdominal injuries (Barkin & Marx, 1999). Crush injuries occur when direct energy causes compression of abdominal organs against the posterior ribs and spine, resulting in contusions, lacerations, or disruptions. Shear injuries occur when acceleration and deceleration forces cause the body to stop abruptly but there is continued movement of internal organs. This can result in tearing of viscera and vascular pedicles at fixed structures. Burst injury of hollow viscera results after sudden and pronounced increased abdominal pressure (i.e., by seat belt).

In children younger than 13 years, penetrating injuries are likely to be caused by accidental impalement on objects or accidental discharge of a weapon. In patients older than 13 years, 75% of penetrating trauma injuries are knife or handgun wounds inflicted by an assailant (Barkin & Marx, 1999; Marx, 1994). However, gunshot and stab wounds are becoming increasingly common in children. Compared with blunt trauma, penetrating trauma results in a significantly higher incidence of injury to hollow viscera, particularly to small bowel.

Penetrating wounds are classified as high/medium-energy (from guns) or low-energy (from knives) insults and substantially affect the severity of the wound. Stab wounds to the abdomen cause intraperitoneal organ damage in 30% of cases, with the liver being the most frequently injured organ (Barkin & Marx, 1999; Marx, 1994). Gunshot wounds enter the peritoneal cavity in 85% of cases, causing visceral injury in more than 95% of patients who have intraperitoneal penetration (Barkin & Marx, 1999; Marx, 1994). Penetrating trauma to the lower chest places the abdomen and diaphragm at risk for injury. In patients with penetration of the lower chest, associated injury to the diaphragm or peritoneal cavity occurs in 25% to 40% of cases (Barkin & Marx, 1999; Marx, 1994). The peritoneal cavity can be entered via back or flank wounds; however, this type of injury more likely results in kidney trauma.

PERTINENT ANATOMY AND PHYSIOLOGY

Severe abdominal injury may lead to significant dysfunction of the intraabdominal organs. Knowledge of the structure, location, and functions of these organs is necessary to understanding the impact of the injury.

The abdomen contains structures bordered by the diaphragm superiorly, the pelvis inferiorly, the vertebral column posteriorly, and the abdominal and iliac muscles anteriorly. Figure 17-2 illustrates the locations of the abdominal structures. The contents are further divided into four abdominal quadrants for the purposes of examination. These quadrants are the right upper quadrant (RUQ), left upper quadrant (LUQ), right lower quadrant (RLQ), and left lower quadrant (LLQ). Figure 17-2 also illustrates the division of the four quadrants and the contents of each.

Stomach

The stomach is located in the left upper quadrant of the abdomen. It is a hollow, muscular organ responsible for storing food during eating, secreting digestive juices (hydrochloric acid) and enzymes (pepsin), mixing foods with these juices, and propelling partially digested food into the duodenum of the small intestine. Blood is primarily supplied to the stomach by a branch of the celiac artery.

Spleen

The spleen is located in the left upper quadrant of the abdomen. Blood is supplied to the spleen by the splenic artery, which enters at the hilum. Because the spleen is a highly vascular organ, it is susceptible to acute and delayed bleeding into the peritoneal cavity.

The spleen is the largest of the secondary lymphoid organs. It is a site for red cell production but less significant than that in the liver. The macrophages of the spleen play a role in fighting infection by filtering and cleansing the blood

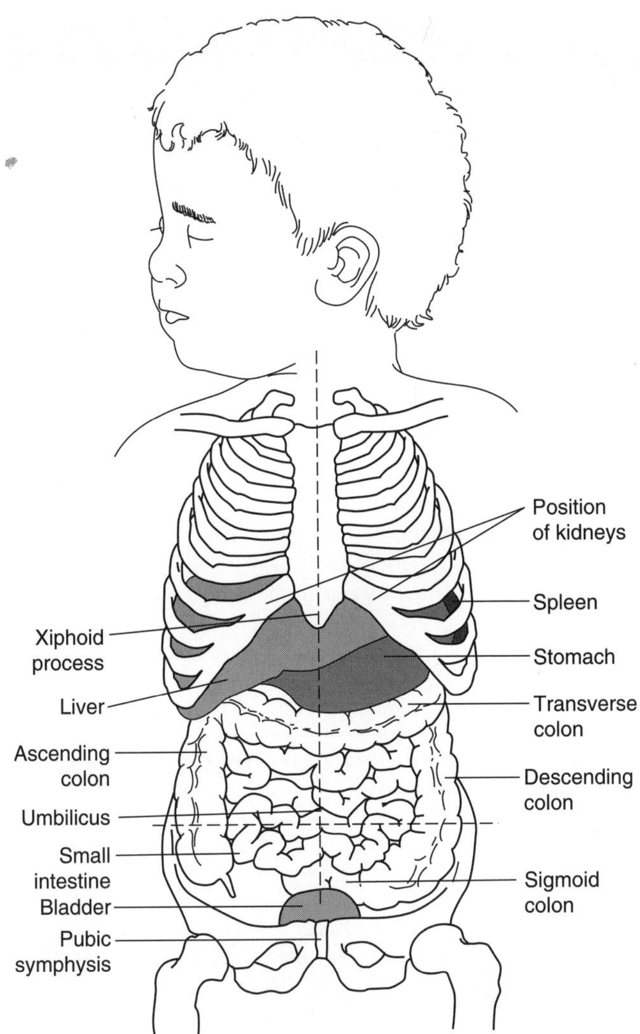

FIGURE 17-2 Abdominal structures. (Redrawn from Mott, S. R., James, S. R., & Sperhac, A. M. [1990]. *Nursing care of children and families* [2nd ed.]. Menlo Park, CA: Addison-Wesley).

through phagocytosis. In addition, its lymphocytes mount an immune response to bloodborne microorganisms.

The spleen is not necessary for life or for adequate hematologic function. However, after a splenectomy, several effects that indicate the various functions of the spleen are seen. For example, decreased levels of iron in the circulation reflect the spleen's role in the iron cycle. Alterations are also seen in the immune function. Antibody production in response to antigens is decreased. There is an increased number of circulating defective red blood cells (RBCs), which is indicative of the role of the spleen in removing these cells.

Liver

The liver is the largest intraabdominal organ. It lies in the right upper quadrant. In the infant and young child, the liver is easily palpable 1 to 2 cm below the right costal margin because of the child's relatively small abdominal cavity compared with that of an adult. The liver is divided into right and left lobes, which are separated by fissures. Between these two lobes is the porta hepatis, where veins, arteries, nerves, and lymphatic tissue enter or leave the liver. Blood supply to the liver is from the portal vein (most) and the hepatic artery.

Because the liver has multiple functions in maintaining homeostasis, any injury to the liver is significant. The liver produces the clotting factors V, VII, VIII, and X; prothrombin; and fibrinogen. It also stores vitamin K, which is necessary for synthesis of factors II, VII, IX, and X. The liver is also responsible for detoxifying drugs and waste products by making them water soluble and capable of being excreted in the urine or bile. In addition, the liver has a primary role in regulation of carbohydrate, protein, and fat metabolism. The liver is the primary synthesizer of plasma proteins that deaminize amino acids and release nitrogen, which is converted to urea for excretion. It is involved in fat metabolism, oxidizing fats as energy sources and forming lipoproteins and phospholipids. Its role in carbohydrate metabolism involves storing glycogen within the hepatocytes and later breaking down glycogen stores to meet the body's needs. It converts glucose, fructose, and galactose to glycogen for storage. During starvation states, it can convert protein and fat to glycogen. Common laboratory tests used to assess liver function are listed in Table 17-1.

Pancreas

The body of the pancreas lies deep in the abdomen, behind the stomach. The head of the pancreas is tucked into the curve of the duodenum, with the tail extending into the left upper quadrant. The pancreas has both exocrine and endocrine functions. The exocrine function is the secretion of enzymes (amylase, lipase, and trypsin), electrolytes, and bicarbonate for digestion and absorption of fats, carbohydrates, and proteins in the small intestine. Trauma to the pancreas can affect digestion of fats, fat-soluble substances, proteins, and carbohydrates. Furthermore, a pancreatic injury may cause leakage of the digestive enzymes into the peritoneal cavity and cause tissue necrosis. Laboratory evaluation of exocrine pancreatic function includes determination of amylase (normal, 0 to 88 IU/L) and lipase (normal, 20 to 180 IU/L) levels.

The endocrine functions of the pancreas are secretion of insulin, glucagon, and gastrin involved in the breakdown and increased utilization of glucose in the liver, as well as stimulation of the digestive process of the stomach. Injury to the pancreas can significantly alter glucose metabolism.

Small Intestine

The small intestine is the primary site for digestion and absorption of fats, amino acids, carbohydrates, and vitamins. It is divided into the duodenum, jejunum, and ileum. The duodenum is the primary site for the absorption of minerals, trace metals, water-soluble vitamins, and carbohydrates. The jejunum is the primary site for the absorption of proteins, carbohydrates, and about 50% of water and electrolytes. Carbohydrates are broken down into monosaccharides (galactose, glucose, and fructose) and absorbed by the

TABLE 17-1 **Liver Function Tests**

Test	Normal Pediatric Value	Interpretation
Alanine aminotransferase (ALT)	Infant: <54 U/L Child: 1-30 U/L	Increases with hepatocellular injury
Aspartate aminotransferase (AST)	Infant: 20-65 U/L Child: 0-35 U/L	Increases with hepatocellular injury
Alkaline phosphatase (ALP)	Infant: 150-420 U/L 2-10 yr: 100-320 U/L 11-18 yr: 100-390 U/L	Increases with biliary obstruction and cholestatic hepatitis
Lactate dehydrogenase (LDH)	Infant: 150-360 U/L Child: 150-300 U/L	Increases with increase in alkaline phosphatase
Glutamyl transpeptidase (GGT)	All ages: <120 IU/L	Increases with biliary obstruction and moderately increases with hepatocellular injury
Bilirubin		
Indirect	All ages: 0.1-0.3 mg/dl	Increases with hemolysis
Direct	All ages: 0.1-1.3 mg/dl	Increases with hepatocellular injury
Total	Infant: <2 mg/dl Child: 0.2-1.3 mg/dl	Increases with biliary obstruction
Prothrombin time (PT)	Infant: 10.1-15.9 sec Child: 10.8-13.9 sec	Increases with vitamin K deficiency or chronic liver disease
Albumin	All ages: 3.8-5.4 g/dl	Reduced with hepatocellular injury (also dependent on protein intake)
Ammonia	Infant: 29-70 μg/dl Child: 0-50 μg/dl	Increases with hepatocellular injury (acute or chronic failure)

From Barone, M. A. (Ed.). (1996). *The Harriet Lane handbook* (14th ed.). St. Louis: Mosby; and Martin, S., & Derengowski, S. (1998). The gastrointestinal system. In M. C. Slota (Ed.), *Core curriculum for pediatric critical care nursing. AACN.* Philadelphia: WB Saunders.

intestinal mucosa through microvilli. Proteins are degraded to amino acids and peptides and absorbed through the microvilli. Protein absorption is impaired if inadequate amounts of pancreatic enzymes are secreted from the pancreas. The enzyme lipase, which is secreted by the pancreas, is responsible for breaking down triglycerides into monoglycerides, free fatty acids, and glycerol. This breakdown allows for intestinal absorption of these components. The ileum is responsible for absorption of bile salts and vitamin B_{12}. The ileocecal valve controls the entry of digested material from the ileum into the large intestine. Blood supply to the small intestine is largely from the superior mesentery artery.

Large Intestine

The large intestine consists of the cecum, appendix, colon (ascending, transverse, descending, and sigmoid), and rectum. The colon is the primary site for water and electrolyte reabsorption.

Abdominal Aorta

The descending aorta passes through the diaphragm to become the abdominal aorta. Several major branches off the aorta supply blood to the abdominal organs. Any injury to the lower chest or abdomen may result in massive hemorrhage and multiorgan dysfunction secondary to hypotension and ischemia.

Genitourinary System

The genitourinary system consists of two kidneys, two ureters, the bladder, and a urethra (Figure 17-3). The kidneys occupy a proportionally larger space in the abdominal cavity and retroperitoneum in children compared with the amount of space in adults. The kidneys are located in the intraperitoneal cavity on either side of the vertebral column. The ureters carry fluid removed from the kidneys to the bladder through peristaltic contractions. The bladder is a muscular organ that stores urine. The infant's bladder has a capacity of 15 to 20 ml, compared with 500 ml in the adult. The bladder gradually descends into the pelvis as the child grows. The female urethra is protected by the symphysis pubis.

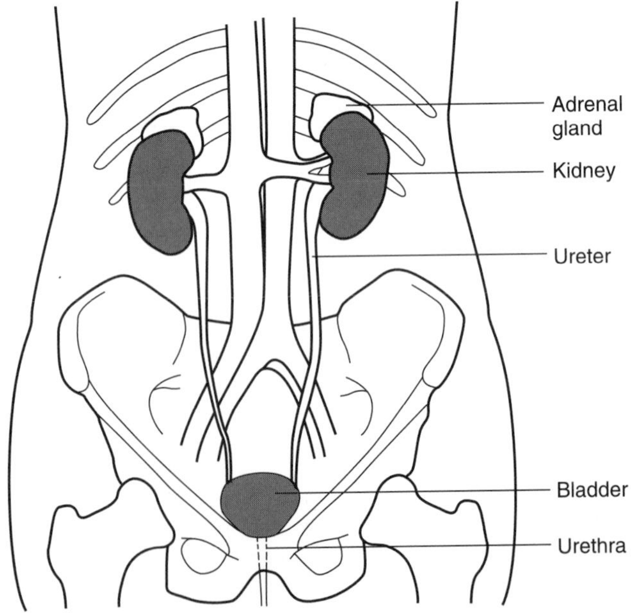

FIGURE 17-3 Components of the urinary system.

The kidneys receive 20% to 25% of the cardiac output. Each kidney receives blood from a single renal artery, which branches from the abdominal aorta. The kidneys are responsible for maintaining homeostasis by filtering the plasma to maintain fluid and electrolyte balance and to eliminate waste products. Renal dysfunction may occur as a result of the injury or decreased renal perfusion secondary to hypovolemia.

ANATOMIC DIFFERENCES IN CHILDREN

There are specific anatomic differences in children that predispose them to injury. Because children are smaller than adults, a greater proportion of their body surface area is subjected to a traumatic force. This force results in multisystem trauma that is seen more commonly in children than in adults (Haller, 1996; Pieper, 1994; Schafermeyer, 1993). In addition, children are more susceptible to abdominal trauma because the small amount of subcutaneous tissue surrounding the organs offers limited protection. Children have relatively poor abdominal muscle tone and a protuberant abdomen compared with adults. A child's rib cage is pliable and difficult to fracture, and it does not provide adequate protection to internal organs. The child may have significant internal injuries with limited signs of external trauma. Children also have proportionally larger solid organs than adults; therefore penetrating injuries are more likely to involve solid organs.

Children are more susceptible to renal injury than adults for several reasons. A child's kidney occupies a proportionally larger space in the abdominal cavity and retroperitoneum. It is located lower in the abdomen and has limited protective fat, which makes it more susceptible to injury. The child's rib cage is more pliable, which allows for greater injury with blunt trauma. The pediatric renal vascular pedicle is more susceptible to shearing forces with rapid deceleration injuries and the renal capsule is less developed, which often results in intraperitoneal bleeding with renal lacerations. Preexisting or congenital renal abnormalities increase the likelihood of injury to the kidney with mild traumatic forces than if the kidney were normal. Hydronephrosis is the most common abnormality and can result in major renal damage after relative minor trauma (McAleer & Kaplan, 1995; Sanchez & Paidas, 1999).

GENERAL ASSESSMENT

The abdominal examination is an important part of evaluating the child with trauma. However, a child who is frightened, is too young to cooperate, or has an altered mental status can make the examination difficult. In addition, significant injuries to the head and extremities may overshadow abdominal injuries. The final component of the primary survey is removal of all of the child's clothing to allow careful inspection of the body. This is extremely important to allow the examiner to identify external evidence of abdominal injury. Whether or not there is a high index of suspicion that a child has incurred an abdominal injury, serial vital signs and abdominal examinations are critical because unrecognized abdominal injuries can cause significant sequelae (Furnival et al., 1996; Rothrock et al., 2000a).

The abdomen, lower chest, and lower back should be examined for abrasions, contusions, lacerations, penetrating wounds (including entry and exit sites), and telltale markings (e.g., tire tracks, seat belt marks). The examination must include log-rolling the patient for adequate inspection of the back. Abdominal distention may be caused by hemoperitoneum or peritonitis, but most often it is caused by gastric distention as a result of swallowing air during crying. Gastric distention may cause pain and hypoventilation, which places the child at risk for aspirating stomach contents. Gastric decompression with the placement of an orogastric (with significant head trauma) or nasogastric tube may assist the examination and prevent vomiting. The gastric contents should be inspected for blood, which indicates upper gastrointestinal injury.

Auscultation and palpation are important aspects of the abdominal examination in the patient without traumatic injury. Although these assessment techniques are frequently inaccurate in the diagnosis of intraabdominal injury, serial measurements may be helpful in determining injury. For example, the presence or absence of bowel sounds does not aid the initial examination, but prolonged ileus may be a sign of continued abdominal injury. Tenderness with palpation or percussion may be due to abdominal wall contusion or may indicate intraabdominal injuries. This clinical finding is seen in up to 90% of patients with intraabdominal injury and alert mental status (Marx, 1993). Abdominal tenderness may by localized to the quadrant of injury (spleen or liver) or it may be diffuse. Rebound tenderness and rigidity, although more specific signs of peritonitis, are less common. Palpation of the chest for rib fractures should be performed and indicates potential liver or splenic injury. The bony prominences of the pelvis must also be palpated for tenderness and instability.

Light palpation is performed first to check for areas of increased muscle tone. Deep palpation is used to evaluate for masses, guarding, tenderness, and rebound pain. Rebound tenderness can be difficult to interpret because it elicits crying and voluntary guarding. Percussion, gentle shaking, or coughing can often elicit rebound tenderness in the child.

Several large studies have shown that the accuracy of the physical examination in diagnosing abdominal injury is 65% at best (Barkin & Marx, 1999). In the hemodynamically stable child with alert mental status and no significant associated injuries, serial examinations may prevent the need for further diagnostic studies. However, in the child with multisystem injuries who has an altered mental status, early diagnostic interventions are indicated.

Bladder rupture commonly occurs with a pelvic fracture, although a distended bladder may rupture alone (McAleer & Kaplan, 1995; Reisman, Naitoh, & Morgan, 1993). Bladder injury should be suspected when the child has lower abdominal pain, hematuria, and inability to void. Urethral injury is suspected when the child has perineal swelling, blood at the meatus, distended bladder, and inability to void. Placement of a Foley catheter is contraindicated because it can cause a partial tear to progress to complete disruption. Rather, a suprapubic tap should be performed to decompress the bladder (McAleer & Kaplan, 1995). The rectal examination evaluates the tone of the anal sphincter, position of the prostate, and integrity of the bony pelvis and bowel wall. Blood in the rectum strongly suggests perforation of the colon or rectum.

DIAGNOSTIC EVALUATION

Radiographic studies are performed only after initial stabilization and when additional diagnostic evaluation is required for management. Plain abdominal radiographs are useful for detecting free intraperitoneal air; however, a normal study does not exclude a perforation. A supine abdomen/pelvis radiograph and a cross-table or left lateral decubitus film should be obtained. The left lateral decubitus radiograph requires the patient to be on his or her side for approximately 10 minutes before the study to mobilize air.

Computed tomography (CT) scanning and ultrasound are often used to further define the extent of abdominal injuries in children. In particular, CT scanning has emerged as the diagnostic modality of choice for definitive radiographic assessment of blunt abdominal trauma in children because of its high sensitivity and specificity (Bond, Eichelberger, Gotschall, Sivit, & Randolph, 1996; Emery, 1997; Rothrock et al., 2000b). CT scanning is also an appropriate diagnostic modality to evaluate multiple organ systems simultaneously. It can be used to identify hepatic, splenic, intestinal, pancreatic, renal, and bladder injuries in children. Taylor, Eichelberger, O'Donnell, and Bowman (1991) found that CT scanning consistently identified abdominal injury if three of the following were present: (1) abdominal abrasions or contusions, (2) abdominal distention, (3) absent bowel sounds, (4) blood in the nasogastric tube, (5) lap belt injury, (6) gross hematuria, (7) assault or abuse as the mechanism of injury, (8) abdominal tenderness, and (9) a trauma score less than 12. Lap belt injury and abuse are two mechanisms of injury associated with significant abdominal injuries that can be documented by CT scanning (Cox & Kuhn, 1996). The disadvantages of the study include the need for contrast, generally both intravenous and oral, and the need to transport the patient. Use of oral contrast has been omitted from some pediatric trauma centers because of delays in evaluation, differences in administration, and risk of aspiration (Cantor & Learning, 1998). Frequent clinical assessments must be performed during the preparation and performance of CT scanning. If there is evidence of deterioration, prompt operative intervention should be performed. Findings on CT scanning that suggest blunt injury are unexplained fluid, solid organ disruption, contrast extravasation, and contrast enhancement of hollow viscus organs (Albanese, Meza, Gardnes, Smith, Rime, & Lynes, 1996; Cox & Kuhn, 1996). The Organ Injury Scaling Committee of the American Association for the Surgery of Trauma has developed a grading system to estimate the extent of abdominal organ injury (Moore, Shackford, Pachter, McAninch, Browner, & Champion, 1989; Moore et al., 1990). This grading system is based on CT findings and is discussed with specific organ injuries later in this chapter.

Ultrasound is another modality used to evaluate the abdomen in children. Although ultrasound may accurately identify intraperitoneal free fluid and thus may strongly suggest the presence of an abdominal injury, it does not reliably demonstrate the specific solid or hollow viscus injury (Coley et al., 2000; Katz, Lazar, Rathaus, & Erez, 1996; Nordenholz, Rubin, Gularte, & Liang, 1997; Pearl & Todd, 1996). Focused abdominal sonography for trauma (FAST) is a rapid diagnostic tool to identify intraabdominal injury in the unstable patient with blunt abdominal trauma, the unstable patient with chest trauma, or the patient requiring emergency surgery for head trauma who needs immediate assessment of the abdomen (Coley et al., 2000; Levins, 2000; Udobi, Rudriquez, Chiu, & Scalea, 2001). In adults, FAST has replaced diagnostic peritoneal lavage (DPL) as a method to diagnose free peritoneal fluid, although it is not as specific as CT scanning in defining extent of injury. However, FAST has limited sensitivity in identifying abdominal injury in children (Coley et al., 2000).

DPL has largely been replaced by ultrasound in the adult population, but it remains a safe and extremely sensitive (98%) method of detecting intraperitoneal hemorrhage. However, it is not organ or injury specific, and it is not useful in the assessment of retroperitoneal injury. It is rarely used in children, except to identify bowel injuries in a child with head trauma who requires immediate surgical intervention or to quickly determine the presence or absence of hemoperitoneum in the hemodynamically unstable patient (Colucciello, 1993; McAnena, Marx, & Moore, 1991; Rothrock, et al., 2000b; Sanchez & Paidas, 1999). Box 17-1 identifies the criteria for a positive DPL.

A battery of laboratory tests is indicated in any patient suspected of having trauma. Immediate type and crossmatching of the patient's blood is required for a patient suspected of having a significant injury. Additional tests include complete blood count (CBC), liver transaminase levels, amylase, electrolytes, lactate, coagulation studies, arterial blood gas, urinalysis, and toxicologic screen (if substance abuse is

BOX 17-1 Positive Diagnostic Peritoneal Lavage Criteria

Hemorrhage
- Gross blood aspirated
- >100,000 RBCs/mm^3 in effluent

Perforation
- Obvious enteric contents (i.e., bile or stool)
- >500 WBCs/mm^3 in effluent
- Amylase >175 mg/dl in effluent

RBCs, Red blood cells; *WBCs*, white blood cells.

suspected). Elevated liver transaminase levels are indicative of liver injury. Hyperamylasemia is suggestive of pancreatic or small bowel injury, but a normal value does not rule out injury. Urine should be evaluated for the presence of blood, which indicates kidney or bladder injury. Hematocrit is obtained on admission and followed throughout the period of observation. If hemorrhage is acute, a normal initial hematocrit may be misleading. Changes in the hematocrit reflect the patient's blood volume and rate of blood loss; therefore a decreasing hematocrit suggests ongoing blood losses. Arterial blood gas determinations are helpful in the evaluation of pulmonary injuries and to monitor for persistent metabolic acidosis when volume resuscitation is inadequate. Leukocytosis (white blood cell elevation) occurs within several hours of the injury and may last for several days. It is a nonspecific response to injury. Prolonged leukocytosis may be seen with visceral injury and bacterial or chemical peritonitis. Serial laboratory tests should be performed to assess for progression of injury and/or resolution.

INITIAL MANAGEMENT

Successful management of the pediatric trauma patient requires a systematic approach to assessment and management (see Chapter 6). Prompt, efficient assessment with simultaneous treatment of potentially life-threatening conditions (e.g., airway obstruction, tension pneumothorax, pericardial tamponade, obvious external sources of bleeding) is necessary because failure to do so may significantly increase morbidity and mortality.

Assessment of the abdomen is generally considered part of the secondary survey. Unless the abdomen is the cause of life-threatening injury, it is evaluated after any respiratory, circulatory, and neurologic compromise. The critically ill child requires intubation and mechanical ventilation for stabilization of airway and breathing. Circulatory stabilization requires the placement of large-bore intravenous lines. Once the patient is transported to the pediatric intensive care unit (PICU), central venous pressure (CVP) and arterial blood pressure lines are placed to allow close monitoring of the patient's intravascular volume and blood pressure and frequent monitoring of laboratory tests. Management of abdominal injury is based on hemodynamic stability. If the cardiovascular status fails to improve after initial volume resuscitation and abdominal injury is suspected as the cause, immediate laparotomy should be considered. Other indications for surgical exploration include (1) massive fluid resuscitation (more than 40 ml/kg of blood transfusions or 50% of estimated blood volume); (2) penetrating trauma; (3) physical signs of peritonitis; and (4) radiographic evidence of pneumoperitoneum, diaphragmatic injury, bladder rupture, or renovascular pedicle injury (Barkin & Marx, 1999). Stauffer (1995) developed an approach to nonoperative abdominal injury management, which is shown in Figure 17-4.

Most deaths related to intraabdominal injuries in the acute resuscitative phase (transport and emergency department resuscitation) are related to intraabdominal hemorrhage (Fackler et al., 1999). Volume resuscitation and the application of a pneumatic antishock garment, also known as *military antishock trousers* (MAST), are lifesaving. These pneumatic garments are available for children older than 4 years. MAST is particularly useful for stabilizing pelvic, hip, and long-bone fractures of the lower extremities and as a method to tamponade hemorrhaging arterial and venous vessels in these organs. The garment should not be removed until hemodynamic stability is ensured or the patient is transported to the operating room for laparotomy.

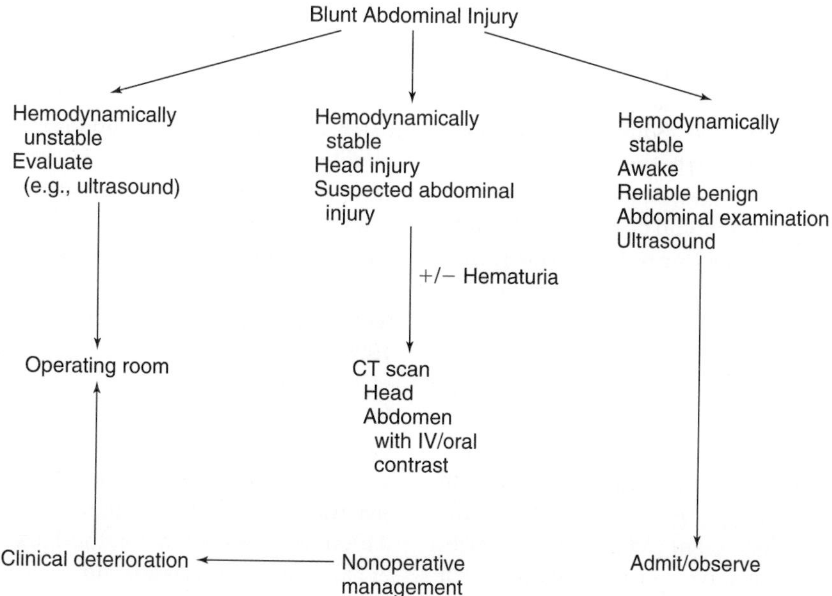

FIGURE 17-4 Algorithm for blunt abdominal injuries with and without multisystem trauma. (From Stauffer, U. G. [1995]. Surgical and critical care management of children with life-threatening injuries. *Journal of Pediatric Surgery, 30*[7], 903-910.)

The extent of intraabdominal injury is often difficult to determine because of the lack of external signs of injury. Nursing care for patients with an abdominal injury includes serial monitoring of vital signs and abdominal girth. Signs of hypovolemia and ongoing bleeding, such as tachycardia, low CVP, weak pulses, prolonged capillary refill time (more than 2 seconds), cool extremities, and decreased urine output, must be anticipated and corrected rapidly with volume resuscitation. Although mental status is a critical parameter in assessing a child's perfusion status, often mental status is already altered as a result of an associated head injury. Initially, crystalloid or colloid fluid may be given as a dose of 20 ml/kg and repeated as necessary. However, there is no substitute for blood if bleeding is ongoing and blood is readily available. The arterial blood pressure may be normal until as much as 25% of total blood volume has been lost, which is indicative of decompensated shock. Therefore, after the initial resuscitative phase, additional volume and blood transfusions should be titrated based on all perfusion parameters. Reassessments are crucial in the identification of progression of abdominal injuries and initially should be performed at 15-minute intervals. Children with abdominal trauma require decompression of the stomach with insertion of a nasogastric tube. This facilitates the abdominal examination, relieves the discomfort associated with an ileus, and allows assessment of stomach contents for presence of blood or bile. Urinary catheterization is indicated to decompress the bladder, monitor urine output, and assess for hematuria. Urine output of 1 ml/kg/hr should be maintained and fluid therapy titrated as needed. Urine catheterization is contraindicated in patients suspected of having a urethral injury.

SPECIFIC INJURIES

SPLENIC INJURY

The spleen is the most commonly injured intraabdominal organ. Boys are three times more likely to sustain a splenic injury than girls (Scorpio & Wesson, 1993). Most of these injuries are the result of trauma from motor vehicle–pedestrian accidents, followed by falls, bicycle crashes, and sports injuries. Penetrating injuries are extremely rare.

In children the rib cage is pliable and does not extend into the abdominal cavity; this leaves the spleen inadequately protected. In addition, the highly vascular anatomy of the spleen places it at significant risk for hemorrhage into the peritoneal cavity.

CLINICAL FINDINGS

Children with splenic injuries usually have nonspecific signs and symptoms. Common clinical findings are presented in Box 17-2. *Kehr sign* refers to the presence of free blood in the abdomen that irritates the diaphragm and the phrenic nerve. The pain is referred along the nerve, causing pain in the left shoulder, which indicates splenic injury. *Cullen sign* refers to the presence of periumbilical ecchymosis caused by intraabdominal bleeding. Cullen sign is a rare manifestation that indicates a ruptured spleen. *Grey-Turner sign* refers to the presence of flank ecchymosis, which indicates retroperitoneal hemorrhage.

BOX 17-2 Clinical Findings Associated With Splenic Injury

Generalized abdominal pain/tenderness
Localized pain/tenderness to LUQ
Abdominal distention/rigidity
Nausea and vomiting
Bruising or abrasion to LUQ
Left shoulder pain (Kehr sign)
Ecchymosis in the left flank (Grey-Turner sign)
Ecchymosis in the umbilical region (Cullen sign)
Dyspnea
Unexplained hypotension

LUQ, Left upper quadrant.

DIAGNOSTIC EVALUATION

Laboratory analysis is often normal in a child with a splenic injury. Abnormalities may include a falling hematocrit and significant leukocytosis (greater than 20,000 mm^3). Chest and abdominal radiographs may show signs suggestive of splenic injury, such as an elevated left hemidiaphragm, left lower rib fractures (uncommon in infants and children), pneumoperitoneum, and dilation or medial displacement of the stomach (Emery, 1997; Scorpio & Wesson, 1993). Abdominal CT scanning is the gold standard for definitive diagnosis in hemodynamically stable children (Colucciello, 1993; Emery, 1997; Turnock, Sprigg, & Lloyd, 1993). CT scanning is the test of choice in most children because it is readily available, it provides specific details of injury, and it can determine multiorgan injury. However, it usually requires the administration of intravenous and oral contrast.

The hemodynamically unstable child with signs of intraabdominal bleeding requires urgent laparotomy without further diagnostic evaluation. However, hemodynamically unstable children without signs of intraabdominal bleeding may benefit from DPL. In general, DPL is not indicated for cases of suspected splenic trauma but rather to assess trauma to other intraabdominal organs in unstable patients. Other diagnostic tests to evaluate splenic injury include nuclear medicine scintigraphy and ultrasonography, which have limited utility (Emery, 1997; Scorpio & Wesson, 1993).

CLASSIFICATION OF INJURY

Classification systems for splenic injury in adults have been developed and applied to children. Table 17-2 shows a modification of the Organ Injury Scaling Committee of the American Association for the Surgery of Trauma (Moore et al., 1989). This classification is based on the location and extent of the injury. However, the usefulness of the system in the treatment of children has not been evaluated (Scorpio & Wesson, 1993).

TABLE 17-2 Grading of Splenic Injury

Grade	Description
1	Capsular tear or subcapsular hematoma
2	Parenchymal laceration (<3 cm deep)
3	Deep parenchymal laceration
4	Multiple lacerations or burst injury

Patient Care Management

Management of splenic injuries is largely supportive. However, surgery is required for children who demonstrate persistent hypotension, rapidly increasing abdominal girth, or a low or falling hematocrit (less than 30%) despite adequate resuscitation (including transfusion of up to 20 ml/kg of packed red cells). Surgery may include a splenectomy or splenorrhaphy. In most circumstances suturing the injury (splenorrhaphy) results in salvage of the spleen. Massive parenchymal damage requires a splenectomy. Postoperative care for these children is the same as for all patients undergoing major abdominal surgery. Monitoring for potential complications include atelectasis, pneumonia, bleeding, ileus, infection, and pain. All patients have a postoperative ileus, and a nasogastric tube should remain in place until the ileus is resolved.

Children who undergo a splenectomy are at risk for overwhelming sepsis and must be protected with the use of prophylactic antibiotics and vaccines. The syndrome of overwhelming postsplenectomy infection (OPSI) occurs in 1.5% of children who have undergone splenectomy after trauma and has a 50% mortality rate (Stylianos, 1998). The incidence of infection is higher in young children, particularly in the years immediately after splenectomy. The vaccines required to protect against invasive disease include Pneumovax, *Haemophilus influenzae* type B, and meningococcal vaccine. Because vaccine failure can occur, penicillin prophylaxis should also be used until the child reaches adolescence. Infections may occur despite the use of antibiotic prophylaxis and vaccination; therefore parents should be taught to recognize signs of infection and to seek medical attention immediately.

Nonoperative treatment of isolated splenic injuries in hemodynamically stable patients is the standard of practice in pediatric surgery (Bond et al., 1996; Coburn, Pfeifer, & Deluca, 1995; Stauffer, 1995; Stylianos, 1995). This conservative treatment is used because of the spleen's important role in cellular and humoral immunity. A frequent surgical finding in children with splenic injury is that bleeding has stopped spontaneously (Bond et al., 1996). The rate of successful nonoperative treatment in pediatric trauma centers exceeds 90% (Morse & Garcia, 1994; Shafi et al., 1997; Stylianos, 1995). Nonoperative management includes strict bed rest, frequent monitoring of vital signs and physical examinations, and serial hematocrits until the child has not required any blood transfusions for more than 48 hours. The child may then begin ambulating but should remain hospitalized for 5 to 7 days to allow evaluation for potential rebleeding of the injury.

Abdominal CT scanning has been used to follow children with healing spleens. A study evaluating 37 children who had nonoperative management of CT-documented blunt splenic injuries revealed healing by 4 months for grade I and II injuries, 6 months for grade III, and up to 11 months for grade IV (Benya, Bulas, Eichelberger, & Sivit, 1995). A similar study evaluating 25 children who had nonoperative treatment with CT-documented blunt splenic injuries revealed healing in 10 of 13 (77%) grade I and II injuries 6 weeks after injury, whereas only 1 of 12 (8%) grade III or IV injuries were healed (Pranikoff, Hirschl, Schlesinger, Polley, & Coran, 1994). In general, the child and parents should be instructed that the child is to refrain from sports or activities that may result in further bleeding or injury to the spleen for at least 8 weeks (Benya et al., 1995).

Hepatic Injury

Blunt liver trauma is the most common fatal abdominal injury (Barkin & Marx, 1999; Torres & Garcia, 1993). Mechanisms of injury are similar to those seen with splenic trauma, with injury from motor vehicle–pedestrian accidents being the most common. The mechanism of injury also commonly results in multiorgan involvement, most often of the head, chest, and musculoskeletal system. Although the incidence of penetrating trauma is low, it is increasing in frequency in areas where drug and gang wars prevail. The liver is the organ most commonly injured in penetrating intraabdominal trauma (Barkin & Marx, 1999; Marx, 1993).

Clinical Findings

Clinical findings may not reliably predict liver injury. Often, there is multiple organ involvement with altered sensorium. External signs of trauma, such as abrasions, ecchymosis, seat belt markings, and entrance and exit wounds, must be noted. Hypotension and abdominal distention with or without tenderness indicate severe injury. Associated injuries to the head, long bones, ribs, and pelvic girdle should raise the level of suspicion for concomitant significant intraabdominal injury.

Diagnostic Evaluation

Studies have shown that elevated serum transaminase levels (aspartate aminotransferase [AST] and alanine aminotransferase [ALT]) correlate with liver injury. Torres and Garcia (1993) found an elevated AST (greater than 450 IU) and ALT (greater than 250 IU) on patient admission resulted in a 62% correlation of CT demonstrable hepatic injury. These liver transaminase levels appear to be useful guidelines indicating the need for further diagnostic evaluation with abdominal CT imaging. The degree of liver enzyme elevation above these levels, however, does not correlate with the severity of injury or predict a child's clinical course.

Although abdominal radiography is a necessary study for evaluation of abdominal trauma, it is not sensitive or specific for liver injury. DPL is of limited use because it is not organ specific. The preferred diagnostic modality is abdominal CT scanning with double contrast (intravenous and oral). Indicators for abdominal CT scanning include (1) history or physical examination findings consistent with intraabdominal injury, (2) elevated AST (greater than 450 IU) and ALT (greater than 250 IU) upon admission, (3) hematuria, and (4) head injury or altered sensoria that render the results of abdominal examination unreliable (Coant, Kornberg, Brody, & Edwards-Holmes, 1992; Hennes, Smith, Schneider, Hegenbarth, Duma, & Jona, 1990; Sahdev, Garramone, Schwartz, Steelman, & Jacobs, 1991; Torres & Garcia, 1993). However, children who are hemodynamically unstable are not suitable candidates for CT scanning and instead should undergo DPL or ultrasonography for diagnostic evaluation.

Classification of Injury

Injuries are graded according to increasing severity. Grading varies based on the scale used. Table 17-3 shows a modification of the Organ Injury Scaling Committee of the American Association for the Surgery of Trauma (Moore et al., 1989). This classification is based on the location and extent of the injury. It also is based on adult liver injuries. Its usefulness in the treatment of children has not been evaluated (Torres & Garcia, 1993).

Patient Care Management

Management of the child with hepatic injury is similar to the treatment of splenic injury. Nonoperative management is indicated for the child who is hemodynamically stable, requires blood transfusion of less than 50% of blood volume (approximately 40 ml/kg), and does not have physical signs of peritonitis (Bond et al., 1996; Coburn et al., 1995; Haller, Papa, Drugas, & Colombani, 1994). Nonoperative management requires frequent monitoring of vital signs and physical examinations in the PICU. Potential complications of nonoperative management include continued bleeding, hepatic necrosis, abscess formation, and missed diagnosis of bowel perforation (Bond et al., 1996). Fever, leukocytosis, and abdominal tenderness remote from the abdominal injury indicate an occult injury. Serial hematocrits, coagulation studies, and liver transaminase levels should be monitored until they are stable. When the liver transaminase levels return to normal, the patient may begin ambulating; however, activity must be restricted until complete healing as documented by CT evaluation has occurred.

TABLE 17-3 Grading of Liver Injuries

Grade	Injury Description
I	Subcapsular hematoma capsular tears
II	Minor lacerations of the parenchyma
III	Deep parenchymal lacerations (>3 cm deep)
IV	Burst liver injury, parenchymal destruction involving 25%-75% of hepatic lobe
V	Burst liver injury, parenchymal destruction involving >75% of hepatic lobe
VI	Hepatic avulsion

Patients with moderate to severe injury may experience significant liver dysfunction. They require close monitoring of liver functions, most importantly coagulation profile and ammonia, transaminases, bilirubin, serum protein, albumin, and glucose levels. The patient may require albumin replacement until protein synthesis is adequate. Vitamin K supplementation or blood product infusion may be necessary to assist in the formation or replacement of clotting factors. Close monitoring of serum glucose is essential, with adequate intravenous glucose administration. Evaluation and adjustment of all medications administered to the patient are necessary because liver dysfunction may cause accumulation.

Patients are monitored closely for ongoing bleeding secondary to liver lacerations or coagulopathy. Blood loss can be detected by serial monitoring of vital signs and abdominal examination, including serial abdominal girth measurements. Vital signs, including heart rate, blood pressure, CVP, and urinary output, are monitored to ensure adequate perfusion and cardiovascular stability. Ongoing bleeding is suspected if a fluid challenge initially produces correction of cardiovascular parameters with subsequent return to prehydration parameters.

Abscess formation is a potential complication of liver injury. Signs of abscess include fever, localized right upper quadrant or diffuse abdominal pain, and nausea and vomiting. Physical examination may reveal hepatomegaly, increased work of breathing secondary to enlarged liver, and jaundice. Laboratory data reveal leukocytosis, hyperbilirubinemia, low total protein, and hypoalbuminemia. CT scanning defines the location and extent of abscess. Medical treatment includes surgical exploration, drainage, and administration of broad-spectrum antibiotic until the specific pathogen is identified by culture.

Gastrointestinal Injury

Hollow organ injury is rare but occurs more frequently in patients with lap belt injuries (Schafermeyer, 1993; Stylianos, 1998). Physical signs of stomach injury include an abrasion or contusion to the upper abdomen, bloody gastric drainage, and free air or abnormal position of the nasogastric tube on abdominal radiograph. A perforated stomach produces a boardlike abdomen and severe pain. Diagnostic evaluation should consist of supine and decubitus abdominal radiographic views. Perforation leads to signs and symptoms of peritonitis within hours and requires surgical repair.

Small and large intestinal injuries rarely occur in children. They are usually associated with penetrating trauma (Ford & Senac, 1993). Blunt intestinal rupture may occur as a result of bursting of fluid-filled bowel loops when they are subjected to sudden increases in intraluminal pressures, compression of bowel against the spine, or rapid deceleration injury (i.e., from the lap belt). Another distinctive pattern of injury resulting from lap belt use is characterized by a triad of injuries that includes abdominal bruising, intestinal and mesentery contusion, and lumbar spine fracture (Chance fracture). The underlying mechanism is a rapid deceleration injury with a sudden forward flexion of the upper body.

Acute perforation (within 24 to 48 hours) is the most common intestinal injury in children after lap belt trauma (Stylianos, 1998). Physical signs may be subtle initially, although signs of peritonitis will develop in all of these patients and necessitate surgical repair. Signs and symptoms of peritonitis include severe abdominal pain, tenderness, distention and/or rigidity, involuntary guarding, absent bowel sounds, fever, leukocytosis (greater than 20,000/µl initially), respiratory distress, and nausea and vomiting. Repeated assessment is extremely important and is the most reliable indicator of enteric disruption. Antibiotic treatment and supportive therapy for dehydration, shock, and acidosis are critical. Surgical repair and peritoneal lavage are indicated.

Management of both gastric and intestinal injuries includes monitoring for potential gastrointestinal bleeding secondary to stress and mucosal breakdown. Low gastric pH, coffee ground or frank blood aspirate, decreasing hematocrit, abdominal pain, and melena (dark, tarry stools) are indications of mucosal erosion. Nursing management is aimed at prevention with the administration of H_2 inhibitors, antacids, and sedatives. Stress ulceration, if not effectively treated, can lead to gastrointestinal hemorrhage necessitating saline lavage, volume resuscitation, and ultimately surgical repair.

Patients who have sustained seemingly minor intestinal injury may return 1 month after lap belt injury with signs and symptoms of partial or complete bowel obstruction (abdominal pain, bilious emesis, and abdominal distention). This delayed presentation is secondary to the development of ischemic intestinal strictures as a result of the blunt injury or unrecognized contained perforations (Lynch, Albanese, Meza, & Weiner, 1996).

Rectal injuries are uncommon, but when they occur are usually caused by penetrating trauma. Evaluation includes a thorough rectal examination to rule out the presence of blood within the rectum, to assess sphincter tone, and to ensure that there has been no disruption of the lower urinary tract. Absence of sphincter tone may indicate spinal cord injury.

Pancreatic Injury

Blunt trauma is the leading cause of pancreatitis in children. The most common mechanism is compression of the pancreas against the vertebral column due to a rapid deceleration force after a motor vehicle accident (Rescorla & Grosfeld, 1993). Other common mechanisms of injury include compression by bicycle handlebars and assault. Early clinical diagnosis of pancreatic injury may be difficult because of the retroperitoneal location of the pancreas. However, because of its location, associated injuries occur in 90% of all children and commonly involve the stomach, duodenum, biliary system, and spleen (Buntain, 1995).

Clinical Findings

Signs and symptoms of pancreatic injury include diffuse abdominal tenderness, deep epigastric pain radiating to the back, bilious vomiting, and findings of associated injuries. However, because of the retroperitoneal location of the pancreas, the patient may initially have limited symptoms.

Diagnostic Evaluation

Laboratory analysis for pancreatic injury includes serum amylase and lipase levels. The extent of increase does not correlate with the severity of injury. A threefold increase above normal values (0 to 88 IU/L) suggests injury, and a rising level indicates significant injury. However, the amylase level may not rise until 24 hours or more after the injury. Hyperamylasemia is a nonspecific finding that may occur with blunt injury in the absence of pancreatic injury.

CT scanning may help identify severe pancreatic injury and reveal pancreatic edema as an early indication of trauma, but it is not as helpful in determining management as it is in other abdominal injuries (Siegel & Sivit, 1997). Ultrasound may be more useful for pancreatic injuries but is unlikely to change the early management (Katz et al., 1996; Pearl & Todd, 1996).

Classification of Injury

A number of injury severity classifications systems can be used to grade pancreatic trauma. Classification of injury is based primarily on the presence of injury to the gland, major ductal system, or duodenum. Table 17-4 shows a classification system used to determine operative procedure (Jurkovich & Carrico, 1990; Rescorla & Grosfeld, 1993).

Patient Care Management

Isolated pancreatic injuries rarely require emergent laparotomy, except in instances of ductal disruption and penetrating trauma. Placement of a nasogastric tube for suction and initiation of parenteral nutrition are necessary to rest the bowel. Pain management is also important. The age of the patient, cardiovascular status, and associated injuries play a role in determining the appropriate agents to use.

Nursing Management for the Child With Abdominal Injuries

Nursing interventions for patients with abdominal injuries after the resuscitation phase should primarily address the following problems: (1) fluid volume deficit, (2) ineffective breathing pattern, (3) alteration in gas exchange, (4) potential for infection, (5) alteration in nutrition, (6) pain, and (7) ineffective wound healing.

TABLE 17-4 Classification of Pancreatic Injury

Type	Injury Description
1	Contusion and laceration without ductal injury
2	Distal transection or parenchymal injury with duct injury
3	Proximal transection or parenchymal injury with probable ductal injury
4	Combined pancreatic and duodenal injury

Fluid Volume Deficit

Depending on the severity of abdominal injury, children may experience decreased fluid volume secondary to bleeding and third spacing. Nursing interventions are directed primarily at monitoring for signs of hypovolemia, promptly notifying the physician, and administering fluids as needed. Hypovolemia is evidenced by tachycardia, decreased pulses, decreased capillary refill time, low CVP, decreased urine output, and ultimately hypotension and metabolic acidosis if left untreated. Fluid resuscitation begins with 20 ml/kg per dose of crystalloid or colloid fluid and is repeated as needed, with monitoring of perfusion parameters. After approximately 40 to 60 ml/kg of total fluid, administration of blood products is necessary. Required blood transfusions of greater than 40 ml/kg indicate ongoing bleeding and the need for surgical exploration.

Ineffective Breathing Pattern

The child who has sustained an abdominal injury may experience respiratory failure necessitating mechanical ventilation. In the resuscitation phase, shock is often the cause of respiratory failure. In the critical care phase, abdominal distention or ascites may significantly compromise diaphragmatic excursion and produce rapid, shallow, ineffective respirations. Nursing management for the child with abdominal injury and respiratory failure is the same for all mechanically ventilated patients. However, the nurse must closely monitor ventilatory settings for signs of decreased lung compliance secondary to parenchymal injury or abdominal distention. Depending on the mode of ventilation, peak inspiratory pressure (PIP) or expiratory volumes (the parameter is not set) should be monitored to assess changing compliance. A mode of ventilation called *pressure-regulated volume control* is effective for patients with significant abdominal distention secondary to abdominal injury. This control mode allows for lower PIPs while guaranteeing a set tidal volume. This type of ventilation is thought to decrease the risk of barotrauma; however, the patient must be chemically paralyzed to ensure tolerance.

Alteration in Gas Exchange

Abdominal distention, immobility, and postoperative pain all can cause ventilation/perfusion mismatch secondary to atelectasis. Patients are at risk for pleural effusion secondary to hypoalbuminemia, low oncotic pressure, increased abdominal distention, and hydrostatic pressure. Patients also are at risk for pneumonia secondary to the traumatic injury and potentially prolonged intubation. Prolonged shock secondary to hemorrhage predisposes the child to acute respiratory distress syndrome (ARDS). Patients with ARDS have severe hypoxemia, decreased lung volume and compliance, diffuse alveolar collapse, and ventilation/perfusion mismatching.

The goals of mechanical ventilation are to support alveolar ventilation and arterial oxygenation, decrease ventilation/perfusion mismatching, and improve functional residual lung capacity. Several new modes of ventilation are aimed at reducing the risk of barotrauma. Nurses must be familiar with these modes of ventilation and closely monitor ventilatory parameters. In addition, continuous pulse oximetry, frequent arterial blood gases, and daily chest radiographs are necessary for the clinician to interpret the child's respiratory status and intervene appropriately. Prone positioning, a common therapy for ARDS, is contraindicated in children with abdominal trauma. Therapeutic rotating beds are an effective alternative for immobile patients.

Potential for Infection

Children with abdominal injury are primarily at risk for infection as a result of peritonitis or abscess formation. Secondary peritonitis may occur from blunt or penetrating trauma. Penetrating wounds introduce bacteria into the peritoneal space from the penetrating object (e.g., knife, gun) and cause the release of endogenous substances from injured organs. Blunt trauma may rupture viscera or alter blood supply, resulting in bacterial or chemical peritonitis.

Physical signs include diffuse abdominal pain or tenderness, abdominal distention or rigidity, rebound pain, fever, and decreased or absent bowel sounds. Abdominal pain and distention can compromise respiratory effort, resulting in hypoventilation.

Abdominal radiography establishes the diagnosis; the radiographs may reveal inflammation and edema of the intestinal wall and free air if the viscera has been perforated. CBC shows evidence of leukocytosis with a bandemia (increased immature white blood cells). Visceral perforation in the infant or young child causes signs and symptoms of acute sepsis and/or shock. The child can rapidly become hypovolemic secondary to third spacing of fluids. Visceral perforation requires surgical repair after the patient is stabilized.

Management begins with intubation and mechanical ventilation to effectively manage respiratory status. Volume resuscitation is administered to treat the hypovolemia and titrated by monitoring perfusion parameters, electrolytes, and arterial blood gases. A nasogastric tube is placed for gastric decompression, and a Foley catheter is placed for accurate measurement of urine output. Broad-spectrum antimicrobials are administered to cover common gram-negative, gram-positive, and anaerobic pathogens until specific infecting organisms are identified. Postoperatively, adequate fluid and electrolyte replacement is essential secondary to continued third space losses. Serial monitoring of vital signs, perfusion parameters, electrolytes, and arterial blood gases is indicated. The patient also requires parenteral nutrition for adequate caloric intake.

Injury to intraabdominal organs can lead to abscess formation. These organs release blood, enzymes, and other fluids, providing an appropriate medium for abscess formation unless they are drained adequately. An abscess is a localized infection and inflammatory process. Purulent exudate is walled off by leukocytes and may expand or deepen as leukocytes are drawn to the area, organisms are killed, and necrotic tissue is dissolved. The exudate may be autolyzed and reabsorbed by the body, thereby avoiding the need for surgical intervention. Rupture of an abscess may occur and cause further contamination. After rupture, a fistula tract can form to an organ or the skin and spread infectious exudate. Bacteremia, septicemia, cellulitis, or peritonitis may follow.

An abdominal abscess may manifest itself through signs of peritonitis. Abdominal radiograph reveals displaced organs or diaphragm. CT scanning defines the location and extent of the abscess. Therapy includes drainage of the abscess, antimicrobial therapy, and adequate nutrition.

Alteration in Nutrition

After cardiovascular stability is ensured, nutrition should be instituted as soon as possible, ideally within 24 to 48 hours after admission. Early nutrition is important to maintain gut mucosa, prevent infection, and promote wound healing (Stechmiller, Treloar, & Allen, 1997; Trocki, Michelini, Robbins, & Eichelberger, 1995). Children have increased caloric demands secondary to developmental needs, stress response to injury, and complications of the traumatic injury. Research supports early enteral nutrition in adults after abdominal surgery and traumatic injuries; however, there is a paucity of research substantiating its use in children (Kudsk et al., 1992; Moore et al., 1992; Stechmiller et al., 1997; Trocki et al., 1995). Research in adults suggests that initiating trophic feeds (generally considered less than 5 ml/hr in children) promotes gut integrity and hormonal balance. When enteral feeds are given, nurses play a critical role in monitoring for feeding intolerance. Interventions include performing serial abdominal girth measurements, observing for abdominal distention and emesis, and monitoring serum glucose. Feedings should be discontinued and intravenous fluids initiated when signs of intolerance are present.

Parenteral nutrition requires a central line to deliver adequate calories. Nurses are responsible for administering total parenteral nutrition (TPN) per institutional guidelines and monitoring for complications. There are many potential metabolic complications of TPN. The most common complication is hyperglycemia secondary to glucose overinfusion. Nursing interventions with initiation of TPN include serial urine dipsticks, bedside glucose measurement, and determination of serum electrolytes. TPN should never be discontinued abruptly, especially in infants, because it can cause hypoglycemia. Rather, TPN should be weaned gradually while bedside glucose values are monitored. Other nursing interventions include strict monitoring of intake and output and daily weights. See Chapter 12 for review of nutritional support in the pediatric trauma patient.

Nutrition is commonly altered because of a paralytic ileus. An ileus may develop secondary to the initial shock, sepsis, surgical manipulation, premature removal of a nasogastric tube, narcotic administration for pain control, and/or neuromuscular blockade administration secondary to respiratory failure with multisystem injury. Decreased peristalsis results in abdominal distention and decreased to absent bowel sounds. Abdominal radiograph reveals either absent bowel gas or diffuse distended bowel. Treatment includes NPO (nothing per os) status, nasogastric tube for gastric decompression, parenteral nutrition for adequate caloric intake, and serial abdominal girth measurements and abdominal assessments until return of normal bowel function is evident. Once normal function returns, enteral feeds should be instituted and advanced slowly, with close monitoring for signs of feeding intolerance.

Pain

Pain after abdominal trauma may be caused by the incision, organ injury, surgical procedure, or the presence of invasive drains and devices. Uncontrolled pain can lead to respiratory compromise and paralytic ileus. Assurance of adequate intravascular volume is critical because narcotic administration may cause hypotension. Nurses are primarily responsible for assessing the patient's pain, administering pharmacologic and nonpharmacologic pain relief measures, and assessing for adequate effect (see Chapter 11). Parents are the single most powerful nonpharmacologic method of pain relief, and it is essential that all efforts be made to involve parents in the care of the child.

Ineffective Wound Healing

Wound healing after an abdominal injury is affected by many factors, such as the type of abdominal injury, associated injuries, time from injury to treatment, and the patient's preexisting health status. Traumatically induced wounds commonly are contaminated either through the penetrating injury itself or from visceral perforation after blunt injury. This often results in the need for healing through secondary closure (i.e., the wound is left open and allowed to heal by granulation and reepithelialization). When contamination is not evident and the wound is closed, suture line disruption and dehiscence may occur later because intraabdominal tissue is unable to hold the suture.

Care of the wound includes aseptic technique with saline-soaked wet-to-dry dressing changes (Garvin, 1997). Nurses are responsible for monitoring the wound for changes in size, depth, drainage, color, odor, redness, edema, and presence or absence of granulation tissue. If an infection is present, the patient may have additional symptoms of fever, tachycardia, leukocytosis, and bandemia (increased immature white blood cells). Cultures are obtained from the wound, blood, and other potential sources (e.g., sputum, urine). Patients must be monitored closely for bacterial translocation.

Kidney Injury

The incidence of traumatic genitourinary injuries in adults has been reported to range from 10% to 30%. A review of pediatric trauma patients found the incidence of injuries to the urogenital tract was less than 3% (Brown, Elder, & Spirank, 1998). The kidney is the organ most commonly injured in the urogenital tract. Typically, it occurs in association with other injuries that are life threatening and require immediate intervention. Although isolated kidney injuries rarely are life threatening, they may be a significant cause of morbidity if they are not recognized early.

Blunt forces are the most common mechanism of injury. They cause more than 90% of all injuries in pediatric patients (Brown, Elder, & Spirank, 1998; McAleer & Kaplan, 1995). Motor vehicle accidents are responsible for 47% to 82% of blunt kidney injuries, followed by falls, sports injuries, and child abuse (Brown, Elder, & Spirank, 1998). The injury occurs when acute deceleration forces crush the kidney against the vertebrae, resulting in parenchymal lacerations or contusions. In addition, rapid deceleration may disrupt the renal parenchyma or the major vessels, such as the renal arteries.

The incidence of penetrating injuries inflicted by knives or guns have risen dramatically (McAleer & Kaplan, 1995). Fatal firearm injuries in children increased by 21% in homicides and 30% in suicides (Barkin & Marx, 1999; Marx, 1993). Penetrating injuries to the chest, abdomen, flank, and lumbar regions should be assumed to have caused renal injury. Associated bowel injury is also more likely with penetrating injuries.

Clinical Findings

During the initial physical examination, the abdomen and flanks are assessed for tenderness, masses, abrasions, contusions, and flank ecchymosis (Grey-Turner sign), all of which indicate retroperitoneal hemorrhage. The lower rib cage and pelvis should be examined for fractures. Signs of shock indicate massive bleeding and strongly suggest associated injuries. Specific physical signs of genitourinary injury are presented in Box 17-3.

BOX 17-3 Physical Signs of Genitourinary Injury

Renal

- Hematuria
- Flank or abdominal pain
- Flank abrasion, contusion, or ecchymosis
- Previous renal abnormality

Ureteral

- Hematuria
- Flank pain
- Deceleration injury with hyperextension
- Penetrating injuries

Bladder

- Hematuria
- Abdominal pain
- Inability to void
- Pelvic fracture
- Renal injury

Urethral

- Hematuria
- Blood at urethra
- Lower abdominal or pelvic pain
- Inability to void
- Scrotal hematoma or perineal swelling
- High-riding prostate

Modified from Mayer, T. (1985). *Emergency management of pediatric trauma* (p. 343). Philadelphia: WB Saunders.

Diagnostic Evaluation

Initial diagnostic evaluation of all patients with suspected abdominal or genitourinary trauma should consist of a urine dipstick and a urinalysis. A positive dipstick value is obtained if hemoglobin or myoglobin is in the urine. False-positive values occur when urine is contaminated with povidone-iodine (Betadine) or hexachlorophene. Hematuria is the most common manifestation of urogenital injury. Microscopic hematuria (greater than 5 RBCs/high-power field [HPF]) identified on urinalysis is present in 85% to 90% of all genitourinary injuries, with greater than 20 RBCs/HPF considered significant for genitourinary trauma (McAleer & Kaplan, 1995; Schafermeyer, 1993). The degree of hematuria, however, does not correlate with the severity of injury.

Positive clinical findings or a significant mechanism of injury suggesting genitourinary injury warrants radiologic evaluation. A chest radiograph should be examined for fractures of the lower ribs. Pelvic radiographs may reveal bladder displacement or fracture. A kidney, ureter, and bladder (KUB) view should be examined for vertebral fractures, free intraperitoneal or retroperitoneal air, psoas shadow obliteration, or elevation of a hemidiaphragm (Allshouse & Betts, 1993).

Abdominal CT scanning with contrast is the gold standard for initial evaluation of trauma, because it allows visualization of all solid organs in both intraperitoneal and retroperitoneal injuries. If isolated urogenital trauma is suspected, the intravenous pyelogram (IVP) is the study of choice because it allows visualization of all genitourinary structures and is readily available and relatively inexpensive (Morey, Bruce, & McAninch, 1996). Ultrasound is less specific than CT scanning, but it can be useful as a rapid initial screening tool in the assessment the abdominal organs and retroperitoneum.

Classification of Injury

Several classification systems for renal injuries have been described in the literature. The degree of injury has been graded as minor and major and in groups of contusions, lacerations, and tears. CT scanning has made the evaluation of renal trauma much more precise. A more recent classification system that may predict management strategy is shown in Figure 17-5 (Rowe, 1995). Typically, conservative therapy is used with grades I, II, and III injuries. Certain grade IV injuries may also be managed conservatively, although many are managed operatively. Grade V injuries require surgical intervention.

Patient Care Management

Management of the patient with renal trauma is undertaken after adequate resuscitation and management of life-threatening injuries. Most blunt injuries can be managed nonoperatively. Nonoperative management consists of bed rest; frequent monitoring of vital signs; serial measurement

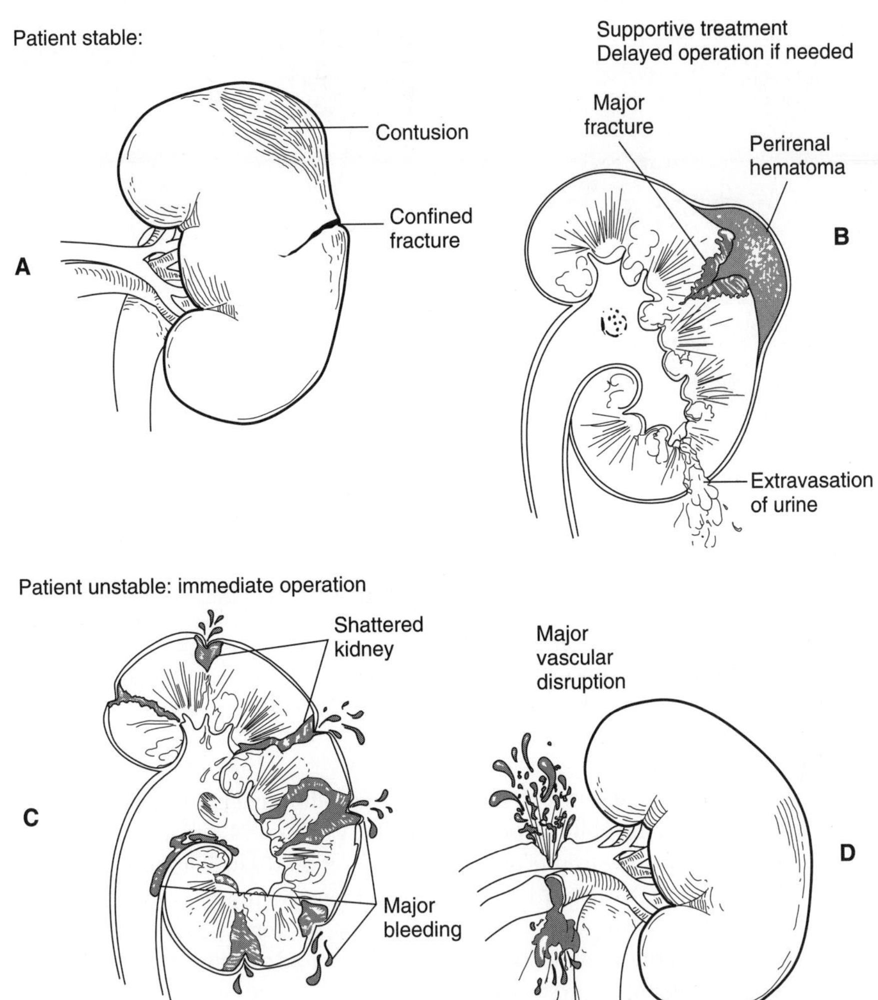

FIGURE 17-5 Types of blunt renal trauma. Types A and B often respond to nonoperative treatment. Types C and D usually operative management. Type D requires emergency surgical intervention or loss of kidney will result. (From Rowe, M. I. [1995]. *Essentials of pediatric surgery.* St. Louis: Mosby.)

of hematocrit, blood urea nitrogen (BUN), and creatinine levels; and urinalysis for resolution of hematuria. Selective severe injuries can be managed nonoperatively with CT staging of injury, frequent monitoring of vital signs and urine output, serial hematocrit measurements, and administration of broad-spectrum antibiotics. Close monitoring is essential to evaluate for complications secondary to renal trauma, which include acute tubular necrosis, delayed bleeding, infection secondary to urinary extravasation and abscess, and secondary hypertension.

Indicators for surgical management include ongoing blood loss; prolonged ileus; poorly controlled urinary extravasation; devitalized renal segments; and associated bowel, urethral, or pancreatic injuries (Allshouse & Betts, 1993). Most cases of penetrating trauma require surgical management, primarily to treat associated injuries. Isolated renal injuries may be treated nonoperatively. These patients are monitored closely for signs of ongoing injury.

Children who have experienced a renal injury receive ongoing outpatient evaluations for delayed sequelae. The number of patients who experience posttraumatic hypertension is small. However, there is an increased risk for secondary hypertension; thus patients must be monitored closely for potential sequelae. Other complications include hydronephrosis and loss of renal parenchyma secondary to ischemia. Abdalati, Bulas, Sivit, Majd, Rushton, and Eichelberger (1994) studied 35 children and found that injury graded by CT scanning correlated with the frequency of complications and the rate of healing. Minor renal contusions and small parenchymal lacerations healed without complications after 3 months. All children with renal lacerations extending into the collecting duct developed mild to severe loss of renal function, but the wounds healed progressively over 4 months. Children with vascular pedicle injury developed severe renal dysfunction.

Ureteral Injury

Blunt traumatic disruption of the ureter or ureteropelvic junction is rare but more common in children than in adults (McAleer & Kaplan, 1995). Figure 17-6 shows the lower genitourinary structures in the pediatric male. The mechanism of injury is usually extreme hyperextension of the trunk

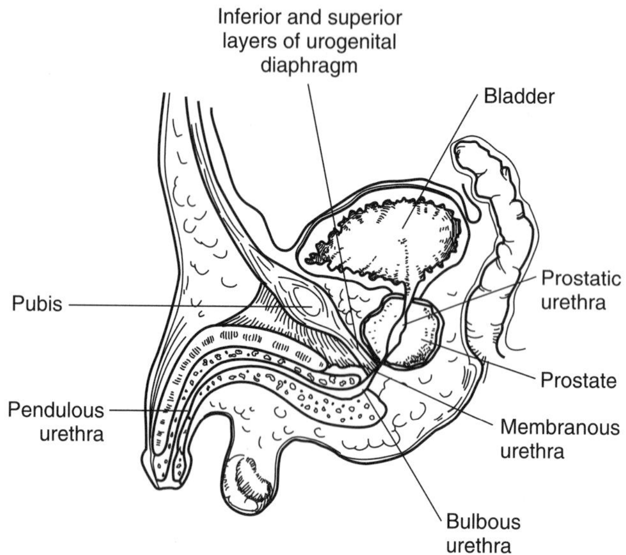

FIGURE 17-6 Anatomy of the male lower genitourinary system. (Redrawn from Zbaraschuk, I., Berger, R. E., & Hedges, J. R. [1991]. Emergency urologic procedures. In J. R. Roberts & J. R. Hedges [Eds.], *Clinical procedures in emergency medicine* [2nd ed.]. Philadelphia: WB Saunders.)

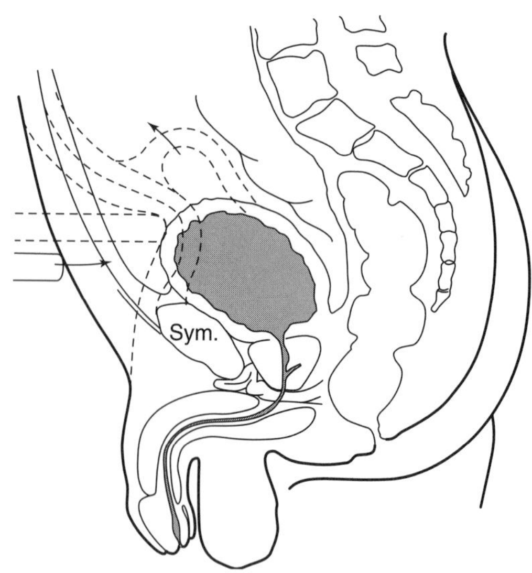

FIGURE 17-7 The bladder in the infant is more susceptible to injury because of the bladder's abdominal location. (Redrawn from Gonzales, E. T., & Guerriero, W. G. [1985]. Genitourinary trauma in children. In P. P. Kelalis, L. R. King, & A. B. Belman [Eds.], *Clinical pediatric urology* [2nd ed.]. Philadelphia: WB Saunders.)

caused by sudden deceleration, as seen in motor vehicle accidents. The elasticity and mobility of the child's spine places the child at risk for this type of injury. Avulsion commonly occurs at the ureteropelvic junction. Partial or complete transection of the ureter may result from penetrating trauma, but this is rare. Delayed recognition of ureteral injuries is not uncommon because hematuria can be absent or transient (Allshouse & Betts, 1993). An abdominal CT scan may raise the suspicion for ureteral avulsion, but an IVP or retrograde pyelogram is usually necessary to make the definitive diagnosis (Morey et al., 1996). Delayed symptoms include fever, ileus, hematuria, and flank or abdominal pain. Management of ureteral injuries is always operative, regardless of the cause of injury. Kidney salvage rate is greater than 95%; however, when diagnosis is delayed, nephrectomy is often necessary (Allshouse & Betts, 1993). Complications of delayed diagnosis include fistula, ureteral stricture, and abscess.

Bladder Injury

The bladder is the second most commonly injured genitourinary organ. In children the bladder is an abdominal organ rather than a pelvic organ and is especially susceptible to trauma. Approximately 15% of patients with pelvic fractures have bladder injuries (McAleer & Kaplan, 1995).

Most bladder injuries are the result of severe blunt trauma, but penetrating injuries to the suprapubic area may lacerate the bladder. The bladder may rupture intraperitoneally or extraperitoneally. Infants and children have an intraabdominal bladder. As children age, the intraabdominal bladder descends into the pelvis. As a result, intraperitoneal rupture occurs more commonly in young children and is associated with a full bladder (Figure 17-7). Physical signs include abdominal pain and tenderness, hematuria, and difficulty voiding. Bladder injuries are often overlooked because of associated injuries and subtle clinical presentation. Often, the injury is not diagnosed until signs of peritonitis and renal dysfunction are present. Signs of extraperitoneal rupture are variable and often subtle. They may include suprapubic pain and tenderness, difficulty voiding, hematuria, and decreased urine output.

Bladder rupture should be considered in children with abdominal trauma if there is gross hematuria, blood at the meatus, and inability to void (see Box 17-3). A cystogram is the radiographic study of choice for suspected bladder rupture and is extremely accurate in identifying bladder injury (Morey et al., 1996). A cystogram involves the instillation of a contrast dye into the bladder via a catheter. However, abdominal CT scanning is performed before the cystogram to evaluate associated injuries and to avoid inaccurate findings secondary to potential extravasation of dye from the bladder.

Urinary catheterization should not be attempted until after diagnostic evaluation with a cystogram. Management of extraperitoneal bladder injuries includes suprapubic catheter or Foley catheter drainage for 7 to 14 days. Intraperitoneal rupture requires surgical exploration, repair, debridement, and bladder drainage. Postoperative management includes a suprapubic catheter for urinary drainage.

Urethral Injury

Children may sustain blunt urethral injuries while they are participating in sports activities, straddling bicycle handlebars, or jumping fences. Automobile-pedestrian accidents resulting in pelvic fractures may result in urethral injuries. However, these injuries are relatively rare in children because of the mobility of the urethra and flexibility of the pelvis.

Classic signs of urethral injury include an inability to void and presence of blood at the urethral meatus (see Box 17-3). A rectal examination must be performed in patients with suspected urethral injuries to evaluate for a high-riding prostate or the presence of bony fragments from a pelvic fracture.

Diagnosis of a urethral tear is confirmed by retrograde urography. CT scanning is not useful in the diagnosis of urethral injuries; however, it is necessary to evaluate associated injuries. Although urinary catheter insertion is a routine nursing care procedure during resuscitative management, patients with signs and symptoms of urethral injury should undergo retrograde urethrogram before insertion of a Foley catheter. In the stable trauma patient with no evidence of pelvic or urethral injuries, it is recommended to wait for spontaneously voided urine before inserting a urinary catheter.

Contusions to the urethra do not require treatment unless the patient is unable to void, in which case a Foley catheter is carefully inserted. Minor tears can often be managed with suprapubic drainage for 10 to 14 days (McAleer & Kaplan, 1995). Severe tears and complete disruption of the urethra require surgical repair. Postoperative management includes insertion of a suprapubic catheter for urinary drainage.

Children who sustain urethral contusions usually heal without sequelae. Some urologists recommend a follow-up urethrogram 4 to 6 months after injury to exclude stricture formation. Potential complications of urethral tears include strictures, incontinence, and impotence. Patients with partial urethral tears require prompt recognition, and manipulation should be avoided to prevent complete tears and increased morbidity.

Genital Injury

Trauma to the external genitalia in females is uncommon. When it occurs, sexual abuse should always be considered (Grisoni, Hahn, Marsh, Volsko, & Dudgeon, 2000). Straddle injuries, falls, impalements, and motor vehicle accidents are other causes of injury.

Injury to the external genitalia in males may occur as the result of blunt trauma, such as falls or kicks, or from penetrating trauma, such as falls onto sharp objects. Zipper injuries are a common cause of injury to the penis. Testicular injury can occur when a child is hit or kicked in the scrotum.

Dysuria, discharge, and lower abdominal pain are common signs of genital injury. Isolated injuries are most often recognized by the parents because the child brought it to the parents attention. Careful inspection for the extent of injury and the presence of foreign bodies is necessary. The anal area should be examined for signs of trauma. Diagnostic studies are not required unless sexual or child abuse is suspected.

Small lacerations can be allowed to heal by secondary intention. Large lacerations require irrigation and suturing. Hematomas are usually self-limiting and respond to conservative treatment with rest and cold packs.

Pelvic Injury

Pelvic fracture is uncommon in children and occurs as a result of blunt trauma from motor vehicle–pedestrian accidents. Unlike in adults with pelvic fractures, mortality from massive hemorrhage or sepsis is unusual in children (Ismael, Bellemare, Mollitt, DiScala, Koeppel, & Tepas, 1996; Moront, Williams, Eichelberger, & Wilkinson, 1994). Death is most often a direct consequence of coexisting central nervous system injury (Koeppel & Tepas, 1996). The presence of multiple pelvic fractures is commonly associated with intraabdominal injury. Most children sustain an isolated pelvic fracture, with the occurrence of intraabdominal injury unlikely.

Nursing Management for the Child With Genitourinary Trauma

Nursing interventions for the child with genitourinary trauma are similar to those for abdominal trauma, in part because of multisystem trauma. Therefore only nursing interventions associated with renal failure related to genitourinary injury are discussed.

Alteration in Elimination

Children with genitourinary injury have altered urinary output related to impaired wound healing or renal parenchymal dysfunction. Nurses are primarily responsible for observing for signs of acute renal failure (ARF), which is characterized by a sudden decrease or loss of kidney function. The effects of ARF are seen in the inability of the kidneys to regulate water, electrolytes, acid-base balance, and waste products. The causes of ARF are divided into three groups: prerenal, intrarenal, and postrenal. ARF in the trauma victim is commonly a prerenal cause. Renal perfusion is compromised as a result of decreased intravascular volume secondary to hemorrhage without actual parenchymal damage. This leads to a severe reduction or loss of glomerular filtration rate.

Intrarenal failure can occur with injury to the cortex (outer layer) or to the medulla (middle layer). Figure 17-8 is a cross section of the kidney showing the structures of the kidney, including the medulla and cortex. The cortex is the vascular portion of the kidney. It contains glomeruli and the distal convoluted tubules of the nephrons. Injury occurs by vascular, infectious, or inflammatory processes, which result in swelling at the capillary bed. Injury to the medullary tissue of the kidneys results in damage to the collecting tubules, ducts, and loops of Henle of the nephrons. Nephrotoxic agents (i.e., aminoglycosides) or rhabdomyolysis are potential causes of injury. Rhabdomyolysis causes destruction of large muscles that release myoglobin into the circulation, resulting in tubular obstruction and ultimately renal failure. Prolonged prerenal or postrenal problems can result in parenchymal damage.

Postrenal failure results from an obstruction in the drainage system. Examples include ruptured bladder, disruption of a ureter or the urethra, pressure from hematomas, neurogenic bladder, and urinary tract infection.

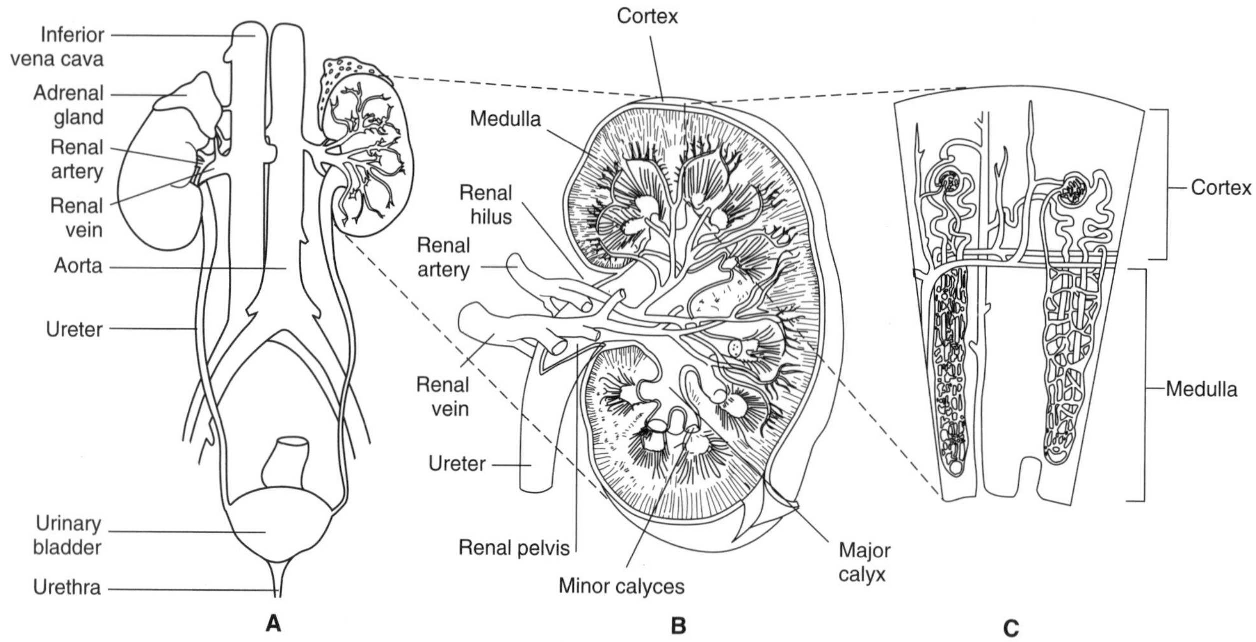

FIGURE 17-8 **A,** The urologic system. **B,** Cross section of the kidney. **C,** Nephrons in the renal cortex and medulla. (From Motts, S. R., James, S. R., & Sperhac, A. M. [1990]. *Nursing care of children and families* [2nd ed.]. Menlo Park, CA: Addison-Wesley.)

TABLE 17-5 Differential Diagnosis of Prerenal and Intrarenal Failure

Laboratory Values	Prerenal	Intrarenal
Urine specific gravity	>1.020	<1.010
Urine osmolality	High (>500)	Low (<300)
Urine sodium	<20 mEq/L	>40 mEq/L
Urinary sediment	Normal (hyaline casts)	Abnormal (cellular casts and debris)
BUN/creatinine ratio	20-40:1	10-15:1
FE_{NA}	≤1%	>1%

BUN, Blood urea nitrogen; FE_{NA}, fractional excretion of filtered sodium.

Nursing management includes monitoring for the development and progression of ARF. Laboratory data are characterized by a BUN greater than 40 mg/dl and a serum creatinine greater than 1.5 mg/dl. Differentiating between reversible prerenal or postrenal ARF and intrarenal failure resulting from renal parenchymal damage is important. Table 17-5 outlines the laboratory tests used to differentiate between prerenal and intrarenal failure and the kidney's ability to conserve sodium and concentrate urine.

ARF can lead to multiple organ insults and further intensify the complexity of patient care management. Thorough and frequent physical examinations are necessary to assess the progression of renal dysfunction. The child's mental status may be altered because of azotemia (excess of urea in the bloodstream) and electrolyte imbalances. Altered fluid volume may greatly affect the cardiovascular and respiratory systems. Intrarenal failure results in fluid overload and may cause congestive heart failure and respiratory failure if the fluid is not adequately removed. Signs and symptoms of fluid overload include increased blood pressure, pulses, cardiac output, and CVP (greater than 8 mm Hg); gallop on cardiac auscultation; crackles on respiratory auscultation; decreased level of consciousness; weight gain; and generalized edema. Prerenal failure results in low cardiac output secondary to hypovolemia and results in decreased perfusion to all body organs and ultimately multisystem failure if not treated adequately. Signs and symptoms of hypovolemia include decreased level of consciousness, blood pressure, pulses, CVP (less than 5 mm Hg), and capillary refill time; tachycardia; cool extremities; weight loss; dry mucous membranes; and poor skin turgor.

Management is aimed at restoring fluid balance and appropriate intravascular volume and correcting electrolyte imbalances and acidosis. Nursing interventions include closely monitoring intake and output, notifying the physician if urine output is less than 1 ml/kg/hr or if fluid intake greatly exceeds output, assessing patency of the urinary catheter, administering diuretics (e.g., furosemide), and monitoring patient response. Patients with ARF are at risk for electrolyte (i.e., hyperkalemia, hyperphosphatemia, hypocalcemia) and acid-base (i.e., metabolic acidosis) disturbances. Blood gases and electrolytes are monitored every 4 to 6 hours until their levels are stable. Patients with serum potassium concentration greater than 7.0 mEq/L and/or clinical signs of hyperkalemia, including peaked T waves or arrhythmias, should be treated emergently with sodium bicarbonate (1 to 3 mEq/kg), intravenous infusion of 1 to 2 ml/kg of 25% glucose and 0.1 U/kg of regular insulin, and 10 ml/kg of 10% calcium chloride. Kayexalate administered rectally is also ordered for patients with mild hyperkalemia; however, it is not effective in rapidly decreasing serum potassium in life-threatening hyperkalemia. Hyperphosphatemia (greater than 7.0 mmol/L) causes hypocalcemia, which can lead to neuromuscular or cardiovascular dysfunction. Significant hyperphosphatemia should be treated before the patient develops hypocalcemia. Treatment includes oral phosphate binders (e.g., calcium carbonate). Significant metabolic acidosis depresses enzymatic and cellular mitochondrial function and ultimately causes cardiovascular dysfunction. Mechanical ventilatory support with mild hyperventilation is important to buffer acidosis. Once adequate ventilation is ensured, sodium bicarbonate can be administered to treat the metabolic acidosis. It is important to note that sodium bicarbonate produces carbon dioxide and will worsen respiratory acidosis if ventilation is not adequate before sodium bicarbonate is administered. The dose of sodium bicarbonate usually is 1 mEq/kg or based on the base deficit (mEq sodium bicarbonate = base deficit × kg body weight × 0.3).

Nursing management includes treatment of hypertension secondary to hypervolemia and increased plasma renin activity. Severe hypertension can lead to neurologic complications such as hypertensive encephalopathy and cardiovascular compromise and therefore must be treated aggressively. Antihypertensive agents commonly administered include nifedipine (calcium channel blocker), sodium nitroprusside (vasodilator), labetalol (β-blocker), and furosemide (diuretic). Drugs and dosages are titrated based on the patient's response.

In the presence of renal dysfunction, drugs whose primary route of elimination is renal require adjustments in their dosages or intervals. Use of normal drug dosages in the face of renal dysfunction can result in toxicity.

If the child with ARF continues to deteriorate despite aggressive medical management, renal replacement therapies must be considered. Dialysis or hemofiltration is indicated for the child with uncontrolled hypervolemia, hypertension, hyperkalemia, hyperuricemia, or acidosis despite aggressive medical management. The reader is referred to the chapter Renal Critical Care Problems in the textbook *Critical Care Nursing of Infants and Children* (Grehn, Kline, & Weishaar, 2001) for an in-depth review of renal replacement therapies. Children with ARF present a unique challenge to nursing care secondary to the complexity of the multisystem complications and management.

SUMMARY

Although trauma is the leading cause of injury in children, abdominal and genitourinary trauma is relatively infrequent in children. Unrecognized injuries are associated with increased mortality and require close monitoring for signs of injury. Initial management is the same for all trauma victims and is tailored based on identified injuries. Nurses play a primary role in assessing and managing these patients and monitoring for complications to promote positive outcomes.

BIBLIOGRAPHY

Abdalati, H., Bulas, D. I., Sivit, C. J., Majd, D. M., Rushton, H. G., & Eichelberger, M. R. (1994). Blunt renal trauma in children: Healing of renal injuries and recommendations for imaging follow-up. *Pediatric Radiology, 24*(8), 573-576.

Albanese, C. T., Meza, M. P., Gardnes, M. J., Smith, S. D., Rime, M. I., & Lynes, J. M. (1996). Is computed tomography a useful adjunct to the clinical examination for the diagnosis of pediatric GI perforation from blunt abdominal trauma in children? *Journal of Trauma, 40*(3), 417-421.

Allshouse, M. J., & Betts, J. M. (1993). Genitourinary injury. In M. R. Eichelberger (Ed.), *Pediatric trauma: Prevention, acute care, and rehabilitation.* St. Louis: Mosby.

Barkin, R. M., & Marx, J. A. (1999). Abdominal trauma. In R. M Barkin & P. Rosen (Eds.), *Emergency pediatrics* (5th ed.). St. Louis: Mosby.

Benya, E. C., Bulas, D. I., Eichelberger, M. R., & Sivit, C. J. (1995). Splenic injury from blunt abdominal trauma in children: Follow-up evaluation with CT. *Radiology, 195*(3), 685-688.

Bond, S. J. (1993). Pelvic fracture and retroperitoneal hematoma. In M. R. Eichelberger (Ed.), *Pediatric trauma: Prevention, acute care, and rehabilitation.* St. Louis: Mosby.

Bond, S. J., Eichelberger, M. R., Gotschall, C. S., Sivit, C. J., & Randolph, J. G. (1996). Nonoperative management of blunt hepatic and splenic injury in children. *Annals of Surgery, 223*(3), 286-289.

Brown, S. L., Elder, J. S., & Spirank, J. P. (1998). Are pediatric patients more susceptible to major renal injury from blunt trauma? A comparative study. *Journal of Urology, 160*(1), 138-140.

Buntain, W. L. (1995). *Management of pediatric trauma.* Philadelphia: WB Saunders.

Cantor, R. M., & Learning J. M. (1998). Evaluation and management of pediatric major trauma. *Emergency Medical Clinics of North America, 16*(1), 229-256.

Coant, P. N., Kornberg, A. E., Brody, A. S., & Edwards-Holmes, K. (1992). Markers for occult liver injury in cases of physical abuse in children. *Pediatrics, 89*(2), 274-278.

Coburn, M. C., Pfeifer, J., & Deluca, F. G. (1995). Nonoperative management of splenic trauma and hepatic trauma in the multiply injured pediatric and adolescent patient. *Archives in Surgery, 130,* 332-338.

Coley, B. D., Mutabagani, K. H., Martin, L. C., Zumberge, N., Cooney, D. R., Caniano, D. A., Besner, G. E., Groner, J. I., & Shiels, W. E., II. (2000). Focused abdominal sonography for trauma (FAST) in children with blunt trauma. *Journal of Trauma: Injury, Infection, & Critical Care, 48*(5), 902-906.

Colucciello, S. A. (1993). Blunt abdominal trauma. *Emergency Medicine Clinics of North America, 11*(1), 107-123.

Cooper, A., Barlow, B., DiScala, C., & String, D. (1994). Mortality and truncal injury: The pediatric perspective. *Journal of Pediatric Surgery, 29*(1), 33-38.

Coran, A. G. (1993). Abdominal trauma. In E. J. Reisdorff, M. R. Roberts, & J. G. Wiegenstein (Eds.), *Pediatric emergency medicine.* Philadelphia: W.B. Saunders.

Cox, T. D., & Kuhn, J. P. (1996). CT scan of bowel trauma in the pediatric patient. *Radiologic Clinics of North America, 34*(4), 807-818.

Emery, K. (1997). Splenic emergencies. *Radiologic Clinics of North America, 35*(4), 831-843.

Fackler, J. C., Arnold, J. H., Nichols, D. G., & Rodgers, M. C. (1996). Acute respiratory distress syndrome. In M. C. Rodgers (Ed.), *Textbook of pediatric intensive care* (3rd ed.). Baltimore: Williams & Wilkins.

Fackler, J. C., Yaster, M., Davis, R. J., Tait, V. F., Dean, J. M., Goldberg, A. L., & Rodgers, M. (1999). Multiple trauma. In M. C. Rodgers & M. A. Helfaer (Eds.), *Handbook of pediatric intensive care* (3rd ed.). Baltimore: Williams & Wilkins.

Ford, E. G., & Senac, M. O. (1993). Clinical presentation and radiographic identification of small bowel rupture following blunt trauma in children. *Pediatric Emergency Care, 9*(3), 139-142.

Furnival, R. A., Woodward, G. A., & Shunck, J. (1996). Delayed diagnosis of injury in pediatric trauma. *Pediatrics, 98*(1), 56-62.

Garvin, G. (1997). Wound and skin care for the PICU. *Critical Care Nurse Quarterly, 20*(1), 62-71.

Gilbert, J. C., & Bailey, P. V. (1998). Abdominal trauma in pediatric critical care. In B. P. Fuhrman & J. J. Zimmerman (Eds.), *Pediatric critical care* (2nd ed.). St. Louis: Mosby.

Grehn, L. S., Kline, A., & Weishaar, J. (2001). Renal critical care problems. In M. A. Q. Curley & P. A. Moloney-Harmon (Eds.), *Critical care nursing of infants and children* (2nd ed., pp. 731-764). Philadelphia: WB Saunders.

Grisoni, E. R., Hahn, E., Marsh, E., Volsko, T., & Dudgeon, D. (2000). Pediatric perineal impalement injuries. *Journal of Pediatric Surgery, 35*(5), 702-704.

Haley, K. (1998). Multiple trauma management. In T. E. Soud & J. S. Rodgers (Eds.), *Manual of pediatric emergency nursing.* St. Louis: Mosby.

Haller, J. A. (1996). Blunt trauma to the abdomen. *Pediatrics in Review, 17*(1), 29-31.

Haller, J. A., Papa, P., Drugas, G., & Colombani, P. (1994). Nonoperative management of solid organ injuries in children. *Annals of Surgery, 219*(6), 625-631.

Hennes, H. M., Smith, D. S., Schneider, K., Hegenbarth, M. A., Duma, M. A., & Jona, J. Z. (1990). Elevated liver transaminase levels in children with blunt abdominal trauma: A predictor of liver injury. *Pediatrics, 86*(1), 87-90.

Ismael, N., Bellemare, J. P., Mollitt, D. L., DiScala, C., Koeppel, B., & Tepas, J. J., III. (1996). Death from pelvic fracture: Children are different. *Journal of Pediatric Surgery, 31*(1), 82-85.

Jurkovich, G. J., & Carrico, C. J. (1990). Pancreatic trauma. *Surgical Clinics of North America, 70*(3), 575-593.

Katz, S., Lazar, L., Rathaus, V., & Erez, I. (1996). Can ultrasonography replace computed tomography in the initial assessment of children with abdominal trauma? *Journal of Pediatric Surgery, 31*(5), 649-651.

Kirelik, S. B. (1999). Genitourinary trauma. In R. M. Barkin & P. Rosen (Eds.), *Emergency pediatrics* (5th ed.). St. Louis: Mosby.

Kudsk, K. A., Croce, M. A., Fabian, T. C., Tolley, E. A., Poret, H. A., Kuhl, M. R., & Brown, R. O. (1992). Enteral versus parenteral feeding: Effects on septic morbidity after blunt and penetrating trauma. *Annals of Surgery, 215*(5), 503-513.

Levins, T. I. (2000). The use of ultrasound in blunt trauma. *Journal of Emergency Nursing, 26*(1), 15-19.

Lynch, J. M., Albanese, C. T., Meza, M. P., & Weiner, E. S. (1996). Intestinal stricture following seal belt injury in children. *Journal of Pediatric Surgery, 31*(10), 1354-1357.

Marsden, C., & Jackimczyk, K. (1993). Genitourinary trauma. In E. J. Reisdorff, M. R. Roberts, & J. G. Wiegenstein (Eds.), *Pediatric emergency medicine.* Philadelphia: WB Saunders.

Marx, J. A. (1993). Penetrating abdominal trauma. *Emergency Medicine Clinics of North America, 11*(1), 125-135.

Marx, J. A. (1994). Abdominal trauma. In R. M. Barkin & P. Rosen (Eds.), *Emergency pediatrics: A guide to ambulatory care* (4th ed.). St. Louis: Mosby.

McAleer, I. M., & Kaplan, G. W. (1995). Pediatric genitourinary trauma. *Urologic Clinics of North America, 22*(1), 177-188.

McAleer, I. M., Kaplan, G. W., Packer, M. G., & Lynch, F. P. (1993). Genitourinary trauma in the pediatric patient. *Urology, 42*(5), 563-568.

McAnena, O. J., Marx, J. A., & Moore, E. E. (1991). Contribution of peritoneal lavage enzyme determinations to the management of isolated hollow visceral abdominal injuries. *Annals of Emergency Medicine, 20*(8), 834-837.

Moore, E. E., Cogbill, T. H., Malangoni, M. A., Jurkovich, G. J., Champion, H. R., Gennarelli, T. A., McAninch, J. W., Pachter, H. L., Shackford, S. R., & Trafton, P. G. (1990). Organ injury scaling II: Pancreas, duodenum, small bowel, colon, and rectum. *Journal of Trauma, 30*(11), 1427-1429.

Moore, E. E., Shackford, S. R., Pachter, H. L., McAninch, J. W., Browner, B. D., & Champion, H. R. (1989). Organ injury scaling: Spleen, liver, kidney. *Journal of Trauma, 29*(12), 1664-1666.

Moore, F., Feliciano, D., Andrassy, R., McArdle, A. H., Booth, F. V., Morgenstein-Wagner, T. B., Kellum, J. M., Welling, R. E., & Moore, E. E. (1992). Early enteral feedings, compared with parenteral reduces postoperative septic complications: The results of a meta-analysis. *Annals of Surgery, 216*(2), 172-183.

Morey, A. F. Bruce, J. E., & McAninch, J. W. (1996). Efficacy of radiographic imaging in pediatric blunt renal trauma. *Journal of Urology, 156*(6), 2014-2018.

Moront, M. L., Williams, J. A., Eichelberger, M. R., & Wilkinson, J. D. (1994). The injured child: An approach to care. *Pediatric Clinics of North America, 41*(6), 1201-1225.

Morse, M. A., & Garcia, V. F. (1994). Selective nonoperative management of pediatric blunt splenic trauma: Risk for missed associated injuries. *Journal of Pediatric Surgery, 29*(1), 23-27.

Newman, K. D. (1993). Gastric and intestinal injury. In M. R. Eichelberger (Ed.), *Pediatric trauma: Prevention, acute care, and rehabilitation.* St. Louis: Mosby.

Newman, K. D., Bowman, L. M., Eichelberger, M. R., Gotschall, C. S., Taylor, G. A., Johnson, D. L., & Thomas, N. (1990). The lap belt complex: Intestinal and lumbar spine injury in children. *Journal of Trauma, 30*(9), 1133-1140.

Nordenholz, K. E., Rubin, M. A., Gularte, G. G., & Liang, H. K. (1997). Ultrasound in the evaluation and management of blunt abdominal trauma. *Annals of Emergency Medicine, 29*(3), 357-366.

Orsborn, R., Haley, K., Hammond, S., & Falcone, R. E. (1999). Pediatric pedestrian versus motor vehicle patterns of injury: debunking the myth. *Air Medical Journal, 18*(3), 107-109.

Osberg, J. S., & DiScala, C. (1992). Morbidity among pediatric motor vehicle crash victims: The effect of seat belts. *American Journal of Public Health, 82*(3), 422-425.

Pearl, W. S., & Todd, K. H. (1996). Ultrasonography for the initial evaluation of blunt abdominal trauma: A view of prospective trials. *Annals of Emergency Medicine, 27*(3), 353-361.

Pieper, P. (1994). Pediatric trauma: An overview. *Nursing Clinics of North America, 29*(4), 563-584.

Polhgeers, A., & Ruddy, R. M. (1995). An update on pediatric trauma. *Emergency Medicine Clinics of North America, 13*(2), 267-1364.

Pranikoff, T., Hirschl, R. B., Schlesinger, A. E., Polley, T. Z., & Coran, A. G. (1994). Resolution of splenic injury after nonoperative management. *Journal of Pediatric Surgery, 29*(10), 1366-1369.

Reisman, J., Naitoh, J., & Morgan, A. S. (1993). Genitourinary trauma. *Topics in Emergency Medicine, 15*(2), 22-39.

Rescorla, F. J., & Grosfeld, J. L. (1993). Pancreatic injury. In M. R. Eichelberger (Ed.), *Pediatric trauma: Prevention, acute care, and rehabilitation.* St. Louis: Mosby.

Rothrock, S. G., Green, S. M., & Morgan, R. (2000a). Abdominal trauma in infants and children: Prompt identification and early management of serious and life threatening injuries. Part 1: Injury patterns and initial assessment. *Pediatric Emergency Care, 16*(2), 106-115.

Rothrock, S. G., Green, S. M., & Morgan, R. (2000b). Abdominal trauma in infants and children: Prompt identification and early management of serious and life threatening injuries. Part II: specific injuries and ED management. *Pediatric Emergency Care, 16*(3), 189-195.

Rowe, M. I. (1995). *Essentials of pediatric surgery.* St. Louis: Mosby.

Sahdev, P., Garramone, R. R., Jr., Schwartz, R. J., Steelman, S. R., & Jacobs, L. M. (1991). Evaluation of liver function tests in screening for intra-abdominal injuries. *Annals of Emergency Medicine, 20*(8), 238-241.

Sanchez, J. I., & Paidas, C. N. (1999). Trauma care in the new millennium. *Surgical Clinics of North America, 79*(6), 1505-1535.

Schafermeyer, R. (1993). Pediatric trauma. *Emergency Medicine Clinics of North America, 11*(1), 187-205.

Scorpio, R. J., & Wesson, D. E. (1993). Splenic trauma. In M. R. Eichelberger (Ed.), *Pediatric trauma: Prevention, acute care, and rehabilitation.* St. Louis: Mosby.

Shafi, S., Gilbert, J. C., Carden, S., Allen, J. E., Glick, P. L., Caty, M. G., & Azizkhan, R. G. (1997). Risk of hemorrhage and appropriate use of blood transfusions in pediatric blunt splenic injuries. *Journal of Trauma, 42*(6), 1029-1032.

Siegel, M. J., & Sivit, C. J. (1997). Pancreatic emergencies. *Radiologic Clinics of North America, 35*(4), 815-830.

Stauffer, U. G. (1995). Surgical and critical care management of children with life-threatening injuries. *Journal of Pediatric Surgery, 30*(7), 903-910.

Stechmiller, J. K., Treloar, D., & Allen, N. (1997). Gut dysfunction in critically ill patients: A review of the literature. *American Journal of Critical Care, 6*(3), 204-209.

Stylianos, S. (1995). Controversies in abdominal trauma. *Seminars in Pediatric Surgery, 4*(2), 116-119.

Stylianos, S. (1998). Late sequelae of major trauma in children. *Pediatric Clinics of North America, 45*(4), 853-859.

Taylor, G. A., Eichelberger, M. R., O'Donnell, R., & Bowman, L. (1991). Indications for computed tomography in children with blunt trauma. *Annals of Surgery, 213*(3), 212-218.

Torres, A. M., & Garcia, V. F. (1993). Hepatobiliary trauma. In M. R. Eichelberger (Ed.), *Pediatric trauma: Prevention, acute care, and rehabilitation.* St. Louis: Mosby.

Trocki, O., Michelini, A., Robbins, S. T., & Eichelberger, M. R. (1995). Evaluation of early enteral feeding in children less than 3 years old with smaller burns (8-25 per cent TBSA). *Burns, 21*(1), 17-23.

Turnock, R. R., Sprigg, A., & Lloyd, D. A. (1993). Computed tomography in the management of blunt abdominal trauma in children. *British Journal of Surgery, 80*(8), 982-984.

Udobi, K. F., Rudriquez, A., Chiu, W. C., & Scalea, T. M. (2001). The role of ultrasonography in penetrating abdominal trauma: A prospective clinical study. *Journal of Trauma: Injury, Infection & Critical Care, 50*(3), 475-479.

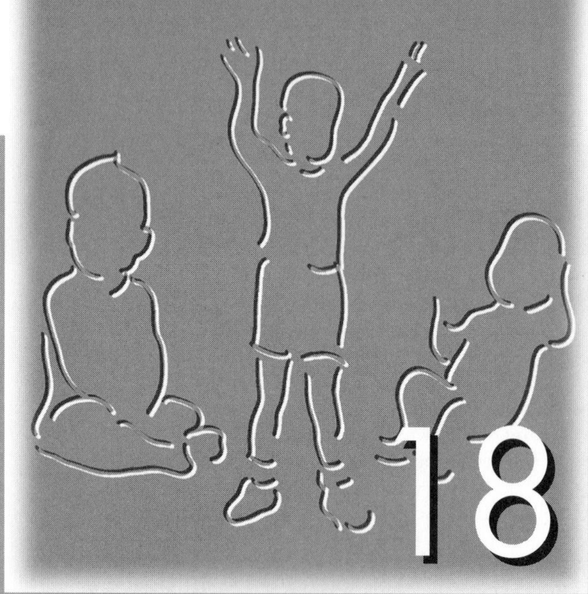

18 Pediatric Musculoskeletal Trauma

Kimberly J. Mason

Musculoskeletal trauma includes injury to the soft tissues and bones of the extremities, as well as bony injury to the spinal column and pelvis. The diagnosis and management of musculoskeletal trauma are challenging.

The musculoskeletal system serves several essential functions, including the means for mechanical support and protection for other body systems and vital organs, a source of essential minerals, a locus for the production of blood components, and the means for locomotion and manipulation (Valadian, Porter, Carroll, & Neuhauser, 1977). The musculoskeletal system is composed of five different types of tissue, each with different physiologic and biomechanical properties: muscle, tendon, ligament, cartilage, and bone. These tissues are often in direct contact with each other, and the interface of different tissue is often an area vulnerable to injury. Because the bones are enveloped in soft tissue, injury to the bone usually includes injury to soft tissues.

SCOPE OF PROBLEM

Childhood trauma is secondary only to acute infection as leading cause of morbidity. The largest proportion of childhood injuries are sprains (39.1%), followed by lacerations (35.4%), fractures excluding the skull (12.0%), intracranial injuries (4.7%), internal injuries (0.2%), and other injuries (8.6%) (Loder, Warschausky, Schwartz, Hensinger, & Greenfield, 1995). In reality, the problem is probably much larger because these statistics are based on injuries that are reported. Many injuries to the musculoskeletal system, such as strains or contusions, may go uncounted because they are managed without contact with a health care provider.

Boys have significantly higher risk for injury than girls do in nearly all age groups (Schiedt et al., 1995). The greatest differences occur during the adolescent years, when boys 13 to 17 years are 1.85 times more likely to be injured than girls in the same age group. Young children have the lowest overall rate and proportion of serious injury (17.1%), whereas adolescents 14 to 17 years have the highest overall rate and proportion of serious injuries (38.7%). Of all injuries, 44% occur at home and 19% at school. Falling, being struck, or being cut with an object accounts for approximately half of all reported causes of injury. Injuries involving sports or recreation, bikes, skates, or transportation accounted for a considerable proportion. Younger school-age children (5 to 8 years) are at particular risk for injury related to playground equipment, despite safety standard measures to reduce the risk for falls, which are the cause of 93% of playground injuries (Roseveare, Brown, McIntosh, & Chalmers, 1999).

Considering pediatric musculoskeletal trauma overall, injuries to the upper extremity are more common than injuries to the lower extremity. Most pediatric fractures occur in the upper extremity, with fractures of the distal forearm being the most common fracture in childhood (Cheng, Ng, Ying, & Lam, 1999; Landin, 1997; Lyons et al., 1999). Most upper extremity injuries are managed in ambulatory settings or in the emergency department and do not require hospitalization. Injuries to the upper extremities are of particular concern because injuries to the upper limb may affect prehensile functioning, fine movements, and important sensory requirements (Gershuni, 1985).

There is increasing concern that intentional injuries to children are underreported. In children with intentional injuries, 51% present with a cutaneous injury (excluding burns) and 17% present with a fracture (Sinal & Stewart, 1998). Up to 55% of abused children have fractures, and more than half of those have multiple fractures. Of fractures in abused children, 8% are found in infants younger than 18 months, but only 2% of accidental fractures are found in this age group. In fact, 85% of fractures in nonabused children occur in those older than 5 years. The most common child abuse fracture is the diaphyseal fracture.

CHALLENGES FOR THE ACUTE CARE NURSE

Considering the frequency of musculoskeletal injuries, a fairly small proportion of patients require hospitalization. Children hospitalized with musculoskeletal trauma generally need a surgical procedure or have serious injuries with a high risk for complications. In addition, musculoskeletal injuries are often part of the constellation of injuries in a child with multisystem injuries. A child with multisystem injuries may need treatment for a musculoskeletal injury that is normally managed in an acute care setting. Even though the musculoskeletal injury may not be the most significant injury, it will affect the care of the child. Musculoskeletal injury has been shown to have a high rate of long-term morbidity, second only to head injury (Wesson et al., 1992).

ANATOMIC AND PHYSIOLOGIC CONCERNS

TENDONS

Tendons are fibrous bands of connective tissue that connect muscle to bone. Collagen is the major constituent of tendons, with a relative paucity of cells (Woo, An, Arnoczky, Wayne, Fithian, & Meyers, 1994). Tendons receive blood supply from vessels in the perimysium, the insertion on the periosteum of the bone and the surrounding tissue. Tendons are sheathed in delicate fibroelastic connective tissues, except at the point of attachment. A tendon may cross a joint for effective origin or insertion of muscles. Tendons have one of the highest tensile strengths of any soft tissue in the body, in part because of collagen and in part because of the arrangement of collagen fibers parallel to tensile force (Woo et al., 1994). Although tendons are strong and flexible, they are relatively inelastic. If a tendon is stretched outside of its range of motion, the fibers or the entire tendon can be torn. Tendons in children are more elastic than those in adults because the stiffness of tendons increases with age.

LIGAMENTS

Ligaments attach bone to bone. Ligaments consist of fibrous bands. They bind joints together and bind bone and cartilage. A primary component is collagen, a unique protein with very high tensile strength that is mainly responsible for the mechanical strength of the soft connective tissues (Woo, Gomez, & Akeson, 1985). Slightly elastic, ligaments stretch to permit joint motion, but they are designed for stability. Ligaments and tendons are capable of supporting very large forces with minimal deformation.

In ligament trauma, failure mechanisms are related to the rate of loading (Woo et al., 1985). A slow rate of loading causes avulsion failure at the ligament insertion to the bone. A rapid rate of loading will cause a midsubstance tear. Joint injuries, dislocations, and ligamentous disruptions are less common in young children, whose ligaments are more elastic. Ligaments grow increasingly stiff with age; by the school-age and adolescent years, joint injuries become more common.

MUSCLES

Muscle tissue makes up the largest portion of the body, and its growth dominates that of the body as a whole (Valadian, Porter, Carroll, & Neuhauser, 1977). Skeletal muscle is responsible for voluntary movement. Muscles also protect joint structures from injury (Kirkendall & Garrett, 1999). Muscle tissue grows by cell hypertrophy, not cellular replication. Muscle tissue does not consist solely of muscle fibers; it also contains connective tissue that carries blood vessels, nerves, and lymphatic channels, which are essential for nourishing and controlling the muscle. Growth and development of muscle tissue are influenced by a complex set of factors that involve hormones, metabolism, and the environment. Although it generally is thought that the number of muscles fibers does not increase after birth, there is evidence that some postnatal increase in fiber number may occur (Valadian et al., 1977).

Although trauma to muscle has far less serious consequences than injury to bone, joints, or ligaments, if muscle tissue is damaged, it can have a functional and cosmetic impact. Muscles are virtually always involved when injury to an extremity occurs (Howard, Porat, Bar-On, Nyska, & Segal, 1998). Muscle strain injuries occur at the muscle-tendon junction (Kirkendall & Garrett, 1999), where the interface of two different tissues is vulnerable because of their different biomechanical properties.

Injuries to muscles can cause nerve and vascular injury. In addition, all fractures and dislocations, especially those produced by high-impact injuries, result in vascular injury. Vascular injuries can range from compression or occlusion to puncture or laceration by bone fragments. Vascular injuries associated with most musculoskeletal trauma rarely require vascular surgical repair, although missed or delayed diagnosis of significant vascular injury can lead to a high complication rate. Severed nerve endings do not regenerate, although some can be repaired surgically. Injured nerves may recover, but the process is very slow. Muscles may atrophy before the nerve can recover, so the child may still have poor function.

JOINTS

Joints are a crucial part of the musculoskeletal system. A joint is a junction between two or more bones. Some joints are movable; some are immovable. Joints are classically enclosed by a fibrous capsule, which contains protective fluid. In the appendicular skeleton, which is composed primarily of movable joints, the joint surfaces are protected by articular cartilage. Articular cartilage lines the ends of long bones and acts as a cushion for joint movement.

Cartilage is a nonvascular supporting connective tissue comprised of various cells and fibers. Articular cartilage has poor ability for repair and healing. In addition to lacking blood vessels, cartilage lacks undifferentiated cells within the tissue that can participate in the repair process (Mankin, Mow, Buckwalter, Iannotti, & Ratcliffe, 1994). The majority of joints in the body, and those most commonly injured, are freely movable diarthroses. The articular surfaces in hinge joints are held together and guided by ligaments.

Normal joint motion depends on the strength and integrity of the muscle and on the normal interaction of its surfaces and controls (Frank, Amiel, Woo, & Akeson, 1985). Injury to the joint structure can lead to mechanical dysfunction and ultimately to joint degeneration. Less mobile joints have greater intrinsic stability and are relatively resistant to external forces (Frank et al., 1985). The more rigid the joint, the more likely it is to sustain high-energy injury through either fracture or a combination of fracture and dislocation; this results because the joint cannot compensate for traumatic forces by moving. Peripheral joints are more predisposed to repetitive trauma, particularly with common activities. Peripheral joints suffer acute types of injuries, such dislocations, with various combinations of damage to bones and soft tissues, particularly ligaments. Failure to restore joint anatomy and function acutely leads to deterioration of the joint over time.

Unique Characteristics of Musculoskeletal System in Children

Active Growth Plate

Children's bones have are actively growing. The physis, or growth place, which is located between the metaphysis and the epiphysis, is the center of longitudinal bone growth. The physis is composed of cartilage cells that are converted to bone. Cartilage cells grow continually on the side of the physis facing the epiphysis of a long bone. Cartilage on the metaphyseal side continually breaks down and is replaced by bone (Canale, 1998). The cartilage cells of the physis are permanently converted to bone during adolescence, under the influence of hormones, so the physis does not exist in the bones of older adolescents or adults. Once the physis cells are converted to bone, the physis is "closed" and longitudinal bone growth is no longer possible. In females the physis closes about 1 year after the first menstrual period. Males will not achieve skeletal maturity until their late teens, which is why males are generally taller and have heavier skeletons.

Because the junction between the metaphysis and the physis is a junction between bone and cartilage, it is a vulnerable interface. Injuries to the physis can have long-term consequences for the growth of the bone, depending on the age of the child and how much growth is remaining. Injury to the growth plate can cause length discrepancies or angular deformities if one area of the physis is damaged and stops growing but the rest of the physis keeps growing normally.

The epiphysis is a secondary ossification center at the end of long bones. The epiphyses are important for bone growth. At birth, most epiphyses are completely cartilaginous structures. The epiphyses gradually become ossified over the growing years, and they are completely bone at skeletal maturity. The sequence of ossification and the pattern of development for each bone are universal, but the rate at which skeletal maturation proceeds varies from person to person (Valadian et al., 1977). When the epiphysis is completely cartilaginous, in young children, the physis is almost completely protected from injury (Jones, 1998) because the cartilage of the epiphysis can absorb some of the energy from a traumatic force. In the school-age child, more of the epiphysis is ossified, so the physis is more vulnerable to injury. When the epiphysis is nearly all bone, it is subject to bony injury.

Rapid Healing

Bone healing in children is usually rapid, primarily because of the thickened, extremely osteogenic periosteum (Jones, 1998). In children the periosteum is a thick biologically active layer with a good blood supply that plays a role in the circumferential growth of bones. It may remain intact with bony injury so that the blood supply to the bone is maintained, which enhances healing. In addition, pediatric bone is penetrated by more vascular channels than adult bone (Jones, 1998) and has a steady supply of nutrients and minerals. Because the mechanisms for bone growth are active in children, the components and mechanisms for bone healing are readily at hand when injury occurs.

The age of the child directly affects the rate of healing of any fracture. The younger the child is, the more rapidly the fracture heals. In the newborn a femoral shaft fracture heals in 3 or 4 weeks, whereas in an adolescent the same fracture heals in 12 to 16 weeks. As the child ages, the healing rate approaches that of an adult (Jones, 1998).

Rapid healing affects the management of bony injury, when compared with adults. Young children, who heal quickly because of their active growth and a ready supply of blood and nutrients, can be treated with casts for relatively short periods. Treatment modalities such as internal fixation are not necessary to provide stabilization for a long duration. Adolescents, whose musculoskeletal structures are approaching maturity, need to be immobilized for longer periods and may require more intensive rehabilitation because of the stiffness of tendons and ligaments.

Bones Are More Plastic

Bone tissue in young children is weaker when measured by bending strength and less stiff than bone tissue in adults (Currey & Butler, 1975). A lower ash content and increased porosity indicate less mineralization, such that the bone has increased plasticity and less energy is needed for bone failure (Wilber & Thompson, 1998). The pediatric skeletal system can absorb more energy before fracture than adult bone. Young bone has the ability to undergo plastic deformation before breaking (Currey & Butler, 1975). The mineral content will change as the child matures so that by skeletal maturity, the ratio is the same as that of an adult.

As children grow and mature, the tissues in the musculoskeletal system acquire the same properties as those of an adult. Mineralization in bone increases so that bones become harder. Soft tissues such as tendons and ligaments become less resilient so that injury to tendon and ligament occurs more commonly in adults than in children.

Healing Bones Tend to Overgrow

Injuries in certain parts of long bones can result in increased growth, so a bone with a healed fracture will be longer than the contralateral, uninjured side. Fractures in children 7 to 13 years seem to have fairly constant overgrowth of 1 cm, regardless of age, whereas fractures in patients older than 13 years do not overgrow (Stephens, Hsu, & Leong, 1989). Longitudinal overgrowth is thought to be attributable to the vascularity associated with healing rather than a compensatory mechanism (Stephens et al., 1989). Most overgrowth occurs in the first 18 months after the injury. The tendency toward overgrowth is considered when treating bony injuries.

Remodeling Potential

Bone is a living tissue that responds to biomechanical forces. As bone is subjected to the stresses of use during normal activity, it remodels appropriately for those activities by laying down bone in areas of stress and removing bone from low-stress areas. In children, bone tissue is undergoing constant modeling and remodeling to accommodate growth and changing physical demands. Because it is actively modeling and remodeling, a child's bone will remodel significantly faster than an adult's bone after a bony injury. Therefore a less-than-perfect alignment of bone fragments can be accepted in certain situations.

The potential for remodeling after a fracture depends on the age of the child, the distance from the end of the bone, and the amount of angulation of the fracture fragments. Remodeling occurs far less readily, if at all, for rotational deformity and any angular deformity that is not in the plane of the joint. Most bone remodeling occurs in the metaphyseal region of bone after fracture (Jones, 1998). The younger the child is, the greater is the amount of remodeling that can be expected.

GENERAL MANAGEMENT OF MUSCULOSKELETAL INJURIES

Regardless of the type of the type of tissue injured, most musculoskeletal injuries are treated based on similar principles with a potential for similar problems. For the most part, the care and management of the different tissues cannot be separated. Management of musculoskeletal injuries includes immobilization and/or stabilization of injured tissues, neurovascular assessment and management, pain management, mobilization, discharge planning, and rehabilitation.

Immobilization and/or Stabilization

Most kinds of musculoskeletal injury require some form of immobilization to permit healing, although different tissues may heal differently. There is increasing evidence that long-term immobilization is actually detrimental to the healing of tendon and ligament (Woo et al., 1994). However, when these tissues are injured in conjunction with bone, the extremity will be immobilized to facilitate healing of the bony injury. Treatment modalities for musculoskeletal injury range from comfort measures such as rest, ice, compression, and elevation (RICE) to surgical intervention and the placement of internal fixation. Treatment modalities can be used across the continuum of care, alone or in combination.

Methods of Immobilization and/or Stabilization

Rest, Ice, Compression, and Elevation. Rest is necessary to prevent continued injury to soft tissues and to allow time for healing. Ice is used to promote vasoconstriction of injured blood vessels and to minimize edema. The inflammatory response plays a role in the healing of tissues, but excessive swelling can cause a injury to neurovascular structures. Compression is used to limit swelling. Compression can be applied by an elastic bandage, a splint, or in some cases, a cast. Elevation of the injured extremity above the level of the heart uses gravity to increase the flow of blood and fluids back to the central system. RICE should be continued for at least 48 to 72 hours after the injury is sustained.

Soft Goods. Soft goods are used to provide comfort and occasional immobilization of a soft tissue injury. In some cases they provide stabilization and support for healing tissues. Soft goods include items such as slings and knee immobilizers. Soft goods are generally not used for long-term immobilization of bony injuries in children, although there are some exceptions. A shoulder immobilizer may be used for certain types of humerus fractures because of the location of the injury and the speed of healing. An advantage of soft goods is that they can be loosened or removed for skin assessment and care. On the downside, however, they do not control motion in all planes, and their ease of removal is a major disadvantage for use in children, who do not always follow directions.

Traction. Traction is the application of a pulling force, generally along the long axis of a bone. Traction can be used to reduce a fracture or dislocation or to maintain alignment of fracture fragments during healing. For patients with musculoskeletal trauma, skin traction is generally used as an interim measure in preparation for more definitive treatment, such as casting or surgery. In the past, skeletal traction was used as a definitive treatment, with the child remaining in traction until the bone healed. Because of the changing economics of health care and the high cost of inpatient care, it is used most often as an interim measure until the child is stable enough for casting or surgery.

Traction permits access to most, if not all, of the skin. The conscious child has some in-bed mobility, even while he or she is in traction. However, even though the child has full range of motion of almost all body parts, a child in traction is at risk for the complications of immobility. Patients in traction need careful skin assessment because they undergo extended periods of supine positioning. In some children, helping maintain good position and alignment while they are in traction may be more challenging that preventing skin breakdown.

A child in skeletal traction requires care of the pin sites, where the skeletal pin pierces the skin. Pin care is controversial, ranging from no cleansing to frequent cleansing with antiseptic solutions such as half-strength hydrogen peroxide. Although the studies have been small, there is no clear evidence to support aggressive cleaning of pin sites (Goldberger, Kruse, & Stender, 1987; Jones-Walton, 1988; Sproles, 1985). Pin sites are assessed for signs of infection, including redness, tenderness, and purulent drainage. Patients have some serous drainage from pin sites, which serves as a lubricant for the tissue sliding over the pin. The amount of drainage varies, depending on the amount of soft tissue movement over the pin and the motion of joints near the pin. Drainage can be managed by covering the pin sites with gauze squares or wrapping the pins with soft bandage roll. Serosanguineous drainage may be noted from the pin sites if the pin is jostled or banged.

Casting. Casts are the most common type of musculoskeletal immobilization used in children. Casting provides a rigid external shell that helps control the displacement of fracture fragments by a hydraulic effect on the soft tissue envelope around the bone (Gershuni, 1985). Casts are used to provide temporary immobilization to maintain, support, and protect realigned bone and to promote healing and early weight bearing. Casts also allow early mobility, whether mobilization consists of the child getting out of bed to a chair because fracture fragments are stabilized or the child learning to ambulate safely with crutches because an injury is protected by a hard cast. In general, a cast incorporates the joint above and below the fracture to provide rotational stability to the fracture fragments (Gershuni, 1985). As previously discussed, rotational malalignment of the fracture fragments will not remodel, resulting in a permanent problem.

Most casts are made of synthetic casting materials. Synthetic casting materials make a strong, light cast, which dries very quickly and often is ready for weight bearing within 15 to 20 minutes. Synthetic casting materials do not require any special positioning or handling once they are dry. Synthetic casting material also comes in an array of colors and patterns, which can make it more acceptable to children.

Plaster casts do have some advantages over synthetic casts. Plaster casting provides better molding to body contours and absorbs bloody drainage. Because synthetic casts may be less able to accommodate swelling than plaster, synthetic casts can increase the risk for compartment syndrome and pressure injury to the skin under the cast (Davids, Frick, Skewes, & Blackhurst, 1997). Plaster casts dry slowly, requiring attention to positioning and handling of the cast, which is the major disadvantage.

Although casts are commonly used, they are not the first choice for immobilization in some situations. Because the cast is applied over the entire extremity, skin assessment and wound care is not possible. Although surgical wounds are not a problem because they are created and covered under the controlled conditions of an operating room, traumatic injuries generally require more active intervention. Casts may cause skin problems, the most minor being skin irritation at the cast edges and the most severe being full-thickness pressure ulcers over bony prominences under the cast. Neurovascular assessments are complicated by a cast because distal pulses usually are not palpable. A cast should be used only with extreme caution in an unconscious patient because the patient cannot clearly communicate discomfort or pain, which is the first sign of a problem beneath the cast.

Depending on the type of cast, mobility and activities of daily living may be difficult. Showering, bathing, and washing one's hair may be hampered by the cast. The cast should not get wet because the cast padding is difficult to dry. Children with long leg casts may need assistance with ambulation. The patient may have difficulty riding in a car or returning to school because of the size and/or location of the cast.

External Fixation. An external fixator consists of a rigid external bar or frame attached to metal pins inserted into the bone. The configuration of the external fixation device attached to the skeletal pins provides a rigid external support structure. Pins are inserted through a skin incision to prevent pulling or tenting of the skin at the pin site. External fixators are used to provide anatomic reduction of bony fragments, particularly fragments, which cannot be adequately stabilized in a cast. The skeletal pins can "spear" each fragment and fix the position once attached to the external bar or frame. External fixators are generally applied in the operating room with the patient under general anesthesia, although they can be applied at the bedside with adequate sedation in critical situations.

Generally accepted indications for external fixation include pelvic fractures; high-energy open fractures, usually of the tibia; multiple injuries involving the head, thorax, and abdomen; and failure of conservative treatment where it was not possible to maintain alignment or reduction by traction or casting (Hull & Bell, 1997). External fixators are also particularly useful for the patient who has a soft tissue injury because the extremity is uncovered. External fixators can be used in the treatment of traumatic bone loss and bone length discrepancies. Complications of external fixation includes pin tract infections, delayed fracture healing, refracture when the pins are removed, limb overgrowth, and joint stiffness, although this is less problematic than in adults.

External fixators permit good patient mobility. External fixators do not restrict joint motion and permit early mobility. Depending on surgeon preference, patients may be permitted to shower or bathe with an external fixator, which may not be possible with a cast. Depending on the location of the external fixator, patients may have difficulty using a toilet or finding clothing. Patients learn pin site assessment and care, which is similar to the care of skeletal pins used for traction. In general, pin site care at home does not require sterile supplies because of the decreased risk for nosocomial infection.

Halo Immobilization. A halo is a circular ring attached to the skull with special skeletal pins. It is designed to penetrate the outer layers of the skull but no other tissues, such as the dura mater. The circular halo ring is connected to four posts that are attached to a vest that is worn over the torso. The vest usually consists of two pieces of molded plastic that are connected at the sides with straps and lined with real or synthetic sheepskin. A halo is used to immobilize the cervical spine after bony or ligamentous injury. A halo limits almost 95% of cervical spine motion (Garfin & Katz, 1985).

Sometimes referred to as *halo traction,* halo immobilization can be considered a type of external fixation because pins are inserted into bone through soft tissue and connected to an external stabilizing device. The position of the head is fixed in relation to the shoulders and torso so that proper alignment of the cervical spine is maintained. Patients in a halo need to be assessed for cervical nerve impingement or a stretch injury to the lower cranial nerves (Jobes, 1982).

Although patients can be mobile while they are in a halo vest, they may find daily activities difficult because of the fixed position of the head and torso. Some children need assistance with ambulation because of the weight and size of the halo apparatus. In addition, some children have difficulty sleeping, bathing, dressing, and finding appropriate clothing. Although showers and tub baths are prohibited, washing one's hair over the sink or tub is permitted, depending on the surgeon's preference.

Surgery. Although most children's fractures can be managed without operative techniques, increasing surgical management of children's fractures is due to improved technology, the ability to use minimal or short-term internal fixation, and financial pressures (Wilkins, 1998). Surgical management is considered standard treatment for certain injuries, such as certain epiphyseal and articular fractures; displaced supracondylar elbow fractures; femur and tibia fractures, especially in a child with multiple injuries; or severe vascular injury associated with a fracture (Chung, 1986).

Not all children who undergo surgery for management of a musculoskeletal injury have an incision. A child may go to the operating room for closed reduction of a fracture, open reduction of a fracture, internal fixation of a fracture, or wound management. Fracture reduction is the manipulation of bone fragments to realign the bone. When a closed reduction is done, the fragments are manipulated without making an incision. Although this usually is done with sedation in the emergency department or an outpatient setting, the child may require general anesthesia because careful manipulation or fluoroscopic imaging is needed to visualize the position of the bone fragments. During an open reduction, a surgical incision is made to permit direct manipulation of the fragments. If the fragments cannot be adequately stabilized, a stabilizing device, such as internal fixation or external fixation, may be needed.

Internal fixation is the application of hardware directly onto the bone. There are numerous types of hardware, ranging from pins to screws, to plates on the outside of the bone, to rods and nails that are inserted into the marrow cavity. Internal fixation is usually not necessary to manage bony injury in children because most pediatric fractures consist of two large fragments that heal readily when they are stabilized in a cast. Internal fixation may be required when the fracture is comminuted or when the child cannot tolerate another treatment modality because of other injuries or medical conditions. Historically, hardware used for internal fixation in children was removed in a second operation because of concerns about the safety of implants left in situ for a lifetime (Black, 1988; Kahle, 1994). With advances in the composition and design of internal fixation devices, removal of hardware may cease to be common practice.

Neurovascular Concerns

Precise and sequential assessments of the neurovascular status of the injured extremity are important to evaluate the status of the tissues and to minimize complications. Neurovascular injury in musculoskeletal trauma can be caused by direct trauma to the soft tissues or by bone fragments moving within the extremity. Injury can also be caused by surgical intervention or severe swelling. In some cases the child may suffer neurovascular injury at the time of injury, or neurovascular compromise may develop as edema progresses, with the risk for development of a compartment syndrome. Elevating the extremity above the level of the heart can help control swelling in an injured extremity. Attention to neurovascular status is an essential part of caring for a patient with musculoskeletal injury because a delay in treatment can result in permanent deficit.

A complete neurovascular assessment includes an assessment of color, temperature, capillary refill, edema, pulses, sensation, and pain (Box 18-1). Neurovascular assessments continue until at least 48 hours after injury, when edema has

BOX 18-1 Neurovascular Assessment

Color

Pink, pale, cyanotic, mottled

Temperature

Warm, cool, cold

Capillary refill

Rapid, sluggish, absent (measured in seconds)

Edema

Absent, mild, moderate, pitting

Pulses

Strong, weak, not palpable, audible by Doppler

Sensation

Normal, hyperesthetic (increased sensation, tingling), hypoesthetic (decreased sensation)

Pain

Constant, intermittent, sharp, dull, burning, aching, with activity, at rest peaked. Sequential assessments are important to detect subtle changes that require intervention. Nerve function is assessed by evaluating motion and sensation. Capillary refill is a good screening tool for circulation, but pulses should be palpated whenever possible or auscultated by Doppler if necessary.

Fractures with an obvious deformity and lacking pulse or motion are reduced emergently without radiographs. Neurovascular assessment should be recorded before and after splinting. Fractures with neurovascular deficit are often reduced in the operating room because open reduction and internal fixation of the fracture fragments may be necessary. Exploration of vessels or nerves may be needed if function does not improve after stabilization. Careful neurovascular assessment continues postoperatively. Referral to physical and occupational therapy should be initiated promptly. The child and family will need ongoing support because the long-term prognosis of a vascular or neurologic injury may be difficult to predict in the immediate postoperative period.

Pain Management

Analgesics and Comfort Measures. Musculoskeletal injuries are painful because of damaged tissue, stretched or injured nerves, ischemia, or surgical wounds. The movement of fracture fragments impinges on soft tissues. Injured muscles tend to spasm. Pain does not automatically stop with fracture reduction and immobilization, although the pain of a fracture should be reduced once the bone fragments are stabilized. Immobilization itself can cause discomfort because of stiffness and the inability of the patient to easily shift position for comfort. Immobility may also limit the patient's ability for self-distraction through activity.

The child's pain should be assessed using an age-appropriate tool, such as the faces scale for young children or a numerical scale for older children. Most children with severe musculoskeletal injury require opiates for pain. Initially, pain medications are administered intravenously until the child is able to eat and drink. Oral opiates can cause nausea, particularly if the child is not eating. The transition to oral analgesics should include equianalgesic dosing around the clock for several days. The need for pain medication usually decreases in about 5 to 7 days as tissues start to heal. It is important to remember that opiates cause constipation, which is already a problem in an immobilized child. A child who is taking opiates should drink plenty of fluids, should avoid constipating foods (e.g., cheese), and may need a daily stool softener.

Muscle spasms result from muscle injury, changes in anatomic relationships in the skeleton, and the shifting position of bone fragments. Muscle spasms can occur before or after fracture reduction. The pain from muscle spasm is characterized as a sudden, sharp, laciniating pain, as opposed to the dull ache of bone and muscle of a stabilized fracture. Some children complain that muscle spasms are worse than any other pain they have experienced. A child who is having muscle spasms requires a muscle relaxant such as diazepam. Muscle spasms are often undertreated because of concerns about the sedative effects of benzodiazepines in a child who is already receiving opiates for pain relief.

Other comfort measures for the child with musculoskeletal injury include application of ice to the injury site. Ice applied over a cast will provide some relief. Elevation can decrease swelling, which can cause a throbbing pain. The nurse should be attentive to positioning the child to prevent pressure on bony prominences and to facilitating frequent changes in position. Lying or sitting in one position for an extended period can cause discomfort, as can lying on an arm or leg and being unable to shift position. As the acute pain diminishes, distraction measures, such as books, music, and video games, become increasingly important in managing the lingering discomfort of the injury and being immobilized. A mild analgesic may be helpful at night because small discomforts are often exaggerated at night, making sleep difficult.

A child with a musculoskeletal injury may experience pain from different treatments or therapeutic procedures. A child with a fracture may undergo a closed reduction, where the fracture fragments are repositioned manually before being immobilized. A child with a fracture may also undergo insertion of traction pins or adjustment of traction.

Most children will need an intravenous sedative, such as morphine, midazolam, or a combination thereof, to manage the pain and anxiety of a fracture reduction. A child who receives intravenous sedation requires close monitoring of vital signs, pulse oximetry, and level of consciousness both during and after the procedure until all measures return to baseline. The need for additional pain medication after administration of sedation medications should be assessed. A 50:50 mixture of inhaled nitrous oxide and oxygen has been used successfully to provide analgesia during fracture reduction, particularly in emergency departments (Evans, Buckley, Alexander, & Gilpin, 1995).

A child with severe soft tissue injury may require painful or uncomfortable procedures, such as dressing changes, on a daily basis. Although these procedures may be done in the operating room, they may take place on the inpatient unit as the injury heals to minimize exposure to anesthetics and cost. Administering oral pain medications 30 to 45 minutes before the planned procedure is an important intervention to promote comfort and cooperation during the procedure. Some children benefit from participating in the procedure and can assist by removing old dressings or handing supplies to the nurse or family member performing the procedure. Some children tolerate the procedure better when they are distracted by a family member, television program, or video game. It is important to collaborate with the child, family, and physician to develop a strategy for managing repeated painful procedures.

Mobilization

Any type of musculoskeletal injury causes impaired physical mobility. Independent mobility may be further complicated by multiple fractures because the child literally may have no good limb. For the most part, mobility is equated with ambulation. However, mobility may be better thought of as movement to change position and the weight of gravity on the body. Simply changing the position relieves pressure on the skin and bony prominences, facilitates pulmonary mechanics, and promotes comfort. The nurse is responsible for the mobility of some children, such as those who are comatose and who cannot move themselves. Some children, such as those in traction, will move readily around in their beds, even though they cannot get out of bed. Transferring a patient from the bed to a chair is a form of mobilization.

The patient care goal should be to maximize mobility. Range-of-motion exercises of unaffected joints and extremities, with or without physical therapy, should be started as soon as possible to prevent contractures. Options include bed mobility with overbed trapeze, wheelchair, walker, or crutches. The patient should be out of bed, at least to a chair, as soon as possible. The patient should participate in activities of daily living and move around in bed to promote mobility of unaffected areas when ambulation is not possible.

Ambulatory assistive devices range from a cane, which is used for balance when the child can put weight on both lower extremities, to crutches or a walker, which provides support to a child who may have to limit the amount of weight put on one of the lower extremities. Generally, children older than 6 years can be successfully taught how to use crutches for ambulation. Children younger than 6 years may be able to use a walker. For the child who cannot bear weight on either lower extremity or who cannot use an assistive device because of injuries to the upper extremities, mobilization may be best achieved with a wheelchair and transfer training.

POTENTIAL COMPLICATIONS

Infection. Infection can occur soon after the initial injury or later during recovery. The highest potential for infection is related to open injuries, with direct inoculation of debris and bacteria into a wound or the development of necrotic tissue. In addition, the use of skeletal pins for traction or external fixation increases the patient's risk for infection. Surgical wounds present a potential source of infection, but in general they are not a problem because they are created in a controlled environment. Late infection is a problem with open fractures, seen as either infection of soft tissue wounds or the development of osteomyelitis.

Patients with open fractures should receive prophylactic treatment with a broad-spectrum antibiotic for at least 48 hours after injury. If an infection develops later, cultures are obtained so that an organism-specific antibiotic can be prescribed. Wound infection also requires local care, as per the physician's order. Pin tract infections are usually managed with local care, although antibiotics may be necessary. If a pin tract infection is severe, the pin may need to be removed.

Compartment Syndrome. *Compartment syndrome* refers to local muscle ischemia and contracture resulting from edema and increased pressure within osteofascial compartments (Mubarak & Owen, 1975). It is a caused by increased pressure within a limited anatomic space that can compromise neurovascular structures. A compartment is an anatomic entity comprised of muscles, nerves, and blood vessels surrounded by fascia. Fascia is a nonelastic connective tissue that normally enhances the contractility of muscle fibers. Increased pressure within a compartment can be caused by the increased volume of intracompartmental contents or the decreased size of the compartment due to external forces, such as a tight cast or constricting dressings. Contents may be increased by hemorrhage after soft tissue injury or fracture and increased capillary permeability after burns (Willis & Rorabeck, 1990). Compartment syndrome may be caused by prolonged limb compression after a drug overdose (Mubarak & Owen, 1975) or reperfusion of a limb after vascular repair.

After a musculoskeletal injury, bleeding and inflammation occur at the site of the injury. The blood and edema increase the contents of this closed space, causing an increase in intracompartmental pressure. Normal compartment pressures, when read by transducer, are 0 to 10 mm Hg. Increased tissue pressure eventually leads to obstruction of venous outflow, leading to further swelling and increased compartment pressure. Once the pressure rises above the arteriolar pressure to the muscles and nerves, no further blood enters the capillary anastomosis and muscle and nerve ischemia occurs (Willis & Rorabeck, 1990).

The presence of an open fracture does not preclude compartment syndrome, because even though one compartment may be violated, another compartment in the extremity may be intact. There are three compartments in the forearm: the superficial flexor, the deep flexor, and the dorsal or extensor anterior. There are four compartments in lower leg: the anterior, the lateral (peroneal), the superficial posterior, and the deep posterior. Compartment syndrome in the lower leg, following tibial shaft fracture, and compartment syndrome in the forearm, following supracondylar fracture of the humerus, are most common (Wilber & Thompson, 1998).

Signs of compartment syndrome include swelling, tenseness in the compartment, exaggerated pain with passive stretch, and paresthesia. A pulse is initially present in acute compartment syndrome because pressure within the compartment is not great enough to occlude or obstruct major arterial vessels (Willis & Rorabeck, 1990). Compartment measurements should be taken in all children with signs of compartment syndrome. Uncooperative children or those with head injuries should be evaluated carefully because they may lack, or be unable to communicate, the usual symptoms.

Initially, the extremity should be positioned at the level of the heart to facilitate both arterial and venous blood flow. All tight, constrictive dressings should be removed. The orthopedic surgeon may need to split the cast on one (univalve) or both (bivalve) sides to relieve the compression of the cast. Compartment pressure measurements are taken. If the compartment pressure readings are 30 mm Hg or higher, the patient will need surgical decompression of the compartment by a fasciotomy, in which the fascia is slit to relieve the pressure. Fasciotomy is the only known reliable method to decompress a compartment and stop the edema-ischemia cycle (Mubarak & Owen, 1975).

During fasciotomy, all necrotic tissue is removed. The wound is left open, although it is covered with a bulky dressing, and is examined in the operating room within 24 to 48 hours. At that point, any additional necrotic tissue is debrided. Repeated debridements may be necessary as the areas of necrotic tissue are demarcated. Once the remaining tissue is pink and healthy, the wound is closed. Depending on the amount of edema remaining and the extent of the tissue damage, skin grafting may be necessary to cover the wound.

Vascular and Nerve Injuries. Injuries to vessels and nerves may occur as a result of treatment in addition to the trauma. Nerves and vessels may be entrapped by percutaneous pins used for fracture stabilization or by fracture fragments, before or after reduction. Generally, neurovascular injury caused by mechanical means such as entrapment is quickly apparent. Neurovascular injury from a compartment syndrome or gradual loss of blood supply may become apparent only over time. The importance of complete and sequential assessments of neurovascular status cannot be overemphasized.

Signs of vascular compromise include an absent distal pulse, lower skin temperature, and poor skin circulation with diminished capillary refill. Capillary refill may be adequate if the collateral circulation is adequate to preserve the pulse. Even so, the collateral circulation may not be sufficient to maintain perfusion through specific muscle groups (Hensinger, 1998). When possible, the examiner should palpate a pulse or use a Doppler to evaluate the status of the pulse in an affected extremity. Diagnosis of vascular injury may require an angiogram. Treatment depends on the cause of the problem.

Signs of nerve injury include paresthesias, diminished sensation, and/or diminished or absent muscle function along the nerve pathway. It is important to test all of the nerves in the affected extremity both before and after surgery and to document the findings. Diagnosis of nerve injury relies on clinical examination. Treatment depends on the cause and the location of the injury. Many nerve injuries will recover, and most authors recommend waiting at least 1 year before obtaining an electromyelogram.

Superior Mesenteric Artery Syndrome (Cast Syndrome). Superior mesenteric artery syndrome consists of acute gastric dilation and vomiting caused by the mechanical obstruction of the third portion of the duodenum by the superior mesenteric artery. Children treated in hip spica or body casts are at risk for developing superior mesenteric artery syndrome, especially if their position in the cast is hyperlordotic. The syndrome has been recognized in patients who are in traction for extended periods; after spine surgery, particularly for kyphosis; and after severe traumatic brain injury (Hensinger, 1998). The syndrome is often associated with weight loss and a decrease in the fat protecting the superior mesenteric artery from the duodenum. If not treated aggressively, superior mesenteric artery syndrome can become difficult to manage, with progressive weight loss, hypokalemia, electrolyte abnormalities, and dehydration. Treatment includes passing a feeding tube past the obstruction or total parenteral nutrition. Patients should be positioned in the side-lying position to encourage duodenal drainage.

Fat Embolism Syndrome. Fat embolism has been associated with long-bone fractures, particularly in adults. Many children have fat emboli after injury, but few develop the clinical syndrome (Hensinger, 1998). Fat embolism syndrome is a posttraumatic respiratory distress syndrome that occurs within 72 hours of skeletal trauma. Its earliest manifestations are elevation of pulse, temperature elevation greater than 100° C, and a falling $Pa{O_2}$ (Evarts, 1984). The cause of the fat emboli is unclear. They may be caused by dissolution of normal circulating fat (Hensinger, 1998). The incidence of fat embolism syndrome in adults has been markedly decreased by immediate stabilization of long bone fractures.

A child with fat embolism syndrome has respiratory distress, tachypnea, and deterioration in blood gas values, particularly oxygen saturation. The child appears restless and confused. Petechiae may develop on the chest, base of neck, and axilla, although they are transient and may be missed. Laboratory findings include decreased $Pa{O_2}$, decreasing hematocrit on serial complete blood counts (CBCs), and thrombocytopenia less than 150,000/mm^3 (Evarts, 1984). Chest radiographs reveal interstitial edema and increased peripheral vascular markings. If untreated, fat embolism syndrome can cause death. Treatment includes supportive respiratory care, restoration of blood volume, and maintenance of fluid and electrolyte balance.

Growth Disturbances. Growth disturbances can result from musculoskeletal injuries, particularly injuries to the physis, which is the center for longitudinal bone grown. If the cartilage cells of the physis are damaged, growth in the bone will be altered. Bone length discrepancies and angular deformities can occur. The younger the child is when the injury is sustained, the greater is the potential for deformity because many years of growth remain. An injury that may cause disabling sequelae in a young child may result in little or no impairment in an adolescent who is nearing the end of skeletal growth.

Increased blood flow to the injured area can result in accelerated growth of the injured bone (as well as surrounding bones), which can lead to overgrowth (usually associated with the femur or humerus) (Jones, 1998). Growth can produce deformity if trauma has altered muscle forces on an extremity, as it does it a child with a head injury (Jones, 1998). Growth disturbances often present late and are progressive because the child is still growing and the normal growth patterns have been disrupted (Wilber & Thompson, 1998). Long-term follow-up, until skeletal maturity, is necessary to determine the ultimate functional outcome and growth of extremities.

Rehabilitation

The goal of rehabilitation after musculoskeletal trauma is the restoration of function in muscles and joints, including both strength and motion. In children rehabilitation generally is not a problem. A shorter period of immobilization results in less stiffening of tendons and ligaments. Children are more aggressive about self-physical therapy, and they generally are more willing to push themselves beyond pain and discomfort. Older children who are immobilized for longer periods may benefit from physical therapy to regain strength and motion when the cast or external fixator is removed. A child with multiple musculoskeletal injuries or multisystem trauma may need inpatient rehabilitation, which can provide more intensive, multiple therapies.

Home Management/Discharge Planning

Most children with a musculoskeletal injury have an altered ability to independently perform activities of daily living because of the injury itself or prescribed immobilization. Although some of the problems with self-care are obvious when a child is in a body cast, even a short arm cast can restrict a person's ability to dress himself or herself, eat without assistance, or write. It is important to collaborate with the child and family to develop a plan for self-care. One should maximize what the child is expected to do for himself or herself and allow the child to do it, no matter how long it takes. Home care equipment, such as a hospital bed with an overbed trapeze or a sliding board to assist with transfers to a wheelchair, can promote independence in daily activities.

If home care equipment or ambulatory assistive devices are needed, the family will need to adjust the home environment for safety and to promote independence. Furniture and rugs may need to be moved so that the child can ambulate safely with a walker or crutches. If a hospital bed is needed at home, the family should consider placing it in an area such as the family room, rather than a bedroom, so that the child can participate more readily in family activities. Needs for special equipment, such as prism glasses, flexible straws, slant boards for writing, and overbed tables, to facilitate self-care and promote independence should be assessed. Occupational and physical therapy are resources for ideas and equipment.

In some situations, children being treated for musculoskeletal injury may not be able to return to school, most commonly because of the need to recover from injuries or because of a body cast or external fixator. Plans for continuing school should be discussed earlier rather than later because requests for tutoring can take several weeks to process. For some children the return to school can be delayed because of transportation problems.

Transportation in general can be a problem, depending on how the child is being immobilized. A small child in hip spica casts may require a special car seat for safe transportation. An older child in a spica cast may need ambulance transportation because the fixed position of the legs and torso may prohibit the child from sitting in a car with adequate restraint. Families who usually rely on public transportation also need assistance. Transportation needs should be assessed early during the hospitalization and insurance coverage investigated because a lack of transportation can delay discharge and prevent appropriate follow-up care.

SOFT TISSUE INJURIES

Description and Pathophysiology

The major function of the soft tissues is to connect muscles to bone or bone to bone, which permits joint motion (Woo et al., 1985). Soft tissue injuries can occur in isolation or in conjunction with other musculoskeletal or multisystem trauma. With the increased interest in athletic activities and increased use of high-speed, energy-efficient transportation, soft tissue injuries are occurring more frequently (Woo et al., 1994). Soft tissue injuries are found in most patients with multiple trauma because the soft tissue often bears the impact of the traumatic force. Even in children with no obvious musculoskeletal injury, soft tissue injuries, such as strains and contusions, may be present.

Soft tissue injuries include abrasions, contusions, lacerations, and soft tissue avulsion injuries. Muscles, tendons, arteries, veins, and nerves, in addition to the skin, may be damaged. The apparent severity of the soft tissue injury can be misleading: Serious injuries to tendons and nerves may occur beneath deceptively small skin lacerations (Chung, 1986). Commonly missed injuries include median or ulnar nerve lacerations at the wrist and tendon lacerations in the hands and feet (Chung, 1986). Soft tissue injuries produce both acute and chronic disability and, although once thought to be of minor consequence, have been shown to lead to joint degeneration over time (Woo et al., 1994). A comprehensive review of all soft tissue injuries is beyond the scope of this chapter, so the discussion here focuses on the common soft tissue injuries that affect musculoskeletal function.

Strain

A strain is damage to the muscle or the attachment of the tendon as a result of overstretching, misuse, or overexertion. The degree of injury ranges from gradual onset of pain and stiffness to a sudden tearing or snapping. Strains can occur in isolation, as a result of exercise or working to excess, or in conjunction with more serious musculoskeletal injury (e.g., a motor vehicle accident). The patient history may include whether the patient braced himself or herself for impact, such as in a motor vehicle accident, for example. Strains are characterized by painful, stiff muscles. The usual treatment is ice and rest, although RICE may be necessary for more severe strains.

Sprain

A sprain is the tearing of ligaments around a joint, most commonly around the ankle, knee, or elbow (Chung, 1986).

Ligaments are damaged by excessive stretching or exertion. The degree of injury ranges from only a few ligamentous fibers torn or separated to a complete tear. A sprain is usually caused by a joint being stretched beyond its normal range of motion, such as a sudden, twisting movement or forcible hyperextension. Cervical extension sprains are generally caused by rear-end motor vehicle accidents. Signs and symptoms include pain, usually on one side of a joint after a fall; painful, discolored tissue around a joint; and swelling in the soft tissue adjacent to the joint. Treatment consists of RICE and immobilization to promote healing and to protect the joint. Most sprains heal in 10 to 21 days, with complete recovery expected. Sprains can require surgery to reapproximate the torn ends of the ligament.

Dislocation

A dislocation is a disruption of a joint that results in the articulating surfaces no longer being in contact. A subluxation occurs when the articulating surfaces lose partial contact. Dislocations occur when force is applied to the joint, either directly or indirectly. Dislocations are characterized by extreme pain and obvious deformity. Neurovascular structures are stretched, which may result in paresthesias and pallor. Treatment consists of early anatomic reduction to minimize neurovascular compromise. Reduction of the dislocation is easier when edema is not extreme. The joint is usually immobilized after reduction to permit soft tissue healing.

Contusion

A contusion is caused by the impact of a blunt object on soft tissue, which causes damage to skin; subcutaneous tissue; and underlying muscles, tendons, and neurovascular structures. Hemorrhage and the severity of tissue damage are functions of the force of impact. A contusion varies from a bump and bruise to hematoma resulting from large amounts of blood. A hematoma can produce pressure and functional impairment of neurovascular structures (Kennedy, 1993). A contusion is characterized by soft tissue swelling, often progressive, and ecchymosis at the site. Contusions near or on joints warrant special attention because they can indicate ligament damage. Treatment of contusions consists of the application of ice and in some cases the application of a compressive dressing. Serial measurements of limb circumference can assist with monitoring the progression of the contusion. Neurovascular assessments are important to determine an impending compartment syndrome.

Trauma to muscle generally has less serious consequences that injury to bones, joints, and ligaments. Although muscle injuries always resolve, myositis ossificans can occur (Howard et al., 1998). Myositis ossificans is the formation of bone in the soft tissue by periosteal bone formation, usually in the part of the muscle in closest proximity to the shaft. The cause of myositis ossificans is unknown. The true incidence is also unknown because few contusions without fracture are followed radiographically (Howard et al., 1998). Myositis ossificans may be misdiagnosed as osteomyelitis or malignancy and usually is diagnosed by ultrasound (Howard et al., 1998). Myositis ossificans is usually pain free. However, there may be associated pain if the bone formation puts pressure on surrounding tissues or the lesion is in a location that makes it susceptible to repetitive trauma or irritation from surrounding muscle or tendon motion (Kennedy, 1993).

Crush

Crush syndrome refers to the systemic manifestations of muscle necrosis, including myoglobinuric renal failure, shock, and cardiac sequelae of acidosis and hyperkalemia (Mubarak & Owen, 1975). A crush injury results from prolonged compression of a muscle mass. Crush syndrome has been reported in earthquake survivors (Shimazu et al., 1997), in patients who underwent a severe beating over more than 5% of the body (Knottenbelt, 1994), and in people who were trapped in crushed vehicles. Crush syndrome may be associated with other injuries, such as pelvic fractures with hemorrhage, bowel or abdominal injuries, other fractures, or burns (Shimazu et al., 1997).

Rhabdomyolysis may be part of the spectrum of injury in any severely injured limb (MacLean & Barrett, 1993). Muscle damage may be caused by direct injury with crush, laceration, or contusion, or it may be the result of ischemia through prolonged compression at time of injury or later as a result of increased compartmental pressure. Regardless of the cause, rhabdomyolysis results from an alteration in cell membranes, which allows release of the intracellular contents. Development of crush syndrome does not appear to be related to the area involved or the duration of compression (MacLean & Barrett, 1993). Systemic effects can range from mild to severe: crush injury, with mild hyperkalemia, hypocalcemia, myoglobinemia and elevated creatinine phosphokinase to crush syndrome, including hypovolemic shock, cardiac arrhythmias and acute myoglobinuric renal failure (MacLean & Barrett, 1993).

With crush syndrome, fluid leaves the circulatory system and shifts into the third space of the injured muscle tissue. As the fluid volume in the extremity increases, a compartment syndrome develops. Because most crush victims have hypotension, their arteriolar-perfusion pressure is less than normal and the danger of muscle tamponade is aggravated (Better & Stein, 1990).

Rhabdomyolysis is caused by increased serum myoglobin resulting from extensive muscle damage. Myoglobin is the oxygen-carrying pigment of muscle cells. Only small amounts of myoglobin are found normally in the plasma because it is excreted readily by the kidneys. Systemic effects become apparent once a sufficient amount of muscle has become necrotic (Mubarak & Owen, 1975). As high amounts of myoglobin are released by damaged muscle cells, the urine turns a red-brown. The myoglobin can block the renal tubules, causing acute tubular necrosis and necessitating dialysis. Cardiac arrhythmias develop as a result of metabolic acidosis, hyperkalemia, and hypovolemia.

Physical findings include swollen, tense extremity; intact pulses, although they may be diminished; good capillary refill; and skin pressure bullae or vesicles (Mubarak & Owen, 1975). The signs of a crush injury are deep unremitting pain, often poorly localized; a tense, swollen extremity; and deep red-brown urine. Laboratory findings include increased serum potassium, hematocrit, and white cell count. Creatinine, blood urea nitrogen (BUN), and enzyme levels (serum glutamic oxaloacetic transaminase, lactate dehydrogenase, creatinine phosphokinase [CPK]) are usually elevated. Most patients with crush syndrome show elevation of muscle enzymes, such as serum CPK. Urine is tested for myoglobin and specific gravity.

Immediate management is directed at treatment of hypovolemic shock and oliguria. Early detection and correction of life-threatening hyperkalemia, acidemia, and hypocalcemia is critical (MacLean & Barrett, 1993). If intravenous volume replacement is inadequate or delayed for more than 6 hours, acute renal failure will develop (Better & Stein, 1990). Intravenous fluids containing bicarbonate, such as Ringer's lactate, are infused. The lactate is broken down to bicarbonate in patients who are not in shock (Knottenbelt, 1994). Fluids are administered to maintain adequate urinary output. Whole blood is not recommended because the patient is already hemoconcentrated; however, if the patient has sustained a blood loss, whole blood may be indicated. Diuretics, such as furosemide and mannitol, are administered as indicated.

The optimal approach to the local injury of the crushed limb is controversial. If the injury is a closed one, management should be conservative (Better & Stein, 1993). The skin has an extraordinary ability to withstand pressure and may still serve as a barrier against infection even though it is damaged. The urge to surgically explore limbs with traumatic rhabdomyolysis should be resisted unless there is an overriding reason to do so (Better & Stein, 1993). Fasciotomy is not considered first-choice treatment for compartment syndrome in a patient with crush syndrome. Although it can remove necrotic muscle, it is associated with significant fluid loss from the open wound and an increased risk for infection (Shimazu et al., 1997). With adequate resuscitation and dialysis, the primary cause of morbidity is sepsis (MacLean & Barrett, 1993). Patients who survive the crush syndrome and acute renal failure ultimately recover completely, even those who require long-term hemodialysis (Better & Stein, 1990).

BONY INJURY

Bone is a living tissue. The skeleton is designed to withstand the demands of daily activities. The ability of cancellous bone to absorb significant energy during compressive forces is one of the most important characteristics of skeletal tissues (Carter, 1985). The size and shape of a bone is a reflection of the forces that act on it. As previously discussed, the bone of a child is different than the bone of an adult. This difference makes a child more susceptible to certain types of injuries but protects the child from others.

When bone is injured, the bone, periosteum, and soft tissues (mostly muscle) around the fracture begin to bleed. Hematoma collects at the fracture site, both inside and outside of the bone, which is essential for the release of bioactive molecules, such as growth factors and cytokinins. The hematoma will evolve into a scaffolding of fibrovascular tissue that supplies the collagen fibers that eventually become part of the primary callus around the fracture. The temporary bridge of collagen fibers is converted into bone as the bone is revascularized from the surrounding tissue and the fracture site is stressed.

During healing the fracture callus is not as well mineralized as normal. The distribution of the callus around the shaft tends to compensate for this lack of material integrity and is an important factor is establishing stability at the fracture site. As the fracture heals, the fracture callus becomes progressively more mineralized and gradually increases in strength (Carter, 1985). Clinical union has occurred when the fracture site does not move during gross examination, when attempts to move the fracture do not cause pain, and when radiographs demonstrate bone across the fracture. At this point, the bone may be clinically stable, and the bone is usually strong enough that the patient can begin to use the extremity in a more normal way, although some plastic deformation is still possible with appropriate forces.

During remodeling, the callus decreases and is replaced with the bone that has formed at the fracture site by endochondral ossification. Once the bone is clinically stabilized, the ongoing stresses and strains on the bone are responsible for remodeling the callus. As bone is subjected to the stresses of use during normal activities, the bone remodels appropriately. Because a child's bone is actively changing and continually responding to growth and physical stress, a child's bone will remodel significantly faster than an adult's bone. The bone usually returns to normal both radiographically and clinically. Unlike the soft tissues, which heal by replacing the injured tissue with collagen scar tissue, bone heals by replacing the injured area with normal bony tissue (Jones, 1998).

It is important to note that cartilage does not heal in the same phases as bone. When the physis is injured, it does not heal by formation of callus. There are inflammatory and reparative phases in cartilage healing but no remodeling phase (Jones, 1998), which has implications for physeal injuries.

FRACTURES

DESCRIPTION/PATHOPHYSIOLOGY

The most common type of bony injury is a fracture, which is a break or disruption in the continuity of the bone (Figure 18-1). Fractures occur when the bone is subjected to more stress than it can absorb. Bending is the most common mode for failure in long bones (Wilber & Thompson, 1998). Stress on the tension side of bone initiates a fracture that is followed by compression on the opposite side. As bending continues, the fracture line eventually travels the entire width of the bone. In general, fractures are described in relation to how the fracture line intersects the long axis of the bone: spiral, oblique, or transverse.

Transverse – Results from angulation force or direct trauma.

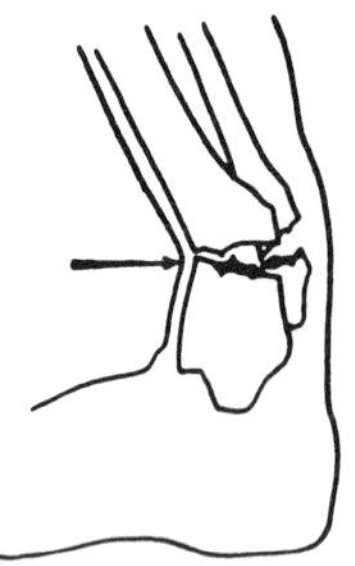

Impacted – Results from severe trauma causing fracture ends to jam together.

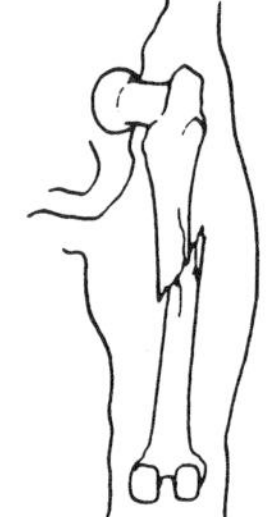

Oblique – Results from twisting force.

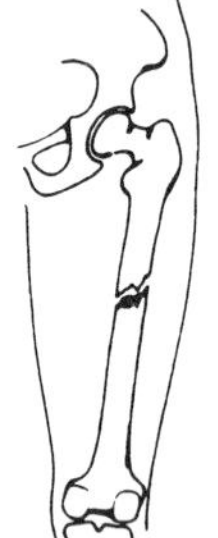

Compressed – Results from severe force to top of head or os calcis or acceleration/deceleration injury.

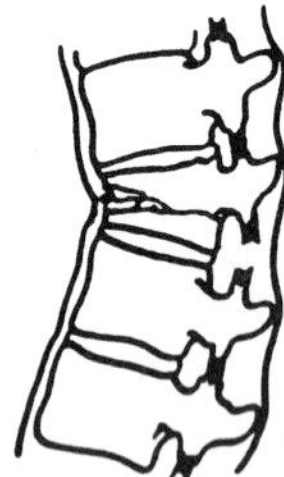

Spiral – Results from twisting force with firmly planted foot.

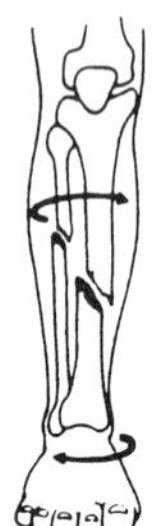

Greenstick – Results from compression force; usually occurs in children younger than 10 years of age.

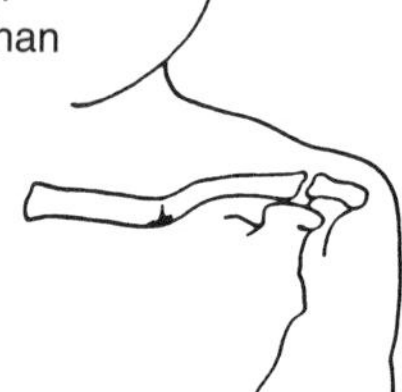

Comminuted – Results from severe direct trauma; has more than two fragments.

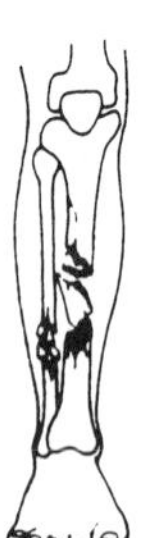

Avulsion – Results from muscle mass contracting forcefully, causing bone fragment to tear off at insertion.

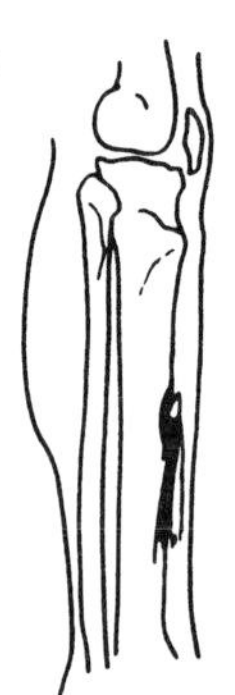

FIGURE 18-1 Types of fractures. (From S. Budassi-Sheehy [Ed.]. [1990]. *Manual of emergency care.* St. Louis: Mosby.)

Pediatric bone is weaker than adult bone, but it has a greater capacity to undergo plastic deformation than adult bone does. Because pediatric bone yields at lower force, less energy is needed to fracture. Different fracture patterns are seen in children because of the material properties of child's bone: compression (torus), incomplete tension-compression (greenstick), and plastic or bend deformities (Wilber & Thompson, 1998). Comminuted fractures (fractures where there are more than two bone fragments) are unusual in young children.

With greenstick fractures, the bone does not break completely. Greenstick fractures occur in children because of increased porosity of the bone, as well as the thick periosteum. Depending on the amount of energy to be absorbed, the large pores in growing bone may stop the propagation of the fracture line, which may leave a portion of the cortex intact on the compression side (Jones, 1998).

Pathologic fractures occur in bone that is weak or lacks normal biomechanical properties (Robertson, 1998). A bone weakened from a generalized bone disorder or a bone tumor may break with only minor trauma. The abnormal weakness allows the bone to fail under stresses that it normally would tolerate. A stress fracture is a variant of a pathologic fracture (Robertson, 1998). It occurs when exceptional repetitive force is exerted on bone that has not had a chance to remodel physiologically to accommodate these forces.

Incidence/Mechanisms of Injury

Fractures are a common childhood injury. Closed fractures, fractures in which the skin is intact, are the most common.

Most series report fractures as 17% to 20% of all childhood injuries (Cheng et al., 1999). The high incidence of fractures in children is attributable to the lower breaking strength of bone than in adults and the physically active lifestyle of children (Hansson & Hirsch, 1997). Most fractures occur in the upper extremity, with fractures of the distal forearm being the most common fracture in childhood (Cheng et al., 1999; Landin, 1997; Lyons et al., 1999).

The risk for a fracture increases as children grow older, in part because of their exposure to different activities. The highest number of fractures is caused by sports and leisure activities (36%), followed by assaults (3.5%) and road traffic incidents (1.4%) (Lyons et al., 1999). Boys have a higher incidence of fracture than girls, particularly after the age of 12 years (Landin, 1997).

Fractures in young children are often the first sign of child abuse. Of abused children, 17% present with a fracture as the initial manifestation of child abuse and 53% of these children will have multiple fractures (Sinal & Stewart, 1998). When a child younger than 2 years presents with a fracture, the index of suspicion for abuse should be high. A detailed history, a complete physical examination, and appropriate radiographic investigation are required to rule out child abuse.

Several mechanisms of injury can cause fractures in children. A direct injury occurs when the force is applied directly, as when a person is struck by an automobile bumper or falls on an object. High-velocity forces are associated with more severe injuries. An indirect injury occurs when the force is applied at a distance from the break, such a distal radius fracture caused by a fall on the outstretched arm. Sudden muscle contractions can avulse or pull a small piece of bony away from the muscle origin or insertion (avulsion fracture). Avulsion fractures in the metaphyseal areas are encountered at sites of major ligamentous and tendinous attachments, such as the ischial tuberosities of the pelvis.

Outcomes/Complications

Malunion is the healing of the bone fragments in incorrect position. It is caused by inadequate stabilization of bony fragments during the healing process. It is most common with the supracondylar fracture of the humerus, producing a cubitus varus, or when the forearm angled away from the body (Hensinger, 1998). Malunion in the lower extremity occurs frequently in the child with a head or spinal cord injury because muscle spasticity often displaces or angulates fractures. Although remodeling can improve some angular malunion, some patients require surgical osteotomy to realign the bone.

Isolated Injuries That Require Acute Care Management

Supracondylar Humerus Fractures

Description/Pathophysiology. Supracondylar humerus fractures are one of the most common fractures of the elbow (Figure 18-2). Supracondylar humerus fractures were classified by Garland based on the degree of displacement of the fracture fragments (Wilkins, 1997). Type I fractures have insignificant displacement and can be treated with simple immobilization without manipulation. Type II fractures have enough displacement to require manipulation. Type II fractures can be treated with a cast or some type of supplementary fixation, depending on the stability of the fracture when the elbow is flexed to 120 degrees. Type III fractures are completely separated with no cortical contact, either posteromedially or posterolaterally. Displacement of bone fragments may cause nerve or vascular injury. Type III

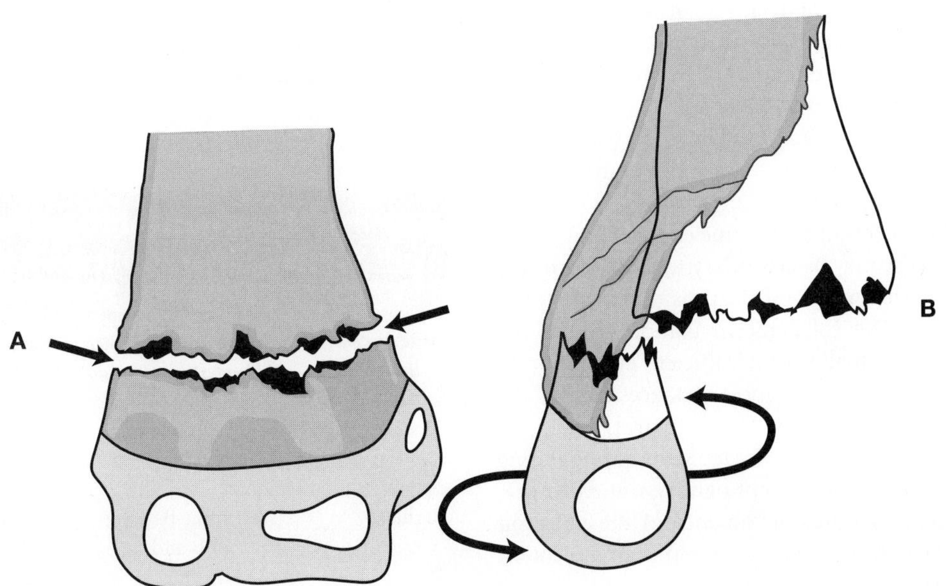

FIGURE 18-2 **A,** Supracondylar fracture of the distal humerus. **B,** Distal fragment often rotates significantly. (From R. J. Touloukian [Ed.]. [1990]. *Pediatric trauma* [2nd ed.]. St. Louis: Mosby.)

fractures generally require reduction and pinning of the fracture fragments.

Supracondylar fractures of the humerus are associated with vascular and neural injury (Farnsworth, Silva, & Mubarak, 1998). The nerves injured are the radial nerve, the ulnar nerve, and median nerve. Injury to the anterior interosseous nerve, a motor branch of the median nerve, may be more common than previously thought (Dormans, Squillante, & Sharf, 1995a). Compromise of the arterial supply may be due to spasm, intimal tears, or a complete rupture of the artery (Ray, Ivory, & Beavis, 1991). Injury to the brachial artery is the most common (Sabharwal et al., 1997).

Incidence/Mechanisms of Injury. Supracondylar fractures are reported to account for 55% to 80% of all elbow fractures (Farnsworth et al., 1998). The mechanism of injury is usually a fall on an outstretched arm (98% to 99% cases) or on a flexed elbow (1% to 2% cases) (Farnsworth et al., 1998) caused by falling from a height or during bicycle crashes. The ability to hyperextend the elbow is believed to direct the force from the fall on the outstretched hand to the anatomically weak olecranon fossa, which results in a supracondylar humerus fracture (Green, 1998). Because ligamentous laxity is greatest in the young, the peak incidence of this fracture is in the first decade of life.

There is a relatively high risk for nerve injury association with supracondylar fracture of the distal humerus in children, between 7% and 15.5% according to published reports of all supracondylar fractures (Green, 1998). The risk for neurovascular injury is highest in patients with type III fractures. Although the consequences of vascular injury associated with supracondylar fracture of the distal humerus may be significant, permanent vascular compromise of the extremity occurs in less than 1% of all supracondylar fractures of the distal humerus (Green, 1998).

Assessment. A supracondylar humerus fracture tends to have a large amount of pain and swelling (Green, 1998). A complete neurovascular examination of the arm is essential because of the risk for neurovascular injury. The vascular status of the extremity is judged by skin color, temperature of the extremity, functioning of the arm, amount of pain, and radial pulse (Green, 1998).

The radial pulse is absent at the time of the initial evaluation. An absent pulse may be secondary to tethering of the artery over the anterior surface of the proximal fragment of the distal humerus. The collateral circulation around the elbow is extensive, which allows for sufficient circulation to the arm to maintain viability, in most instances, even if the artery is damaged (Green, 1998). The forearm is examined carefully to determine circulatory status. Signs of impending ischemia include pain, compartment tightness, and decreasing motor and sensory function. Absence of the pulse on palpation and by Doppler is significant and is an indication for arterial exploration (Green, 1998).

The neurologic examination should include a motor and sensory check of the medial ulnar and radial nerves, as well as injury to the anterior interosseous nerve, which is a motor branch of the median nerve. Preoperative functional documentation of each individual nerve is essential as a means of assessing postoperative changes (Table 18-1).

On radiographs, the use of fat pad signs on the lateral radiographs is helpful in localizing the trauma to the region of the elbow (Green, 1998). Two elbow fat pads are located between the elbow joint capsule and the distal humerus: one anterior and the other posterior. With elbow effusion, one or both become elevated from the surface of the distal humerus as seen on the lateral x-ray film. The appearance of an elevated fat pad is not conclusive for a fracture, but it can aid in localizing the area of injury in the presence of other signs and symptoms (Green, 1998).

Management

Stabilization. Treatment methods include closed reduction with percutaneous pinning, open reduction with internal fixation, and closed reduction only. Skeletal traction has been used to reduce and stabilize displaced supracondylar fractures, but its use has declined as the benefits of surgical methods, such as closed reduction and percutaneous pinning, have been determined. Best results are obtained after closed reduction and two smooth mediolateral percutaneous pins are crossed at the fracture site (Wilkins, 1997). Percutaneous pins are now standard for stabilization when a cast alone is inadequate. Open reduction has gained acceptance for certain supracondylar humerus fractures. Indications for open reduction include open fractures, when there is circulatory compromise or neurologic loss during or after closed reduction, and when adequate closed reduction cannot be obtained (Green, 1998).

Displaced supracondylar fractures of the humerus historically have been regarded as urgent or emergent operative cases, that is, requiring surgery as soon as possible. However, Iyengar, Hoffinger, and Townsend (1999) reported that an overnight delay did not cause negative outcomes when the need for open reduction, clinical appearance, range of motion, or nerve function was evaluated.

TABLE 18-1 Assessment of Nerve Function With Supracondylar Humerus Fractures

Nerve	Sensory Area	Motor Function
Anterior interosseous	(None; purely motor nerve)	Flexion of distal phalanges of thumb and index finger
Median	Distal surface of index finger	Opposition of thumb and little finger Wrist flexion
Radial	Web space between thumb and index finger	Hyperextension of thumb Wrist extension
Ulnar	Distal end of small finger	Abduction of fingers

Neurovascular Concerns. Severely displaced supracondylar fractures of humerus may be complicated by arterial injury due to spasm, intimal tear, or complete rupture of the brachial artery, resulting in loss of pulse and a pale, cool hand (Ray et al., 1991). Lack of palpable radial pulse may be misleading because there may be low, although adequate, flow and/or collaterals keeping the limb viable.

If there is still no pulse auscultated by Doppler after reduction and stabilization of the fracture fragment and signs of vascular insufficiency are present, then the vessels are explored and compartment pressures measured (Wilkins, 1997). Pulse oximetry can be used because it gives a rapid, quantitative estimate of peripheral perfusion (Ray et al., 1991). Pulse oximetry alone is not an accurate measurement of the adequacy of oxygenation to muscles because adequate oxygenation depends on the flow of blood to the muscles as well as the level of oxygenation (Singh, 1992). Surgical arteriotomy is the mainstay of relieving any vascular obstruction. If the median nerve is injured, it may mask signs of vascular insufficiency.

Iatrogenic nerve injuries can occur during percutaneous pinning and open reduction/internal fixation. Postoperative nerve palsies can be result of unrecognized preoperative palsy, manipulation during surgery, or damage to a nerve by one of medial pin placements (Lyons, Ashley, & Hoffer, 1998). Most nerve palsies are recognized on the day of surgery or in the immediately postoperative phase, although a nerve palsy may be noted when the cast is removed. Options for treating nerve palsy include exploration, medial (ulnar) or medial (radial) pin removal, or observation. There is little evidence to suggest that immediate exploration is helpful (Lyons et al., 1998).

Outcomes/Complications. Numerous series demonstrate that patients will have complete return of nerve function, even if nothing is done (Brown & Zinar, 1995; Dormans et al., 1995a; Lyons et al., 1998). Other complications include claudication and cold intolerance if the brachial artery remains obstructed (Wilkins, 1997).

Cubitus varus, an angular deformity, can occur as a result of malreduction or loss of reduction of supracondylar fractures. Because of the anatomy of the distal humerus, a near-anatomic reduction of a supracondylar fracture is necessary to allow provide fracture stability and to prevent the medial tilt of the distal fragments that causes cubitus varus (Green, 1998). Although undesirable in appearance, cubitus varus does not limit function. Surgical correction by wedge osteotomy is required to prevent a late ulnar nerve palsy, which has been reported in patients with uncorrected cubitus varus.

Diaphyseal Femur Fractures

Description/Pathophysiology. Diaphyseal femur fractures are commonly isolated injuries or are associated with minor trauma, such as abrasions or contusion (Routt, 1998). Femur fractures generally require hospitalization for stabilization. The large muscular cuff of the thigh can pull fracture fragments out of alignment and make reduction and stabilization difficult, particularly in older children. Unopposed muscle contractions across the fracture site produce deformity and displacement of the fracture fragments (Routt, 1998).

Incidence/Mechanisms of Injury. The origin of most pediatric femoral shaft fractures is accidental blunt trauma (Routt, 1998). In a study of a population of children in Switzerland, Buess and Kaelin (1998) found that the cause of femur fractures varied with age. In children aged 0 to 4 years, the primary cause was falls. In children aged 6 to 10 years, the majority were caused by traffic crashes. In children aged 13 to 15 years, the majority were sports related. It is important to note that femoral shaft fractures in small children may be result of abuse and should be investigated carefully (Routt, 1998).

Assessment. Routine anteroposterior and lateral radiographs of the femur, including the hip and knee, are generally adequate to diagnose a pediatric femoral shaft fracture. The initial films are usually obtained without traction of any type, including a Hare splint, to assess shortening and deformity (Routt, 1998). Computed tomography (CT) scanning may be useful in certain situations to better identify associated physeal and intraarticular fractures.

Management

Stabilization. Treatment of femoral shaft fractures has become increasingly dependent on age and the location of the injury. Younger children with isolated femoral shaft fractures are managed by a variety of closed techniques. Older children receive more aggressive intervention because of their lower potential for remodeling (Routt, 1998).

Patients younger than 11 years are usually treated with immediate spica casting or traction, followed by casting for closed isolated injuries (Yandow, Archibeck, Stevens, & Shultz, 1999). Early spica cast application for femoral shaft fractures consistently produces satisfactory outcomes in patients younger than 6 years (Stans, Morrissy, & Renwick, 1999). External fixators are a treatment option, but they usually reserved for treating femur fractures in children with multiple injuries.

Flexible intramedullary (IM) nails are another option for stabilizing femur fractures in younger children. Flexible nails are prebent to conform to the anatomic curves of the involved bone, inserted to provide three-point fixation, and then anchored in the proximal and distal metaphyses. Secondary muscles provide additional support. Slight movement at the fracture site stimulates callus formation (Wilber & Thompson, 1998). In children aged 5 to 12 years, the flexible IM nail provides good reduction without overriding of the fracture and major angular deviation, which in turn limits the amount of overgrowth (Buess & Kaelin, 1998).

Patients 12 years and older who are skeletally mature have less remodeling potential, making the potential problems of malunion, shortening, and loss of knee motion less desirable. In older patients, early spica cast application has resulted in leg length discrepancies as a result of shortening at the fracture site (Stans et al., 1999). Traction followed by casting has resulted in poor outcomes in older children. An external fixator may be used, although not as commonly as other treatment options.

Femoral shaft fractures in children older than 14 years may be treated with rigid, reamed IM rods. Reaming the medullary canal to the inner cortical diameter permits the use of a large rod and allows it to function as an internal splint, which obviates the need for external splinting (Routt, 1998). A reamed IM rod can be locked proximally, distally, or both, to help control rotation of the bone fragments. There have been reports of avascular necrosis of the femoral head, which limits their use to children older than 13 years (Wilber & Thompson, 1998).

Mobilization. Mobilization of a child with diaphyseal femoral fractures depends on the type of immobilization or stabilization. A child in a spica cast is limited to a bed or chair because the position of the cast is designed to preclude weight bearing. Patients treated with IM nails or rods are usually able to bear weight with an ambulatory assistive device, such as crutches, within days of surgery and can bear full weight within 4 to 8 weeks (Buess & Kaelin, 1998).

Rehabilitation. Children will limp (average of 4.5 weeks) after cast removal regardless of their age (Czertak & Hennrikus, 1999). A child may need physical therapy for gait training with a walker or crutches or therapy to regain strength and motion if casting or traction is used.

Discharge Planning. The child discharged in a spica cast will benefit from equipment at home to facilitate care. A hospital bed can facilitate positioning because the head and knees can be adjusted easily. An overbed trapeze can assist with positioning and maintaining strength in the upper extremities. Depending on the child's size, a wheelchair with a reclining back can be used to get the child out of bed. If the child is older and the cast is large, the family should be instructed on safe transfer techniques to prevent back injuries. Most children in a spica cast will need ambulance transportation because they are difficult to restrain safely in car. Plans for home tutoring should be initiated early because most schools will not take children in spica casts for transportation and safety reasons.

Outcomes/Complications. Complications of spica casting include loss of reduction, usually rotation or shortening, and poor alignment (Buess & Kaelin, 1998). Rotational malunion does not remodel, although soft tissues will accommodate rotational changes so that foot progression angles are symmetrical (Czertak & Hennrikus, 1999). Complications of the flexible IM nail include skin irritation or perforation at nail portals and excess external rotation (Buess & Kaelin, 1998). Complications with the rigid rod include hematoma in the thigh (Buess & Kaelin, 1998).

Overgrowth of a fractured femur seems to most prominent in patients treated between the ages of 8 and 10 years; therefore some shortening in the original reduction (in the range of 1.5 to 2 cm) is allowable (Routt, 1998). The phenomenon is unpredictable in older children and adolescents and does not seem to be prominent with open reduction. Limb length inequality is the most common complication of femoral shaft fractures in children, producing limb and compensatory scoliosis. Growth disturbances have been reported in as many as 30% of patients younger than 13 years, in part because more growth is remaining at the time of injury.

Tibial Fractures

Nonphyseal fractures involving the tibia and fibular are among the most common injuries involving the lower extremities in children and adolescents and constitute approximately 15% of all pediatric fractures (Thompson & Behrens, 1998). Falls, sports, and motor vehicle accidents are common mechanisms of injury. Treatment methods for tibial fractures depend on the location of the injury. Most are treated with closed reduction and casting, usually with a long leg cast to control the position of the bone fragments and to prevent rotation.

Children with tibial fractures are often admitted to the hospital to monitor the development of compartment syndrome. The anterior compartment syndrome occurs most often after a fracture of the tibial shaft (Thompson & Behrens, 1998), although other compartments may also be involved. Incipient compartment syndrome should be suspected in a child who complains of inordinate pain under the cast, even though no signs of compartment syndrome are present.

Physeal Injury

Description/Pathophysiology

Physeal injuries are unique to the bones of children because the cartilage cells of the physis are converted to bone in adolescence and the physis no longer is present. Skeletal age is an important factor in the consideration of injuries in children. The closer the child is to the end of growth, the less prominent is the role of the growth plate in the treatment of the injury (Jones, 1998). Because the physis is the center for longitudinal growth, physeal injuries can have a long-term impact on the child. The Salter-Harris classification system describes injuries to the physis by their radiographic appearance and potential for long-term injury to the physis (Table 18-2). The injuries most commonly associated with physeal fractures are injuries to the neurovascular and ligamentous structures near the physis (Canale, 1998).

Incidence/Mechanisms of Injury

The incidence of physeal injuries in long bones has been reported to range from 18% to 30% (Mann & Rajmaira, 1990; Mizuta, Benson, Foster, Paterson, & Morris, 1987). The distal radial physis is the most commonly injured physis (Canale, 1998). Physeal damage can result in progressive angular deformity, limb length discrepancy, or joint incongruity.

TABLE 18-2 **Salter-Harris Classification of Physeal Injuries**

Type	Description	Treatment Options	Potential for Long-Term Consequences
I	Fracture lines runs along the physis to separate the epiphysis from the metaphysis	• Closed reduction and casting • Internal fixation may be required after open or closed reduction	• Low risk for growth disturbance • Cartilage cells of the physis are intact
II	Fracture line runs along the physis and then into the metaphysis	• Closed reduction and casting	• Fairly low risk for growth disturbance • Cartilage cells of the physis are intact
III	Fracture line runs along the growth plate and then into the epiphysis	• Open reduction and internal fixation with smooth pins to restore joint congruity	• Risk of growth disturbance depends on the age of the child • Cartilage cells in the physis can be damaged, resulting in localized conversion of the cartilage cells to bone
IV	Fracture line runs through the epiphysis, through the physis and into the metaphysis	• Open reduction and internal fixation with smooth pins to restore joint congruity	• Risk of growth disturbance depends on the age of the child • Cartilage cells in the physis can be damaged, resulting in localized conversion of the cartilage cells to bone
V	Injuries to the cartilage cells of the physis other than a fracture For example, crushing injuries to the weight-bearing physis at the ankle, electrical injuries from high voltage wires, radiation, or frost bite	• Rarely diagnosed acutely • Treatment is delayed until the development of a bony bridge across the physis is apparent	• By definition, type V injuries always result in growth arrest in the affected bone

From Joy, C. (1989). *Pediatric trauma nursing.* Rockville, MD: Aspen Publishers.

The physes appear to be the weakest area in children's bone, and they are the structures that must be preserved if normal growth is to occur (Canale, 1998). Injuries involving the growth plate usually occur at the junction of calcifying cartilage cells and at those cells that are uncalcified. Damage to the physis can occur by crushing, vascular compromise to the physis, or bone growth bridging from the metaphysis to the bony portion of the epiphysis. The physis is more susceptible to injury by rotation than by angulation or traction.

Assessment

Because of the chondro-osseous nature and irregular contours of the physes, some acute physeal injuries are not seen clearly on plain radiographs (Canale, 1998). Two views taken at 90-degree planes to each other may help delineate the fracture, along with comparison films of the opposite extremity, and help determine whether physeal injury has occurred. Oblique views may be helpful in injuries of the forearm or lower leg. Varus and valgus stress views are useful for injuries about the knee and elbow to demonstrate gapping between the epiphysis and the metaphysis. Magnetic resonance imaging may be helpful in evaluating physeal injuries (Ohasi, Brandser, & El-Khoury, 1997).

Management

Stabilization. All physeal injuries must be treated as gently as possible to avoid injuring the cartilage cells of the physis. Multiple closed reductions of epiphyseal fractures are contraindicated because they may damage the physis (Wilber & Thompson, 1998). If the fracture cannot be reduced with a closed reduction, then open reduction is warranted.

Displaced type III and IV fractures require anatomic reduction, usually by open reduction and internal fixation, to restore alignment to the physis and to the articular surface of the joint (Wilber & Thompson, 1998). The prognosis is usually good, provided the vascularity to the fragment remains intact and the reduction is anatomic.

Outcomes/Complications

Problems after injury to the growth plate are not common, but the potential for deformity exists whenever the physis is injured (Jones, 1998). The most obvious and catastrophic consequence of physeal injury is disruption of longitudinal growth of the bone. Complete growth arrest may result in significant limb length inequality, with functional impairment (Canale, 1998). Partial growth arrest may result in angular deformity or progressive shortening. The arrest occurs when a bridge of bone forms across the physis from the metaphysis to the epiphysis, tethering growth. All bony bars result from damage to the physeal cells, most commonly from fracture.

Multiple Musculoskeletal Injuries

The majority of musculoskeletal injuries are simple isolated injuries from which children readily recover. Most serious musculoskeletal injuries are the result of high-velocity forces, such as motor vehicle accidents, which cause injury to other body systems. Life-threatening orthopedic injuries include multiple long-bone fractures, pelvic fractures, and cervical spine instability and are often part of multisystem trauma. High-priority extremity injuries include major joint dislocations, open joint injuries, open fractures, and fractures associated with vascular injury (Wilber & Thompson, 1998).

In children, certain types of musculoskeletal injury should be considered indicators of high-energy trauma and warrant careful evaluation. Fractures of the first rib have been designated as a "hallmark of severe trauma" in both children and adults because the force required to break the first rib often results in other serious injuries (Harris & Soper, 1990). Fractures of the first rib occur as a result of a large amount of energy transference to thoracic skeleton, which is particularly significant in a child whose rib cage is more compliant than that of an adult. Multiple rib fractures are a marker of severe trauma in children. Of children younger than 3 years with multiple rib fractures, 63% are the victims of abuse (Wilber & Thompson, 1998).

The standard trauma radiographic series consists of a lateral view of the cervical spine, a supine anteroposterior view of the chest, and an anteroposterior view of the pelvis. The lateral view of the cervical spine has been reported to be 98% accurate in diagnosing cervical spine injury, but it cannot be considered definitive in the unconscious or comatose child (Wilber & Thompson, 1998). The anteroposterior radiograph of the pelvis screens for fractures of the pelvis and can be used to assess for fractures or dislocations of the hips and proximal femur. Pelvic CT scanning is warranted if an injury to the sacrum, sacroiliac joints, or acetabulum is suspected clinically or by standard radiographs. Radiographs of the extremities are based on clinical evaluation, including palpation.

Multiple Fractures

Multiple fractures, without injury to other body systems, may be life threatening because of blood loss. Broken bones bleed into soft tissue and bone fragments can injury blood vessels, leading to increased blood loss. Multiple fractures may be limb threatening, particularly if they occur in the same extremity, such as an ipsilateral femur and tibia fracture, commonly referred to as a *floating knee*. When multiple fractures occur, they are usually the result of high-velocity incidents. Significant soft tissue injuries can also be expected.

Stabilization

Multiple fractures are an indication for surgical stabilization, including external fixators and IM nails. For the patient with ipsilateral fractures in the same extremity, it is recommended that at least one of the fractures be rigidly stabilized by either internal or external fixation (Wilber & Thompson, 1998). Surgical options include IM nails for both the upper and lower extremities, external fixation, and plating.

Discharge Planning

Multiple fractures affect home care and discharge planning. Fractures of the upper and lower extremities limit the child to wheelchair mobility because the upper extremities cannot bear weight for crutches or a walker. Bilateral fractures of the upper extremities drastically limit the child's ability to eat or dress independently. Because mobility and the ability for self-care may be severely limited, the family may find equipment such as a hospital bed helpful. Family members should receive instruction on body mechanics and patient transfers to prevent back injuries. The child and family may need assistance with transportation and home tutoring arrangements.

Open Fractures

Description/Pathophysiology

Open fractures are one of the most serious musculoskeletal injuries (Wilber & Thompson, 1998). An open fracture is a fracture associated with injury to the skin, subcutaneous tissue, or muscle. With concomitant soft tissue and bony injury, the essential prerequisites for fracture healing—a blood supply and stability of the fracture fragments—are compromised (Gustilo, Merkow, & Templeman, 1990). Extensive soft tissue injury and disruption of blood supply around fracture site contribute to prolonged healing time and increase the incidence of delayed union and nonunion (Buckley, Smith, Sponseller, Thompson, & Griffin, 1990).

Open fractures are classified according to the mechanism of injury, the degree of soft tissue damage, the configuration of the fracture, and the level of contamination (Gustilo et al., 1990) (Box 18-2). The risk of primary or secondary amputation is increased with open fractures that require vascular repair. Vascular injuries associated with open fractures include occlusion, transection, avulsion, and pseudoaneurysm (Brinker & Bailey, 1997). No statistically significant relationship between fracture healing and number of vessels injured, type of injury, or vascular procedure exists, except for unrepaired injury to the posterior tibial artery, which has an increased risk of delayed union or nonunion.

Some severe open fractures are better managed with amputation rather than extensive reconstructive procedures that leave the patient with a minimally functional extremity. Amputation may be required if the extremity is deemed nonviable because of massive injuries to bone, soft tissue, or neurovascular structures or because of uncontrollable wound infection (Brinker & Bailey, 1997). Various severity scores have been developed to provide guidance when deciding between limb salvage and amputation, considering the age of the child, extent of injury, and extent of limb ischemia (Gregory et al., 1985).

Some closed fractures caused by violent forces may result in extensive destruction of the soft tissue sleeve surrounding the limb without resulting in an open fracture. These injuries are characterized by skin contusions, deep abra-

BOX 18-2 Classification of Open Fractures

Type I
- Wound <1 cm long
- Usually moderately clean puncture through which a spike of bone has pierced the skin
- Little soft tissue damage
- No sign of crushing injury
- Fracture usually is simple, transverse, or short oblique with little comminution

Type II
- Laceration is >1 cm long
- No extensive soft tissue damage, flap, or avulsion
- Slight or moderate crushing injury
- Moderate comminution of fracture
- Moderate contamination

Type III
- Extensive damage to soft tissues, including muscles, skin, and neurovascular structures
- High degree of contamination
- Great deal of comminution and instability as a result of high-velocity trauma

Type IIIA
- Soft tissue coverage of bone is adequate despite extensive laceration, flaps, or high-energy trauma
- Includes segmental or severely comminuted fractures from high-energy trauma regardless of size of wound

Type IIIB
- Extensive injury to or loss of soft tissue, with periosteal stripping and exposure of bone
- Massive contamination
- Severe comminution from high-velocity trauma
- After irrigation and debridement, a segment of bone is exposed
- Local or free flap is needed for coverage

Type IIIC
- Any open fracture associated with arterial injury that must be repaired, regardless of degree of soft tissue injury

sions, burns, or frank separation of cutis from subcuticular tissue, which can result in partial- or full-thickness tissue loss and secondary infections of the fracture site. These injuries are best treated as open fractures (Behrens, 1998).

Incidence/Mechanism of Injury

Open fractures are rare in children younger than school age because of their small body mass, large amount of subcutaneous fat, and limited exposure to high-risk activities (Behrens, 1998). Violent traffic and other incidents are responsible for more that 80% of open fractures in children older than 2 years. Because open fractures are caused by high-velocity forces, the child may have associated injuries, including other fractures, head injury, abdominal injuries, and chest injuries, such as pulmonary contusion.

Lawnmower incidents are involved in a higher percentage of open fractures in children and warrant special attention. The average age of children injured in most series of lawnmower injuries is approximately 5 years (Dormans, Azzoni, Davidson, & Drummond, 1995a; Farley et al., 1996). Injuries result from direct contact with the blade or from objects being thrown by the blade and striking the child (Alonso & Sanchez, 1995). Dormans et al. (1995b) reported in their series that 69% of the injuries were to bystanders or nonoperators. Riding lawnmower injuries are more severe than manual lawnmower injuries (Vosburgh, Gruel, Herndon, & Sullivan, 1995). The injuries themselves range from fractures, often comminuted, to primary or secondary amputations and head and eye injuries. The tragedy is that these serious injuries are completely preventable by prohibiting children younger than 14 years from being in the vicinity of a lawnmower when it is in use.

Assessment

Initial assessment of a patient with an open fracture includes a careful assessment of the neurologic and vascular status of the extremity and of the soft tissue injuries. Documentation of the neurovascular status of limb is crucial (Gustilo et al., 1990). Determining the vascular status of an extremity with an open fracture is a priority because the ability to preserve or restore blood flow to the extremity is key to preserving the extremity.

Cardinal signs of arterial injury are pulselessness, pain, pallor, paresthesias, and paralysis. Presence of palpable pulses or Doppler-documented flow does not rule out arterial injury (Wilber & Thompson, 1998). If arterial injury is suspected or diagnosed clinically, an arteriogram should be done. Ischemic time should also be determined. Experimental and clinical data suggest that more than 6 to 8 hours of warm ischemia time prohibits survival despite revascularization (Pilcher, Seligson, & Davis, 1994).

Arteriography should be reserved for use in identifying patients with abnormal results on vascular examination and an uncertain level of arterial injury in the lower extremities. Angiography is more important in the upper extremity because collateral circulation around the shoulder and elbow can often maintain palpable pulses and show evidence of pulsatile flow by Doppler examination (Seligson, Ostermann, Henry, & Wolley, 1994).

Management

Goals of treatment of open fracture are prevention of infection, healing of the fracture, and restoration of function to the extremity (Gustilo et al., 1990). Based on experience in many centers, the process for treating open fractures has been fairly standardized (Box 18-3). Multisystem, life-threatening problems are recognized and addressed before operative treatment of an open fracture.

The general operative approach is divided into three phases (Gregory et al., 1985): (1) reduction and fixation of fractures and dislocations, usually with an external fixator; (2) identification and repair of vascular (arterial and venous) injuries; and (3) wound management, which requires concentrated attention to debridement and wound coverage. Primary or secondary nerve repair is performed on

BOX 18-3 Chronology of Treatment of Open Fractures (Gustilo, Merkow, Templeman)

1. Treat all open fractures as an emergency.
2. Perform thorough evaluation to diagnose other life-threatening injuries.
3. Begin appropriate antibiotic therapy in the emergency department or at latest in the operating room and continue for only 2-3 days.
4. Immediately debride wound using copious irrigation; for type II and III injuries, repeat in 24-72 hours.
5. Stabilize fractures.
6. Leave wound open for 5-7 days.
7. Perform early autogenous bone grafting.
8. Rehabilitate the involved extremity.

a case-by-case basis. For an extremity obviously threatened by ischemia, arterial and venous exploration and repair combined with debridement of nonviable tissue remain the quickest method to restore viability (Odland, Gisbert, Gustilo, Ney, Blake, & Bubrick, 1990).

Stabilization. Successful treatment of open fractures requires skeletal stabilization of the bony injury and careful management of associated soft tissue injuries (Brinker & Bailey, 1997). Bony stability reduces the rate of infection and protects the integrity of the remaining soft tissues to promote wound healing (Gustilo et al., 1990). Stabilization of fractures is accomplished during the initial operative debridement, when possible. Fracture stabilization has priority over vascular repair if it can be done quickly because reduction maneuvers can damage a vascular anastomosis (Seligson et al., 1994). For most children with open fractures, the first choice for fracture stabilization is an external fixator. The external fixator can be replaced by a cast when soft tissue healing is completed (if the fracture is stable), or the external fixator can be maintained until there is evidence of fracture stability (Buckley et al., 1990).

Neurovascular Concerns. Hemorrhage from the extremity is controlled early (Odland et al., 1990). Ischemic time greater than 6 hours interferes with limb salvage. Treatment options for vascular injuries include observation, ligation, interpositional vein graft, and vessel repair (Brinker & Bailey, 1997). A fasciotomy is mandatory after vascular repair to prevent postanatomic compartment syndrome (Seligson et al., 1994).

Primary nerve repair can be performed if indicated. Massive neurologic injury is an indication for amputation because a denervated extremity will be nonfunctional. As always, careful, sequential assessment of neurovascular status is essential.

Wound Management. In the operating room the surgeon attempts to determine the extent of the real injury, which often exceeds the apparent injury by a factor of 2 to 3 (Behrens, 1998). Debridement is a carefully planned and systematic process that removes all foreign or dead material from the wound (Behrens, 1998). Wound edges are extended liberally to allow unobstructed access. All necrotic or contaminated tissues are debrided, including subcutaneous tissue, fat, fascia, and muscle. Muscle viability is assessed using "the four *C*'s" (*c*onsistency, *c*ontractility, *c*olor, and *c*apacity to bleed) but they are not always reliable (Behrens, 1998). Capacity to contract with pinch and presence of arterial bleeding seem to be best signs of viability. Debridement is accompanied by irrigation of the wound, using copious amounts of fluid to cleanse the wound and remove debris and contaminants. Because the extent of necrosis is often underestimated, the wound should be left open and reevaluated in 48 to 72 hours.

Soft tissue coverage can prevent infection and create a better milieu for healing by obliterating dead space. Early soft tissue reconstruction (within 5 to 7 days) is desirable if a clean, stable wound has been achieved (Gustilo et al., 1990). Wounds can be managed with primary delayed primary closure, healing by secondary intention, split-thickness skin grafting, and free tissue transfers, depending on the fracture classification and the degree of soft tissue injury. Blood vessels in children younger than 2 years are often too small to permit microvascular anastomosis but older children with larger vessels are good candidates for microvascular free tissue transfers (Horowitz, Nichter, Kenney, & Morgan, 1985).

Antibiotic Therapy. The risk for infection is increased with open fractures because of direct inoculation of microorganisms and debris into the wound. In addition, open injuries can be overlooked, particularly if the skin injury is small. Because the skin and soft tissues are elastic, the fracture itself is not a clear indication of the extent of injury. The severity of soft tissue injury is the most important predictor of infection.

Of open fractures, 70% are contaminated at the time of injury with gram-negative and aerobic gram-positive organisms (Gustilo et al., 1990). The risk for infection depends greatly on the severity of the soft tissue wounds. Open fractures are treated with a cephalosporin and an aminoglycoside for at least 48 hours. Infection usually becomes evident within the first month, the majority within first 7 days (Gustilo & Anderson, 1976). If a wound becomes infected, a Gram stain and culture along with immediate debridement and irrigation are warranted.

Outcomes/Complications. Children with open fractures have a higher incidence of delayed union than children with closed fractures in the same bone. The same factors that predispose adults to delayed union or nonunion (degree of displacement, comminution, soft tissue damage, and periosteal stripping) also contribute to delayed unions and nonunions in children (Cramer, Limbird & Green, 1992). Children with open fractures are at increased risk for acute wound infection, pin tract infections from external fixation devices, and osteomyelitis.

A high percentage of open fractures caused by lawnmower accidents result in amputation (Dormans et al., 1995b). Although limb salvage may be appropriate in some patients, inappropriate attempts at limb salvage may contribute to long hospitalizations, a higher incidence of surgical complications, and increased pain and expense compared with early amputation.

Bone Loss

Bone loss resulting from injuries in children is unusual. Most bone loss is associated with violent injury, such as motor vehicle accidents or incidents involving power mowers or machinery and therefore is accompanied by extensive soft tissue injury. Bone loss can be a segmental bone loss or occur through a traumatic amputation.

Segmental Bone Loss

A segmental bone loss is a type of open fracture in which a portion of the bone is missing, with distal and proximal parts intact. Primary management is similar to the management of an open fracture. The surgeon attempts to save as much periosteum and skeletal components as possible while stabilizing the remaining skeletal elements. As with all open fractures, the wound is left open until the status of the bone and soft tissue is clear.

With advances in science and technology, the potential for reconstruction with bone grafts or bone transport is increased. Historically, amputation was often the best option for a child with a segmental bone loss because replacing the lost segment was not feasible. With the introduction of circular external fixators, such as the Ilizarov external fixator, bone transport has become a reasonable option for some children.

With a bone transport procedure, a segment of the remaining bone is moved slowly and gradually until it is in contact with the bone at the other end of the missing segment. As the bone segment is transported, the body forms new bone behind it, similarly to the development of callus in bone healing. Once the segments are in contact, the bone heals. Patients and families are taught how to perform the daily adjustment to the circular external fixator, as well the routine daily management. Families need ongoing support and assistance during the very lengthy process.

Traumatic Amputation

Traumatic amputations are classified as complete and incomplete. A *complete amputation* is the complete separation of the body part as a result of the injury. The term *incomplete amputation* is used to describe every other degree of disruption, short of complete separation. An incomplete amputation is a type III open fracture.

Emergency management of an incomplete amputation includes controlling the bleeding, cleaning the tissue margins, and cooling the extremity to maximize tissue viability for reconstruction. When a child has a complete amputation, every effort is made to find and preserve all body parts. Body parts should be covered with a moist cloth and placed in a plastic bag, which is submerged in ice water. In some cases replantation may be possible, but in any case, the tissues can be used for grafting and reconstruction.

Surgical interventions, which include replantation, amputation, and refinement of a traumatic amputation, are undertaken so that there is adequate soft tissue coverage over the end of the bone in the residual limb. Amputation is appropriate treatment for an extremity deemed nonviable because of massive injuries to bone, soft tissue, or neurovascular structures or because of uncontrollable wound infection (Brinker & Bailey, 1997). Bone fragments can be stabilized with internal or external fixation (Loder, Brown, Zaleske, & Jones, 1997).

Neurovascular assessments for the patient with a replantation include specific assessments of arterial and venous circulation. A sign of arterial occlusion is a pale, cool extremity with poor turgor. On a dermal stick, serum is obtained and there should be brisk bleeding. A sign of venous occlusion is a cyanotic, cool extremity with tense turgor. The extremity should be elevated unless there are signs of arterial compromise. Cold temperatures should be avoided; otherwise, the vessels constrict. Assessments of nerve function are equally important, although there may be little immediate improvement.

Postoperative care for the patient with an amputation or refinement of a traumatic amputation includes wound care and dressing changes. As with any open injury, the wound may be left open for reassessment and debridement, depending on the condition of the skin and tissue. The patient receives antibiotics, depending on the results of the wound cultures taken in the operating room. Although elevation is important to prevent wound edema, the extremity should be elevated for only 12 hours per day to prevent muscle contractures. Range-of-motion exercises should be performed on the residual limb. Ambulation should begin when the wound is closed.

Femur Fracture With Closed Head Injury

Management of femoral fractures in child with a head injury presents special problems. Spasticity and restlessness are the main problems in children with moderate to severe head injuries. Traction is insufficient to control the fracture fragments, which increases the risk for malunion. Early casting in a child with a femur fracture and head injury prevents assessment of skin injury or compartments because problems cannot be communicated by the child. Traction or casting can lead to malunion, osteomyelitis, skin breakdown, excessive shortening, and rotational deformities (Routt, 1998). Options for a stabilizing femur fracture in a patient with head injury include IM fixation, external fixation, and plating.

External fixation for a femur fracture in a child with a head injury provides good control of fracture fragments without extensive surgery and permits neurovascular and skin assessments. External fixation has the capability to stabilize adjacent joints to prevent excessive soft tissue movement and contractures (Tolo, 1990).

Internal fixation methods include IM nails and compression plating. As discussed previously, there are two types of IM nails: flexible and rigid. Flexible IM nails tend to have poor rotatory control, necessitating supplementary casting. Reamed IM nailing is preferable in patients older than 12 years in whom there is less risk for injury to the growth plate. IM nailing can present a danger to growth areas, particularly the apophysis of the trochanter of the femur.

Compression plating provides good control of bone fragments, high rate of union, low risk for infection, ease of mobilization, and low risk for functionally important limb length discrepancy, but plate removal requires another operation and the long scar has a poor cosmetic appearance (Kregor, Song, Routt, Sangeorzan, Liddell, & Hansen, 1993). In most cases casting is not necessary. Problems with plate fixation include the invasiveness of the procedure, which requires a long incision; plate breakage; risk for a stress fracture after plate removal; and lack of consensus regarding plate removal.

Mobilization

Mobilization of a child with a femur fracture and closed head injury is affected by the child's neurologic status. The stabilization methods used for femur fracture in a child with a head injury permit mobility with crutches or a walker. However, depending on the child's neurologic status and recovery from head injury, ambulation with as assistive device may not be possible. The child may be restricted to a wheelchair.

Outcomes/Complications

Ectopic bone formation is reported to appear around major joints, most often the hip, elbow, and knee, particularly in a patient with head injury (Hensinger, 1998). It is more common in teenagers, although any age group is at risk. Inflammation and tenderness near a joint in an area of soft tissue and bony trauma usually precede ectopic bone formation. Laboratory findings include elevated serum alkaline phosphate level before ossification and during active bone formation. Bone formation is evident on radiographs 3 to 4 weeks after injury.

Joint movement may cause some resorption. Symptomatic ectopic bone formation may restrict hip or knee motion and require excision (Routt, 1998). Surgical excision should be delayed until the process is completely mature, about 1 year after injury. Pharmacologic agents such as salicylates and indomethacin may be helpful. Most children can be managed successfully with observation (Hensinger, 1998). Prophylaxis is strongly considered, especially in children with associated craniocerebral trauma (Routt, 1998).

Pelvic Fractures

Description/Pathophysiology

Pelvic fractures are defined as fractures of the bones of the pelvis or a separation of one of the two immobile joints in the pelvis, sacroiliac joint, or symphysis pubis. Pelvic bony fractures in children are uncommon, except for avulsion fractures. Pelvic fractures are considered a life-threatening orthopedic injury in a patient of any age because of the close proximity to internal organs and large vessels, the large marrow cavities, and the expansile peritoneal cavity, which can disguise bleeding into the abdomen. Pelvic fractures, other than avulsion fractures, result from high-energy trauma and are often accompanied by injury to other organ systems and additional skeletal disruptions (Rieger & Brug, 1997).

Open pelvic fractures are defined as direct communications between pelvic fractures and vaginal, rectal, perianal, or other skin lacerations (Reiger & Brug, 1997). Rectal and perianal wounds need to be treated aggressively to prevent contamination of the fracture.

The stability of the bony fragments is important for determining the treatment of a pelvic fracture. Numerous classification systems have been developed to describe the type of injuries to the adult pelvis and the stability of the fracture. Torode and Zieg (1985) classified pediatric pelvic fractures based on an entire spectrum of injuries associated with the fracture, not the bony injury alone (Table 18-3). Unlike adults, joint laxity allows single fractures in the pelvic ring in children (Garvin, McCarthy, Barnes, & Dodge, 1990). A large diastasis of the pubic symphysis can occur in children without any resultant instability of the sacroiliac joints posteriorly (Torode & Zieg, 1985).

Many children with pelvic bony injury have associated injuries to the musculoskeletal system, abdomen, and thorax. The most common constellation of injuries is central nervous system, intraabdominal, and musculoskeletal injuries (Vazquez & Garcia, 1993). Musculoskeletal injuries are very common, including fractures of the femur, tibia, femoral neck, clavicle, humerus, radius, and ulna (Garvin et al., 1990). A child with a pelvic fracture may also have multiple contusions and soft tissue injuries.

A child's pelvis is able to accommodate more energy before fracture than an adult's pelvis. The contents of the pelvis are more susceptible to injury because energy passes through the bony structures (Garvin et al., 1990). Because of the significant energy involved in producing fractures of the pelvis, the major consequences are from associated visceral injuries (Swiontkowski, 1998). Injuries to other organ systems include bladder/urethral injury and neurologic injury, particularly injury to the lumbosacral plexus with sacroiliac disruptions or sacral fractures.

Patients with pelvic fracture are at risk for hemorrhage from multiple sources, including osseous, vascular, and visceral structures. The energy of injury is absorbed only partially by pelvis. The remainder of the energy is absorbed by soft tissues (Failinger & McGanity, 1992). Displaced pelvic fractures can injure paravaginal, superior gluteal, and internal iliac arteries, which can compromise the viability of the lower extremity if the fractures are not recognized and treated promptly. Bleeding usually occurs from small vessels rather than major arteries (Wilber & Thompson, 1998).

Incidence/Mechanism of Injury

When pelvic bony injuries occur, they are the result of high-energy trauma, primarily motor vehicle accidents involving a pedestrian, bicyclist, or occupant. Severely displaced pelvic

TABLE 18-3 Torode and Zieg Classification of Pediatric Pelvic Fractures

Classification	Definition	Management
Type I avulsion fractures	• Avulsion of bony elements of the pelvis, usually a separation through or adjacent to cartilaginous growth place	• Excellent prognosis without operative intervention • Usually do not require hospital admission • Treated symptomatically with crutches, occasionally bed rest
Type II iliac wing fractures	• Fracture of the iliac wings causing a disruption of iliac apophysis or an infolding fracture of wind of ilium	• Often admitted to hospital, primarily for observation of associated injuries • Good results with short period of bed rest until comfortable, then prompt mobilization, occasionally with crutches or walker
Type III simple ring fractures	• Fracture of pubic rami or disruption of pubic symphysis • Generally not clinically unstable, even if displaced	• Often admitted to hospital, primarily for observation of associated injuries • Good results with short period of bed rest until comfortable, then prompt mobilization, occasionally with crutches or walker • May be treated with spica or pelvic sling, although external fixation may be better
Type IV ring disruption fractures	• Fracture or joint disruption creating an unstable segment of pelvic ring • Bilateral pubic rami fractures (straddle fractures) • Fractures of either right or left pubic ramus or pubic symphysis *and* fracture through posterior elements or disruption of the sacroiliac joint • Fractures of anterior and posterior structures of pelvic ring	• Higher association with visceral injuries and increased morbidity: neurologic, genitourinary, abdominal injuries, and hemorrhage • External or internal fixation • Increased incidence of long-term bony complications, including nonunion of pubic rami, triradiate cartilage injury, displacement of normal pelvic ring

fractures have a 63% to 75% incidence of associated injuries, including head injuries, other fractures, hemorrhage, genitourinary injuries, abdominal injuries (including rectal lacerations, intestinal tears, and visceral ruptures of the liver, spleen, and kidneys) (Wilber & Thompson, 1998). Additional injuries are more common in children because they are more likely to be struck by a motor vehicle as an unprotected pedestrian (Garvin et al., 1990).

Pediatric pelvic fractures have a death rate of 8% compared with adult mortality rates, which range from 10% to 20% (Torode & Zieg, 1985). Mortality is more likely related to injuries of other organ systems, particularly the central nervous system (Reiger & Brug, 1997).

Assessment

Clinical signs of a pelvic fracture are often noted after the patient is stabilized. Abrasions and contusions on contiguous structures should alert the trauma team to a potential pelvic fracture (Failinger & McGanity, 1992). A limb length discrepancy or obvious rotational deformity of pelvis or lower extremity may also indicate pelvic fracture.

Hematuria (the inability to void), blood at the urethral meatus, or an abnormal prostatic examination should prompt further evaluation (Reiger & Brug, 1997). Careful rectal and vaginal examinations are necessary to rule out an open pelvic fracture. Rectal injury is evaluated in patients with sacral fractures because fragments of bone frequently traverse the rectal wall (Failinger & McGanity, 1992).

If the child has a suspected pelvic fracture, careful clinical and radiologic assessments are necessary to evaluate pelvic stability. Abdominal, rectal, vaginal, and neurologic examinations, as well as urinalysis, are necessary (Reiger & Brug, 1997). A single anteroposterior view of the pelvis is a standard part of the trauma evaluation. Inlet and outlet views should be obtained on hemodynamically stable patients. Obturator and iliac oblique acetabular radiographs are obtained on children with suspected acetabular fractures or with triradiate cartilage disruptions. CT scans can show posterior sacroiliac complex and are standard for acetabular fractures (Reiger & Brug, 1997).

Instability should be suspected if there is severe displacement on visual inspection, gross instability of hemipelvis with manual manipulation, any evidence of major posterior injury, or an open wound or posterior bruising (Failinger & McGanity, 1992). Stability of the pelvis is determined through palpation and bimanual compression and distraction of the iliac wings (Failinger & McGanity, 1992) because an unstable pelvis may appear reduced on the initial radiographs.

Management

Emergency management includes immobilizing the pelvis with sand bags, evaluating associated injuries, and assessing for subtle signs of abdominal bleeding. The goal of treatment for pelvic fractures is anatomic reduction and maintenance of a symmetric pelvis (Reiger & Brug, 1997). Conservative treatment for pelvic fractures includes bed rest, pelvic sling, skeletal traction, or hip spica cast. Most children achieve favorable results with minimal treatment (Reiger & Brug, 1997).

Stabilization. Unstable pelvic ring disruptions should be reduced and stabilized. Pelvic stability requires an intact posterior weight-bearing arch with stable linkage of iliac wings to the sacrum and spine (Failinger & McGanity, 1992). Early reduction and stabilization of the pelvis by external fixation can reduce loss from retroperitoneal bleeding, especially bleeding from cancellous bone surfaces (Reiger & Brug, 1997). However, external fixation does not provide adequate stabilization of vertically unstable fractures to allow weight bearing (Failinger & McGanity, 1992). Indications for internal fixation include a purely posterior ligamentous injury, failed reduction or continued displacement, associated acetabular fractures, multiple injuries, open posterior wound without perineal contamination, and vertically unstable fractures. Fractures of other bones, particularly of the femur and lower extremity, should be treated operatively (Reiger & Brug, 1997).

Neurovascular Concerns. Treatment of hemorrhage includes sufficient replacement of fluid and blood. If vital signs are not stabilized, the child should be evaluated for a source of intraabdominal bleeding, usually by peritoneal lavage (Failinger & McGanity, 1992). Hemorrhage can be difficult to control because there are multiple sites of bleeding, particularly in open pelvic fractures. Early skeletal immobilization can control hemorrhage by limiting pelvic volume and stabilizing bony fragments to maintain retroperitoneal tamponade (Carrillo, Wohltmann, Spain, Schmieg, Miller & Richardson, 1999).

When the child has major vascular injuries to the lower extremities, hemorrhage control and immediate restoration of vascular perfusion are necessary to prevent permanent damage to the extremity (Carrillo et al., 1999). Hemipelvectomy in childhood should be considered in patients with uncontrollable hemorrhage and extensive disruption of soft tissue, iliac vessels, or nerves (Reiger & Brug, 1997).

Outcomes/Complications

Long-term morbidity is generally not attributed to bony injury but to associated pelvic injuries (Reiger & Brug, 1997). No morbidity related to sacroiliac joint disruption or triradiate cartilage disruption has been reported in most patients (Garvin et al., 1990). Acetabular fractures have a relatively higher rate of morbidity because injury to triradiate cartilage, which is the growth center of the acetabulum, can result in a growth disturbance in the acetabulum (Reiger & Brug, 1997). Late complications of unstable fractures include pain, leg length discrepancy, scoliosis, gait abnormalities, and difficulty sitting (Failinger & McGanity, 1992).

Vertebral Fractures

Description/Pathophysiology

The vertebral column consists of 24 individual vertebrae joined by intervertebral discs, ligaments, and skeletal muscle. Any part of the vertebral column can be injured. The bony vertebra can be fractured and ligaments can be torn. The presence of spinal fracture at any level in a child with multiple trauma is associated with a greater incidence (5% to 10%) of noncontiguous fracture at other levels of the spine (Wilbur & Thompson, 1998). The traumatic force can be transmitted over multiple segments because of the increased cartilage/bone ratio and the increased laxity of a child's skeleton compared to that of an adult.

When the vertebral column is injured, the spinal cord is subject to injury from the traumatic force itself, from impingement by the bony fragments, or from a damaged blood supply. Fractures to the vertebra can occur with or without neurologic injury. Although neurologic injury is an important issue, the stability of the spinal column after the fracture is equally important. In the short term, fragments from the vertebral bodies could cause neurologic injury. In the long term, scoliosis can develop in an unstable vertebral column.

The three-column classification system was developed to describe the stability of the vertebral column (Denis, 1984). Although its relevance to the pediatric spine has not been confirmed (Sullivan, 1998), the system provides a model for understanding the circumstances in which the vertebral column is unstable. The classification system divides the bony elements and supporting ligaments of the vertebral column into three columns. The posterior column is formed by the posterior bony complex and posterior ligaments. The middle column is formed by the posterior longitudinal ligament, posterior annulus fibrosis, and posterior wall of the vertebral body. The anterior column is formed by the anterior longitudinal ligament, anterior annulus fibrosis, and anterior part of the vertebral body. If the bony elements are disrupted as the result of a fracture or because the supporting ligaments are damaged, the column is considered disrupted. If only one of the three columns is disrupted, the vertebral column as a whole is considered stable. If two or more of the three columns are disrupted, the vertebral column is considered unstable. Spinal injury is discussed in detail in Chapter 15.

SUMMARY

Musculoskeletal injury provides a challenge for the pediatric trauma nurse. Injuries can range from mild to life threatening. The nurse uses astute assessment skills to determine the type of injury and works with the multidisciplinary team to successfully manage the child while minimizing complications.

BIBLIOGRAPHY

Alonso, J. E., & Sanchez, F. L. (1995). Lawn mower injuries in children: A preventable impairment. *Journal of Pediatric Orthopaedics, 15,* 83-89.

Behrens, F. F. (1998). Fractures with soft tissue injuries. In N. E. Green & M. F. Swiontkowski (Eds.), *Skeletal trauma in children* (2nd ed., Vol. 3, pp. 103-119). Philadelphia: WB Saunders.

Better, O. S., & Stein, J. H. (1990). Early management of shock and prophylaxis of acute renal failure in acute traumatic rhabdomyolysis. *New England Journal of Medicine, 322,* 825-829.

Black, J. (1988). Does corrosion matter? *Journal of Bone and Joint Society, 70B*, 517-520.

Brinker, M. R., & Bailey, D. E. (1997). Fracture healing in tibia fractures with an associated vascular injury. *Journal of Trauma, 42*, 11-19.

Brown, I. C., & Zinar, D. M. (1995). Traumatic and iatrogenic neurological complications after supracondylar humerus fractures in children. *Journal of Pediatric Orthopaedics, 15*, 440-443.

Buckley S. L., Smith, G., Sponseller, P. D., Thompson, J. D., & Griffin P. P. (1990). Open fractures of the tibia in children. *Journal of Bone and Joint Surgery, 72A*, 1462-1469.

Buess, E., & Kaelin, A. (1998). One hundred pediatric femoral fractures: Epidemiology, treatment attitudes, and early complications. *Journal of Pediatric Orthopaedics, 7*, 186-192.

Canale, S. T. (1998). Physeal injuries. In N. E. Green & M. F. Swiontkowski (Eds.), *Skeletal trauma in children* (2nd ed., Vol. 3, pp. 17-58). Philadelphia: WB Saunders.

Carrillo, E. H., Wohltmann, C. D., Spain, D. A., Schmieg, R. E., Jr., Miller, F. B., & Richardson, J. D. (1999). Common and external iliac artery injuries associated with pelvic fractures. *Journal of Orthopaedic Trauma, 13*, 351-355.

Carter, D. R. (1985). Biomechanics of bone. In A. M. Nahum & J. Melvin (Eds.), *The biomechanics of trauma* (pp. 135-165). Norwalk, CT: Appleton-Century-Crofts.

Cheng, J. C. Y., Ng, B. K., Ying, S. Y., & Lam, P. K. W. (1999). A 10-year study of the changes in the pattern and treatment of 6493 fractures. *Journal of Pediatric Orthopaedics, 19*, 344-350.

Chung, S. M. K. (1986). *Handbook of pediatric orthopaedics*. New York: Van Nostrand Reinhold.

Cramer, K. E. (1995). The pediatric polytrauma patient. *Clinical Orthopaedics and Related Research, 318*, 125-135.

Cramer, K. E., Limbird, T. J., & Green, N. E. (1992). Open fractures of the diaphysis of the lower extremity in children: Treatment, results and complications. *Journal of Bone and Joint Surgery, 74A*, 218-232.

Currey, J. D., & Butler, G. (1975). The mechanical properties of bone tissue in children. *Journal of Bone and Joint Surgery, 57A*, 810-814.

Czertak, D. J., & Hennrikus, W. L. (1999). The treatment of pediatric femur fractures with early 90-90 spica casting. *Journal of Pediatric Orthopaedics, 19*, 229-232.

Davids, J. R., Frick, S. L., Skewes, E., & Blackhurst, D. W. (1997). Skin surface pressure beneath an above-the-knee cast: Plaster compared with fiberglass casts. *Journal of Bone and Joint Surgery, 79A*, 565-569.

Denis, F. (1984). Spinal instability as defined by the three-column spine concept in acute spinal trauma. *Clinical Orthopaedics and Related Research, 189*, 65-76.

Dormans, J. P., Azzoni, M., Davidson, R. S., & Drummond, D. S. (1995a). Major lower extremity lawn mower injuries in children. *Journal of Pediatric Orthopaedics, 15*, 78-82.

Dormans, J. P., Squillante, R., & Sharf, H. (1995b). Acute neurovascular complications with supracondylar humerus fractures in children. *Journal of Hand Surgery, 20A*, 1-4.

Ehara, S., El-Khoury, G. Y., & Sato, Y. (1988). Cervical spine injury in children: Radiologic manifestations. *AJR American Journal of Roentgenology, 151*, 1175-1178.

Evans, J. K., Buckley, S. L., Alexander, A. H., & Gilpin, A. T. (1995). Analgesia for the reduction of fractures in children: A comparison of nitrous oxide with intramuscular sedation. *Journal of Pediatric Orthopaedics, 15*, 73-77.

Evarts, C. M. (1984). The fat embolism syndrome. In M. H. Meyers (Ed.), *The multiply injured patient with complex fractures* (pp. 67-70). Philadelphia: Lea & Febiger.

Failinger, M. S., & McGanity, P. L. J. (1992). Unstable fractures of the pelvic ring. *Journal of Bone and Joint Surgery, 74A*, 781-791.

Farley, F. A., Senunas, L., Greenfield, M. L., Warschausky, S., Loder, R. T., Kewman, D. G., & Hensinger, R. N. (1996). Lower extremity lawn-mower injuries in children. *Journal of Pediatric Orthopaedics, 29*, 669-672.

Farnsworth, C. L., Silva, P. D., & Mubarak, S. J. (1998). Etiology of supracondylar humerus fractures. *Journal of Pediatric Orthopaedics, 18*, 38-42.

Frank, C. B., Amiel, D., Woo, S. L-Y, & Akeson, W. H. (1985). Joints: Clinical and experimental aspects. In A. M. Nahum & J. Melvin (Eds.), *The biomechanics of trauma* (pp. 369-397). Norwalk, CT: Appleton-Century-Crofts.

Garfin, S. R., & Katz, M. M. (1985). The vertebral column: Clinical aspects. In A. M. Nahum & J. Melvin (Eds.), *The biomechanics of trauma* (pp. 301-340). Norwalk, CT: Appleton-Century-Crofts.

Garvin, K. L., McCarthy, R. E., Barnes, L., & Dodge, B. M. (1990). Pediatric pelvic ring fractures. *Journal of Pediatric Orthopaedics, 10*, 577-582.

Gershuni, D. H. (1985). Clinical aspects of extremity fractures. In A. M. Nahum & J. Melvin J (Eds.), *The biomechanics of trauma* (pp. 413-446). Norwalk, CT: Appleton-Century-Crofts

Goldberger, D. K., Kruse, L., & Stender, R. (1987). A survey of external fixator pin care techniques. *Clinical Nurse Specialist, 1*(4), 166-169.

Green, N. E. (1998) Fractures and dislocations about the elbow. In N. E. Green & M. F. Swiontkowski (Eds.), *Skeletal trauma in children* (2nd ed., Vol. 3, pp. 259-317). Philadelphia: WB Saunders.

Gregory, R. T., Gould, R. J., Peclet, M., Wagner, J. S., Gilbert, D. A., Wheeler, J. R., Snyder, S. O., Gayle, R. G., & Schwab, C. W. (1985). The mangled extremity syndrome (M.E.S.): A severity grading system for multisystem injury of the extremity. *Journal of Trauma, 25*, 1147-1150.

Gustilo, R. B., & Anderson, J. T. (1976). Prevention of infection in the treatment of one thousand and twenty-five open fractures of long bones. *Journal of Bone and Joint Surgery, 58A*, 453-458.

Gustilo, R. B., Merkow, R. L., & Templeman, D. (1990). The management of open fractures. *Journal of Bone and Joint Surgery, 72A*, 299-304.

Hansson, G., & Hirsch, G. (1997). Fractures in children. *Journal of Pediatric Orthopaedics, Part B, 6*, 77-78.

Harris, G. J., & Soper, R. T. (1990). Pediatric first rib fractures. *Journal of Trauma, 30*, 343-345.

Hensinger, R. N. (1998). Complications of fractures in children. In N. E. Green & M. F. Swiontkowski (Eds.), *Skeletal trauma in children* (2nd ed., Vol. 3, pp. 121-147). Philadelphia: WB Saunders.

Hope, P. G., & Cole, W. G. (1992). Open fractures of the tibia in children. *Journal of Bone and Joint Surgery, 74B*, 546-553.

Horowitz, J. H., Nichter, L. S., Kenney, J. G., & Morgan, R. F. (1985). Lawnmower injuries in children: Lower extremity reconstruction. *Journal of Trauma, 25*, 1138-1146.

Howard, C. B., Porat, S., Bar-On, E., Nyska, M., & Segal, D. (1998). Traumatic myositis ossificans of the quadriceps in infants. *Journal of Pediatric Orthopaedics, 7*, 80-82.

Hull, J. B., & Bell, M. J. (1997). Modern trends for external fixation of fractures in children: A critical review. *Journal of Pediatric Orthopaedics Part B, 6*, 103-109.

Iyengar, S. R., Hoffinger, S. A., & Townsend, D. R. (1999). Early versus delayed reduction and pinning of type III displaced supracondylar fractures of the humerus in children: A comparative study. *Journal of Orthopaedic Trauma, 12*, 51-55.

Jaicks, R. R., Cohn, S. M., & Moller, B. A. (1997). Early fracture fixation may be deleterious after head injury. *Journal of Trauma, 42*, 1-6.

Jobes, R. D. (1982). Cranial nerve assessment with halo traction. *Orthopaedic Nursing, 1*(4), 11-15.

Jones, E. (1998). Skeletal growth and development as related to trauma. In N. E. Green & M. F. Swiontkowski (Eds.), *Skeletal trauma in children* (2nd ed., Vol. 3, pp. 1-16). Philadelphia: WB Saunders.

Jones-Walton, P. (1988). Effects of pin care on pin reactions in adults with extremity fracture treated with skeletal traction and external fixation. *Orthopaedic Nursing, 7*(4), 29-33.

Kahle, W. K. (1994). The case against routine metal removal. *Journal of Pediatric Orthopaedics, 14*, 229-237.

Kathol, M. H. (1997). Cervical spine trauma. *Radiology Clinics of North America, 35*, 507-532.

Kennedy, J. P. (1993). Soft tissue injury. In J. P. Kennedy & F. W. Blaisdell (Eds.), *Extremity trauma* (pp. 16-28). New York: Thieme Medical Publishers.

Kirkendall, D. T., & Garrett, W. E. (1999). Muscle strain injuries: Research findings and clinical applicability. *Mediscape Orthopaedics and Sports Medicine, 3,* 2.

Knottenbelt, J. D. (1994). Traumatic rhabdomyolysis from severe beating: Experience of volume diuresis in 200 patients. *Journal of Trauma, 37,* 214-219.

Kregor, P. J., Song, K. M., Routt, M. L., Jr., Sangeorzan, B. J., Liddell, R. M., & Hansen, S. T., Jr. (1993). Plate fixation of femoral shaft fractures in multiply injured children. *Journal of Bone and Joint Surgery, 75A,* 1774-1780.

Landin, L. A. (1997). Epidemiology of children's fractures. *Journal of Pediatric Orthopaedics Part B, 6,* 79-83.

Lui, T. N., Lee, S. T., Wong, C. W., Yeh, Y. S., Tzan, W. C., Chen, T. Y., & Hung, S. Y. (1996). C1-C2 fracture-dislocations in children and adolescents. *Journal of Trauma, 40,* 408-411.

Loder, R. T., Brown, K. L. B., Zaleske, D. J., & Jones, E. T. (1997). Extremity lawn-mower injuries in children: Report by the Research Committee of the Pediatric Orthopaedic Society of North America. *Journal of Pediatric Orthopaedics, 17,* 360-369.

Loder, R. T., Warschausky, S., Schwartz, E. M., Hensinger, R. N., & Greenfield, M. L. (1995). The psychosocial characteristics of children with fractures. *Journal of Pediatric Orthopedics, 15*(1), 41-46.

Lyons, J. P., Ashley, E., & Hoffer, M. M. (1998). Ulnar nerve palsies after percutaneous cross-pinning of supracondylar fractures in children's elbows. *Journal of Pediatric Orthopaedics, 18,* 43-45.

Lyons, R. A., Delahaunty, A. M., Kraus, D., Heaven, M., McCabe, M., Allen, H., & Nash, P. (1999). Children's fractures: a population based study. *Injury Prevention, 5,* 129-132.

MacLean, J. G. B., & Barrett, D. S. (1993). Rhabdomyolysis: A neglected priority in the early management of severe limb trauma. *Injury, 24,* 205-207.

Mankin, H. J., Mow, V. C., Buckwalter, J. A., Iannotti, J. P., & Ratcliffe, A. (1994). Form and function of articular cartilage. In S. R. Simon (Ed.), *Orthopaedic basic science* (pp. 1-44). Chicago: American Academy of Orthopaedic Surgeons.

Mann, D. C., & Rajmaira, S. (1990). Distribution of physeal and nonphyseal fractures of long bones in children aged 0 to 16 years. *Journal of Pediatric Orthopaedics, 10,* 713-716.

McGrory, B. J., Klassen, R. A., Chao, E. Y., Staeheli, J. W., & Weaver, A. L. (1993). Acute fractures and dislocations of the cervical spine in children and adolescents. *Journal of Bone and Joint Surgery, 75A,* 988-995.

Mizuta, T., Benson, W. M., Foster, B. K., Paterson, D. C., & Morris, L. L. (1987). Statistical analysis of the incidence of physeal injuries. *Journal of Pediatric Orthopaedics, 7,* 518-523.

Moskowitz, A. (1989). Lumbar seatbelt injury in a child: A case report. *Journal of Trauma, 29,* 1279-1282.

Mubarak, S., & Owen, C. A. (1975). Compartmental syndrome and its relation to the crush syndrome: A spectrum of disease: A review of 11 cases of prolonged limb compression. *Clinical Orthopaedics and Related Research, 113,* 81-89.

Odland, M. D., Gisbert, V. L., Gustilo, R. B., Ney, A. L., Blake, D. P., & Bubrick, M. P. (1990). Combined orthopedic and vascular injury in the lower extremities: Indications for amputation. *Surgery, 108,* 660-666.

Ohasi, K., Brandser, E. A., & El-Khoury, G. Y. (1997). Role of MR imaging in acute injuries to the appendicular skeleton. *Radiologic Clinics of North America, 35,* 591-613.

Orenstein, J. B., Klein, B. L., Gotschall, C. S., Ochsenschlager, D. W., Klatzko, M. D., & Eichelberger, M. R. (1994) Age and outcome in pediatric cervical spine injury: 11-year experience. *Pediatric Emergency Care, 10*(3), 132-137.

Orenstein, J. B., Klein, B. L., & Ochsenschlager, D. W. (1992). Delayed diagnosis of pediatric cervical spine injury. *Pediatrics, 89,* 1185-1188.

Pilcher, D. B., Seligson, D., & Davis, J. H. (1994). Prolonged warm ischemia and limb survival: A case report. *Journal of Trauma, 37,* 941-943.

Poole, G. V., Miller, J. D., Agnew, S. G., & Griswold, J. A. (1992). Lower extremity fracture fixation in head-injured patients. *Journal of Trauma, 32,* 654-659.

Ray, S. A., Ivory, J. P., & Beavis, J. P. (1991). Use of pulse oximetry during manipulation of supracondylar fractures of the humerus. *Injury, 22,* 103-104.

Reynolds, M. A., Richardson, J. D., Spain, D. A., Seligson, D., Wilson, M. A., & Miller, F. B. (1995). Is the timing of fracture fixation important for the patient with multiple trauma? *Annals of Surgery, 222,* 470-481.

Rieger, H., & Brug, E. (1997). Fractures of the pelvis in children. *Clinical Orthopaedics and Related Research, 336,* 226-239.

Robertson, W. W. (1998). Pathologic fractures and tumors. In N. E. Green & M. F. Swiontkowski (Eds.), *Skeletal trauma in children* (2nd ed., Vol. 3, pp. 159-170). Philadelphia: WB Saunders.

Roseveare, C. A., Brown, J. M., McIntosh, J. M. B., & Chalmers, D. J. (1999). An intervention to reduce playground equipment hazards. *Injury Prevention, 5,* 124-128.

Routt, M. L. C. (1998). Fractures of the femoral shaft. In N. E. Green & M. F. Swiontkowski (Eds.), *Skeletal trauma in children* (2nd ed., Vol. 3, pp. 405-429), Philadelphia: WB Saunders.

Sabharwal, S., Tredwell, S. J., Beauchamp, S. D., Mackenzie, W. G., Jakubec, D. M., Cairns, R., & LeBlanc, J. G. (1997). Management of pulseless pink hand in pediatric supracondylar fractures of humerus. *Journal of Pediatric Orthopaedics, 17,* 303-310.

Schiedt, P. C., Harel, Y., Trumble, A. C., Jones, D. H., Overpeck, M. D., & Bijur, P. G. (1995). Epidemiology of nonfatal injuries among US children and youth. *American Journal of Public Health, 85,* 932-938.

Seligson, D., Ostermann, P. A. W., Henry, S. L., & Wolley, T. (1994). The management of open fractures associated with arterial injury requiring vascular repair. *Journal of Trauma, 37,* 938-940.

Shimazu, T., Yoshioka, T., Nakata, Y., Ishikawa, K., Mizushia, Y., Morimoto, F., Kishi, M., Takacka, M., Tanaka, H., Iwai, A., & Hiraide, A. (1997). Fluid resuscitation and systemic complications in crush syndrome: 14 Hanshin-Awaji earthquake patients. *Journal of Trauma, 42,* 641-646.

Shoemaker, B. L., & Ose, M. (1997). Pediatric lap belt injuries: Care and prevention. *Orthopaedic Nursing, 16*(5), 15-22.

Shook, J. E., & Lubicky, J. P. (1997). Paralytic scoliosis. In K. H. Bridwell & R. L. DeWald (Eds.), *The textbook of spinal surgery* (pp. 837-880). Philadelphia: Lippincott-Raven.

Sinal, S. H., & Stewart, C. D. (1998). Physical abuse of children: A review for orthopedic surgeons. *Journal of Southern Orthopaedic Association, 7,* 264-276.

Singh, D. (1992). Pulse oximetry and fracture manipulation [Letter to the editor]. *Injury, 23,* 70.

Skak, S. V., Overgaard, S., Nielsen, J. D., Andersen, A., & Nielsen, S. T. (1996). Internal fixation of femoral shaft fractures in children and adolescents: A 10- to 21-year follow-up of 52 fractures. *Journal of Pediatric Orthopaedics Part B, 5,* 195-199.

Sproles, K. J. (1985). Nursing care of skeletal pins: A closer look. *Orthopaedic Nursing, 4*(1), 11-19.

Stans, A. A., Morrissy, R. T., & Renwick, S. E. (1999). Femoral shaft fracture treatment in patients age 6 to 16 years. *Journal of Pediatric Orthopaedics, 19,* 222-228.

Stephens, M. M., Hsu, L. C. S., & Leong, J. C. Y. (1989). Leg length discrepancy after femoral shaft fractures in children: Review after skeletal maturity. *Journal of Bone and Joint Surgery, 71B,* 615-618.

Sullivan, J. A. (1998). Fractures of the spine in children. In N. E. Green & M. F. Swiontkowski (Eds.), *Skeletal trauma in children* (2nd ed., Vol. 3, pp. 343-368). Philadelphia: WB Saunders.

Swiontkowski, M. F. (1998). Fractures and dislocations about the hip and pelvis. In N. E. Green & M. F. Swiontkowski (Eds.), *Skeletal trauma in children* (2nd ed., Vol. 3, pp. 369-404). Philadelphia: WB Saunders.

Thompson, G. H., & Behrens, F. (1998). Fractures of the tibia and fibula. In N. E. Green & M. F. Swiontkowski (Eds.), *Skeletal trauma in children* (2nd ed., Vol. 3, pp. 459-503). Philadelphia: WB Saunders.

Tolo, V. T. (1990). External fixation in multiply injured children. *Orthopaedic Clinics of North America, 21,* 393-400.

Torode, I., & Zieg, D. (1985). Pelvic fractures in children. *Journal of Pediatric Orthopaedics, 5,* 76-84.

Valadian, I., Porter, D., & Carroll, L. (1993). Muscles. In I. Valadian & D. Porter (Eds.), *Physical growth and development: From conception to maturity* (pp. 153-168). Boston: Little, Brown.

Valadian, I., Porter, D., Carroll, L., Neuhauser, E. T. (1977). The skeletal system. In I. Valadian & D. Porter (Eds.), *Physical growth and development: From conception to maturity* (pp. 63-98). Boston: Little, Brown.

Vazquez, W. D., & Garcia, V. F. (1993). Pediatric pelvic fractures combined with an additional skeletal injury is an indicator of significant injury. *Surgery, Gynecology & Obstetrics, 177,* 468-472.

Vosburgh, C. L., Gruel, C. R., Herndon, W. A., & Sullivan, J. A. (1995). Lawn mower injuries of the pediatric foot and ankle: Observations on prevention and management. *Journal of Pediatric Orthopaedics, 15,* 504-509.

Ward, W. T., Levy, J., & Kaye, A. (1992). Compression plating for child and adolescent femur fractures. *Journal of Pediatric Orthopaedics, 12,* 626-632.

Wesson, D. E., Scorpio, R. J., Spence, L. J., Kenney, B. D., Chipman, M. L., Metley, C. T., & Hu, X. (1992). The physical, psychological, and socioeconomic costs of pediatric trauma. *Journal of Trauma, 33,* 252-257.

Wilber, J. H., & Thompson, G. H. (1998). The multiply injured child. In N. E. Green & M. F. Swiontkowski (Eds.), *Skeletal trauma in children* (2nd ed., Vol. 3, pp. 71-102). Philadelphia: WB Saunders.

Wilkins, K. E. (1997). Supracondylar fractures: What's new? *Journal of Pediatric Orthopaedics Part B, 6,* 110-116.

Wilkins, K. E. (1998). Operative management of children's fractures: Is it a sign of impetuousness or do the children really benefit? *Journal of Pediatric Orthopaedic, 18,* 1-3.

Willis, R. B., & Rorabeck, C. H. (1990). Treatment of compartment syndrome in children. *Orthopaedic Clinics of North America, 21,* 401-412.

Woo S. L.-Y., An, K.-N., Arnoczky, S. P., Wayne, J. S., Fithian, D. C., & Meyers, B. S. (1994). Anatomy, biology, and biomechanics of tendon, ligament, and meniscus. In S. R. Simon (Ed.), *Orthopaedic basic science* (pp. 45-87). Chicago: American Academy of Orthopaedic Surgeons.

Woo, S.-Y., Gomez, M. A., & Akeson, W. H. (1985). Mechanical behaviors of soft tissues: Measurements, modifications, injuries and treatment. In A. M. Nahum & J. Melvin J (Eds.), *The biomechanics of trauma* (pp. 109-133). Norwalk, CT: Appleton-Century-Crofts

Yandow, S. M., Archibeck, M. J., Stevens, P. M., & Shultz, R. (1999). Femoral-shaft fractures in children: A comparison of immediate casting and traction. *Journal of Pediatric Orthopaedics, 19,* 55-59.

SECTION

MULTISYSTEM ISSUES

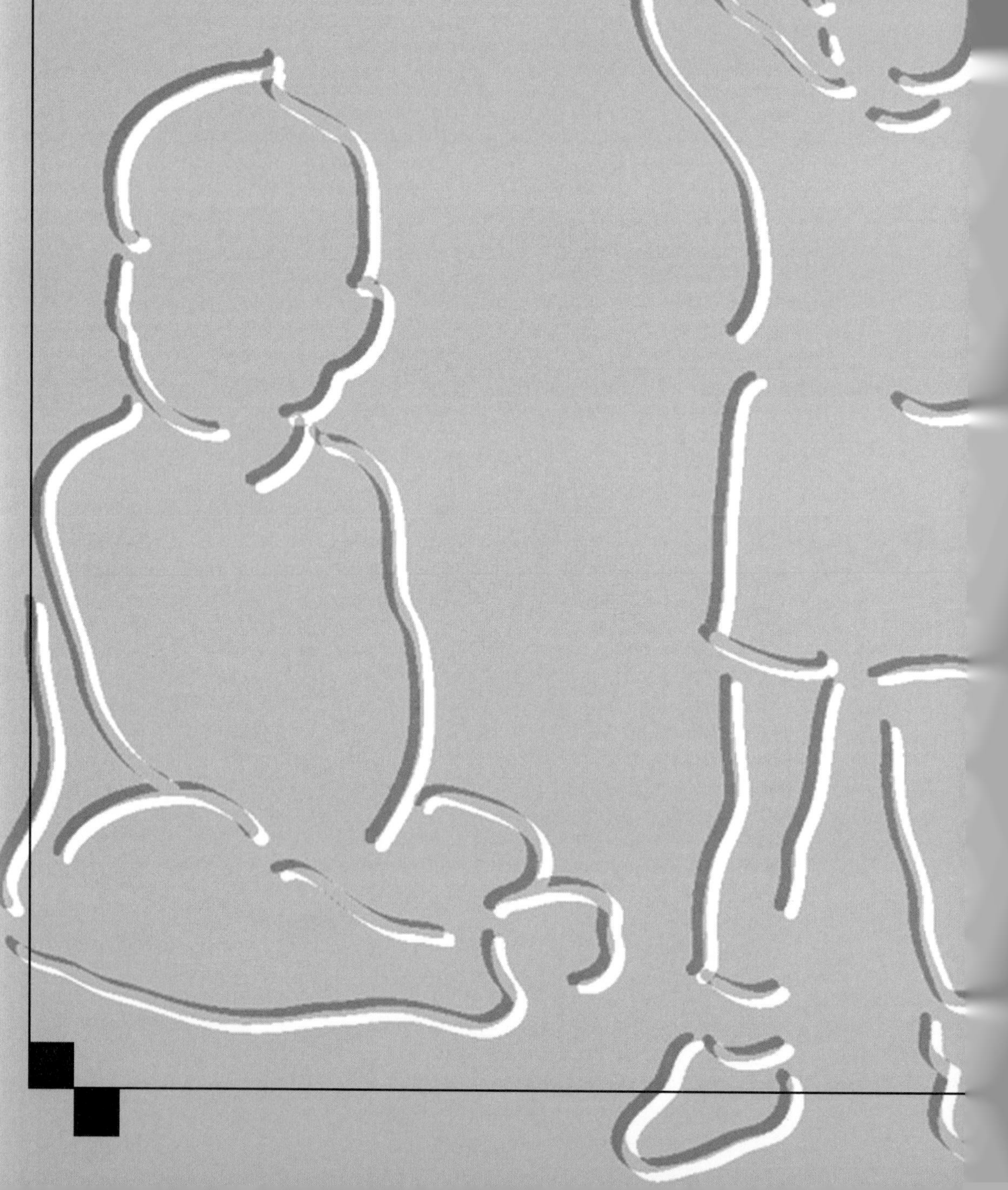

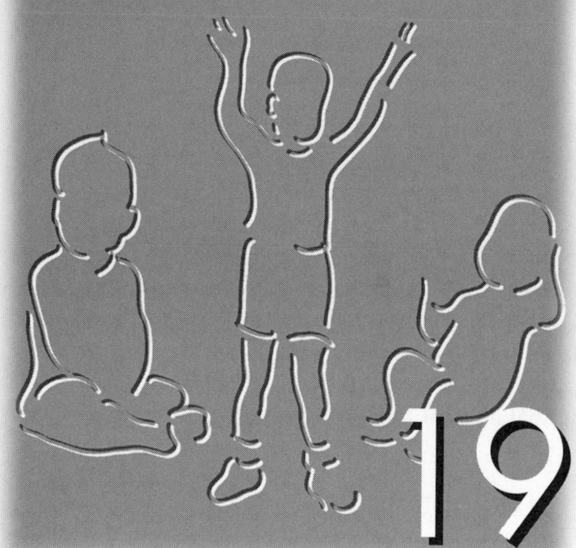

19 Thermal Injuries

Carolyn M. Perry

A burn injury dramatically changes a child's life in an instant. The child endures the shocking experience of the burn; pain and suffering in the acute care setting; and long-term disability, rehabilitation, and disfigurement. This type of catastrophic injury is devastating to both the child and the family. Fortunately, significant declines in the incidence of burn injury have been made. This progress coincides with the increased national attention to burn prevention, widespread use of smoke alarms, burn prevention education, regulation of consumer product safety, and establishment of burn treatment centers. Fewer than 10 hospitals specialized in burns in the United States during the 1950s. Today, approximately 125 specialized burn care centers exist to provide the most current care (American Burn Association [ABA], 2000). The first burn care management specifically targeted to children appeared in Galveston, Texas, at Shriner's Hospital for Crippled Children Burn Institute in 1962. This and the other Shriner's Burn Centers in Cincinnati, Boston, and Sacramento have significantly advanced the understanding and management of pediatric burn injuries.

Pediatric nurses manage thermal injuries in children during the acute phase through the rehabilitative phase. Burn victims often require intensive care to manage multisystem failure, and all require wound care management specific to the type of wound and stage of healing. Nurses are responsible for much of the teaching necessary to prevent or minimize the risk of thermal injury to families with children. This chapter provides a discussion of the risk factors, patterns of thermal injury, pathophysiology, management, and interventions for prevention of burns in the pediatric population.

EPIDEMIOLOGY

Each year more than 1 million persons in the United States sustain significant burns. Approximately 700,000 emergency department visits each year result from burn-related injuries (ABA, 2000). In 1999 an estimated 99,500 children 14 years and younger were treated in hospital emergency departments for burn-related injuries. Of these injuries, 62,580 were thermal burns, 23,620 were scald burns, 9,430 were chemical burns, and 2,250 were electrical burns. In 1999 nearly 3800 children 14 years and younger were treated in hospital emergency departments for fireworks-related injuries. The death rate from fire and flame injury among children 14 years and younger declined 56% from 1987 to 1998 (National Safe Kids Campaign, 2000d).

Victims of burn belong to one of four etiologic categories. The first are victims of their own actions, such as those who played with matches. The second category includes innocent bystanders, such as victims of structure fires. The third category includes victims of preexisting illnesses, such as may occur with epilepsy and injury during a convulsion. Finally, fire-rescue victims are those who tried to save individuals or personal property from a fire (Feldman, Slater, & Goldfarb, 1986).

Unintentional Thermal Injuries

Unintentional injuries cause more deaths in childhood than all other causes combined. Burns are the fifth leading cause of unintentional injury-related death in children younger than 1 year, outranked by suffocation, motor vehicle occupant injury, choking, and drowning. Burns are the fourth leading cause of unintentional injury in children 1 to 4 years old, behind drowning, vehicular injuries, and pedestrian injury. Among children 5 to 14 years old, fire and burns are the fifth leading cause of unintentional injury-related deaths, preceded by motor vehicle occupant injury, drowning, pedestrian injury, and bicycle injury (National Safe Kids Campaign, 2000c). More specifically, scald burn injury (caused by hot liquids or steam) is the most common type of burn-related injury among young children. Hot liquid scalds are responsible for most minor and major burns in children younger than 4 years, accounting for 85% of total injuries. Flame burns account for 13% and most commonly are reported in older children (Herrin & Antoon, 1996).

Thermal injuries are the leading cause of home-related death in children, surpassing drowning, suffocation, choking, unintentional firearm injury, poisoning, and falls (National Safe Kids Campaign, 2000e). The house fire is the most lethal cause of burns in children. Of all fire-related deaths, 75% result from smoke inhalation, caused by the toxic gases produced by fires. Young children are at greatest risk for injuries in the home because they spend the majority of their time there. Children have an additional risk for injury because they may not be able to escape a dangerous situation. They experience a prolonged duration with the burn source, resulting in a deep burn injury. As children grow older and spend less time in the home, the percentages of both fatal and nonfatal unintentional injuries occurring in the home decrease (National Safe Kids Campaign, 2000e).

The kitchen is a primary site of pediatric thermal injury. Cooking activities present numerous hot liquid hazards and usually result in partial-thickness burns (Hill & Strange, 1996). Hot liquid scalds often occur when children younger than 3 years reach for and tip over hot liquids on a stove or counter. Health care providers should be familiar with the characteristic patterns of unintentionally inflicted scald injuries. These include burns on the face, neck, anterior torso, and dominant arm (Hansbrough & Hansbrough, 1999). Contact with hot objects is the second most common burn mechanism in young children. A child can sustain a moderate burn injury by bumping or reaching for an object around heated sources such as a hot stove, oven door, clothing iron, or curling iron (Hansbrough & Hansbrough, 1999).

Water temperature from the faucet can be hot enough to create significant thermal injuries in children. The thermostats of hot water tanks in apartment houses are often set between 140° and 160° F because of the heavy demand for hot water (Hansbrough & Hansbrough, 1999). Thermostats should be set at 120° F. Children will sustain a full-thickness burn from 130° F water in 10 seconds, in 1 second from 140° F water, and 0.5 second from 149° F water (Hill & Strange, 1996). The duration of exposure to hot water may become significant in suspected child abuse cases if the examiner finds inconsistencies in the history of how the burn occurred.

Flame burns occur more often than scalds in children older than 3 years. Children who play with fire account for more than one third of preschool deaths by fire (Nortrade Medical, Inc., 2000). The preschooler is more likely to play alone in the bedroom with matches or lighters. Older boys are usually with friends and out of adult sight when playing with matches and gasoline (Parish, 1997). Flammable fabrics, space heaters, matches, outdoor fires, and house fires are the most common causative factors involved in flame burns. Flame burn injuries account for most major fatal burns (National Safe Kids Campaign, 2000b).

Intentional Thermal Injury

Burns may also result from intentional injury to a child. From 20% to 30% of all pediatric burns in the United States may be caused by child abuse (Crawley, 1996). Most of these injuries occur in children younger than 3 years (Bennett & Gamelli, 1998). Abused burned children often require longer hospitalizations (Hultman, Priolo, Cairns, Grant, Peterson, & Meyer, 1998) and may be more likely to require skin grafting than are nonabused children (Andronicus, Oates, Peat, Spalding, & Martin, 1998). Immersion in hot water is the most commonly reported injury, followed by contact burns with hot objects such as cigarettes. The patterns, site of injury, and inconsistency with history are important clues to intentional thermal injury. Chapter 14 presents information about child abuse.

Common Characteristics of Burn Victims

Although children up to 5 years old represent 9% of the U.S. population, they sustain nearly 20% of all fire-related deaths in the home and are more than twice as likely as the rest of the population to die in a fire. Children have a limited perception of danger, less control of their environment, and limited ability to react promptly and properly to a fire or burn situation (National Safe Kids Campaign, 2000b). Low-income families are at greatest risk for fire-related death and injury because of factors such as lack of functional smoke alarms, substandard housing, economic constraints to enable adequate adult supervision, and use of alternative heating sources. Home fires and home fire–related death are more likely to occur during cold-weather months when there is a significant increase in the number of deaths because of the use of portable or area-heating equipment such as fireplaces, space heaters, and wood stoves.

Children living in rural areas have a dramatically higher risk of dying in a residential fire. Death rates in rural areas are more than twice the rates in large cities and three times higher than rates in large towns and small cities. Native American children are twice as likely as white children to die in a fire, and the risk of death in African American children is tripled. Boys have a higher rate of fire-related death and injury than do girls because boys are nearly twice as likely as girls to play with fire (National Safe Kids Campaign, 2000a). Girls have three times as many microwave-related burns as boys (Powell & Tanz, 1993).

Thermal injuries are some of the most expensive traumatic injuries to treat. The annual cost of fire-related deaths and injuries among children younger than 14 years is $1.2 billion. Children younger than 4 years account for more than half of this annual cost, $555 million. The total annual cost of scald-related deaths and injuries among children 14 years and younger is approximately $2.1 billion, with children younger than 4 years accounting for more than 60% of the total costs ($1.3 billion). Total charges for pediatric admissions to burn centers average $22,700 per case (National Safe Kids Campaign, 2000a).

CLASSIFICATION AND DEFINITION OF BURNS

Burn management depends on the severity of thermal injury. The ABA has classified burn injuries into minor, moderate,

BOX 19-1 Classification of Burn Severity Children

Minor Burn Injury

<10% BSA in children

2% BSA, full-thickness injury without cosmetic or functional risk to eyes, ears, face, hands, feet, or perineum

Moderate Burn Injury

10%-20% BSA mixed partial- and full-thickness injury in children <10 years of age

10% or less BSA full-thickness injury that does not present serious threat of functional or cosmetic impairment of the eyes, ears, face, hands, feet, or perineum

Major Burn Injury

>20% BSA in children

10% or greater BSA full-thickness injury

All burns to face, eyes, ears, hands, feet, or perineum likely result in functional or cosmetic impairment

All burn injuries complicated by inhalation injury or major trauma

Data from Thomas, D. O. (1991). *Quick reference to pediatric emergency nursing*. Gaithersburg, MD: Aspen.
BSA, Body surface area.

and major categories (Box 19-1). Minor burns in a child can usually be treated on an outpatient basis. In infants younger than 6 months, however, even minor burns may be physiologically significant and hospitalization should be considered. Children with moderate burns should be treated in a burn unit or general hospital. Major burns should be treated in a specialized burn center. Burn severity depends on the type of burn incurred, depth and extent of the burn, patient age, and associated illness or injury. The ABA specifies burns that require referral to a specialized burn center (Box 19-2). Subtle differences in assessment will provide the pediatric trauma nurse with information that is critical in determining the appropriate nursing interventions for the patient and family.

Causes of Burns

Burns can be caused by thermal agents such as scalds and flames; chemical agents such as acids, alkali, and organic compounds; electrical agents; or radioactive agents such as x-rays or ultraviolet radiation. In addition, frost bite injuries and toxic epidermal necrolysis share many characteristics of burns. Most burn injuries are caused by thermal agents (97%). Scalds account for 65% to 85% of all burns (Uitvlugt & Ledbetter, 1995). The intensity of the heat source, the duration of contact, and the age of the child determine the extent of tissue damage in a thermal burn. Normal skin can tolerate temperatures up to 40° C (104° F) without injury, but higher temperatures will produce burns.

Characteristics of Burns

The severity of a burn injury is expressed using the percentage of total body surface area (TBSA) involved and the depth of skin injury. The severity of destroyed tissue correlates directly with the physiologic responses, initial management, and prognosis. Other contributing factors in determining the seriousness of injury are the age of the child, location of wounds, causative agent, presence of respiratory involvement, general health of the child, and presence of concomitant injuries (Baker, 1999).

BOX 19-2 American Burn Association's Criteria for Burn Injuries Requiring Referral to a Burn Center

1. Second- and third-degree burns >10% TBSA in patients <10 years or >50 years of age
2. Second- and third-degree burns >10% TBSA in other age groups
3. Second- and third-degree burns that involve the face, hands, feet, genitalia, perineum, and major joints
4. Third-degree burns >5% TBSA in any age group
5. Electrical burns, including lightning injury
6. Chemical burns
7. Inhalation injury
8. Burn injury in patients with preexisting medical disorders that could complicate management, prolong recovery, or affect mortality
9. Any patients with burns and concomitant trauma (e.g., fractures) in which the burn injury poses the greatest risk of morbidity or mortality (In such cases, if the trauma poses the greater immediate risk, the patient must be treated initially in a trauma center until stable before being transferred to a burn center. Physician judgment will be necessary in such situations and should be in concert with the regional medical control plan and triage protocols.)
10. Hospitals without qualified personnel or equipment for the care of children, in which case children with burns should be transferred to a burn center with these capabilities
11. Burn injury in patients who will require special social/emotional and/or long-term rehabilitative support, including cases involving suspected child abuse and substance abuse.

From Ford, E. G., & Andrassy, R. J. (Eds.). (1994). *Pediatric trauma: Initial assessment and management.* Philadelphia: WB Saunders.
TBSA, Total body surface area.

Depth of Burn

The depth of a burn may determine the patient's eventual appearance and function. Most initial burn assessments overestimate body surface area (BSA) and underestimate depth. Burns have traditionally been classified as first-, second-, and third-degree burns. However, a more descriptive terminology relating to the extent of skin destruction is also used.

First-degree, or superficial partial-thickness, burns involve only the outer layers of the epidermis. They are typically bright red in appearance and painful. Pain is the primary symptom and usually resolves in 48 to 72 hours. Tissue damage is minimal, edema is barely perceptible, and skin integrity is maintained. Damaged epithelium often peels off in 5 to 7 days, without blister formation or scarring. First-degree burns are not included in TBSA calculations because they heal so rapidly. First-degree burns may result from sunburn, scalding fluids, or flash burns secondary to explosions (Parish, 1997).

Second-degree burns are subclassified into superficial and deep partial-thickness injuries. Superficial partial-thickness injuries involve only the epidermis. Wounds appear blistered; blanch to pressure; and are mottled pink or red, moist, hypersensitive to touch, and extremely painful. Capillaries are damaged, and increased local vascular permeability leads to plasma leak into the interstitial space, forming blisters. Wounds heal spontaneously in 7 to 14 days, with minimal scarring. Examples of superficial partial-thickness burns are flash burns, scaldings, and brief contact with hot objects.

Deep partial-thickness burns involve the entire epidermis and dermis, but the epidermal appendages necessary for epidermal regeneration are spared (Lyebarger & Kadilak, 2001). They are often scattered among third-degree burns and can be difficult to identify. These injuries have a mottled appearance with waxy white areas. The surface of the burn is dry. Pain is present but is less than that seen in superficial injuries. Blister formation is unusual, although fluid loss from damaged vessels is significant. Fluid losses and metabolic effects are similar to those of third-degree burns. A deep partial-thickness injury heals slowly in 4 to 6 weeks by regeneration from the epithelial lining of skin appendages, sweat glands, and hair follicles. Hypertrophic scarring often occurs if the wound heals by primary closure rather than skin grafting.

Third-degree or full-thickness burns involve the entire epidermal and dermal layers, and they extend to the subcutaneous tissue. They may appear white and pale, red, black, charred, and leathery. Blisters may or may not be present. Thrombosed blood vessels may be visible. The dry, leathery appearance of the wound results from destruction of the elasticity of the burned dermal layer. Pain is notably absent, and there is no sensation to touch because of destruction of dermal nerve endings. The total absence of pain differentiates full-thickness from partial-thickness burns. However, most full-thickness burns have superficial and partial-thickness burned areas at the periphery of the burn, where nerve endings are intact and exposed. Also, excised eschar and donor sites expose nerve endings. The dead avascular tissue provides an ideal environment for bacterial growth. If tissue is not grafted, new granulation tissue forms on the wound bed. The wound heals slowly from the edges, with a high risk of infection and severe scarring. A full-thickness burn is usually caused by a flame, high-intensity flash, chemical, electricity, or prolonged contact with any source of heat (Baker, 1999; Parish, 1997).

Extent of Burn

The extent of injury is expressed by the percentage of body surface burn in relation to TBSA. Several methods have been devised to calculate the percentage of BSA burned. Only second- and third-degree burns are included in the calculations.

Lund and Browder Chart. Lund and Browder (1944) first documented the importance of accurate proportionate BSA as a guide to treatment. They compiled direct measurements of BSA for different ages and related them to burn areas. Modifications of their charts are the most commonly used methods for accurately estimating burn size. Infants and children younger than 14 years have larger heads and shorter lower extremities compared with adults (Figure 19-1).

Rule of Nines. The rule of nines is applied by assigning 9% or multiples of 9 of the BSA to each portion of the body as follows: 18% each for the front and back surface of the trunk (36% total), 9% each for the front and back surface of each leg (18% each leg, 36% total), 9% total for each arm (18% total), 9% for the head, and 1% for the genitalia. The rule of nines enables rapid estimation of the injury. These figures apply to the adult. They may also be used in children older than 14 years but require adjustment for the pediatric population (Herrin & Antoon, 1996). For children in the first year of life, 18% of the body surface consists of the head and neck, and each lower extremity is 14%. With each year of age, 1% is subtracted for the head and neck and added to the lower extremity (Helvig, 1993) (Table 19-1).

Rule of Palm. In small burns of less than 10% BSA or in oddly shaped wounds, the rule of palm provides a rapid estimation of burn size. The examiner superimposes the patient's palm (from the wrist crease to finger crease) over the burned area and counts the number of palms it takes to cover the injury. The palmar area of any given patient is usually 1% of total skin surface.

PATHOPHYSIOLOGY

A thermal injury is similar to other forms of pediatric trauma in that it causes damage to tissues, resulting in an inflammatory reaction with both local and systemic effects (Davey, Wallis, Perkins, & Tingay, 1995; Parish, 1997). A review of local and system effects of thermal injury in the pediatric patient follows.

Local Effects

Anatomy of the Skin

The skin is the largest organ of the body, ranging from 0.25 m^2 in the newborn to 1.0 m^2 in the adult. The skin consists of two layers: the epidermis and the dermis (Figure 19-2). The epidermis is a thin avascular layer that acts as a protective barrier against the environment. The thickness of the epidermis varies. It is thickest over the palmar surfaces of the hands and the plantar surfaces of the feet. When the epidermal is thin (as over the ears, genitalia, and medial portions of upper extremities and in very young patients), even a brief exposure to a heat source may result in a full-thickness burn. The epidermis itself is composed of five layers, the deepest of which is a single layer of basal cells capable of producing new skin cells that move to the skin's surface to replace lost cells. The number of basal cells that survive after injury determines the extent to which regeneration is possible.

The dermis is formed by connective tissue and contains collagen and elastic fibers. The two-layered dermis contains

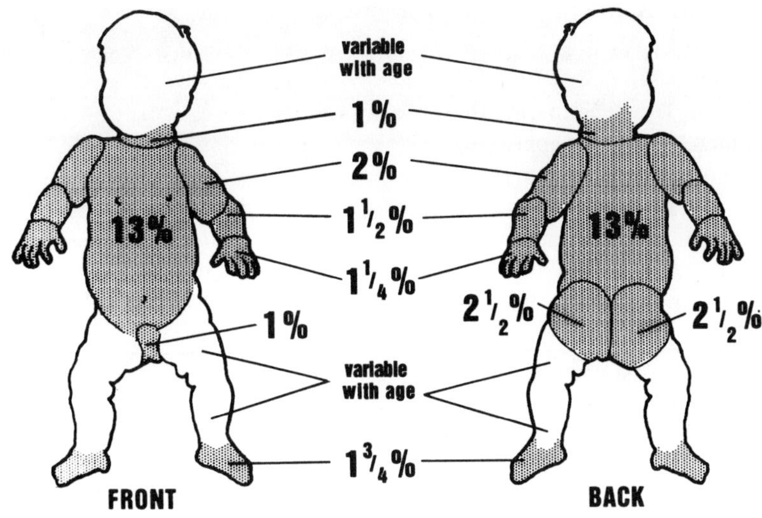

Lund and Browder Chart

	Age - Years						Burn Depth		
	Birth	1	5	10	15	Adult	partial	full	Total Burn
Head	19	17	13	11	9	7			
Neck	2	2	2	2	2	2			
Ant Trunk	13	13	13	13	13	13			
Post Trunk	13	13	13	13	13	13			
R Buttock	2.5	2.5	2.5	2.5	2.5	2.5			
L Buttock	2.5	2.5	2.5	2.5	2.5	2.5			
Genitalia	1	1	1	1	1	1			
RU Arm	4	4	4	4	4	4			
LU Arm	4	4	4	4	4	4			
RL Arm	3	3	3	3	3	3			
LL Arm	3	3	3	3	3	3			
R Hand	2.5	2.5	2.5	2.5	2.5	2.5			
L Hand	2.5	2.5	2.5	2.5	2.5	2.5			
R Thigh	5.5	6.5	8	8	9	9.5			
L Thigh	5.5	6.5	8	8	9	9.5			
R Leg	5	5	5.5	6	6.5	7			
L Leg	5	5	5.5	6	6.5	7			
R Foot	3.5	3.5	3.5	3.5	3.5	3.5			
L Foot	3.5	3.5	3.5	3.5	3.5	3.5			
								Cumulative Total	

FIGURE 19-1 Modified Lund and Browder chart. The shaded areas remain relatively constant for all age groups. (From Uitvlugt, N. D., & Ledbetter, D. J. [1995]. Treatment of pediatric burns. In R. M. Arensman [Ed.], *Pediatric trauma: Initial care of the injured child* [p. 179]. New York: Raven Press.)

blood vessels, nerve endings, sweat glands, sebaceous glands, lymph vessels, and hair follicles. The dermis supplies nutrition to the epidermis. The dermis is not capable of reepithelialization and requires surgical excision and grafting to close the wound (Baker, 1999). Under the dermis is a layer of subcutaneous tissue comprised of fat and connective tissues. The dermis contributes to retention of body fluids and body heat.

The functions of the skin are important to consider when caring for burn patients. The skin prevents loss of body fluids, controls body temperature, synthesizes vitamin D upon exposure to sunlight, and determines identity. Most important, the skin is the primary protective barrier against invasive infection, preventing penetration of microorganisms into the subcutaneous tissues. Burn wound infection is a major cause of mortality and morbidity. Sweat glands help maintain body temperature by controlling the amount of heat lost by evaporation. Infants have thinner epidermal layers and insulating subcutaneous tissue than older children and adults. They tend to lose more water and heat at a faster rate compared with adults. Their thin layers of skin increase their susceptibility to serious burn injuries. Children have a higher mortality rate than do adults for the same TBSA and severity of burn injury (Parish, 1997). The skin also contributes to appearance and individual identity, which is a major readjustment problem for severely burned victims.

Zones of Burn Injury

Tissue injury from burns results in coagulation and altered inflammatory response because of vascular changes. When skin is destroyed, edema forms and evaporative fluid loss increases. There are three zones of burn injury based on the extent of local tissue damage (Figure 19-3).

Zone of Hyperemia. The outermost zone, the zone of hyperemia, is characterized by an intact epidermis and

TABLE 19-1 **Pediatric Modified Rule of Nines**

Body portion	Age (yr) 1	2	3	4	5
Head and neck	18%	17%	16%	15%	14%
Anterior leg	14%	14.5%	15%	15.5%	16%
Posterior leg	14%	14.5%	15%	15.5%	16%
Anterior trunk	18%	18%	18%	18%	18%
Posterior trunk	18%	18%	18%	18%	18%
Anterior arm	9%	9%	9%	9%	9%
Posterior arm	9%	9%	9%	9%	9%

During the first year of life, the child's head and neck make up 18% of the body surface, and each lower extremity is 14%. As age progresses each year, subtract 1% for the head and neck and add it to the lower extremity.

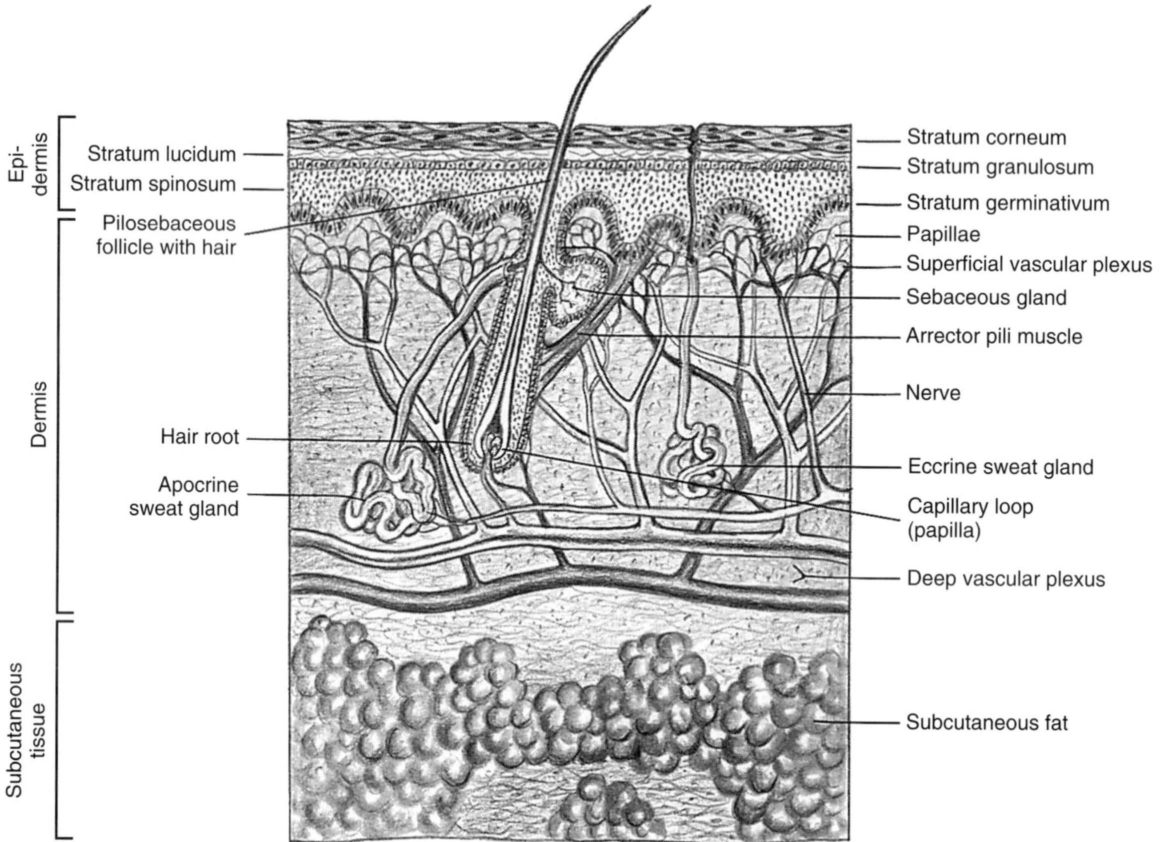

FIGURE 19-2 Schematic cross-sectional representation of the skin. (From Thompson, J. M., McFarland, G. K., Hirsch J. E., & Tucker, S. M. [2001]. *Mosby's manual of clinical nursing* [5th ed.]. St. Louis: Mosby.)

dilated microvasculature with increased blood flow. The increased blood flow is one of the consequences of the inflammatory response. The skin heals without scarring (Kirelik & Hawk, 1997).

Zone of Vascular Stasis. The zone of vascular stasis is the area surrounding the zone of coagulation and is characterized by compromised capillary blood flow and diminished perfusion. Tissue is severely damaged from heat but is not coagulated. Tissue in this zone can be saved with prevention of further injury and with adequate perfusion (Baker, 1999).

Zone of Coagulation (Necrosis). The innermost zone where capillary blood flow has ceased as a result of hypercoagulation and tissue destruction is the zone of coagulation. Tissue destruction in this zone is irreversible. The area appears pale white and is unaffected by digital pressure. The tissue temperature in this zone reaches at least 45° C (113° F) during the thermal injury. The zone of coagulation may continue to develop up to 24 hours after the burn (Lazear, 1993).

Systemic Effects

Although all major organ systems are affected by burn injury, the skin is the first organ affected. Injury to the skin unfolds

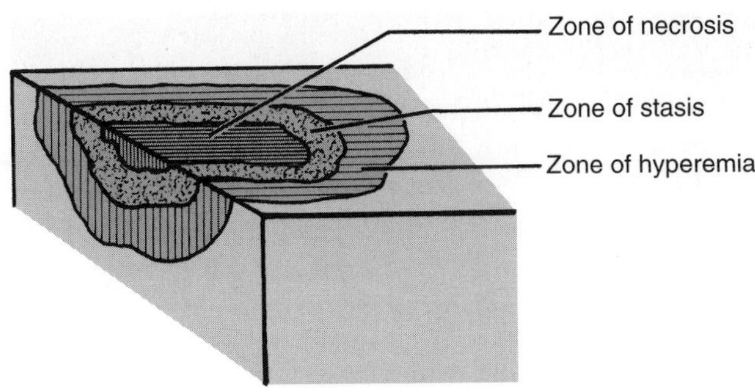

FIGURE 19-3 Zones of burn injury. (From Wong, D. L., Hockenberry-Eaton, M., Wilson, D., Winkelstein, M. L., Ahmann, E., & Divito-Thomas, P. A. [Eds.]. [1999]. *Nursing care of infants and children* [6th ed.]. St. Louis: Mosby.)

a series of events that can cause serious damage to other organs if early and aggressive resuscitation is not initiated.

Cardiovascular System

Burn shock is caused by dramatic alterations in circulation and is apparent immediately after the thermal injury. Cardiac output decreases by approximately 50% of the preburn value and is attributed to several factors. Myocardial depressant factor is associated with severe burn injury and directly affects the contractility of the heart (Baker, 1999). This factor combines with increased capillary permeability to cause massive leaks and vasodilation, which result in rapid reduction in circulating blood volume. Burns covering more than 15% to 30% of the BSA cause a generalized fluid leak throughout the body, not just at the site of the injury. This process occurs for 24 hours after the injury and then begins to resolve. If adequate fluid resuscitation is provided, cardiac output returns to normal in 24 to 36 hours. If fluid is not replaced, cardiac output continues to decrease, resulting in inadequate perfusion, organ dysfunction, and ultimately death (Baker, 1999).

Renal System

Renal function is affected immediately by thermal injury via two mechanisms. First, peripheral circulatory failure occurs as cardiac output decreases, which decreases blood flow to the kidneys. Second, the kidneys respond to the stress of decreased blood flow by increasing circulating levels of antidiuretic hormone, which further decreases urine output. Acute tubular necrosis results from the combination of these powerful physiologic mechanisms (Baker, 1999; Cortiella & Marvin, 1997). Oliguria may persist for 48 to 72 hours after the burn occurred, even when the intravascular volume has been replenished (Carvajal, 1994). Urinalysis reveals elevated blood urea nitrogen and creatinine levels, a result of tissue breakdown and decreased circulating volume. The hematuria present is caused by the hemolysis of red blood cells. Cell destruction releases large amounts of myoglobin, which occludes kidney tubules. Tubules that are blocked are unable to produce urine and eventually die. Myoglobinuria is observed predominantly in electrical trauma but is also present in thermal injuries (Cortiella & Marvin, 1997).

By the time an infant reaches 1 year of age, renal function is comparable to that of the adult. Infants younger than 6 months, however, have limited osmolar concentrating capacity, and free water clearance by the kidney is less efficient as demands from thermal injury are compounded. For these reasons, infants are prone to fluid retention, which is reflected as peripheral edema and pulmonary impairment. Pulmonary edema is caused more frequently by hydrostatic pressures and, in the absence of an inhalation injury, is almost diagnostic of fluid overload. Management of overhydration should include pharmacologic diuresis.

Pulmonary System

Pulmonary complications are the leading cause of death from burn injury. The pulmonary effects that result from burn injury include inhalation injury, hot liquid aspiration, hypoxia, pneumonia, pulmonary edema, and acute respiratory distress syndrome (ARDS). Specific pulmonary complications are often linked to the cause of the thermal injury.

Inhalation injury increases the risk of mortality and length of hospitalization (Schiller, 1996). Inhalation injuries commonly occur in patients who are burned in a closed space such as a small building, basement, or mobile home. Inhalation injuries should be suspected in children with fire burns, but the injuries are not always obvious or recognized in scald injuries. Patients often have burns of the face, singed nasal hairs, hoarseness or wheezing, or carbonaceous sputum. Inhalation of steam, hot liquid, smoke, or other irritants produces edema, erythema, and blistering in the upper airway. Progressive edema may cause upper airway obstruction. Smoke, hot particle inhalation, or hot liquid aspiration may cause mucosal sloughing, atelectasis, bronchiolar plugging, and infection. Upper airway damage usually is related to heat injury, whereas lower airway injury is related to chemical or toxic effects (Cortiella & Marvin, 1997). Inhaling heated air may cause damage to the upper airway but usually does not damage tissue below the vocal cords. Upon inspiration the heat is cooled in the upper airway before reaching the trachea. Reflex closure of the cords and laryngeal spasm prevent full inhalation. Toxic chemical inhalation affect the lower respiratory tract and can cause pulmonary edema and alveolar-capillary defects (Cortiella & Marvin, 1997). Several stages of pulmonary injury associated with inhalation injuries are observed (Table 19-2). The mortality rate increases to 100% if acute pulmonary insufficiency exists. Occurrence of pulmonary edema within 48 to 72 hours is associated with a 50% mortality rate. Bronchopneumonia occurring 5 to 7 days after the burn occurred is associated with a 30% to 40% mortality rate (Cot, Ryan, Todres, & Goudsouzian, 1993).

Although rarely reported, aspiration of hot liquid can occur in conjunction with upper-body scalds, leading to acute compromise of the small pediatric airway by rapidly progressive mucosal edema and airway occlusion with clinical features similar to those of acute infectious epiglottitis. Aspiration of hot liquid should be suspected in children with burns in or around the mouth, particularly if there are

TABLE 19-2 Stages of Pulmonary Injury

	Physical Examination	Bronchoscopic Evidence
First	Singed nasal hairs, eyebrows	Potentially normal; may have slight edema in upper airway, epiglottis and arytenoids; could have soot in airway passages
Second	24 hours: stridor, dyspnea, and tachypnea	Upper airway edema, particularly arytenoids, epiglottis; and erythematous
Third	72 hours if not intubated: worsening stridor; tachypnea	Not intubated: worsening of above
	If intubated: bronchorrhea; tachypnea	Intubated; edematous with increasing blood vessel markings, possible cast formation, increasing secretions

From Cortiella, J. (1997). Management of the pediatric burn patient. *Nursing Clinics of North America, 32*(2), 316.

any subtle signs of upper airway edema. Stridor and excessive salivation are common symptoms occurring with hot water inhalation burns (Hudson, Jones, & Rode 1994). When hot liquid aspiration is suspected in the child with respiratory distress, immediate endotracheal intubation should be performed. If this complication is suspected in the child without respiratory distress, direct laryngoscopy in the operating room is done (Sheridan, 1996).

Smoke inhalation is another common cause of pulmonary complications in the pediatric patient. The composition of the smoke depends on the substance burning, the temperature and rate at which the smoke is being generated, and the amount of oxygen present in the burning environment. As the child inhales, smoke and soot particles enter the respiratory tract. The size of the particles directly influences the severity of the lung injury. Larger particles are filtered in the upper airway and do not enter the lower airway. However, accumulation of debris and secretions can cause airway obstruction, atelectasis, and impaired ciliary clearance. Smoke inhalation may extend to the alveoli, causing edema and atelectasis.

Inhaling toxic chemicals caused by combustion can cause trauma to the tracheobronchial tree. Chemicals formed via combustion and incomplete combustion can be toxic when inhaled (Table 19-3). The process of combustion consumes oxygen. Victims of fires in closed spaces, such as a house or a car, will inhale air that has an oxygen concentration of less than 21%. The reduction in the fraction of inspired oxygen (FiO_2) leads to arterial hypoxemia.

TABLE 19-3 Chemicals Resulting From Combustion and Incomplete Combustion That Can Be Toxic When Inhaled

Burning Source	Toxic Substance
Organic materials	Carbon monoxide
Polyurethane	Hydrogen cyanide ammonia, halogen acids
Rubber	Sulfur dioxide
Upholstery	Hydrogen chloride
Wool, silk	Hydrogen cyanide, hydrogen sulfide
Polyvinyl chloride	Phosgene

From Emergency Nurses Association. (1995). *Trauma nursing core course: Provider manual* (4th ed.). Park Ridge, IL: Author.

Inhalation of carbon monoxide (CO) is the leading cause of death from house fires. CO is present in the smoke resulting from combustion of organic materials such as wood, coal, and gasoline. CO is also released when the available oxygen to support combustion is consumed and incomplete combustion occurs. When inhaled, CO crosses the alveolar-capillary membrane and binds to the oxygen-binding sites on the hemoglobin molecule. Because CO has an affinity 200 to 300 times greater than oxygen to bind to hemoglobin, the oxygen-carrying capacity of hemoglobin is greatly reduced. CO also affects cardiac muscle by binding with myoglobin, causing changes such as hemorrhage and necrosis of the cardiac muscle. The oxygen remaining on the hemoglobin molecule is not easily released to the tissues. Thus tissue hypoxia is even more serious for patients who have preexisting cardiac or pulmonary conditions. The presence of CO on hemoglobin does not affect the patient's partial pressure of oxygen (PaO_2) but does affect the oxygen content (O_2 content = oxygen combined with hemoglobin in physical solution) (Nunn, 2000). The patient will have a low oxygen saturation (SaO_2), as calculated from an arterial blood gas sample. The oxygen saturation obtained by pulse oximetry may be inaccurate because the pulse oximeter cannot accurately discriminate between oxyhemoglobin and carboxyhemoglobin. Because PaO_2 remains normal, the chemoreceptors are not stimulated to increase ventilation and the patient sustains tissue hypoxia (Flynn, 2002). Sustained lung damage causes increased pulmonary arterial pressure, resulting in right-sided heart failure and tissue organ failure. These two effects contribute to the multisystem organ failure common in burn patients (Cortiella & Marvin, 1997).

Pulmonary edema may be observed in patients who have sustained thermal injury to the skin with or without inhalation injury. Pulmonary edema is observed in patients with toxic chemical inhalation as a result of fluid overload or in conjunction with ARDS (Baker, 1999; Cortiella & Marvin). Burned children with ARDS have a higher mortality rate than pediatric trauma patients with ARDS (Scannell, Waxman, & Tominaga, 1995). This syndrome results from pulmonary damage and fluid leak into the interstitial spaces of the lung. Loss of compliance and interference with oxygenation are the consequences of pulmonary insufficiency in conjunction with systemic sepsis (Baker, 1999). Respiratory failure in pediatric burn patients can be caused by pneumonia secondary to sepsis, airway injury, or contamination from intubation. Most pulmonary infections in the early postburn period result from nosocomial exposure, immobility, and abdominal distention. Pulmonary infections from sepsis that occur from a septic burn wound or phlebitis from an intravenous catheter occur later in the postburn period.

Full-thickness burns encircling the chest can cause edema and inelastic eschar formation, restricting chest wall excursion and ventilation. It becomes increasingly difficult for the child to ventilate. Escharotomy of the chest relieves this pressure and improves ventilation. The full-thickness burn of eschar is sharply incised to the subcutaneous tissues. Bilateral incisions are made in the anterior axillary lines and connected across the anterior surface by a subcostal incision (Figure 19-4). This technique is also applicable to circumferential extremity burns when neurovascular compromise develops from progressive tissue edema.

Central Nervous System

Hypoxemia, sepsis, and hypovolemia all have devastating effects on the brain. These complications can result in encephalopathy, a relatively common occurrence. Manifestations of encephalopathy include hallucinations, personality changes, delirium, seizures, and coma. A full neurologic recovery is likely, even with prolonged and serious manifestations (Baker, 1999).

Gastrointestinal System

Systemic responses from thermal injuries interrupt the gastrointestinal (GI) system. Poor peripheral circulation is likely to cause an ileus. Gastric motility is usually restored after adequate fluid resuscitation and resolves within 48 to 72 hours. Recurrence of an ileus later in the hospital course suggests developing sepsis (Baker, 1999). Ulcers are a common GI effect from thermal injuries, specifically Curling's ulcer. The GI erosion of this condition is unknown, but it is related to compromised submucosal blood flow in the immediate postburn period and atrophy of the intestinal microvilli because of lack of enteral nutrition (Baker, 1999). Increased levels of gastric acid secretion may also cause ulcers. Treatment with antacids and H_2 blockers decreases acidity in the stomach, prevents ulcer formation, and prevents development of perforation or hemorrhage.

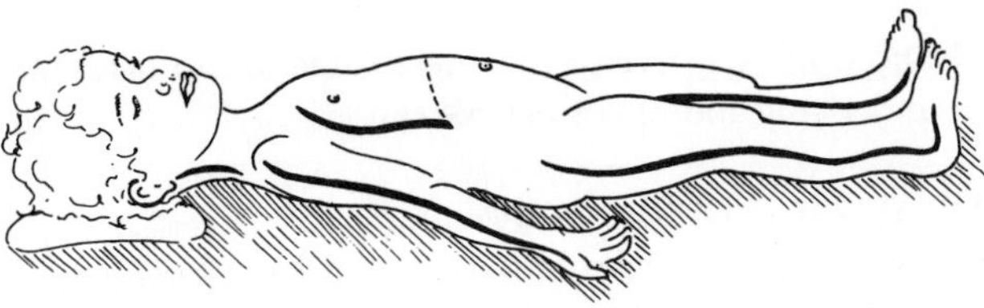

FIGURE 19-4 Escharotomy of the chest relieves pressure and improves ventilation. The full-thickness burn of eschar is sharply incised to the subcutaneous tissues. Bilateral incisions are made in the anterior axillary lines and connected across the anterior surface by a subcostal incision. (Redrawn from Ford, E. G., & Andrassy R. J. [Eds.]. (1994). *Pediatric trauma: Initial assessment and management* [p. 298]. Philadelphia: WB Saunders.)

Endocrine and Metabolic Systems

Stress of the injury causes the sympathetic nervous system to stimulate the adrenal medulla to release epinephrine and norepinephrine, which increase cardiac output. The adrenal cortex produces and releases cortisol to promote tissue repair and wound healing. Adrenocortical hormone levels peak immediately after injury and remain elevated. The stress of the burn injury also accelerates the metabolic rate. Compared with adults, children are already predisposed to a higher basal metabolic rate per kilogram and have limited glycogen stores to provide energy. The extent of the increase in metabolic rate depends on the nature and severity of traumatic insult. Age, ambient temperature, pain, anxiety, patient activity, and infection also influence the rate of metabolism. Increased metabolism in the patient is demonstrated by tachypnea resulting from increased oxygen consumption, tachycardia caused by increased sympathetic response, and low-grade fever (Mozingo, Cioffi, & Pruitt, 1994).

Burn patients have higher caloric needs than patients with any other injury. Patients with a greater than 40% BSA burn may experience metabolic rates two times greater than normal (Herndon, Rutan, Alison, & Cox, 1993). Stress causes glycogen depletion within 12 to 24 hours, after which the body resorts to glyconeogenesis for high-energy needs. Blood glucose levels may be elevated as a result of insulin resistance. Rapid protein breakdown and muscle wasting occur if sufficient protein replacement is not provided (Baker, 1999). These metabolic and hormonal consequences have important effects on nutritional status.

IMMEDIATE LIFESAVING MEASURES FOR BURN VICTIMS

Emergency Care

Immediate management of a burn injury is usually the responsibility of the family or local emergency medical services (EMS). The first consideration is to stop the burning process (Box 19-3). Neutralization of the burning source does not take precedence over rapid assessment of the patient's airway. The child should be transported to the nearest facility for definitive treatment and evaluated for transfer to a specialized burn center. Management of child and family anxiety, although not the highest priority at this stage, is recognized as an important aspect of care.

Stop the Burning Process

Extinguishing the fire is the first critical step. Children have a tendency to panic and run when they are afraid, which is the worst possible action. The emphasis should be on "stop, drop, and roll," using a blanket, rug, coat, or towel to smother the flames while placing the child in a supine position. The risk of facial burns, hair ignition, and inhalation injury is minimized by rapidly placing the blazing

BOX 19-3 Emergency Treatment for Major and Minor Burns

Minor Burns: Stop the Burning Process

- Apply cool water to the burn or hold the burned area under cool running water; do not use ice.
- Do not disturb any blisters that form.
- Do not apply anything to the wound.
- Cover the burn with a clean cloth if there is risk of damage or contamination.
- Remove burned clothing and jewelry.

Major Burns: Stop the Burning Process

- Flame burns: Smother the fire.
- Place the victim in the horizontal position.
- Roll the victim in a blanket or similar object; avoid covering the head.
- Assess for an adequate airway and breathing.
- If the victim is not breathing, begin mouth-to-mouth resuscitation.
- Remove burned clothing and jewelry.
- Cover wound with a clean cloth.
- Keep victim warm.
- Transport the victim to medical aid.
- Begin intravenous and oxygen therapy.

From Wong, D. L., Hockenberry-Eaton, M., Wilson, D., Winkelstein, M. L., Ahmann, E., & Divito-Thomas, P. A. (Eds.). (1999). *Nursing care of infants and children.* St. Louis: Mosby.

victim in a horizontal position (Parish, 1997). All clothing and jewelry are immediately removed from the child. Clothing and jewelry exposed to flames or hot water may retain heat for long periods and continue to be a source of thermal injury. Synthetic fibers may melt when exposed to high temperatures, sticking to the skin and concentrating heat exposure to localized areas. Jewelry can transfer heat from metal to skin, and its constricting nature may enhance the formation of edema. The degree of burn injury is related to the degree of heat and the length of time the burning agent is applied to the skin (Foster & Ford, 1994).

Ensure Airway, Breathing, and Circulation

Neutralization of the burning source does not take precedence over rapid assessment of the patient's airway. Airway, breathing, and circulation should be assessed and prioritized as soon as possible (Box 19-4). If the patient has significant airway compromise or is not breathing, the appropriate airway device should be inserted and ventilation restored. The spontaneously breathing patient should be assessed for adequacy of respiratory effort and gas exchange. The maximum available concentration of oxygen should be administered with humidification, if possible (Gillespie, 1992). The mechanics of respiration are evaluated and the chest wall inspected for loss of integrity. Occasionally, the severely burned patient will have circumferential burns of the torso that prevent effective excursion. An initial evaluation of the circulatory status should confirm the presence of a perfusing cardiac rhythm. A pulseless child will require pediatric advanced life support and further evaluation to determine an underlying and/or correctable cause.

BOX 19-4 Rapid Cardiopulmonary Assessment

Every clinician who works with children should be able to recognize potential pulmonary and circulatory failure and impending cardiopulmonary arrest based on a rapid cardiopulmonary assessment.

A. Airway patency
   - Able to maintain independently
   - Requires adjuncts/assistance to maintain

B. Breathing
   - Rate
   - Mechanics
     - Retractions
     - Accessory muscles
     - Nasal flaring
   - Air entry
     - Chest expansion
     - Breath sounds
     - Stridor
     - Wheezing
     - Paradoxical chest movement
   - Color

C. Circulation
   - Heart rate
   - Blood pressure
   - Volume/strength of central pulses
   - Peripheral pulses
     - Present/absent
     - Volume/strength
   - Skin perfusion
     - Capillary refill time (consider ambient temperature)
     - Temperature
     - Color
     - Mottling
   - Central nervous system perfusion
     - Responsiveness
     - Awake
     - Responds to voice
     - Responds to pain
     - Unresponsiveness
   - Recognizes parents
   - Muscle tone
   - Pupil size
   - Posturing

From American Heart Association. (1997). *Pediatric advanced life support.* Dallas: Author.

Treat the Wound

The use of cool or iced solutions to reduce the pain of a partial-thickness burn may be helpful, but only in burns of greater than 20% TBSA and in environmental temperatures of greater than 50° F (Parish, 1997). The burn can be covered with a clean cloth to minimize external contamination. Covering a burn also alleviates pain by eliminating air contact with the nerve endings. The child with extensive burns should be completely covered to prevent hypothermia.

Topical medication should be not be applied until the child is assessed in an emergency department.

Transport the Child

The child should be transported to the nearest medical facility or emergency department. If this cannot be accomplished within 30 minutes, intravenous access should be attempted with a large-bore catheter (Parish, 1997). Oral fluids should not be given because of the risk of paralytic ileus and to prevent vomiting and subsequent aspiration. All trauma patients require cervical spine immobilization. When the child is moved, the head and body must be held and turned as a unit and the head and neck firmly supported so that the head does not roll, twist, or tilt (American Heart Association, 2000).

Provide Reassurance

The family and child will need reassurance from the persons responding to the initial scene. Communicating with the family at every step of stabilization may help some families, whereas others will be unresponsive because they are in shock. Still others may be combative and disruptive. Using professional judgment in the management of the family may guide clinicians to the best course of action for the situation.

Management of Major Burns

The main priorities upon arrival to the hospital include establishment and maintenance of an adequate airway, evaluation of the cardiopulmonary system, initiation of fluid administration, and evaluation and treatment of the wound. A number of procedures and activities are often initiated on admission (Box 19-5). Patients with severe burn injuries often present as alert and calm and do not act seriously injured. On initial presentation the patient should be questioned about how the burn occurred and about significant medical history. Gaining knowledge about how the burn occurred can assist in determining the extent of the injury.

BOX 19-5 Procedures and Activities Initiated for Patients With Hospital Admissions for Major Burns

1. Ascertain the adequacy of the airway and provide oxygen, intubation, and ventilation support as indicated.
2. Insert a large-bore intravenous line, preferably through unburned skin, to deliver fluids at a sufficiently rapid rate to effect resuscitation.
3. Remove clothing and jewelry and examine for secondary trauma.
4. Obtain an admission weight.
5. Insert a nasogastric tube to empty stomach contents and maintain gastric decompression.
6. Insert an indwelling Foley catheter to obtain specimens and depth of injury.
7. Calculate fluid requirements and establish the appropriate regimen.
8. Provide intravenous medication for control of pain and anxiety only after adequate oxygenation is ensured and fluid resuscitation is initiated.
9. Obtain baseline laboratory studies.
10. Perform escharotomy and/or fasciotomy to the chest and extremities for constricting circumferential eschar or elevated compartment pressures and for impaired circulation.
11. Apply topical antimicrobials and dressings to the burn wounds.
12. Obtain a history regarding the injury and other pertinent data.
13. Administer appropriate tetanus prophylaxis.

From Wong, D. L., Hockenberry-Eaton, M., Wilson, D., Winkelstein, M. L., Ahmann, E., & Divito-Thomas, P. A. (Eds.). (1999). *Nursing care of infants and children.* St. Louis: Mosby.

Airway

Establishment of a patent airway is the main priority. The child's narrow airway is easily obstructed by foreign matter such as blood, mucus, and dental fragments, and it is cleared with suctioning. If the patient has circumferential burns of the neck, the developing edema may compromise the patient's airway. When suspicion for respiratory compromise exists, immediate intubation should be considered. The most important management concerns for upper airway injuries are recognition and realization that inhalation injuries are progressive (Foster & Ford, 1994). Further treatment depends on the extent of the inhalation injury and whether the patient has any previous respiratory problems (Table 19-4). Tracheostomy should be avoided in early burn management (American Heart Association and American Academy of Pediatrics, 2000). The length of time to maintain artificial airway control and ventilation depends on the patient's management course. Tissue edema often begins to resolve in 48 to 72 hours. A predictable decrease in pulmonary function occurs after each debridement or excision of inflamed or infected eschar. Early burn wound excision and grafting may require prolonged intubation because of repeated operations and the use of significant quantities of narcotic analgesics. Decreasing the work of breathing and maintaining mechanical support can reduce metabolic demands.

Fluid Management

The goal of fluid resuscitation in the burned child is to provide enough intravenous fluids to prevent shock without causing pulmonary edema. The objective is to maintain the function of vital organ through adequate support of cardiac output and replacement of plasma volume without producing excessive edema. Fluid resuscitation compensates for water and sodium losses to the traumatized area and the interstitial spaces, replenishing sodium deficits, restoring circulating volume, providing adequate perfusion, correcting acidosis, and improving renal function. Experts agree on the objectives of fluid resuscitation, but controversy exists regarding the quantity, composition, and timing of fluid administration.

Several formulas have been proposed for resuscitation in children, with most based on the weight of the patient, as in

TABLE 19-4 Treatment Algorithms for Pathophysiologic Events Resulting From Mild, Moderate, and Severe Inhalation Injury

Problem	Diagnostic/Treatment	Seen In
Hypoxia	Supplemental oxygen	All injuries
Reactive bronchorrhea, copious secretions	Incentive spirometry, chest physiotherapy, nasotracheal suctioning	All injuries
Inspissated secretions	Humidification, nasotracheal suctioning	Moderate to severe injuries
Wheezing	Diagnostic bronchoscopy to distinguish endobronchial obstruction (plugging) from bronchospasm and edema	Moderate to severe injuries
Plugging (inspissated mucus or mucosal slough)	Humidification, therapeutic bronchoscopy as needed, aerosolized heparin	Moderate to severe injuries
Bronchospasm	Nebulized β_2-agonists; if ineffective, then intravenous aminophylline	Moderate to severe injuries
Respiratory failure	Intubation, mechanical ventilation, permissive hypercapnia, tracheostomy if failure is prolonged (>14 days)	Severe inhalation injury

From Fitzpatrick, J. C., & Cloffi, W. G., Jr. (1996). Diagnosis and treatment of inhalation injury. In D. N. Herndon (Ed.), *Total burn care* (p. 187). Philadelphia: WB Saunders.

TABLE 19-5 Standard Formulas for Estimating Fluid Requirements for Burned Children for the First 24 Hours of Therapy

Formula	Fluid Type*	First 24 hr
Parkland	Electrolyte	4 ml/kg/% burn
	Colloid	None
	Glucose in water	None
Brooke	Electrolyte	0.5 ml/kg/% burn
	Colloid	1.5 ml/kg/% burn
	Glucose in water	2000 ml
Evans	Electrolyte	1 ml/kg/% burn
	Colloid	1 ml/kg/% burn
	Glucose in water	2000 ml
Carvajal (1975)	Electrolyte with 12.5 g human serum albumin per liter	5000 ml/m^2 body surface area burned + 2000 ml per square total body surface area

From Foster, J. E., & Ford, E. G. (1994). Burn injury. In E. G. Ford & R. J. Andrassy (Eds.), *Pediatric trauma: Initial assessment and management* (p. 302). Philadelphia: WB Saunders.
* *Colloid*, Plasmanate, plasma, dextran; *electrolyte*, Ringer's lactate.

adults. The formula may not be accurate in children because of their greater BSA in relation to their weight in comparison with adults; this is because children lose additional fluid through their exposed surface area (Herndon et al., 1993). Several formulas are available, each using a different calculation (weight in kilograms, percentage of BSA burned, square meter of surface area) and each varying slightly depending on the type of fluid administered (Table 19-5). Carvajal (1994) reports that although the Parkland formula and the modified Brooke formula have worldwide popularity, many inaccuracies and major modifications of the initial resuscitation plan have been reported with their use. The main concern with these formulas is that they do not differentiate between maintenance requirements and burn-related fluid losses.

Regardless of the formula used to calculate fluid requirements, it should be remembered that the formulas are only *guides* for fluid administration. Adequacy of resuscitation is assessed and evaluated using objective clinical parameters. Urine output should be greater than 0.5 to 2 ml/kg/hr, and serum electrolytes, osmolarity, and albumin levels should be normal. Pulse rate and pulse pressure should be within normal parameters for age, and adequate capillary refill should be observed in the distal extremities. Arterial, central venous, or pulmonary artery pressure monitoring is necessary only in very complicated or severe cases, such as preexisting disease states of juvenile diabetes or cystic fibrosis (Herndon et al., 1993).

The controversy regarding fluid composition lies in choosing between an isotonic or hypertonic solution and whether colloids need to be added. Herndon et al. (1993) recommend an isotonic solution for initial fluid resuscitation. Advocates of hypertonic solutions believe that intravascular volume can be obtained by osmotically pulling fluid from the interstitial space rather than adding exogenous fluid. Potential hypernatremia, hyperosmolarity, and intravascular dehydration are severe drawbacks to the use of this resuscitation method, especially in children (Herndon et al., 1993).

The use of colloids is criticized on the assumption that colloids administered during the first 24 hours after injury increase protein accumulation in the interstitium and trap water (Demling, 1987). One study demonstrates that albumin added to resuscitation fluids maintains serum albumin levels within the normal range, curtails edema, and improves the general condition of the patient (Carvajal, 1980). The most commonly used colloid is albumin. Herndon et al. (1993) recommend adding albumin 6 hours after injury in amounts to prevent hypoalbuminemia (less than 2.0 g/dl). Whole blood or packed red blood cells should not be given unless the child's hemoglobin or hematocrit level is rapidly falling.

Timing of the fluid resuscitation within the first 24 hours after the burn occurred is critical to prevent shock and maintain organ function. The Parkland burn resuscitation formula suggests that half of the first 24-hour fluid requirement be given in the first 8 hours. Results of a study reported by Puffinbarger, Tuggle, and Smith (1994) support the practice of infusing the first half of the 24-hour fluid requirement over 4 hours instead of the usual 8 hours. These results demonstrate the possible physiologic benefits of rapid resuscitation, including increased normalization of vital signs, increased urine output, normalization of urine specific gravity, and decreased need for ventilator support.

After the first 24 to 48 hours, the capillary seal is restored. Intravenous resuscitation fluid can be tapered as enteral nutrition is increased. Continuous enteral feedings can be started as early as 6 hours after injury and slowly increased over the next 12 hours. By 24 hours after injury, all but the most severely burned patients may be receiving all their fluid needs as enteral feedings (Herndon et al., 1993).

Nutrition

Burn injury induces a catabolic response that qualifies burns as the most physiologically stressful of all disease processes. Nutritional support is essential to promote wound healing, positive nitrogen balance, weight preservation, and improved immune function, as well as for maintenance of host defense mechanisms (Ireton-Jones & Gottschlich, 1993). Energy requirements are directly related to burn size and gradually return toward normal as the wound heals or is physiologically closed. The basal metabolic rate may increase to more than twice the baseline (Hansbrough & Hansbrough, 1999). There is no easy way to predict metabolic demands after burns. A formula based on BSA is an accurate means of calculating caloric requirements in children. The Shriner's Burn Institute in Galveston uses a formula of 1800 kcal/m^2 BSA plus 2200 kcal/m^2 burn per day (Herndon et al., 1993).

The patient's GI tract is the best route for providing calories. If the child is able to eat, a high-protein, high-calorie diet is encouraged as soon as possible. An absence of bowel sounds does not preclude enteral nutrition. Because the small bowel maintains motility and absorptive capabilities, placement of a small-bore feeding tube into the duodenum allows for safe delivery of enteral nutrition during periods of paralytic ileus associated with trauma, sepsis, and anesthesia (Herndon et al., 1993; Jenkins, Gottschlich, & Warden, 1994). Total parenteral nutrition (TPN) is avoided and administered only if the child has GI dysfunction and cannot tolerate enteral feedings (Herndon et al., 1993). Hyperalimentation has detrimental effects on immune function, whereas enteral feeding increases blood flow in the intestinal tract, preserves GI function, and minimizes bacterial translocation by decreasing mucosal atrophy of the intestines (Herndon et al., 1993).

Wound Management

After the initial period of shock and restoration of fluid balance, patient care turns to wound management. Early and aggressive burn wound debridement, frequent daily dressing changes, and early excision with grafting most effectively prevent sepsis. Burn wound sepsis is a major cause of morbidity and mortality in burn victims. Immediately after the burn, burn surfaces are sterile or have low populations of normal skin microflora. Rapid colonization takes place during the first 72 hours after injury. The burn unit itself may be a source of virulent nosocomial organisms (Foster & Ford, 1994). Nosocomial infections are believed to occur more commonly in patients with burns than in other patients undergoing surgery (Weber, Sheridan, Pasternack, & Tompkins, 1997).

Topical Antimicrobials. Burned skin loses its barrier function, and the impaired blood supply of the dead tissue encourages rapid proliferation of bacteria. Topical antibiotic preparations have been developed to assist in preventing bacterial colonization of the wounds. Before the development of effective topical agents, wound sepsis was the major cause of mortality from burn injury (Baker, 1999). The most commonly used topical antibiotics are summarized in Table 19-6.

Dressing Changes. In general, dressings are changed at least every 8 to 24 hours. The wound is cleansed and gently debrided with each dressing change (Herndon et al., 1993). Hydrotherapy is often used to cleanse the wound and involves soaking the patient in a tub or showering the patient for no more than 20 minutes. The water loosens and removes sloughing tissue, exudate, and topical medications. Mesh gauze entraps the exudative slough and is easily removed during hydrotherapy. Debridement is tedious and painful and requires attention to pain management.

Biologic Dressings. Biologic dressings, such as porcine heterograft (i.e., xenograft), human cadaveric allograft (i.e., homograft), and synthetic dressings (e.g., Biobrane, OpSite, and Omniderm), adhere to the wound surface, reduce wound bacterial colony counts, limit fluid and protein loss, reduce pain, increase the rate of epithelialization, and facilitate movement of joints to retain range of motion (Baker, 1999; Herndon et al., 1993) (Box 19-6). These dressings must be applied only to clean wounds that are free of debris. Xenograft skin is obtained from a variety of species, mostly pigs. Pigskin dressings and synthetic skin substitutes, such as Biobrane, OpSite, and Omniderm, are replaced daily or every 2 to 3 days. Homograft skin is obtained from human cadavers and processed by commercial skin banks. Donors are screened for communicable diseases and the skin is tracked much like blood transfusions. The homograft can protect the wound while waiting for the patient's autograft. If the dressing covers areas of heavy microbial contamination, infection occurs beneath the dressing and can deepen the burn injury.

Systemic Antibiotics. Systemic antibiotics are not administered prophylactically to treat burns. Several trials have shown that such practice does not protect against wound infections and may contribute to the development of

TABLE 19-6 **Commonly Used Topical Antibiotics**

Agent	Dressings	Advantages	Disadvantages
Silver nitrate 0.5% ($AgNO_3$)	Open, modified, or occlusive; impedes joint movement; dressings changed twice daily; keep dressing moist, rewet at least every 2 hr	Greatly reduces evaporative losses; does not interfere with wound healing; bacteriostatic action against major burn flora, including *Pseudomonas* and *Staphylococcus;* inexpensive	Does not penetrate eschar; ineffective on established burn wound infections; little effect on *Klebsiella* and *Aerobacter* groups; stains skin, clothing, and linens; makes assessment of the wound difficult because of staining; hypotonicity pulls electrolytes from the wound depleting sodium, potassium chloride, and magnesium; stings on application
Silver sulfadiazine 1% (AgSD)	Occlusive; motion of joints maintained; applied twice daily; do not use in patients with a history of allergy to sulfa	Little pain on application; bactericidal by altering DNA and cell metabolism; effective against gram-positive and gram-negative bacteria; easy to apply; nontoxic	Transient neutropenia; does not penetrate eschar; forms proteinaceous gel on wound surface that is painful to remove; occasional rashes and pruritus; decreases granulocyte formation
Mafenide acetate 10% (Sulfamylon)	Cream: usually open; do not apply to face; apply twice daily Solution: occlusive; keep dressing moist (rewet at least every 2 hr); protect solution from light	Penetrates eschar and diffuses rapidly into burn wound and underlying tissues; effective in deep flame, electrical, and infected wounds; biostatic against many gram-positive and gram-negative organisms, including *Pseudomonas* and *Clostridium*	Difficult and painful to remove cream; pain on application; metabolic acidosis, hypercapnia, and carbonic anhydrase inhibition; inhibits wound healing; hypersensitivity in some patients.
Bacitracin	Open, modified; motion of joints maintained; change dressing twice daily	Bactericidal and bacteriostatic against gram-positive organisms; low toxicity; painless application; ease of application	Limited activity against gram-negative organisms; allergic reaction in sensitive individuals.

From Wong, D. L., Hockenberry-Eaton, M., Wilson, D., Winkelstein, M. L., Ahmann, E., & Divito-Thomas, P. A. (Eds.). (1999). *Nursing care of infants and children.* St. Louis: Mosby.

resistant organisms in the wound and organs (Hansbrough & Hansbrough, 1999; Uitvlugt & Ledbetter, 1995). Children should be examined daily for signs of sepsis, and the presence of any three of the following symptoms should initiate prophylactic administration of systemic antibiotics: obtundation or changed sensorium, hyperventilation, hyperglycemia, thrombocytopenia, hypothermia or hyperthermia, and leukocytopenia or leukocytosis. When these signs are present and colony counts in the wound exceed 10^5 organisms per gram of tissue, systemic antimicrobial therapy should begin specifically for the organism cultured. If the wound appears clean, other sources of sepsis, such as the lungs, genitourinary tract, or thrombophlebitis, should be suspected. Routine cultures of sputum and urine are obtained two to three times each week (Herndon et al., 1993). Otitis media should not be overlooked as a source of fever in the pediatric population (Baker, 1999).

Pain. Pain management is extremely important to the recovery of the child. Pain in burned children depends on the depth of the burn, stage of healing, and pain threshold. Pain control during dressing changes, especially the first change, is extremely important. In some cases a local anesthetic agent, such as dilute 2% lidocaine (Xylocaine) applied in the wound bed about 15 minutes before debridement, may be enough to eliminate pain (Krasner, 1995). If the local anesthetic is not sufficient, some clinicians advocate the use of benzodiazepines in combination with opioids (Senecal, 1999). Burn dressing changes cause a great deal of anxiety in younger children. These medications can be titrated to achieve the desired effects of analgesia, decreased anxiety, and cooperation (Table 19-7). Morphine and fentanyl are reliable parenteral analgesic agents used for dressing changes and difficult physical therapy. The advantage of fentanyl is its quick onset of action and short duration. Small doses (0.3 μg/kg) can be given repeatedly to achieve and maintain an acceptable level of analgesia without oversedating the child (Senecal, 1999). The short half-life ensures neutralization of effects within 1 hour, but often sooner. Ketamine may be considered for its dissociative properties of anesthesia with low risk of hypoxia. Ketamine adds the possibility of airway protection, but some children do not like the dissociative

BOX 19-6 Types of Skin Grafts

Temporary Grafts

1. Allografts (homografts): skin that is obtained from genetically different members of the same species who are free of disease
2. Xenografts (heterografts): skin that is obtained from members of a different species, primarily pigskin

Permanent Grafts

1. Autografts: tissue obtained from undamaged areas of the patient's own body
2. Isograft: histocompatible tissue obtained from genetically identical individuals

Methods of Applying Split-Thickness Grafts

1. Sheet graft: a sheet of skin, removed from the donor site, placed intact over the recipient site and sutured in place
2. Mesh graft: a sheet of skin removed from the donor site and passed through a mesher, which produces tiny slits in the skin; meshing allows expansion of the skin to cover 1.25 to 9 times the area of the sheet graft.

From Wong, D. L., Hockenberry-Eaton M., Wilson D., Winkelstein, M. L., Ahmann, E., & Divito-Thomas, P. A. (Eds.). (1999). *Nursing care of infants and children.* St. Louis: Mosby.

feeling it induces. Propofol has been used for painful procedures, but the anesthesiologist should monitor the patient carefully during its use (Schiller, 1996). Because undertreatment of the pain can escalate anxiety, optimal pain control is necessary. Initial regimens for pain management may include a continuous infusion or around-the-clock intermittent doses of an opioid and additional doses of opioid and benzodiazepine titrated to effect before and during the burn dressing changes. Extensive debridement procedures are often not well managed with conscious sedation and may require general anesthesia (U.S. Department of Health and Human Services, 1992).

Pain management in children requires a multidisciplinary approach using pharmacologic and nonpharmacologic strategies. Senecal (1999) provides an exhaustive list of nonpharmacologic interventions before, during, and after painful procedures for patients at every developmental level. Many nonpharmacologic approaches are effective as adjuvants and include hypnosis, distraction, relaxation, imagery, positive reinforcement, and family participation. Children manage better during dressing changes when their participation and control are maximized. For example, a child may want to help remove the dressing. The time and environment for the dressing change should be predictable to the child. Dressing changes are performed in a separate treatment room so that the child can consider his or her room as a safe place (U.S. Department of Health and Human Services, 1992). Chapter 11 presents in-depth information about pain management.

REHABILITATION

PHYSICAL REHABILITATION

Rehabilitation starts the moment the child is admitted to the hospital with daily visits from physical and occupational therapy. Physical rehabilitation involves the positioning of patients, splinting, passive and active range of motion, and assistance with activities of daily living and gradual ambulation. Children respond to these exercises more enthusiastically if the program is presented as play. Child life specialists are expert at involving the child in play activities that are interesting and fun. Family members should be involved early in the course of treatment so that they are familiar and comfortable with the regimen.

Many patients develop scarring and contractures as the result of burn injuries. Pressure therapy is necessary to reduce hypertrophic scar formation. *Hypertrophic scarring* refers to the development of thickened, raised skin. Constant pressure should be applied 24 hours per day until the scars mature, usually 6 to 8 months after injury (Herndon et al., 1993). These pressure garments are available prefabricated or custom made. They deliver consistent pressure on scarred areas, shorten the time of scar maturation, and decrease the thickness of the scar, as well as the redness and associated itching. Continued adjustments to scarred areas (e.g., scar release, grafting, rearrangement) and multiple minor cosmetic surgical procedures are necessary to produce long-term function and improve appearance. In general, children scar worse than adults, possibly because of the rapid cell

TABLE 19-7 Pain Medications Useful in Pediatric Patients

Drug	Dose	Indications	Outcome
Chloral hydrate	250-500 mg q8h	Preoperative; sleep	Amnesia
Diazepam	1-2 mg q3-4h	Preoperative; anxiety	Dissociation
Midazolam	0.5 mg/kg q3-4h	Anxiety	Sedation/amnesia
Demerol	1-2 mg q2-3h	Operating room; debridement	Analgesia/amnesia
Ketamine	0.2-0.5 mg/kg	Acute pain	Analgesia/amnesia
Morphine sulfate	0.2-0.5 mg/kg q2-3h	Acute pain	Analgesia/amnesia
Fentanyl	1-2 μg/kg q1h	Acute pain	Analgesia/amnesia

From Herndon, D. N, Rutan, R. L., Alison, W. E., Jr., & Cox, C. S., Jr. (1993). Management of burn injuries. In M. R. Eichelberger (Ed.), *Pediatric trauma: Prevention, acute care, rehabilitation* (p. 588). St. Louis: Mosby.

mitosis associated with growth. Patients who have darker skin color tend to develop worse scarring. Scar tissue has no sweat glands, and children with extensive scarring may experience difficulty during hot weather.

Psychosocial Support

The trauma of the injury and being hospitalized in an unfamiliar environment can leave a child bewildered and drained. Responses to hospitalization are related to the developmental stage of the child. Chapter 9 provides discussion of a child's response to hospitalization based on developmental age.

There is growing support that trauma affects not only the victim but also those close to the child. The focus is on the child in any emergency setting, and the parents may feel powerless. They feel responsible for the injury, even if these feelings are unjustified. The family requires assistance through the grief, guilt, and helplessness. The parents are included in the multidisciplinary team and participate in the development of the plan of care. In the acute phase they can hold or read to their child. In later stages parents can assist with feeding and dressing changes and provide the child with some sense of normalcy. The rehabilitation process continues with home therapy and a follow-up program. The effect of the burned child's possible disfigurement and disability can be minimized if the child feels accepted back into normal family activities. Psychologic support may be of benefit for years as the child matures and experiences new social situations. Many burn centers offer support programs in which burn patients and their families have the opportunity to discuss their concerns and share their experiences and feelings. Therapeutic recreational programs such as camps and day trips offer opportunities to associate with others who share these traumatic experiences.

PREVENTION

Pediatric thermal injury prevention begins and ends with education and should be targeted to the community, the patients, and their families. Nursing's role is always significant because nurses have many opportunities to interact with patients and families in all stages of development.

Patient and Family Education

Nurses are responsible for educating parents and children about injury prevention as part of health promotion throughout childhood. Anticipatory guidance regarding normal developmental behaviors helps alert the parent to potential injury occurrences. For example, because preschool children have the motor capability to light matches, they should be supervised in an environment free from matches and lighters. Knowing the different types of burns associated with children at different developmental levels is critical to provide timely teaching to parents.

Teaching scald prevention should be targeted to parents of toddlers and preschoolers because scalds are the most common type of burn in this population. Education to prevent this type of injury should be aimed at everyone responsible for a child's safety, including parents, grandparents, baby-sitters, and older siblings. These small children tend to be underfoot in the kitchen, especially while a parent is cooking. Their natural curiosity draws them to investigate everything within and just out of reach. They overturn cups and cooking pots filled with hot or boiling water in less time than it takes a parent to stop them.

Toddlers grasping for stabilization when learning to walk often grab electric cords of cooking appliances or tablecloths on which hot foods and liquids are resting. Tablecloths should not be used when small children are present. Parents should be warned about potential scalds from foods cooked in the microwave oven, which can cause devastating injuries to the mouth, throat, and esophagus. Parents should know that their daughters are especially at risk for burns from microwave cooked food, and the young girls should be properly instructed and supervised (Powell & Tanz, 1993).

Nurses should educate parents about the need for supervision and an environment free of matches, gasoline, lighters, and all other flammable materials. "Childproofing" the home will minimize potential problems with children playing with matches and lighters. Studies indicate that an estimated 38% of children 6 to 14 years old have played with fire at least once. Home fires caused by tend to begin in a bedroom where children are left alone. Children playing with matches or lighters start nearly 80% of these fires. Parents should be aware that boys are nearly twice as likely as girls to play with fire (National Safe Kids Campaign, 2000d).

The importance of installing and maintaining smoke detectors cannot be overemphasized. Smoke alarms are extremely effective at preventing fire-related death and injury. The chances of dying in a residential fire are cut in half when a smoke alarm is present. Smoke detectors should be installed on every level in the home and in every sleeping area. As of 1997, 94% of homes in the United States had at least one smoke alarm. However, only three fourths of all homes had at least one working smoke alarm. Smoke alarms should be tested every month, and the batteries should be replaced at least once a year or according to manufacturer's recommendations. The alarms must be replaced every 10 years. Ten-year lithium alarms that do not require an annual battery change are available (National Safe Kids Campaign, 2000d).

Families must be instructed to plan and practice several fire escape routes from each room in the home and identify an outside meeting area. Practicing the escape plan may help children who become frightened and confused in a fire to escape to safety. Nearly 40% of residential fire-related deaths among children 9 years and younger occur when the child is attempting to escape, becomes frozen and unable to act, or acts irrationally. Although an escape plan might help reduce these deaths, only 26% of households have developed and practiced such a plan (National Safe Kids Campaign, 2000d). Nurses should teach children and direct the parents to reinforce the "stop, drop, and roll" lesson to decrease the severity of a burn if they are caught in a fire.

LEGISLATION

Many regulations have been designed to prevent unintentional thermal injuries from occurring. All national and regional code-making agencies have amended their plumbing code language to require antiscald technology and a maximum water heater temperature of 120° F in all newly constructed residential units (National Safe Kids Campaign, 2000d). Federal regulations and regional building codes have also established requirements for the design, construction, and installation of windows and approved devices intended to be used for emergency escape or rescue.

A functioning smoke detector is not present in two thirds of the residential fires in which a child is injured or killed. Households without functioning smoke alarms are approximately two and a half times more likely to have a fire than those with smoke alarms. Currently, 32 states and the District of Columbia have laws that require smoke alarms in both new and existing residences, which may reduce the likelihood of death in house fires by 85% (Herrin & Antoon, 1996). Seven states have no comprehensive smoke alarm laws. The remaining 11 states have a variety of laws covering specific limited situations, such as new dwellings or multioccupancy dwellings only.

In 1994 the Consumer Product Safety Commission issued a mandatory safety standard requiring disposable and novelty cigarette lighters to be child resistant. Since this standard has been in effect, the number of fires caused by children playing with lighters has declined 42% and the number of deaths and injuries associated with fires has declined by 31% and 26%, respectively (National Safe Kids Campaign, 2000c). Beginning in 1953, the federal government passed standards regulating the flammability of general wearing apparel, carpets, rugs, mattresses, and children's sleep wear. The federal Flammable Fabric Act was passed in 1972 and is monitored by the Consumer Products Safety Commission. Requiring sleep wear fabric to be flame retardant has reduced the incidence and severity of injury from children igniting fabrics.

SUMMARY

Most pediatric burn victims sustain their injuries from intentional or unintentional sources in their own home. Nearly all thermal injuries in the pediatric population can be prevented with teaching directed at the caregivers of those at risk. Legislation has helped but has not eliminated the problem.

Pediatric trauma nurses who care for burned children and their families require knowledge about the pathophysiology of thermal injury. Because burns are so often implicated in child abuse cases, nurses must be familiar with the characteristics and patterns of intentional and unintentional thermal injuries. Successful resuscitation of the burned child depends on a treatment plan designed specifically for the type of injury, considering the impact on all major body systems. Serious pediatric burns often require referral to a specialized burn treatment center. Interventions performed on the scene can decrease the extent and severity of injuries, including those of smoke inhalation. Mechanical ventilation, fluid replacement, nutritional support, wound management, and pain control are critical aspects of care for survival. Careful positioning to prevent contractures should be incorporated into the plan of care upon admission, followed by constant continuous pressure application after the burn injury is healed. Psychosocial support needs of burned children are addressed upon admission. Communication with the family to include them in the plan of care is a priority and is better managed in a multidisciplinary approach.

BIBLIOGRAPHY

Allwood, J. S. (1995). The primary care management of burn. *Nurse Practitioner, 20*(8), 74-87.

American Burn Association. (2000). *Burn incidence and treatment in the US: 2000 fact sheet.* Accessed June 20, 2001. Available at: http://www.ameriburn.org/pub/factsheet.htm.

American Heart Association and American Academy of Pediatrics. (2000). *Pediatric advanced life support.* Dallas: Author.

Andronicus, M., Oates, R. K., Peat J., Spalding, S., & Martin H. (1998). Non-accidental burns in children. *Burns, 24*(6), 552-558.

Baker, R. A. U. (1999). Burns. In D. L. Wong, M. Hockenberry-Eaton, D. Wilson, M. L. Winkelstein, E. Ahmann, & P. A. Divito-Thomas (Eds.), *Nursing care of infants and children* (pp. 1136-1365). St. Louis: Mosby.

Bennett, B., & Gamelli, R. (1998). Profile of an abused burned child. *Journal of Burn Care Rehabilitation, 19,* 88-94.

Carvajal, H. F. (1980). A physiologic approach to fluid therapy in acutely burned children. *Journal of Surgery, Gynecology and Obstetrics, 150,* 379-384.

Carvajal, H. F. (1994). Fluid resuscitation of pediatric burn victims: A critical appraisal. *Pediatric Nephrology, 8,* 357-366.

Cortiella, J., & Marvin, J. A. (1997). Management of the pediatric burn patient. *Nursing Clinics of North America, 32*(2), 311-325.

Cot, C. J., Ryan, J. F., Todres, I. D., & Goudsouzian, N. G. (1993). *A practice of anesthesia for infants and children.* Philadelphia: WB Saunders.

Crawley, T. (1996). Childhood injury: Significance and prevention strategies. *Journal of Pediatric Nursing, 11*(4), 225-232.

Davey, R. B., Wallis, M. A., Perkins, A., & Tingay, M. (1995). Thermal and electrical injuries. In W. L. Buntain (Ed.), *Management of pediatric trauma* (pp. 431-449). Philadelphia: WB Saunders.

Demling, R. H. (1987). Fluid replacement in burned patients. *Surgical Clinics of North America, 67,* 15-30.

Dimick, A., & Wagner, R. (1992). Burns. In G. R. Schwartz, C. G. Cayton, M. A. Mangelsen, TA. Mayer, & B. K. Hanke (Eds.), *Principles and practice of emergency medicine* (3rd ed., pp. 200-209). Philadelphia: Lea & Febiger.

Emergency Nurses Association. (1995). *Trauma nursing core course: Provider manual* (4th ed., pp. 253-284). Park Ridge, IL: Author.

Fallis, C. (1991). Burns. In J. C. Fallis (Ed.), *Pediatric emergencies: Surgical management* (pp. 21-26). Philadelphia: BC Decker.

Feldman, M., Slater, H., & Goldfarb, I. (1986). The management of burned children in a general hospital burn unit. *Journal Burn Care Rehabilitation, 7,* 244-246.

Fitzpatrick, J. C., & Cloffi, W. G., Jr. (1996). Diagnosis and treatment of inhalation injury. In D. N. Herndon (Ed.), *Total burn care* (p. 187). Philadelphia: WB Saunders.

Flynn, M. B. (2002). Burn injuries. In K. A. McQuillan, K. T. Von Rueden, R. L. Hartsock, M. B. Flynn, & E. Whalen (Eds.), *Trauma nursing: From resuscitation to rehabilitation* (3rd ed., pp. 788-807). Philadelphia: WB Saunders.

Foster, J. E., & Ford, E. G. (1994). Burn injury. In E. G. Ford & R. J. Andrassy (Eds.), *Pediatric trauma: Initial assessment and management* (pp. 291-303). Philadelphia: WB Saunders.

Gillespie, R. W. (1992). *Prehospital advanced burn life support.* Chicago: American Burn Association.

Hansbrough, J. F., & Hansbrough, W. (1999). Pediatric burns. *Pediatrics in Review, 20*(4), 117-124.

Helvig, E. (1993). Pediatric burn injuries. *AACN Clinical Issues, 4,* 433-442.

Herndon, D. N., Rutan, R. L., Alison, W. E., Jr., & Cox, C. S., Jr. (1993). Management of burn injuries. In M. R. Eichelberger (Ed.), *Pediatric trauma: Prevention, acute care, rehabilitation* (pp. 568-589). St. Louis: Mosby.

Herrin, J. T., & Antoon, A. Y. (1996). Burn injuries. In W. E. Nelson, R. E. Behrman, R. M. Kliegman, & A. M. Arvin (Eds.), *Nelson textbook of pediatrics* (15th ed., pp. 270-277). Philadelphia: WB Saunders.

Hill, D. S., & Strange, G. R. (1996). Burns. In G. R. Strange, W. Ahrens, S. Lelyveld, & R. Schafermeyer (Eds.), *Pediatric emergency medicine: A comprehensive study guide* (pp. 603-606). New York: McGraw-Hill.

Hudson, D. A., Jones, L., & Rode H. (1994). Respiratory distress secondary to scalds in children. *Burns, 20*(5), 434-437.

Hultman, C. S., Priolo, D., Cairns, B. A., Grant, E. J., Peterson, H. D., & Meyer, P. A. (1998). Return to jeopardy: The fate of pediatric burn patients who are victims of abuse and neglect. *Journal of Burn Care and Rehabilitation, 19*(4), 366-376.

Ireton-Jones, C., & Gottschlich, M. M. (1993). The evolution of nutrition support in burns. *Journal of Burn Care and Rehabilitation, 14,* 272-280.

Jenkins, M. E., Gottschlich, M. M., & Warden, G. D. (1994). Enteral feeding during operative procedures in thermal injuries. *Journal of Burn Care and Rehabilitation, 15*(2), 199-205.

Kirelik, S. B., & Hawk, W. H. (1997). Management of the burn patient. In R. A. Dieckmann, D. H. Fiser, & S. M. Selbst (Eds.), *Illustrated textbook of pediatric emergency and critical care procedures* (pp. 680-684). St. Louis: Mosby.

Krasner, D. (1995). The chronic wound pain experience: A conceptual model. *Ostomy Wound Management, 41,* 20-25.

Lazear, S. E. (1993). Tissue integrity: Burns. In J. A. Neff & P. S. Kidd (Eds.), *Trauma nursing: The art and science* (pp. 449-475). St. Louis: Mosby.

Lund, C. C., & Browder, N. C. (1944). The estimation of areas of burns. *Surgery, Gynecology and Obstetrics, 79,* 352-358.

Lyebarger, P. M., & Kadilak, P. (2001). Thermal injury. In M. A. Q. Curley & P. A. Moloney-Harmon (Eds.), *Critical care nursing of infants and children* (2nd ed., pp. 981-997). Philadelphia: WB Saunders.

Mozingo, D. W., Cioffi, W. G., & Pruitt, P. A. (1994). Burns. In F. Bongard & D. Sue (Eds.), *Current critical care diagnosis and management* (pp. 2918-2925). Norwalk, CT: Appleton & Lange.

National Safe Kids Campaign. (2000a). *Fire: Why kids are at risk.* Accessed June 20, 2001. Available at: http://www.safekids.org.

National Safe Kids Campaign. (2000b). *Injury facts: Burn injury,* Accessed June 20, 2001. Available at: http://www.safekids.org.

National Safe Kids Campaign. (2000c). *Injury facts: Childhood injury.* Accessed June 20, 2001. Available at: http://www.safekids.org.

National Safe Kids Campaign. (2000d). *Injury facts: Fire injury (residential).* Accessed June 20, 2001. Available at: http://www.safekids.org.

National Safe Kids Campaign. (2000e). *Injury facts: Home injury.* Accessed June 20, 2001. Available at: http://www.safekids.org.

Nortrade Medical, Inc. (2000). *Burn-related injury/death statistics.* Accessed June 20, 2001. Available at: http://www.burnfree.com/burnfact.htm.

Nunn, J. F. (2000). *Nunn's applied respiratory physiology* (4th ed.). London: Butterworth Heinemann.

Parish, R. A. (1997). Thermal injury. In R. M. Barkin, G. L. Caputo, D. M. Jaffe, J. F. Knapp, R. W. Schafermeyer, & J. S. Seidel (Eds.), *Pediatric emergency medicine: Concepts and clinical practices* (pp. 489-496). St. Louis: Mosby.

Powell, E. C., & Tanz, R. R. (1993). Comparison of childhood burns associated with use of microwave ovens and conventional stoves. *Pediatrics, 92*(2), 344-349.

Puffinbarger, N. K., Tuggle, D. W., & Smith E. I. (1994). Rapid isotonic fluid resuscitation in pediatric thermal injury. *Journal of Pediatric Surgery, 29*(2), 339-342.

Scannell, G., Waxman, K., & Tominaga, G. T. (1995). Respiratory distress in traumatized and burned children. *Journal of Pediatric Surgery, 30*(4), 612-614.

Schiller, W. R. (1996). Burn management in children. *Pediatric Annals, 25*(8), 431, 434-438.

Senecal, S. J. (1999). Pain management of wound care. *Nursing Clinics of North America, 34*(4), 847-860.

Sheridan, R. L. (1996). Recognition and management of hot liquid aspiration in children. *Annals of Emergency Medicine, 27*(1), 89-91.

U.S. Department of Health and Human Services. (1992). *Acute pain management: Operative or medical procedures & trauma.* Rockville, MD: Author.

Uitvlugt, N. D., & Ledbetter, D. J. (1995). Treatment of pediatric burns. In R. M. Arensman, M. B. Statter, D. J. Ledbetter, & T. Vargish (Eds.), *Pediatric trauma: Initial care of the injured child* (pp. 173-199). New York: Raven Press.

Weber, J. M., Sheridan, R. L., Pasternack, M. S., & Tompkins, R. G. (1997). Nosocomial infections in pediatric patients with burns. *American Journal of Infection Control, 25*(3), 195-201.

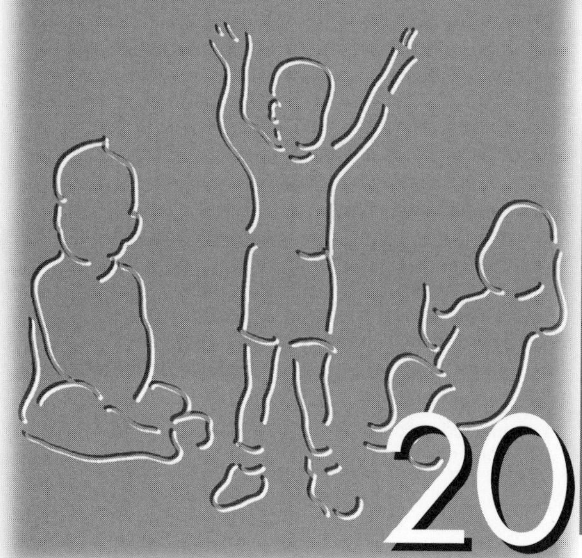

20 Submersion Injury

Rita Giordano

In the United States, drowning is the second leading cause of death and injury in children younger than 15 years and the single leading cause in children younger than 5 years (Baker, O'Neill, Ginsburg, & Li, 1992; Kallas, 2000; Levin, Moriss, Toro, Brink, & Turner, 1993; Rowin, Christensen, & Allen, 1996; Waller, Baker, & Szoeka, 1989). Drowning and near-drowning are catastrophic events that forever change the lives of children and families. The psychologic and emotional stress alone are overwhelming. Innumerable years of productive life are lost as the result of neurologic impairment resulting from submersion injuries. Drowning results in an annual loss of nearly 50,000 years of potential life, and 20% to 40% of children who survive near-drowning incidents never recover normal neurologic function (Allman, Nelson, Pacentine, & McComb, 1986; Biggart & Bohn, 1990; Wintemute, 1990, 1992). The medical costs to families and society can be devastating. Several investigators reported that there are approximately four hospitalizations for every death caused by drowning and approximately four emergency department visits for every hospitalization (Fields, 1992; Spyker, 1985; & Wintemute, 1990). The indirect cost to society is estimated to be \$35 to \$650 million per year, making it the third most costly childhood injury (Guyer & Ellers, 1990; Rowin et al., 1996). This cost is exceeded only by injuries resulting from motor vehicles accidents.

As experience has increased over the years, consistent definitions of submersion injuries have evolved. Historically, *drowning* has been defined as death from asphyxia while a person is submerged in water* or within 24 hours after the submersion occurred (Fields, 1992; Levin et al., 1993). Near-drowning is an event that requires medical treatment and results in survival for at least 24 hours after submersion occurred (Fields, 1992; Kallas & O'Rourke, 1993). Sachdeva (1999) differentiates submersion incidents into immersion syndrome and submersion injury. Immersion syndrome is specific to death after contact with cold water. Subcategories of submersion injuries are drowning, near-drowning, and save. *Drowning* is death within 24 hours after a submersion, *near-drowning* is temporary survival after a submersion, and *save* is water rescue or removal from water. *Secondary drowning* is death that results from complications of submersion 24 hours after the event occurred. Use of consistent definitions enables more accurate comparisons across age groups and builds a foundation for the establishment of best practice.

The tragedy of childhood drowning is all too familiar to medical personnel working in emergency and critical care areas. Emergency and intensive care staff are faced with the challenge of providing a full spectrum of care that includes meeting the physical, psychologic, and spiritual needs of the patient and family. This chapter provides information that will assist staff in meeting these needs and positively affect outcomes.

EPIDEMIOLOGY

Numerous factors place the pediatric population at risk for submersion injuries. Figure 20-1 shows a brief overview of the epidemiology associated with this age group. Major factors include age, gender, and race. Although drowning is the second leading cause of death in all children, the toddler (1 to 4 years old) and the older adolescent (15 to 19 years old) are of particular concern. This increased risk can be correlated to the developmental level and associated skills of these age groups. Physically, toddlers have a large head/body ratio and are developing refined gross motor skills. They can easily lose balance and have great difficulty recovering because of lack of strength, confusion, and poor coordination. The toddler is active, curious, and undaunted in attempts to explore the environment. A body of water, such as a residential pool, ocean, bathtub, or industrial size bucket, holds special appeal for the inquisitive toddler. Constant supervision is required to avert tragedy. Lack of adequate supervision is an important variable associated with submersion injuries

*In this chapter, we use the term *water*, but drownings can occur in any fluid medium.

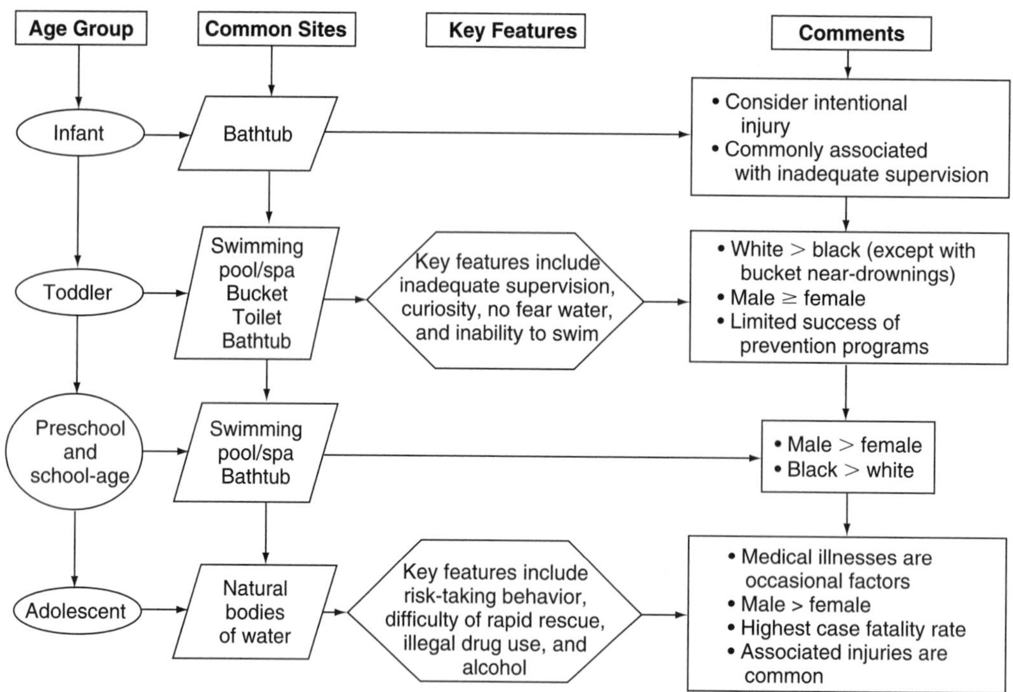

FIGURE 20-1 Submersion injury epidemiology. (From Rowin, M., Christensen, D., & Allen, E. [1996]. Pediatric drowning and near-drowning. In M. Rogers & D. Nichols [Eds.], *Textbook of pediatric intensive care* [3rd ed., pp. 875-891]. Baltimore: Williams & Wilkins.)

for children of various ages (Kallas, 2000; Wintemute, 1990). A study by Nichter and Everett (1989) demonstrated that most toddler drownings occur in the late afternoon or early evening, when parents and caregivers are likely to be distracted by mealtime preparation. Quan, Gore, Wentz, Allen, and Novak (1989) report that a responsible supervising adult could be identified in 84% of toddler drownings but that only 18% of the incidents were witnessed.

The overall pediatric drowning rate has declined since the 1960s, but the rate of swimming pool drownings has steadily increased. Toddlers and preschoolers have an affinity for residential pools. This age group accounts for approximately 50% to 90% of all pool drownings (Rowin et al., 1996). Two thirds of these drownings occur in the child;s home pool where supervision has lapsed for less than 5 minutes (O'Flaherty & Pirie, 1997). Pool devices, such as solar blankets and winter pool covers, contribute to drowning deaths in this age group. Small children are trapped beneath the unsecured solar blanket as they attempt to reach for floating objects. The blanket then covers the child, effectively shielding him or her from sight. The winter pool cover allows water to accumulate on its surface, creating a new body of water and an additional hazard for the child. Although the pool covers are strong enough to hold a child upright, they provide no traction to prevent the child from slipping and falling. Other common drowning sites are large industrial-sized buckets, hot tubs, spas, and bathtubs. Bucket drownings are associated with high mortality rates because of the toddler's inability to escape and the possible ingestion of caustic fluids within the bucket (Kallas, 2000). Bathtubs are a particular threat for children 6 months to 1 year old who can sit but cannot recover after a loss of balance (O'Flaherty & Pirie, 1997). The increasing number of spas and whirlpools in the home present a growing threat to children. Of particular concern are the suction devices in spas and whirlpools, which can entrap hair, clothing, and body parts of the young child.

The incidence of submersion injuries is high in the older adolescent age group (15 to 19 years old). Developmentally, this group is striving for independence and self-expression while longing for peer approval and acceptance. These characteristics often lead to reckless, risk-taking behaviors that take place with little or no adult supervision. Adolescent drowning is linked to water sports, boating, swimming in undesignated or unprotected areas, and voluntary hyperventilation in preparation for prolonged underwater swimming. The high morality rate in teenagers is also affected by the use of illicit drugs and alcohol, which are implicated in approximately 50% of all submersion events (Kallas, 2000; Weinstein & Kreiger, 1996). These injuries are associated with boating activities in natural bodies of water where help is less accessible and prompt rescue and treatment cannot occur for a variety of reasons.

There is an increased incidence of pediatric submersion injuries in the western and Gulf Coast regions that is thought to be due to the warmer climate and large number of in-ground swimming pools. Drowning is the leading cause of death of children in Arizona, California, and Florida (Division of Injury Control, Center for Environmental Health and Injury, Center for Disease Control, 1990; Fields, 1992; Wintemute, 1990). In contrast, the northeastern states have the lowest number of drownings (Rowin et al., 1996).

Regardless of geographic area, most drownings occur during the summer on weekends (Baker et al., 1992; Christensen, 1992; Wintemute, Kraus, Teret, & Wright, 1987). Drowning rates are higher in rural areas than in urban or suburban areas, partly because there is reduced access to emergency medical care in rural areas (Baker et al., 1992).

Other risk factors include gender and race. Males are more likely to drown than females (Kallas, 2000). Drowning rates in boys peak at age 2 years and again at ages 16 to 18 years (Baker et al., 1992; Brenner, Smith, & Overpeck, 1994; Levin et al., 1993). In the toddler age group, boys are less likely to survive a near-drowning and more likely to be found in full arrest than girls (Quan, Wentz, Gore, & Copass, 1990). In girls, high numbers of drowning deaths are seen in the toddler age group but do not peak again in adolescence (Rowin et al., 1996). There is speculation that adolescent girls are less inclined to engage in reckless behaviors, such as drinking, taking drugs, and responding to dares, which decreases their risk of accidental drowning. Submersion injuries occur more commonly in black children than in white children, especially in adolescent boys (DeNicola, Falk, Swanson, Gayle, & Kisson, 1997). This may be attributed to their poorly developed swimming skills, heightened risk-taking behaviors, and drug and alcohol use (DeNicola et al., 1997). Race is a factor that has also been linked to the drowning site. White children sustain injuries more often in residential pools, whereas black children have a greater incidence in natural bodies of water, such as lakes, rivers, ditches, and ponds (DeNicola et al., 1997).

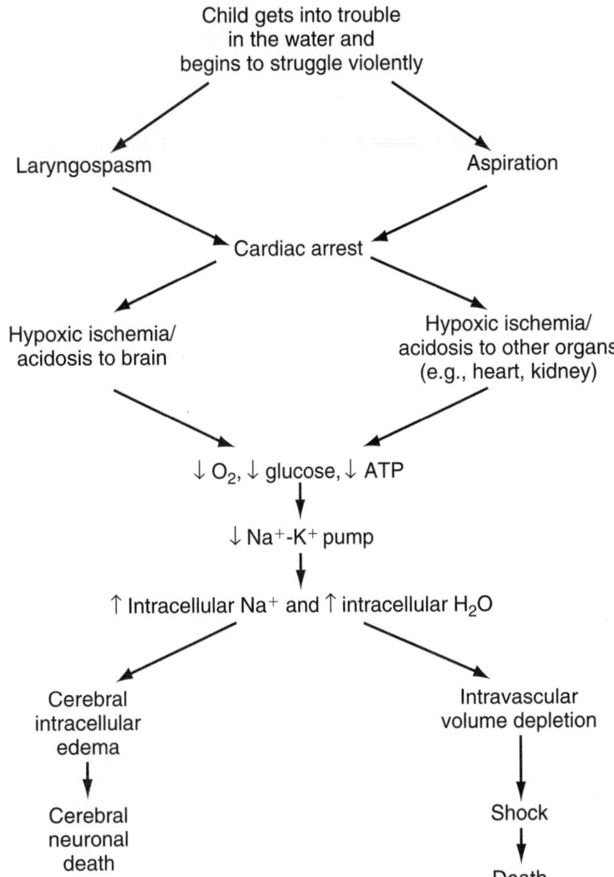

FIGURE 20-2 Near-drowning in children: natural history and pathophysiology. (From Walsh, B., & Ioli, J. [1994]. Childhood near-drowning: Nursing care and primary prevention. *Pediatric Nursing, 20,* 266.)

PATHOPHYSIOLOGY

Tissue hypoxemia is the single most devastating consequence of submersion injuries. The central nervous system (CNS) is particularly sensitive to the effects of hypoxemia. The extent of hypoxic damage to other organ systems varies. The ability of the body to survive with a good neurologic outcome depends on the degree of oxygen deprivation combined with the individual's capacity to sustain and recover from hypoxia. Timely initiation of tissue oxygenation is the most important aspect of therapy and is the most effective method currently used to improve neurologic outcome (Figure 20-2).

Drowning Sequence

After submersion, a sequence of events take place in both animals and humans. Initially, there is a sense of panic associated with ineffective swimming movements. Small amounts of water enter the mouth while breath holding occurs. This involuntary closure of the glottis triggers initial laryngospasm. At this point, two things can happen. With the violent struggle to survive, copious amounts of water may be swallowed, resulting in rapid loss of consciousness. Vomiting with involuntary aspiration occurs next and is sometimes referred to as *wet drowning. Dry drowning* occurs in a small percentage of victims; severe laryngeal spasms persist and prevent pulmonary fluid aspiration. Regardless of the type of drowning, the final consequence of submersion injury is hypoxemia (Weinstein & Kreiger, 1996). Prognosis is affected by a variety of factors, such as length of immersion, temperature of the water, and time until effective cardiopulmonary resuscitation was provided. Even though these factors affect prognosis and have multisystem effects, morbidity and mortality are directly related to the degree of neuronal damage. Only a small percentage of patients die as a result of other organ system failures.

SYSTEMIC EFFECTS

Central Nervous System

The brain often sustains irreparable damage as the result of submersion injuries. Primary injury to the CNS is due to the hypoxic-ischemic insult. The brain relies on constant delivery of oxygen to maintain metabolic activities and energy stores. Many biochemical processes occur within the cerebral tissue as a result of this primary injury. Energy, in the form of adenosine triphosphate (ATP), is depleted after approximately 2 minutes of ischemia (Rowin et al., 1996). Without ATP, cellular metabolism is severely compromised, with the inevitable development of cerebral edema and resultant neuronal death. The primary hypoxic insult initiates a complex cascade of biochemical events within the CNS. This cascade effect is commonly called the *secondary insult.* These biochemical responses include failure of the sodium-potassium pump, increased intracellular sodium and calcium, phospholipid hydrolysis, lipid peroxidation with release of fatty acid metabolites, and oxygen free radical formation. All of these responses are toxic to brain tissue and contribute to the ischemic process (Rowin et al., 1996). Other systemic factors, such as cardiogenic shock, hypovolemia, and pulmonary insufficiency, also contribute to cerebral impairment.

Cerebral edema resulting from the primary and secondary injuries develops between 24 and 72 hours after the submersion event. Intracranial pressure (ICP) may rise quickly, compromising cerebral perfusion. Once adequate systemic circulation and oxygenation have been restored, cerebral damage may persist due to loss of autoregulatory mechanisms. Transient vasodilation, cerebral arterial spasm, and free radical formation appear to contribute to CNS injury in the postresuscitative phase (Rowin et al., 1996).

Pulmonary System

Aspiration of fluid into the lungs is responsible for subsequent pulmonary dysfunction after submersion injury. Aspiration leads to hypoxia, which is primarily caused by increased ventilation/perfusion mismatching, surfactant alteration or loss, pulmonary hypertension, decreased lung compliance, fluid shifts across alveolar membranes, and anatomic changes in alveolar epithelial cells (Levin et al., 1993). Pulmonary surfactant is affected in different ways, depending on the type of water ingested. Freshwater clinically alters surfactant and renders it nonfunctional. Saltwater causes entire surfactant washout from the alveolus. Such changes in surfactant properties cause atelectasis, decreased lung compliance, and increased intrapulmonary shunting (Levin et al., 1993). Infants and young children normally have low lung compliance, which increases their risk of atelectasis and pulmonary edema. In children who appear clinically stable and free of hypoxemia, shunting may take days to resolve. Pulmonary edema is likely to occur as a result of fluid aspiration. Inflammation causing alveolar capillary membrane disruption results in the leaking of plasma-rich exudate into the alveolus (Beyda, 1991). In addition to alveolar effects, pulmonary hypertension occurs because of damage to the airway and pulmonary vasculature. These pathologic disturbances within the lung impair gas exchange and result in hypoxemia, hypercapnia, and acidosis.

Secondary drowning, which can occur 3 to 72 hours after rescue, is an interesting phenomenon in a small group of children (Rowin et al, 1996). This event develops after an initial positive response to pulmonary management. Later, respiratory decline occurs because of surfactant instability, which results in alveolar collapse. Other causes of respiratory impairment after rescue include bacterial infection, barotrauma, chemical pneumonitis, foreign body aspiration, and hypoventilation associated with neurologic decline.

Cardiovascular System

Most children have healthy stable cardiovascular systems, which makes them less prone to sustained myocardial damage after submersion injury. However, infants and children have fewer oxygen reserves than adults. Anything that increases oxygen consumption or reduces oxygen delivery in infants or children can cause decompensation (Hazinski, 1999). The effects on the heart associated with drowning are related to the myocardial ischemia resulting from hypoxia. Life-threatening arrhythmias, such as ventricular tachycardia or fibrillation, may arise as a result of hypoxia and acidosis. Cardiac arrest is a late consequence that is usually preceded by marked bradycardia (Beyda, 1998). Cardiogenic shock may result from myocardial hypoxic damage. Metabolic acidosis can add to the already impaired myocardial performance. It has been suggested that submersion results in a sympathetic storm, and marked elevations of serum catecholamine have been reported in some children (Karch, 1987). The sudden release of catecholamine can cause additional myocardial ischemia and widespread vascular changes. Cytosolic calcium overload and oxygen-derived free radicals have also been associated with myocardial injury after resuscitation from cardiac arrest. Low left ventricular filling pressures are commonly seen after a serious near-drowning episode. This is the result of excessive pulmonary and systemic capillary permeability and results in hypovolemia. These hemodynamic changes only complicate the clinical picture of global ischemia and mandate prompt intervention.

Fluids and Electrolytes

There has been debate surrounding the pathophysiologic effects of freshwater versus saltwater ingestion in the drowning victim. Studies have demonstrated no clinically significant electrolyte imbalances, fluid shifts, or changes in hematocrit in submersion victims, regardless of the tonicity of the water (Modell & Davis, 1969; Orlowski, Abulleil, & Phillips, 1989). Of more concern is the amount of water aspirated during the submersion event. The general therapeutic course is essentially the same for freshwater or saltwater ingestion. Hypervolemia or hypovolemia is routinely seen in these victims. The ingested fluid is rapidly assimilated by pulmonary and gastric circulation, which leads to systemic volume overload. Overzealous fluid replacement will likely result in the development of pulmonary edema in a child who sustains a lung injury. Gastric distention may be present, with associated vomiting and aspiration during initial treatment. Judicious fluid resuscitation is mandated in the early treatment phases to prevent further volume overload. Hypovolemia is a consequence of the hypoxic insult, which damages the endothelium and causes increased capillary permeability. This results in loss of proteinaceous fluid into the third space and depletion of intravascular volume. Drowning victims also experience a variation in glucose metabolism. Hyperglycemia is a frequent problem that may further complicate the neurologic outcome. Accumulation of excessive endogenous circulating catecholamine after the stress of the submersion is thought to be the cause of hyperglycemia (Rowin et al., 1996). Studies have shown that children with a blood glucose level of 350 mg/dl or greater have an increased likelihood of death or poor neurologic outcome compared with children with normal blood glucose levels (Michaud, Rivara, Longstreth, & Grady, 1991). Caution must be used when administering insulin to neurologically compromised patients. If hypoglycemia occurs, the increased cerebral blood flow and elevated ICP further complicate the clinical course and neurologic outcome.

Renal, Hepatic, and Gastrointestinal Systems

The injuries sustained to the renal, hepatic, and gastrointestinal (GI) systems are the result of oxygen deprivation during the submersion event. Renal impairment, as evidenced by albuminuria, hemoglobinuria, hematuria, oliguria, and anuria, is a common finding. Acute tubular necrosis is also present. Liver damage is manifested by elevation of bilirubin and transaminase levels. Coagulant precursors found in the liver may be affected and place the patient at risk for disseminated intravascular coagulation (DIC). The GI mucosal surface can experience sloughing as the result of the hypoxia. These events place the patient at risk for bacterial infections and possible perforation. Changes in bowel patterns occur and bloody, mucus-filled diarrhea stools result.

Hypothermia and the Diving Reflex

Hypothermia, defined as core temperature less than 85° C, and the diving reflex have been considered protective mechanisms for submersion victims. This is especially true for children. Hypothermia is common in pediatric submersion because victims lose heat rapidly because of their large body surface area and their limited subcutaneous fat insulation. The cooling process is escalated further by vigorous swimming movements that result in skeletal muscle vasodilation. As body heat is lost, core temperature continues to decrease, resulting in various systemic aberrations, such as cardiac arrhythmia, hypotension, hypoventilation, apnea, and altered neurologic findings (Kallas, 2000). The most important effect of severe hypothermia is decreased energy utilization. Hypothermia profoundly alters systemic perfusion, decreasing cerebral oxygen consumption and metabolic rates. As a result of this mechanism, hypothermia is thought to be beneficial in preserving brain tissue. Hypothermia also increases blood viscosity, alters white blood cell function, and decreases insulin production (Rowin et al., 1996). For hypothermia to be protective, core body temperature must fall rapidly, decreasing the cellular metabolic rate before significant hypoxemia begins. Kallas (2000) postulates that water temperature must be extremely cold, approximately 5° C, with a core body temperature less than 28° to 30° C to positively affect neurologic survival.

The diving reflex has also been thought to provide protection after a cold-water submersion. This reflex, seen in marine mammals, provides protection by shunting blood to the brain and heart and reducing metabolic requirements. Although the reflex is strong in marine mammals, it is considered weak or nonfunctional in humans (DeNicola et al., 1997). Dramatic recoveries with good neurologic outcomes have been documented after prolonged hypothermia, but persistent hypothermia poses a direct threat to survival.

THERAPEUTIC MANAGEMENT

Prehospital Setting

Prehospital management has a significant effect on the outcome of pediatric submersion victims. Treatment aimed at preventing irreversible tissue injury from prolonged hypoxia and ischemia must be initiated immediately after the child has been removed from the water. Any delay in rescue and resuscitation will lengthen the duration of the submersion, increase the possibility of hypoxemia and acidosis, and negatively affect the child's outcome (Quan, 1999). Although timely intervention is critical, it is extremely important to obtain an accurate history at the scene. The estimated time and duration of the submersion, the temperature and medium of water, and the presence or absence of spontaneous respirations immediately after rescue are important details to include in the history (Luttrell, 1991). Although these details are often difficult to obtain, they are vital in guiding care.

Management begins with assessment of airway, breathing, and circulation (the ABCs) (Figure 20-3). Cardiopulmonary resuscitation (CPR) should be initiated for all near-drowning victims experiencing cardiac arrest and should continue until the child is transferred to an emergency care facility. Establishing an adequate airway is the initial priority. Placing the child in the "sniffing" position without hyperextending the neck will open the airway. A high index of suspicion for cervical spine injury must be maintained because events surrounding the submersion injury are usually unclear. The jaw-thrust maneuver without the head-tilt component should be used to ensure adequate airway protection and stabilization of the cervical spine. Artificial airway devices may be required to maintain an open airway and allow for adequate ventilation. Any child who cannot protect the airway, exhibits a decreasing level of consciousness or deteriorating neurologic examination, is in severe respiratory distress despite supplemental oxygen, or is hypothermic or in full arrest requires tracheal intubation (Rowin et al., 1996).

After a patent airway is established, effective respirations must be maintained or provided by mouth-to-mouth rescue breathing or with a bag-valve-mask device when available. Numerous clinicians recommend that mouth-to-mouth breathing be attempted while the child is still in the water (Levin et al., 1993; Sarnaik & Lich-Lai, 1992; Shaw & Briede, 1989). Because the primary goal is prevention of hypoxia, high-flow oxygen must be delivered as soon as possible. If the child is breathing spontaneously and can maintain a patent airway, 100% oxygen can be delivered by face mask. The effectiveness of respiration must be evaluated frequently. In children who require respiratory assistance,

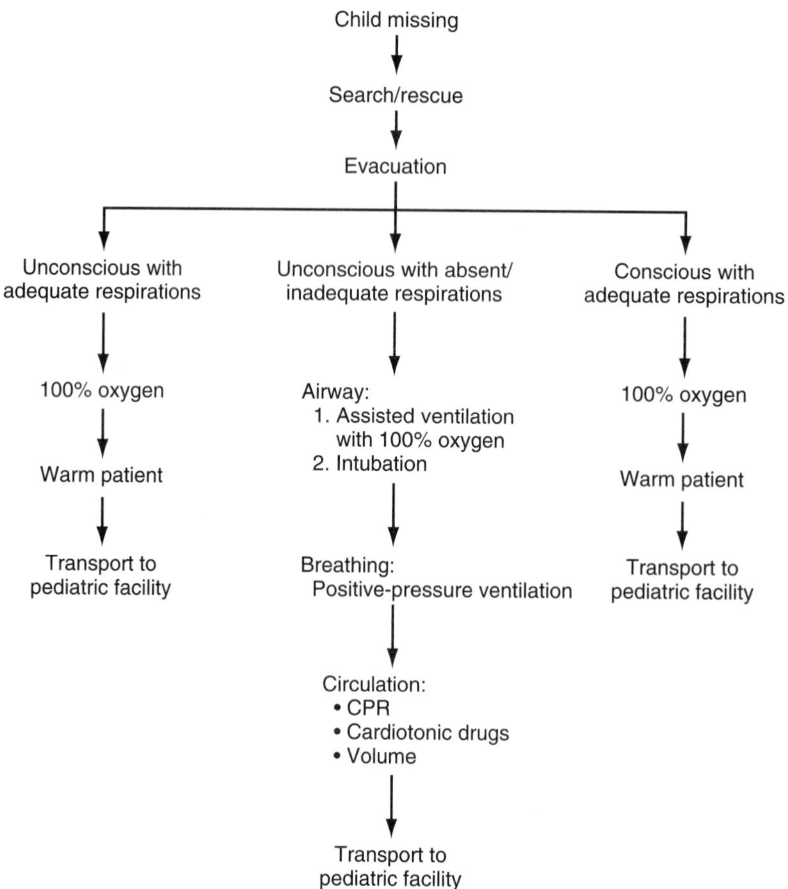

FIGURE 20-3 Prehospital management of a pediatric submersion incident. (From Beyda, D. [1991]. Near-drowning & treatment of the child with a submersion incident. *Critical Care Nursing Clinics of North America, 3,* 282.)

positive-pressure ventilation should be initiated with a self-inflating bag in an attempt to minimize intrapulmonary shunting and improve oxygenation. Noninvasive pulse oximetry and transcutaneous oxygen/carbon dioxide (O_2/CO_2) monitoring will provide ongoing assessment of oxygenation and ventilation at the scene and during transport to an emergency care facility.

In the past, the Heimlich maneuver was recommended to remove water from the lungs. However, the safety of this procedure in children has been challenged (Modell 1993; Rosen, Stoto, & Harley, 1995). There is concern that performing this maneuver may delay resuscitation efforts and increase the risk of aspiration. The American Heart Association (AHA, 1997) currently recommends the use of the Heimlich maneuver *only* in patients with submersion injuries in whom a foreign body is suspected of obstructing the airway or for those not responding appropriately to mouth-to-mouth ventilation.

After the airway is secured and effective respirations established, circulation must be assessed. In the field the child may be cold and mottled, with decreased peripheral pulses and a nonpalpable blood pressure. DeNicola et al. (1997) recommend a thorough search for pulses, which can take up to 1 full minute to assess and should be done before initiating CPR. Stroke volume is small in children, and cardiac output is affected primarily by heart rate. Bradycardia likely will result in decreased cardiac output and subsequent system hypoperfusion. Because significant hypovolemia is likely to occur, it is prudent to obtain vascular access. Use of two large-bore intravenous devices is advocated to deliver initial 20 ml/kg isotonic fluid boluses and subsequent fluid replacement needs if signs of hypovolemia are present. Assessment of peripheral perfusion, pulses, and blood pressure will direct further fluid resuscitation. If intravenous access cannot be established, an intraosseous infusion must be placed. Fluid and cardiac resuscitation in the field should be guided by standard protocols and medical control from the receiving institution. The hypothermic child with cardiac compromise must be handled and treated with passive rewarming measures to decrease the occurrence of possible arrhythmias. Once rescued and initially managed, the child should be rapidly transported to the nearest medical facility for further stabilization and definitive treatment. Complicating conditions, such as seizures, head injuries, neck injuries, and trauma, must be considered during field and transport management.

Hospital Setting: Collaborative Management

Comprehensive management of the pediatric submersion victim requires a well-trained multidisciplinary team of care providers to meet the unique and challenging needs of these patients and their families. Management is varied and depends on the severity of injury and the resulting multisystem effects. The spectrum of care from emergency management to the pediatric intensive care unit (PICU) primarily focuses on the pulmonary, cardiovascular, and neurologic systems.

Emergency Department Management

A systematic approach to care is extremely important in the emergency department and must include a detailed history provided by the emergency medical services (EMS) personnel before they leave. Assessment and care begin with determining the presence or absence of spontaneous respirations, pulses, and blood pressure. If the child was managed emergently in the field, reassessment of the effectiveness of these measures should be performed and modified when necessary. A detailed respiratory assessment must be performed.

Airway. Signs of respiratory distress can be difficult to detect and are often nonspecific. Observation of tachypnea, tachycardia, retractions, nasal flaring, grunting, stridor, wheezing, mottled color, and changes in responsiveness signal the potential for respiratory failure and indicate the need for intervention (Hazinski, 1999). Respiratory deterioration can occur rapidly in the presence of pulmonary disease or injury. Children have small, narrow airways that are easily obstructed by mucus, edema, or airway constriction. Further obstruction of these tiny airways will increase the work of breathing and quickly deplete limited energy reserves. Children have extremely compliant rib cages that allow them to sustain severe chest trauma without rib fractures. If rib fractures are present, intrathoracic injury and pulmonary contusions should be suspected. Increased chest wall compliance results in inspiratory retractions in the presence of pulmonary disease or injury. These retractions can result in decreased tidal volume, increased work of breathing, and fatigue (Hazinski, 1999). Another pediatric-specific pulmonary difference is the child's thin chest wall. This allows breath sounds to be easily transmitted throughout the chest but may contribute to misleading assessment findings and mask the presence of atelectasis, pneumothorax, and hemothorax. Monitoring changes in pitch may be more helpful than focusing on assessing changes in intensity (Hazinski, 1999). Assessment findings such as apnea, gasping, worsening systemic perfusion, bradycardia, and increasingly abnormal arterial blood gases indicate further deterioration and confirm respiratory failure (Hazinski, 1999).

Breathing. High-flow oxygen (100%) given by face mask should be initiated. Ongoing monitoring includes continuous pulse oximetry, capnography, and arterial blood gases. Prompt intubation should be done before signs of severe respiratory distress or hypoxia are evident. Intubation may be necessary to maintain a patent airway, achieve adequate oxygenation and ventilation, or decrease the work of breathing and reduce fatigue (Hazinski, 1999). Elective intubation in the absence of respiratory depression should be considered if the child has lost airway protective reflexes, has a deteriorating neurologic examination, or is severely hypothermic (Rowin et al., 1996). Oral intubation is generally preferred because it can be performed quickly and is associated with few complications. Rapid-sequence intubation is used when possible to reduce the risk of gagging and vomiting. This is particularly important for near-drowning victims because they often have a full stomach.

Once the intubation has been completed, it is necessary to ensure that the tube is in the correct position. This can be done by looking for bilateral chest expansion during positive-pressure ventilation and assessing for equal breath sounds bilaterally. The nurse must be especially diligent in the assessment of breath sounds in children because these sounds are easily transmitted throughout the thoracic cavity and can mask serious injury. It is important to compare the quality and pitch of the breath sounds bilaterally and observe for chest expansion from the head or foot of the bed (Hazinski, 1999). Auscultation should be done under the axilla and over the back to provide a comprehensive assessment. Listening for breath sounds over the stomach is important to rule out esophageal intubation. Most important, signs of clinical improvement are sought as a way to evaluate tube position. If the intubated patient continues to have inadequate respirations and oxygenation, the endotracheal tube must be assessed for displacement, obstruction, or pneumothorax (Hazinski, 1999). If the tube is displaced into the pharynx or esophagus, breath sounds will be decreased and possibly heard over the stomach. A tube in the right mainstem will result in increased breath sounds and chest rise on the right and decreased air movement on the left. Obstruction of the tube results in little or no air movement or chest expansion. A unilateral pneumothorax will produce decreased breath sounds and chest expansion on the affected side. A tension pneumothorax will cause a mediastinal shift away from the leak and may result in decreased cardiac output. Beyda (1991, 1998) advocates the early use of positive end-expiratory pressure (PEEP) in children who have sustained a severe pulmonary injury and are hypoxic in the emergency department. The use of PEEP reduces intrapulmonary shunting caused by atelectasis and improves functional residual capacity (FRC) and gas exchange.

Placement of a nasogastric tube and the resulting decompression of the stomach are important component of respiratory management. This is especially true for near-drowning victims who are at high risk for aspiration. The diaphragm is the chief muscle of respiration and often the only respiratory muscle in young children because of their inadequately developed intercostal muscles. Because of this anatomy, anything that interferes with diaphragmatic movement is likely to contribute to respiratory distress.

Circulation. As airway and breathing are evaluated, the patient's hemodynamic status is simultaneously assessed. Continuous electrocardiography, blood pressure monitoring, capillary refill time, skin temperature, and skin color are important assessment parameters. These findings provide a good indication of the effectiveness of tissue perfusion and the potential for early shock. Fluid resuscitation may be required for the hypovolemic or acidemic patient. The goal of fluid management is to provide adequate tissue perfusion and thereby minimize damage and provide cerebral protection. Although cerebral edema is a concern, judicious fluid management is essential to correct volume loss and promote effective perfusion and oxygenation. Initially, crystalloids are given in boluses of 20 ml/kg with frequent cardiac, respiratory, and neurologic assessments to ensure early identification of complications. Insertion of a urinary catheter should be considered to continuously evaluate urine output.

Numerous arrhythmias, such as asystole, ventricular tachycardia or fibrillation, and bradycardia, may present after a submersion injury (Kallas, 2000). Management of these abnormal rhythms is based on pediatric advanced life support protocols (AHA, 1997). Ventricular fibrillation is associated with hypothermia and is particularly unresponsive to defibrillation. Three defibrillation attempts are acceptable; however, if these attempts are unsuccessful, CPR must be reinstituted and no further attempts made until the child's temperature has been normalized (Kallas, 2000).

The presence of hypothermia renders the initial examination unreliable. The infant may appear dead because of diminished cardiac and neurologic activity. Prompt intervention and determination of core body temperature are critical. Hypothermia should be assumed in all pediatric submersion events, and prompt rewarming measures must be taken. External rewarming is achieved by immediately removing wet clothing, drying the skin, applying warm blankets, and using a radiant heat source. Internally, the core can be rewarmed through the infusion of warmed intravenous fluids; delivery of warmed humidified oxygen; or gastric, rectal, or peritoneal lavage with warmed fluid (DeNicola et al., 1997). With the severely hypothermic patient, hemodialysis and extracorporeal circulation techniques may be a possibility (Kallas, 2000). Rewarming requires careful observation and includes careful evaluation of electrolytes, blood gases, and acid-base status. External rewarming of the extremely hypothermic patient can cause localized burns. Internal rewarming has been associated with cardiac arrhythmias and further cardiac compromise. Because the hypothermic heart is prone to ventricular fibrillation, excessive stimulation should be avoided. Beyda (1991) suggests that core temperature be increased slowly by 1° C per hour to minimize complications. If the hypothermic child requires resuscitation, prudent use of cardiotonic medications is recommended. Excretion of these drugs in the presence of hypothermia is delayed and results in high plasma concentrations (Elixson, 1991). Some drugs, such as epinephrine, lidocaine, and bretylium, may reach toxic levels with repeated administration. If attempts to restore cardiovascular stability cannot be achieved in the emergency department after rewarming, further attempts at resuscitation are futile (DeNicola et al., 1997).

Neurologic Assessment. In addition to assessment and management of the ABCs, a neurologic assessment must be performed. It is important to evaluate the level of consciousness using the Glasgow Coma Scale (GCS) or the Modified Glasgow Coma Scale (MGCS) for infants. It is important to obtain an accurate baseline neurologic measurement because GCS assessments will be performed serially to evaluate trends in the patient's condition. Assessment of brainstem reflexes is useful in determining the degree of neurologic injury. This assessment includes pupil reactivity, corneal response, gag reflex, oculovestibular and oculocephalic reflexes, and the presence of spontaneous respiratory effort. The extent of the evaluation of these reflexes depends on the severity of the impairment. Pupil reactivity can be performed quickly and provides information about increased ICP or severe cerebral damage. Early identification of increased ICP mandates prompt interventions aimed at reducing secondary cerebral injury. Nursing measures are directed toward minimizing increased ICP. Interventions include providing preoxygenation before suctioning, limiting the use and duration of suctioning, maintaining the head in the midline position, avoiding extreme flexion of the hips and neck, and elevating the head of the bed 30 to 15 degrees (Vernon-Levett, 1996). Seizure activity requires prompt management so that increases in cerebral oxygen consumption and blood flow can be minimized (Rowin et al., 1996).

Laboratory and Imaging Studies. Selected diagnostic laboratory and imaging studies are initiated in the emergency department. Baseline serum electrolytes, complete blood count with differential, and renal and hepatic studies may be indicated, depending on the severity of injury. Measurement of serum glucose is particularly important because of the debilitating effects of hypoglycemia. Toxicologic studies are warranted if alcohol or illicit drug use is suspected. Chest radiographs are needed to determine endotracheal tube placement and potential lung damage from aspirated water. Cervical spine radiographs are needed to rule out spinal fractures or deformities. A negative cervical spine radiograph, however, may not be adequate evidence that a cervical injury has not resulted. Submersion victims have a significant potential for trauma and should be cared for with a high index of suspicion for injury. Cervical spine clearance may include neurosurgical consultation and additional diagnostic tests. Computed tomography scanning of the head may be helpful, depending on the mechanism of injury.

Once stabilized, the child must be assessed to identify and treat non–life-threatening injuries. The acronym AMPLE (*a*llergies, *m*edications, *p*ast history, *l*ast meal, and *e*vents pertinent to the injury) helps the clinician quickly gather relevant facts about the patient's history. Information on the possibility of abuse, neglect, homicide, suicide, alcohol, and drug ingestion is included.

Many children who experience submersion injuries are alert and breathing spontaneously at the scene. In these cases submersion time was often brief, with the possibility of a transient period of apnea. These children are relatively asymptomatic on the initial examination, but an observation period to observe for potential complications is critical. Care for these children is often provided in the emergency department. The child who has survived submersion requires continuous pulse oximetry, arterial blood gases, and supplemental oxygen. A baseline chest radiograph is useful for comparison if the child develops symptoms of respiratory distress. Respiratory assessments should be done frequently in an effort to identify tachypnea, diminished or adventitious breath sounds, cough with frothy sputum production, increased work of breathing, and the continued need for supplemental oxygen. These symptoms commonly signal the presence of pulmonary edema (Luttrell, 1991). Most clinicians recommend a minimum of a 24-hour admission for all patients, including those with no symptoms, because they are at risk for abrupt clinical changes (Fiser, 1993; Olshaker, 1992). However, an observation period of 6 to 12 hours may be sufficient for a child who is alert and asymptomatic (Kallas, 2000; Noonan, Howrey, & Ginsburg, 1996; Quan, 1999). Strict criteria for discharge may be more important than defining a rigid observation interval. Before discharge is considered, the child must be able to maintain an oxygen saturation of 95% or greater on room air, have no pulmonary symptoms, and have normal serial neurologic examinations. Once the criteria are met, the child becomes eligible for discharge. If the criteria are met and the parents and caregivers understand the signs and symptoms that require prompt attention, discharge can be considered. If, however, the child requires extensive resuscitation in the field or is unstable in the emergency department, further stabilization is indicated and admission to the PICU becomes necessary.

Pediatric Intensive Care Unit Management

Near-drowning causes various degrees of organ damage that results from the global hypoxic-ischemic event. The primary goal of intensive care management is to reduce secondary brain injury. This is accomplished by using cerebral resuscitation interventions aimed at minimizing secondary damage from hypoxia, ischemia, acidosis, seizure activity, and fluid or electrolyte imbalances. Patients admitted to the PICU require continuous cardiorespiratory monitoring, pulse oximetry, capnography for intubated patients, and careful assessment of intake and input. Unstable patients also need arterial and central venous pressure monitoring. Pulmonary artery monitoring may provide valuable information about cardiac or pulmonary function (Rowin et al., 1996). Currently, serial echocardiograms are being used more frequently in place of this invasive technology. Other essential components of management for these patients are frequent neurologic examinations and assessment of GCS and MGCS scores.

Nursing of the acutely ill pediatric victim of a submersion event requires expert skill. Anticipating patterns of multiorgan system failure and providing timely interventions are essential. Inadequate oxygenation and ineffective breathing patterns must be identified when the subtle signs first appear. Symptoms of intravascular volume instability must be recognized and treated promptly to prevent cerebral complications. Careful titration of intravenous fluids and hourly intake and output are extremely important. All nursing measures must be designed to prevent an increase in cerebral oxygen demand and ICP. Because many near-drowning victims have extended stays in the PICU, they are at risk for complications such as infection, malnutrition, and physical immobility. Nurses must be vigilant in monitoring for these complications and develop plans to maximize outcomes.

Pulmonary Management. The unintubated, spontaneously breathing child who is admitted to the PICU requires close assessment for the subtle signs of respiratory distress. Deterioration of the respiratory system is possible up to 24 to 72 hours after a near-drowning event and results from secondary drowning, adult respiratory distress syndrome, chemical pneumonitis, or pneumonia (Rowin et al. 1996). Administration of oxygen is first-line therapy. Use of continuous positive airway pressure (CPAP) by mask has been suggested in certain situations, including mild to moderate hypoxemia, despite the use of supplemental oxygen in an alert child (Dottorini, Eslami, Baglioni, Fiorenzano, & Todisco, 1996; Modell, 1993). However, this treatment modality has not been widely used or investigated in children with submersion injuries. CPAP improves oxygenation by increasing FRC, and some authors suggest that it may be an easier and less expensive alternative to endotracheal intubation for patients who remain conscious and breathing spontaneously (Dottorini et al., 1996).

The detrimental effects of positive airway pressure include increased intrathoracic pressure resulting in decreased cardiac output (especially with hypovolemia), alveolar hyperinflation with possible air leaks, and impeded cerebral venous return. Gastric decompression is required with CPAP to prevent distention and decrease the work of breathing. Serial respiratory assessments for continued hypoxemia, impaired ventilation, increased work of breathing, or deteriorating mental status may indicate the need for endotracheal intubation.

Inadequate Pao_2 (less than 60 mm Hg while receiving 30% oxygen), decreased oxygen saturation (less than 90%), or increasing respiratory acidosis may indicate the need for intubation and ventilation. Because near-drowning victims are often unresponsive to supplemental oxygen, PEEP may be necessary to improve oxygenation in the intubated patient with severe pulmonary dysfunction. Pressure should be increased gradually, with the goal of maintaining oxygen saturation levels greater than 90% while receiving Fio_2 of 0.5 or less (Hazinski, 1999). PEEP is usually well tolerated, but it can impair cardiac output. Because this is especially evident in hypovolemic patients, normal intravascular volume must be maintained. Patients treated with high PEEP are at risk for barotrauma, such as pneumothoraces and subcutaneous emphysema. As pulmonary dysfunction resolves, PEEP can be weaned rapidly. If conventional modes of ventilation are not effective, more aggressive therapies, such as high-frequency jet ventilation and extracorporeal membrane oxygenation, may be needed (Arensman, Statter, Bastawrous, & Madonna, 1996; Paulson, Spear, & Peterson, 1995). The use of an artificial surfactant, nitric oxide, liquid ventilation, and intratracheal pulmonary ventilation are evolving interventions for patients with pulmonary insufficiency.

Careful monitoring for infection is important because all near-drowning victims are at risk for possible aspiration. Most authors agree that the value of corticosteroids or prophylactic antibiotics for treatment of pulmonary complications in near-drowning victims has not been proven and may be detrimental (Fields, 1992; Levin et al., 1993; Rowin et al., 1996). The use of prophylactic antibiotics should be considered for patients who aspirate grossly contaminated fluid.

Cardiovascular Management. Cardiovascular management is aimed at interventions that will maintain adequate cardiac output and organ perfusion. Although the healthy pediatric heart is resilient to permanent injury after submersion, the hypoxic effects of inadequate cardiac output and perfusion contribute to multiorgan damage. Anoxic or ischemic injury is manifested by nonspecific ST- and T-wave changes with elevation of cardiac isoenzymes. Fluid intake must be calculated carefully to ensure improved end-organ perfusion without increasing the workload of the heart. Administration of excessive fluids compromises cardiac function by increasing the symptoms of left-sided failure and exacerbating cerebral edema (Rowin et al, 1996). Inotropic medications to optimize cardiac contractility may help maintain or improve organ perfusion. Continuous inotropic infusions require meticulous assessment to determine and titrate the effects on cardiac output. A flow-directed pulmonary artery catheter can be helpful in the assessment of cardiac function and oxygen delivery.

Neurologic Management. Effective management of neurologic damage from submersion accidents remains controversial (DeNicola et al., 1997; Rowin et al., 1996; Sachdeva, 1999). In the late 1970s, studies indicated that aggressive therapies used to treat cerebral edema would improve recovery for these patients (Conn, Edmonds, & Barker, 1979, 1980). Interventions were aimed at controlling cerebral edema, evaluating and treating increased ICP, and decreasing cerebral metabolic requirements. However, subsequent studies have shown that these approaches do not prevent secondary neurologic damage after hypoxia and ischemia and may adversely affect outcome (Lavelle & Shaw, 1993; Modell, 1993; Nussbaum & Maggi, 1988; Pfenninger, 1993).

Current neurologic care in the PICU consists of conservative management aimed at preventing secondary brain injury. Interventions are directed at rapidly restoring and stabilizing oxygenation and cerebral circulation (Rowin et al., 1996). Prevention of acidosis, hypotension, hyperthermia, hyperglycemia, uncontrolled seizures, and fluid overload are important for optimal recovery (DeNicola et al., 1997). Mild hyperventilation for short periods, sedation, and head elevation may be helpful in reducing intracranial hypertension. The resulting hypoxic-ischemic brain damage from a submersion injury is irreversible, and efforts must focus on reducing secondary neuronal damage. Experimental therapies are emerging and hold some promise of improving outcome. A detailed discussion of collaborative management for children with hypoxic-ischemic injuries is given in Chapter 14.

Associated System Management. Although cerebral resuscitation and prevention of secondary brain injury are the primary focuses, other organ systems are damaged by hypoxemia and must be carefully evaluated and protected. Decreased blood supply to the GI tract may result in the formation of stress ulcers and GI bleeding. Sloughing of the intestinal mucosa may occur and result in copious bloody diarrhea, which is associated with a poor prognosis (Kallas, 2000). Management of GI symptoms consists of bowel rest, nasogastric decompression, gastric pH monitoring, and the administration of antacids. Parenteral nutritional support is necessary in the severely impaired child.

Acute renal failure (ARF) is the result of the initial hypoxic-ischemic injury. In most cases ARF resolves with appropriate cardiopulmonary management. Diuretics, fluid restriction, or dialysis may be needed if fluid overload or electrolyte abnormalities exist (Kallas, 2000).

Disturbances in the normal serum coagulation patterns may develop and result in DIC. Early detection with supportive care and management directed at the cause is required. Blood products, such as fresh frozen plasma, platelets, or cryoprecipitates, may interrupt the cycle of DIC (Hazinski, 1999).

Psychosocial Management. Psychosocial care of patients with submersion injuries and their parents is extremely important. The unexpected nature and the severity of the event place an enormous burden on the family and patient. Because submersion events are largely preventable, family members experience an overwhelming sense of guilt that may last a lifetime. The critical care nurse is often the health care professional who has the most frequent and intimate contact with the family.

Family-centered care may best facilitate the needs of the pediatric patient. The contemporary family structure is no longer traditional, and assumptions must not be made about the family makeup and roles. Family-centered care operationalizes the belief that the family is the central force in the child's life, responsible for meeting physical, emotional, and social needs. This philosophy enables the health care team to appreciate and respect family diversity in structure, socioeconomic status, and cultural backgrounds (Ahmann, 1994).

Parents experience many stressors that are manifested in a variety of behaviors unique to their culture and previous hospital experiences. The nurse may be confronted with many different responses from patients and families, ranging from intense anger to complete denial. An attitude of nonjudgmental calm that demonstrates respect for individual differences must be conveyed. Collaboration with social work services, child life specialists, and pastoral care will greatly increase the opportunity to benefit the patient, family, and other health care providers.

PROGNOSTIC INDICATORS

The factors that accurately predict which children will survive neurologically intact from a submersion event are not completely known. Although numerous studies have attempted to predict outcome variables, no system is completely accurate. Submersion time has been discussed as an important variable (Orlowski, 1987; Quan & Kinder, 1992; Quan et al., 1990). Submersion times longer than 10 minutes in nonicy water and the need for resuscitation for more than 25 minutes have been associated with poor outcomes (Quan & Kinder, 1992; Quan et al., 1990). Submersion times of less than 5 minutes and the need for resuscitation for less than 10 minutes result in good outcomes. Children found to have a normal sinus rhythm, reactive pupils, and an intact neurologic system are also more likely to have good outcomes. Numerous studies have associated the need for cardiopulmonary resuscitation in the emergency department with poor outcomes (Biggart & Bohn, 1990; Kyriacou, Arcinue, Peek, & Kraus, 1994; Nichter & Everett, 1989). The same association has been shown to be true for patients who require cardiotonic drugs in the emergency department (Nichter & Everett, 1989). Conversely, numerous authors have reported that children who are asystolic upon arrival to the emergency department, who require prolonged CPR, and who receive cardiotonic drugs have made full recoveries (Christensen, Jansen, & Perkin, 1997; Lavelle & Shaw, 1993).

Selected physical findings and initial laboratory data are used as predictors of outcome. Low pH (less than 7.1), coma at initial presentation, and the need for prolonged resuscitation have been used as predictors of poor outcome (Fandel & Bancalari, 1976; Habib, Tecklenburg, Webb, Anas, & Perkin, 1996; Orlowski, 1979). Graf, Cummings, Quan, and Brutocao (1995) documented the association of unreactive pupils, elevated initial serum glucose, and male gender with a poor prognosis. Oakes, Sherck, Maloney, and Charters (1982) reported that good outcomes were related to the patient arriving at the emergency department with a spontaneous heart rate.

The GCS has been widely used to predict outcomes of pediatric near-drowning victims (Bratton, Jardine, & Morray, 1994; Dean & Kaufman, 1981; Lavelle & Shaw, 1993). A score that does not improve in 24 hours predicts an ominous outcome (Bratton et al., 1994; Lavelle & Shaw, 1993). Subsequent researchers have reported use of the Pediatric Risk of Mortality (PRISM) score in both emergency departments and PICUs to predict outcome (Spack, Gedeit, Splaingard, & Havens, 1997; Zuckerman, Gregory, & Damiani, 1998). PRISM is a scoring system that predicts mortality in critically ill children (Pollack, Ruttimann, & Getson, 1988). The basic premise of the PRISM score is that the amount and extent of physiologic dysfunction is related to the patient's risk. By categorizing the patient's condition using physiologic variables and various ranges described in the PRISM score, one can determine a relative score of the patient's severity of illness (Zuckerman et al., 1998). Further analysis allows computation of mortality risk.

Predicting neurologic outcome is a major clinical problem in near-drowning. Many clinicians wish to avoid resuscitation for patients whose outcome is likely to be a persistent vegetative state; however, clinicians are also committed to give all patients a chance for meaningful survival and recovery (DeBoer, 1997). Some clinicians believe that all children initially should be resuscitated aggressively because there is no absolute predicator of outcome, but others disagree. As technology improves and becomes more available, the number of deaths from submersion will decrease and the number of neurologically damaged survivors increase. There are no easy answers for these situations and no current mechanism to accurately predict outcome for these children.

OUTCOME

Historically, pulmonary dysfunction was the leading cause of death of near-drowning victims. Medical advances in cardiopulmonary management have changed this situation. After initial stabilization, the hypoxic insult to the brain and its sequelae determine morbidity and mortality. Outcome data reported by numerous authors indicate that children who survive and are admitted to the PICU have a 50% to 80% chance of surviving with an intact neurologic system. Mortality rates are 25% to 35%, and approximately 10% survive with neurologic damage (Abrams & Mubarak, 1991; Biggart & Bohn, 1990; Jensen, Williams, Thurman, & Keller, 1992; Lavelle & Shaw, 1993; Levin et al., 1993).

The long-term consequences of neurologic impairment can be staggering for the victim and family. Cerebral anoxia is associated with musculoskeletal alterations. The extent of the injury determines the degree of immobility, posturing, spasticity, and contractures (Abrams & Mubarak, 1991). Posturing and spasticity tend to progress rapidly and are especially severe. Near-drowning victims with neurologic impairment tend to have long durations of unconsciousness, decreased verbal skills, and poor cognitive abilities (Wintemute, 1990). The financial, emotional, and social costs to the family are tremendous. The victims often require a level of medical, nursing, and child care that is expensive, time consuming, and emotionally exhausting. Parents may have no time or energy for outside employment or diversional activities. Intense anger and guilt may surface and increase the risk of divorce, separation, and the development of dysfunctional parenting patterns (Borta, 1991). Siblings of the victim suffer from guilt and often display emotional and developmental regression. Aggressive behavior, impaired learning skills, and excessive dependency are common dysfunctional features reported in siblings as they attempt to grieve and cope with the loss of their brother or sister (Borta, 1991). Decisions by the family members and clinicians to withdraw life support for severely impaired near-drowning patients must be handled carefully. These ethical issues are discussed more fully in Chapter 3.

PREVENTION

Undoubtedly, the most important tactic in decreasing the morbidity and mortality associated with submersion injuries is primary prevention. Nurses, physicians, and other health care professionals must take advantage of opportunities to assess potential risk factors for submersion injuries and heighten awareness of patients, parents, and other members of the community. One study of 800 pediatricians in the United States revealed that most pediatricians do not routinely provide information about drowning prevention to their patients' parents (O'Flaherty & Pirie, 1997). Only a small percentage of these physicians were involved in community or legislation efforts directed at drowning prevention. Few of these physicians received formal drowning prevention education during their pediatric residency training, and a large majority believed that further education on prevention of drowning and near-drowning would be useful (O'Flaherty & Pirie, 1997).

Prevention strategies focus primarily on three important areas: adult supervision, CPR education, and water safety and accessibility to water sources (Nieves, Buttacavoli, Fuller, Clarke, & Schimpf, 1996). The lack of constant adult supervision is directly linked to submersion events in children (Quan et al., 1989). Supervision of children enjoying water activities can be enhanced in many ways. Assigning adults to act specifically as observers, without any other responsibilities or distractions, ensures a degree of safety. This is especially true if the activities are associated with a social event that involves alcohol. Given this scenario, an adult must be designated to remain vigilant (Nieves et al., 1996). Portable phones located at poolside with emergency phone numbers nearby will decrease the need to leave the vicinity. Rules for unsupervised swimming should be enforced, with children exiting the pool area if the adult is called away. All toys and flotation devices should be removed from view to decrease the temptation for children to approach the pool or swimming area while they are unsupervised. Flotation devices should never be considered a replacement for adult supervision. The infant and small child are particularly prone to submersion injury and should never be left unattended in a bathtub or near any open standing water, such as toilets, buckets, or wading pools.

Education about submersion has two purposes. The first is to educate the community in general. The second is to teach parents and caregivers specific skills, such as CPR, that can be used at the time of submersion. Raising public awareness about water safety can be achieved through local and national media coverage, community action organizations, public health clinics, and physician offices. Local statistics regarding the morbidity and mortality of childhood drowning can be used as powerful evidence to that help raise public awareness of the devastation that can result from submersion injuries. Public funds are needed to construct barriers, develop supervised swimming areas, and advocate for aquatic education. The American Academy of Pediatrics advocates a national surveillance system to define drowning circumstances so that information focused on preventive strategies for children can be developed. The National Safe Kids Coalition is dedicated to the prevention of injury and the promotion of safety for children. Many local Safe Kids chapters exist and focus on community needs and interactive educational activities directed at prevention. Local hospitals that sponsor health fairs promoting child safety are a source of support. Basic life support and CPR classes are strongly recommended for parents, siblings, and child care workers so that they can initiate easy, lifesaving measures. Opportunities should be available for all teenagers to learn first aid and CPR. Competence in swimming is strongly encouraged for elementary school-age children and should be reinforced frequently. Use of alcohol and drugs while boating or swimming must be strongly discouraged, especially in the male adolescent population. Intervention programs through schools and aquatic recreation areas may help prevent serious injury or death in this age group.

Limiting the child's accessibility to pools and using pool barriers are important preventive tactics to minimize accidental drowning (Wintemute, 1992). Legislation concerning barriers to pool access has been extremely successful in places such as New Mexico, Hawaii, and Australia. Laws requiring pool fences have existed in Arizona, Australia, and New Zealand since the late 1980s and early 1990s. Pool fencing systems have been shown to be most effective if they meet specific criteria, such as being unclimbable, self-closing, self-locking, and at least 5 feet high, with openings between bars of less than 4 inches (Nieves et al, 1996). The fence must isolate the pool from the house and yard to prevent the child from entering the area. Pool alarms and covers are not as effective because they require active participation by the pool owner to ensure that they are functioning properly.

There are no easy solutions for prevention of submersion injuries. Sophisticated medical care and technologies have been developed to care for these victims, and a variety of prevention strategies have been developed around the world to reduce these injuries. The only real hope, however, is that a concerted effort by parents, health care providers, industry, and government will decrease the tremendous loss of children.

BIBLIOGRAPHY

Abrams, R. A., & Mubarak, S. (1991). Musculoskeletal consequences or near-drowning in children. *Journal of Pediatric Orthopedics, 11,* 168-175.

Ahmann, E. (1994). Family-centered care: The time has come. *Pediatric Nursing, 20,* 52-53.

Allman, F., Nelson, W., Pacentine, G., & McComb, G. (1986). Outcome following cardiopulmonary resuscitation in severe pediatric near-drowning. *American Journal, Disabled Child, 140,* 571-575.

American Heart Association. (1994). *Textbook of pediatric advanced life support.* Dallas: Author.

Arensman, R. M., Statter, M. B., Bastawrous, A. L., & Madonna, M. B. (1996). Modern treatment modalities for neonatal, & pediatric respiratory failure. *American Journal of Surgery, 172,* 41-47.

Baker, S., O'Neill, B., Ginsburg, M., & Li, G. (1992) *The injury fact book.* New York: Oxford University Press.

Beyda, D. (1991). Near-drowning, & treatment of the child with a submersion incident. *Critical Care Nursing Clinics of North America, 3*(2), 273-280.

Beyda, D. (1998). Childhood submersion injuries. *Journal of Emergency Nursing, 24*(2), 140-144.

Biggart, M., & Bohn, D. (1990). Effect of hypothermia and cardiac arrest on outcome of near-drowning accidents in children. *Journal of Pediatrics, 117,* 179-183.

Borta, M. (1991). Psychological issues in water-related injuries. *Critical Care Nursing Clinics of North America, 3*(2), 325-328.

Bratton, S., Jardine, D., & Morray, J. (1994). Serial neurologic examinations after near-drowning, & outcome. *Archives of Pediatric Adolescent Medicine, 148,* 167-170.

Brenner, R. A., Smith, G. S., & Overpeck, M. D. (1994). Divergent trends in childhood drowning rates, 1971 thru 1988. *JAMA, 271,* 1606-1608.

Christensen, D. W. (1992). Near-drowning. In M. C. Rogers (Ed.), *Textbook of pediatric intensive care* (pp. 877-880). Baltimore: Williams & Wilkins.

Christensen, D., Jansen, P, & Perkin, R. (1997). Outcome and acute care hospital costs after warm water near-drowning in children. *Pediatrics, 99,* 715-721.

Conn, A., Edmonds, J., & Barker, G. (1979). Cerebral resuscitation in near-drowning. *Pediatric Clinics of North America, 26,* 691-701.

Conn, A., Montes, J., & Barker G. (1980). Cerebral salvage in near-drowning following neurologic classification by triage. *Canadian Anesthesia Society Journal, 17,* 201-209.

Dean, J. M., & Kaufman, N. D. (1981). Prognostic indicators in pediatric near-drowning: The Glasgow coma scale. *Critical Care Medicine, 9,* 536-539.

DeBoer, S. (1997). Neurological outcomes after near-drowning. *Critical Care Nurse, 17,* 19-25.

DeNicola, L., Falk, J., Swanson, M., Gayle, M., & Kisson, N. (1997). Submersion injuries in children and adults. *Critical Care Clinics, 13*(3), 477-502.

Division of Injury Control, Center for Environmental Health and Injury Control, Center for Disease Control. (1990). Childhood injuries in the United States. *American Journal Disabled Child, 144,* 627-646.

Dottorini, M., Eslami, A., Baglioni, S., Fiorenzano, G., & Todisco, T. (1996). Nasal-continuous positive airway pressure in the treatment of near-drowning in freshwater. *Chest, 110,* 1122-1124.

Elixson, E. M. (1991). Cold water drowning. *Critical Care Nursing Clinics of North America, 3,* 287-292.

Fandel, I., & Bancalari, E. (1976). Near-drowning in children: Clinical aspects. *Pediatrics, 58,* 573-579.

Fields, A. I. (1992). Near-drowning in the pediatric population. *Critical Care Clinics, 8,* 113-129.

Fiser, D. H. (1993). Near-drowning. *Pediatric Review, 14,* 148-151.

Graf, W., Cummings, P., Quan, L., & Brutocao, D. (1995). Predicting outcome in pediatric submersion victims. *Journal of Trauma, 22,* 544-549.

Guyer, B., & Ellers, B. (1990). Childhood injuries in the United States. *American Journal of Disabled Child, 144,* 649-652.

Habib, D. M., Tecklenburg, F. W., Webb, S. A., Anas, N. G., & Perkin, R. M. (1996). Prediction of childhood drowning and near-drowning morbidity and mortality. *Pediatric Emergency Care, 12,* 255-258.

Hazinski, M. (1999). Pulmonary disorders. In *Manual of pediatric critical care* (pp. 289-356). St. Louis: Mosby.

Jensen, L. R., Williams, S. D., Thurman, D. J., & Keller, P. A. (1992). Submersion injuries in children younger than 5 years in urban Utah. *Western Journal of Medicine, 157,* 641-644.

Kallas, H. (2000). Drowning and near-drowning. In W. Nelson, R, Behrman, R. Kliegman, & A. Arvin (Eds.), *Textbook of pediatrics* (16th ed., pp. 279-287). Philadelphia: WB Saunders.

Kallas, H. J., & O'Rourke, P. P. (1993). Drowning and immersion injuries in children. *Current Opinions in Pediatrics, 5,* 295-302.

Karch, S. B. (1987). Serum catecholamines in nearly-drowned children. *American Journal of Emergency Medicine, 5,* 261-265.

Kyriacou, D., Arcinue, E., Peek, C., & Kraus, J. (1994). Effect of immediate resuscitation on children with submersion injury. *Pediatrics, 94*(2), 137-142.

Lavelle, J., & Shaw, K. (1993). Near-drowning: Is emergency department cardiopulmonary resuscitation or intensive care unit resuscitation indicated? *Critical Care Medicine, 21,* 369-373.

Levin, D., Moriss, F., Toro, L., Brink, L., & Turner, G. (1993). Drowning and near-drowning. *Pediatric Clinics of North America, 40,* 321-336.

Luttrell, P. (1991). Care of the pediatric near-drowning victim. *Critical Care Nursing Clinics of North America, 3*(2), 293-306.

Michaud, L., Rivara, F., Longstreth, W., & Grady, M. (1991). Initial blood glucose and poor outcome following severe brain injuries in children. *Journal of Trauma, 31,* 1356-1362.

Modell, J. (1993). Drowning. *New England Journal of Medicine, 328,* 253-256.

Modell, J., & Davis, J. (1969). Electrolyte changes in human drowning victims. *Anesthesiology, 30,* 414-420.

Nichter, M., & Everett, P. (1989) Childhood near-drowning: Is cardiopulmonary resuscitation always indicated? *Critical Care Medicine, 17,* 993-995.

Nieves, J., Buttacavoli, M., Fuller, L., Clarke, T., & Schimpf (1996). Childhood drowning: Review of the literature, & clinical implications. *Pediatric Nursing, 22*(3), 206-210.

Noonan, L., Howrey, R., & Ginsburg, C. (1996). Freshwater submersion injuries in children: A retrospective review of seventy-five hospitalized patients. *Pediatrics, 98,* 368-371.

Nussbaum, E., & Maggi, J. (1988). Pentobarbital therapy does not improve neurologic outcome in nearly drowned, flaccid-comatose children. *Pediatrics, 81,* 630-634.

Oakes, D., Sherck, J., Maloney J., & Charters, A. (1982). Prognosis and management of victims of near-drowning. *Journal of Trauma, 22,* 544-549.

O'Flaherty, J. E., & Pirie, P. L. (1997). Prevention of pediatric drowning and near-drowning: A survey of members of the American Academy of Pediatrics. *Pediatrics, 99,* 169-174.

Olshaker, J. S. (1992). Near-drowning. *Emergency Medicine Clinics of North America, 10,* 339-350.

Orlowski, J. (1987). Drowning, near-drowning, and ice-water submersions. *Pediatric Clinics of North America, 34,* 75-92.

Orlowski, J. P. (1979). Prognostic factors in pediatric cases of drowning and near-drowning. *Journal American College of Emergency Physicians, 8,* 176-179.

Orlowski, J. P., Abulleil, M. M., & Phillips, J. M. (1989). The hemodynamic and cardiovascular effects of near-drowning in hypotonic, isotonic, or hypertonic solutions. *Annals of Emergency Medicine, 18,* 1044-1049.

Paulson, T. E., Spear, R. M., & Peterson, B. M. (1995). New concepts in the treatment of children with acute respiratory distress syndrome. *Journal of Pediatrics, 127,* 163-175.

Pfenninger, J. (1993). Neurologic intensive care in children. *Intensive Care Medicine, 19,* 243:250.

Pollack, M., Ruttimann, U., & Getson, P. (1988). Pediatric risk of mortality (PRISM) score. *Critical Care Medicine, 16,* 1110-1116.

Quan, L. (1999). Near-drowning. *Pediatrics in Review, 20*(8), 255-259.

Quan, L., & Kinder, D. (1992). Pediatric submersions: Prehospital predictors of outcome. *Pediatrics, 99*(6), 909-913.

Quan, L., Gore, E., Wentz, K., Allen, J., & Novak, A. (1989). Ten-year study of pediatric drowning and near-drowning in Kings County, Washington: Lessons in injury prevention. *Pediatrics, 83,* 1035-1040.

Quan, L., Wentz, K., Gore, E., & Copass, M. (1990). Outcome and predicators of outcome in pediatric submersion victims receiving pre-hospital care in King County, Washington. *Pediatrics, 86,* 586-593.

Rosen, P., Stoto, M., & Harley, J. (1995). The use of the Heimlich maneuver in near-drowning. *Journal of Emergency Medicine, 13,* 397-405.

Rowin, M., Christensen, D., & Allen, E. (1996). Pediatric drowning and near-drowning. In M. Rogers & D. Nichols (Eds.), *Textbook of pediatric intensive care* (3rd ed., pp. 875-891). Baltimore: Williams & Wilkins.

Sachdeva, R. C. (1999). Near-drowning. *Critical Care Clinics, 15*(2), 281-296.

Sarnaik, A. P., & Lich-Lai, M. W. (1992). Near-drowning. In B. R. Furman & J. J. Zimmerman (Eds.), *Pediatric critical care* (pp. 1201-1207). St. Louis: Mosby.

Shaw, K. N., & Briede, C. A. (1989). Submersion injuries: Drowning and near-drowning. *Emergency Medicine Clinics of North America, 7,* 355-370.

Spack, L., Gedeit, R., Splaingard, M., & Havens, P. (1997). Failure of aggressive therapy to alter outcome in pediatric near-drowning. *Pediatric Emergency Care, 13,* 98-102.

Spyker, D. A. (1985). Submission injury: Epidemiology, prevention, and management. *Pediatric Clinics of North America, 32,* 113-125.

Vernon-Levett, P. (1996). Neurologic critical care problems. In M. Curley, J. Smith, & P. Moloney-Harmon. (Eds.), *Critical care nursing of infants and children* (pp. 656-694). Philadelphia: WB Saunders.

Waller, A., Baker, S., & Szoeka, A. (1989). Childhood injury deaths: National analysis and geographic variations. *American Journal of Public Health, 79,* 310-315.

Walsh, B., & Ioli, J. (1994). Childhood near-drowning: Nursing care and primary prevention. *Pediatric Nursing, 20,* 266.

Weinstein, M., & Kreiger, B. (1996). Near-drowning: Epidemiology, pathophysiology, and initial treatment. *Journal of Emergency Medicine, 14*(4), 461-467.

Wintemute, G. (1990). Childhood drowning and near-drowning in the United States. *American Journal of the Disabled Child, 144,* 663-669.

Wintemute, G. (1992). Drowning in early childhood. *Pediatric Annals, 21*(7), 417-421.

Wintemute, G., Kraus, J., Teret, S., & Wright, J. (1987). Drowning in childhood and adolescence: A population-based study. *American Journal of Public Health, 77,* 830-832.

Zuckerman, G. B., Gregory, P. M., & Damiani, S. M. (1998). Predictors of death and neurologic impairment in pediatric submersion injuries. *Archives of Pediatric Adolescent Medicine, 152,* 134-140.

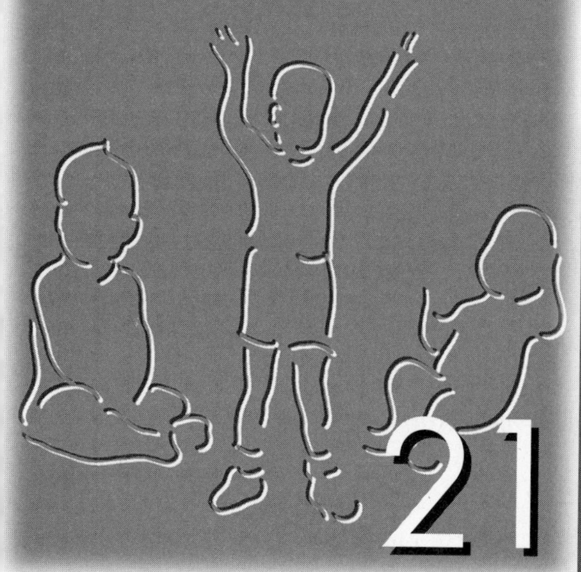

21 The Unborn Infant as Trauma Victim

Paula M. Timoney

The pregnant patient is one of the most challenging patients for the emergency response team. They are treating not only the pregnant woman but also the unborn infant. An understanding of the physiologic changes associated with pregnancy enables the health care team to properly assess and treat the pregnant patient while optimizing outcomes for both the mother and her unborn infant. The knowledge required to provide comprehensive assessment and management of the pregnant trauma patient is beyond the scope of this discussion. A thorough review of the management for a trauma victim is found in the Trauma Nursing Core Course (Emergency Nurses Association [ENA], 1995) and in Chapters 4 and 6 of this book. This chapter provides a brief overview of the unique assessment and management skills necessary to care for a pregnant trauma patient and her unborn infant.

TRAUMA IN PREGNANCY

Trauma is the most common nonobstetric cause of maternal death, accounting for up to 20% of all nonobstetric deaths. The main cause of fetal death is maternal death, with an 80% fetal mortality rate in mothers presenting with shock (Henderson & Mallon, 1998; Troiano, 1991). Noncatastrophic trauma is also associated with injuries to the fetus. The most common cause of fetal death in mothers who survive the trauma is abruptio placenta resulting from blunt trauma to the abdomen (Pimentel, 1991).

Fetal Physiology

The effect of trauma on the fetus depends on the gestational age, type of trauma, and extent of disruption of the normal physiology of both the mother and fetus (Pearlman, Tintinalli, & Lorenz, 1990b). During the first several weeks of gestation, the conceptus implants and the placenta develops. Until week 12 of gestation, the uterus remains a pelvic organ, protected from injury by the pelvic bones. Later in pregnancy, the uterus protrudes into the abdomen. This places the fetus in a compromised position but often protects the mother from serious abdominal injury caused by blunt trauma.

Survival of the fetus depends on adequate perfusion and delivery of oxygen through the placenta. The placental circulation is directly dependent on maternal systemic pressure. Maternal hypotension or shock decreases uterine perfusion and produces hypoxia in the fetus (Oakley & Johnson, 1991; Troiano, 1991). Fortunately, vital fetal organs are protected by a redistribution of fetal cardiac output during episodes of uterine hypoperfusion. The response of the fetus to such an insult varies with gestational age (Pearlman et al., 1990b). Fetal heart rate changes such as bradycardia or tachycardia, decreased or absent variability, or late decelerations indicate compromised uterine perfusion and hypoxia. These changes are often evident in the presence of normal maternal vital signs and may be the first indication of maternal instability and disruption in uterine physiology (Harvey & Troiano, 1992; Pearlman & Tintinalli, 1991; Pearlman et al., 1990b).

Maternal Physiology

It is particularly important to understand the physiologic changes of pregnancy because they can easily be mistaken for pathology resulting from trauma or mask serious injuries (Gregoire, 1997). Table 21-1 lists a summary of physiologic changes of pregnancy and relationship to trauma.

Cardiovascular System

Blood volume in the pregnant woman increases by 20% to 40% to meet the needs of the mother and her growing fetus.

TABLE 21-1 Physiologic Changes of Pregnancy and Relationship to Trauma

System	Change	Significance
Cardiovascular	↑ Volume ↑ Heart rate ↑ Cardiac output ↓ Systemic vascular resistance ↓ Arterial blood pressure	No clinical signs of shock until 30% loss of circulating volume
	Vena caval compression	↓ Uteroplacental perfusion with supine position
Respiratory	↑ Tidal volume ↑ Oxygen consumption ↓ Functional residual capacity ↓ Arterial PCO_2	Chronic compensatory alkalosis
	↓ Serum bicarbonate	↓ Blood buffering capacity Risk of acidosis when normal nonpregnant blood gas values are used to guide ventilation
Gastrointestinal	↓ Gastric motility	Bowel sounds less audible Delayed emptying time
	↓ Gastroesophageal sphincter competency	↑ Risk of aspiration
Renal	↑ Blood flow	
	Dilation or ureters and urethra	↑ Risk of stasis and infection
	Bladder displaced	↑ Susceptibility to injury
Musculoskeletal	Displacement of abdominal viscera	Altered probability of injury Altered pain referral patterns
	Pelvic venous congestion	↑ Risk of hemorrhage with injury
Reproductive	↑ Uterine enlargement ↑ Pelvic vascularity	↑ Vulnerability to injury Potential for significant blood loss with uterine injury

From Troiano, N. H. (1991). Trauma during pregnancy. In C. J. Harvey (Ed.), *Critical care obstetrical nursing* (p. 149). Gaithersburg, MD: Aspen.

This causes an increase in maternal cardiac output and, in the third trimester, an increase in heart rate. Conversely, blood pressure falls in the first and second trimesters and returns to normal before term (Vaizey, Jacobson, & Cross, 1994). The increase in blood volume is a protective mechanism designed to accommodate for blood loss during delivery. However, in the event of a trauma, the pregnant patient may tolerate blood loss of 20% to 35% before demonstrating signs and symptoms of shock. Systemic vascular resistance is decreased because of increased progesterone levels that cause vasodilation of the peripheral vessels and the presence of the low-resistance placenta (Harvey & Troiano, 1992). As the uterus enlarges, the heart is pushed upward and to the left in the chest, causing a left-axis deviation and ST- and T-wave changes on the electrocardiogram (Gregoire, 1997).

From about 20 weeks of gestation, the aorta and inferior vena cava (IVC) are compressed by the uterus when the mother is in the supine position. To increase return blood flow from the lower extremities and enhance uterine perfusion, the preferred position is the left lateral decubitus.

Hematologic System

The increase in plasma volume is greater than the increase in red blood cell volume, which causes a physiologic anemia in the pregnant woman. There is also an increase in white blood cells. The anemia and leukocytosis obscure the initial presentation in the emergency department (Henderson & Mallon, 1998).

Changes in the coagulation cascade are important to consider when treating a pregnant trauma victim. An increase in the level of fibrinogen and factors VII, VIII, IX, and X and a decrease in plasminogen activator levels make pregnancy a hypercoagulable state that predisposes the patient to venous thrombosis (Vaizey et al., 1994). The pregnant trauma patient is more prone to develop disseminated intravascular coagulation (DIC) if abruptio placenta or amniotic fluid embolism occurs (Pearlman et al., 1990b).

Respiratory System

As the uterus enlarges, the diaphragm rises about 4 cm, elevating the rib cage and decreasing the lung capacity. To compensate, respiratory rate and tidal volume increase, causing a decrease in the carbon dioxide level. Normal acid-base balance is maintained by renal excretion of bicarbonate. This creates a chronic state of compensated respiratory alkalosis in the pregnant patient, making the fetus more prone to acidosis and hypoxia in the event of injury (Harvey & Troiano, 1992).

Gastrointestinal System

Reduced gastrointestinal motility and an incompetent gastroesophageal sphincter resulting from hormonal changes contribute to passive regurgitation and aspiration in the pregnant patient (Harvey & Troiano, 1992; Vaizey et al., 1994). A physiologic ileus makes bowel sounds less audible and causes constipation. The liver, appendix, spleen, stomach, and other abdominal organs are displaced by the growing fetus. This serves as a protective mechanism against major abdominal organ injury to the mother but places the fetus at greater risk. Stretching of the abdominal wall decreases sensitivity to pain and may mask the presence of peritonitis in trauma (Vaizey et al., 1994).

Genitourinary System

The ureters and urethra are stretched and dilated, making stasis of urine more common. Toward the end of the pregnancy, the bladder becomes an intraabdominal organ, making it more susceptible to injury (Coleman, Trianfo, & Rund, 1997; Gregoire, 1997; Harvey & Troiano, 1992; Vaizey et al., 1994). As urine volume increases, drugs are excreted more quickly and may not be absorbed completely (Gregoire, 1997).

Musculoskeletal System

Hormonal effects of pregnancy cause softening and relaxation of the interosseous ligaments of many joints. This occurs at the same time the pregnant woman's center of gravity is altered by a growing uterus, thus increasing the chance of falls (Harvey & Troiano, 1992).

TYPES OF TRAUMA

Epidemiology

Women today are more active. They often remain in the workforce throughout their pregnancy, making them more susceptible to trauma. Pregnant women are at risk for motor vehicle accidents, falls, and direct assaults to the abdomen caused by violence (Harvey & Troiano, 1992; Weiss, 1999). It is estimated that between 6% and 7% of all pregnant women will become a victim of trauma during their pregnancy (Agnoli & Deutchman, 1993; Esposito, 1994; Harvey & Troiano, 1992; Henderson & Mallon, 1998; Neufeld, 1993; Pearlman & Tintinalli, 1991; Pimentel, 1991).

The causes of trauma in pregnancy are similar to those in the nonpregnant population (Esposito, Gens, Smith, Scorpio, & Buchman, 1991). The most common types of trauma are blunt trauma, penetrating trauma, electrical injuries, and burns. The gravid abdomen may protect the pregnant woman from serious abdominal injuries and improve maternal survival (Pimentel, 1991). However, as the uterus enlarges with advancing gestational age, the liver and spleen are compressed and may be more susceptible to rupture (Troiano, 1991).

Blunt Trauma

The leading type of trauma in pregnancy is blunt trauma caused by motor vehicle accidents, falls, and assaults (Gabbe, Niebyl, & Simpson, 1996; Poole, Martin, Perry, Griswold, Lambert, & Rhodes, 1996). The amniotic fluid serves as a cushion to protect the fetus. However, abruptio placenta can occur as a result of a direct blow or hypovolemic shock (Gabbe et al., 1996).

Motor Vehicle Accidents

Motor vehicle accidents are the most common cause of blunt trauma in pregnancy (Cunningham et al., 1997; Henderson & Mallon, 1998; Weiss, 1999). Fetal injury most frequently occurs in the third trimester, when the fetus becomes as intraabdominal organ. The severity of fetal injury is directly related to maternal injury, although the absence of maternal injury does not mean the fetus is not in jeopardy. Careful fetal assessment is indicated in all pregnant trauma patients (Towery, English, & Wisner, 1993).

Falls

Falls are the second leading cause of blunt trauma in pregnancy (Oakley & Johnson, 1991). During pregnancy, the woman's center of gravity changes, making her more susceptible to falls. The chance of injury to the fetus is related to the height of the fall and the surface landed upon. There is little chance of fetal injury in patients who do not lose consciousness or do not have obvious bruising.

Assaults

There is an increase in domestic violence and physical assault during pregnancy. A review of the literature by Ribe, Teggatz, and Harvey (1993) identified blows to the abdomen and the setting of domestic violence as two of the three risk factors for fetal demise after a blunt force assault upon a pregnant woman. Third trimester gestation was the third risk factor. Abruptio placenta was reported as the cause of death in all cases of fetal demise. Although risk for injury to the fetus appears to be less with physical assaults than with motor vehicle accidents, the possibility of fetal injury cannot be overlooked (Poole et al., 1996).

Penetrating Trauma

Penetrating injuries consist of gunshot wounds, stab wounds, and injuries related to shrapnel or missiles. The gravid uterus often protects the pregnant woman's major abdominal organs from serious injury caused by penetrating trauma.

Gunshot Wounds

Gunshot wounds are becoming more common during pregnancy as the incidence of violence in our society continues to increase (O'Shaughnessy, 1997). Any body part can be affected, but during pregnancy the uterus occupies a large part of the abdomen, making it more susceptible to penetrating trauma. The incidence for fetal injury resulting from gunshot wounds is 70%, with a 65% fetal mortality rate (Oakley & Johnson, 1991). Patients with gunshot wounds generally require surgical exploration (Grubb, 1992; O'Shaughnessy, 1997).

Stab Wounds

Stab wounds are much less common than gunshot wounds and tend to have a better prognosis for both mother and fetus (Esposito, 1994). Unless there is evidence of intraperitoneal hemorrhage or bowel perforation, conservative management may be indicated (Esposito, 1994; Grubb, 1992). Management of stab wounds depends on several factors: gestational age, location of the wound in the upper abdomen, and condition of the fetus. Grubb (1992) reported the nonsurgical management of a patient with multiple stab wounds resulting in survival of both mother and fetus.

Missiles/Shrapnel

Although uncommon in the United States, high-velocity penetrating wounds from missiles and shrapnel occur in other parts of the world. Awwad, Azar, Seoud, Mroueh, and Karam (1994) reviewed 16 years of data on high-velocity penetrating wounds in Beirut. They found that mortality is most likely the result of maternal pulmonary complications, wound infection and dehiscence, small bowel obstruction, and iatrogenic complications. The recommendation from this group was that with close monitoring of the fetus and mother, surgical exploration can be avoided in the pregnant woman with this type of penetrating trauma.

Electrical Injury

Electrical injury may occur from accidental electrical shock or lightning strikes during pregnancy. The placenta and amniotic fluid are excellent conductors of electricity (Fatovich, 1993; Steer, 1992). Fortunately, reports of electrical shock in pregnancy are rare.

Voltage

Early case studies report a high fetal mortality rate in pregnant women exposed to electrical shock (Fatovich, 1993; Jaffe & Fejgin, 1997). However, in a review of 31 cases, Einarson, Bailey, Inocencion, Ormand, and Koren (1997) report that accidental electrical shock does not result in adverse fetal outcome. Current pathway and amount of voltage are important predictors of fetal and maternal outcome. Electrical current that passes through the uterus is more harmful to the fetus (Einarson et al., 1997). The authors agree that urgent fetal monitoring is important despite apparently trivial cases of accidental shock.

Lightning

Reports of lightning strikes in pregnant woman are rare. Generally, there is a good maternal and fetal prognosis after lightning strikes (Troiano, 1991). However, lightning has been reported to cause immediate fetal death, precipitate the onset of labor, or result in delayed fetal death (Steer, 1992).

Burns

Burn injury is one of the most severe injuries that afflict human beings (Akhtar, Mulawkar, & Kulkarni, 1994). In a review article by Polko and McMahon (1997), the incidence of thermal injuries in pregnant women was reported to be low. These injuries are more common in developing countries. Fetal survival is directly related to gestational age and the extent of maternal injury (Unsur, Oztopcu, Atalay, Alpay, & Turhanoglu, 1996). Akhtar et al. (1994) reported a 100% fetal mortality in women with burns over 60% of the total body surface. Early excision and grafting decreases the incidence of septic complications, which are closely related to poor fetal and maternal outcome (Akhtar et al., 1994; Prasanna & Singh, 1996). Ullmann, Blumenfeld, Hakim, Mahoul, Sujov, and Peled (1997) recommend urgent delivery of the fetus greater than 26 weeks of gestation in women with extensive burns.

COMPLICATIONS

The maternal death rate from trauma in pregnancy is approximately 10% (Esposito, 1994.) Head injury secondary to a motor vehicle accident is the most common cause of trauma-related maternal death. This is similar to the death rate in nonpregnant women of childbearing age (Esposito, 1994; Esposito et al., 1991). Fetal death most often results from maternal death, and the fetal death rate is higher in pregnant trauma patients than other groups of pregnant women (Esposito, 1994).

Unfortunately, there are few studies that identify reliable predictors of fetal mortality. The best predictor of poor fetal outcome is maternal shock and hypoxia (Esposito et al., 1991). Ali, Yeo, Gana, and McLellan (1997) evaluated 68 pregnant trauma patients and found that fetal mortality was very high among those patients with an Injury Severity Score (ISS) greater than 12, despite a low maternal mortality. The major predictor in their study was the presence of DIC. This is in contrast to the study by Dahmus and Sibai (1993), which demonstrated that the presence of DIC was not predictive of poor fetal outcome. Scorpio, Esposito, Smith, and Gens (1992) documented that an ISS greater than 12 and a low serum bicarbonate level correlated with poor fetal outcome.

Biester, Tomich, Esposito, and Weber (1997) found no predictive value in their use of the Revised Trauma Score to determine the risk of adverse fetal outcomes or to indicate the duration of fetal monitoring following maternal trauma. The lack of predictive value in these studies is most likely attributable to the presence of normal vital signs in pregnant trauma victims despite a compromised fetus.

Abruptio Placenta

Abruptio placenta is the most common cause of fetal death other than maternal death (Pearlman, Tintinalli, & Lorenz, 1990a; Pimentel, 1991). It most commonly occurs after blunt trauma to the abdomen and may occur up to 24 hours after injury, even though physical signs of trauma are minimal (Gabbe et al., 1996). Abruptio placenta occurs when the placenta separates from the uterine wall, resulting in loss of perfusion to the fetus. Signs of abruptio placenta are vaginal bleeding, abdominal or uterine tenderness and pain, and uterine contractions (Clark, 1999; Henderson & Mallon, 1998). Although vaginal bleeding is the most common sign, about 10% of affected women present with a concealed hemorrhage and no bleeding (Clark, 1999).

Preterm Labor

Preterm labor is a common response to maternal trauma (Pimentel, 1991). In an evaluation of pregnant women after blunt trauma, Towery et al. (1993) found that premature uterine contractions are the most common complication. However, Pearlman and Tintinalli (1991) found that 90% of contractions resolve spontaneously without tocolytic therapy and result in a normal pregnancy. Contractions that do not stop are an indication of an underlying pathologic condition and warrant further investigation (Neufeld, 1993).

Fetomaternal Hemorrhage

Loss of blood from the fetal to the maternal circulation is four to five times more likely to occur in pregnant trauma patients than in uninjured pregnant patients. This complication is more commonly associated with motor vehicle accidents than with other causes of blunt trauma (Agnoli & Deutchman, 1993). Signs and symptoms include uterine tenderness and fetal distress. Diagnostic confirmation is a positive Kleihauer-Betke stain on maternal blood. The Kleihauer-Betke stain indicates the presence and volume of fetomaternal hemorrhage. In mild cases fetal and neonatal anemia occur and can be prevented by fetal intravascular transfusion (Lipitz, Achiron, Horoshovski, Rotstein, Sherman, & Schiff, 1997). Severe cases may result in fetal exsanguination and death. Rh immune globulin should be given to all pregnant trauma patients who have O-negative blood type. The amount of bleeding may be minimal and still cause maternal Rh isoimmunization (Coleman et al., 1997; Cunningham et al., 1997; Smart, 1994).

Uterine Rupture

Uterine rupture resulting in fetal death is an uncommon complication of maternal trauma (Dittrich, 1996; Lifschultz & Donoghue, 1991; Rowe, Lafayette, & Cox, 1996). Uterine rupture may occur in the most severe accidents that cause maternal abdominal trauma. Fetal mortality from this complication is 100% (Pearlman et al., 1990b). Signs and symptoms indicating uterine rupture are palpable fetal body parts, loss of fetal heart tones, lack of normal orientation and uncertain placental location on ultrasonographic examination, and presence of gross blood on diagnostic peritoneal lavage (Rowe et al., 1996).

Skull Fracture

Direct fetal injuries from maternal blunt trauma are uncommon because of the protection offered by the maternal soft tissues, the uterus, and amniotic fluid (Pearlman & Tintinalli, 1991). However, cranial injuries have been reported (Evrard, Sturner, & Murray, 1989; Hartl & Ko, 1996; Scorpio et al., 1992; Stafford, Biddinger, & Zumwalt, 1988). During the third trimester the fetal head descends into the pelvis and is most vulnerable to cranial injuries (Pearlman et al., 1990b). The fetal skull may be injured as a result of maternal pelvic fracture or by direct compression of the fetal skull by an external force (Stafford et al., 1988). It is often difficult to visualize fetal skull fractures on x-ray film because of the maternal pelvis (Matthews & Hammersley, 1997). In some cases the injury is initially identified when the fetus is delivered with evidence of a healing fracture.

Neurologic Sequelae

There is controversy surrounding the association of maternal trauma with long-term neurologic injury in infants. Several case reports cite maternal trauma as a cause of fetal intracranial hemorrhage and/or cerebral lesions (Anquist, Parnes, Cargill, & Tawagi, 1994; Baethmann, Kahn, Lenard, & Voit, 1996; Eaton, Ahmed, & Dubowitz, 1991; Lifschultz & Donoghue, 1991; Matthews & Hammersley, 1997; Stafford et al., 1988; Viljoen, 1995). The possible cause of neurologic injury is decreased uteroplacental circulation, placental abruption, or placental embolism. However, direct cause and effect has not been proven. This is primarily because of the time delay between the traumatic injury and the onset of abnormal findings. In a large, retrospective review spanning 11 years in Western Australia, Gilles et al. (1996) found no link between maternal trauma and cerebral palsy.

ASSESSMENT

Classification

Pregnant trauma victims fall into one of four classes based on gestational age and clinical presentation as outlined by Henderson and Mallon (1998). The classification is based on gestational age and extent of maternal trauma. Management can be tailored to best meet the needs of the pregnant patient and her unborn infant by using this classification system (Box 21-1).

Initial Assessment

Assessment may be difficult because of the physiologic changes of pregnancy. A pregnant woman may experience blood loss of 20% to 35% without demonstrating signs of shock (Harvey & Troiano, 1992). The practitioner must always consider the possibility that an injured woman of childbearing age is pregnant. When establishing priorities, major efforts initially concentrate on resuscitation of the pregnant woman. Fetal survival is dependent on maternal survival.

In the initial assessment, airway, breathing, circulation are the focus, just as for any other trauma patient (Troiano, 1991). The only evaluation of the fetus as part of the primary assessment is a thorough evaluation of maternal circulation (Henderson & Mallon, 1998). The mother who presents with borderline hemodynamic stability is most likely to have a fetus already in jeopardy (Esposito, 1994).

After initial stabilization procedures, neurologic status should be evaluated. Traumatic brain injury is a major concern, occurring most frequently in young adults between the ages of 15 and 44, which coincidentally are the childbearing years (Jordan, 1994). It is important to remember that pregnancy-induced hypertension may cause signs and symptoms that mimic a head injury (ENA, 1995).

Head-to-Toe Assessment

A detailed history, including obstetric history, is followed by a thorough maternal physical examination and fetal assessment (Rozycki, 1993). It should be kept in mind that physical assessment findings that usually indicate injury may be less evident in the pregnant trauma patient because of decreased peritoneal stimuli (Coleman et al., 1997).

Measurement of fundal height is the quickest way to determine fetal viability. If the uterine size is higher than the umbilicus, the fetus is presumed to be viable (Pimentel, 1991). Figure 21-1 shows uterine size at different weeks of

BOX 21-1 Classification of Pregnant Trauma Patients

Group 1

The patients in this group are women who experience trauma and are not aware they are pregnant. The concern in these patients is the risk of teratogenicity from unnecessary radiographs. Even with modern methods of birth control, contraception is not 100% effective, making history alone unreliable. Therefore it is recommended that a pregnancy test be performed in all women of childbearing age who sustain trauma.

Group 2

At 22 weeks or less of gestation, the fetus is not considered viable. Therefore resuscitation is primarily directed at the pregnant patient without consideration of the fetus. At this time, the fetus is still protected from injury by the pelvis.

Group 3

The most challenging of pregnant trauma patients are women at greater than 23 weeks of gestation. Suddenly, the health care team is presented with two patients instead of one. The diagnosis of fetal distress is critical in the management of these patients because fetal survival may be enhanced by surgical delivery.

Group 4

The final classification of pregnant trauma patients is that of women who present in perimortem condition. Once maternal arrest occurs, survival of the unborn infant is dependent on immediate delivery. Immediate delivery is the final step in resuscitation of the mother and the fetus. Although the presence of the fetus makes resuscitation of the mother difficult, the large amount of blood pooled in the uterus makes return of circulation in the mother near impossible. Therefore delivery of the unborn infant may benefit both the mother and the infant.

From Henderson, S. O., & Mallon, W. K. (1998). Trauma in pregnancy. *Emergency Medicine Clinics of North America, 16*(1), 209-228.

gestation. Fetal evaluation begins with auscultation of the fetal heart rate by stethoscope or Doppler. This should be done early and repeated frequently (Neufeld, 1993). A fetal heart rate monitor should be applied for continuous monitoring. Fetal heart tones should be 120 to 160 beats/min with good variability. The presence of fetal bradycardia or tachycardia may indicate distress.

Physical examination of the mother should include a pelvic examination looking for the presence or absence of amniotic fluid, bleeding, cervical dilation, effacement, and fetal station (Rozycki, 1993). The presence of amniotic fluid or bleeding warrants further investigation. Cervical dilation may indicate that delivery is imminent, and preparation for delivery and neonatal stabilization should occur.

A thorough abdominal assessment should assess for pain, tenderness, tenseness, and seat belt marks. Abdominal pain or tenderness is a sign of abruptio placenta, and further evaluation and intervention is crucial.

One of the most reliable tools for fetal assessment is ultrasonography. It is noninvasive and can be performed rapidly at the bedside. Because of the ease and low cost of the procedure, it should be considered for all pregnant trauma victims. Gestational age, viability, fetal activity, placental location, and the amount of amniotic fluid can be evaluated. Decreased fetal activity noted on ultrasound is an early sign of fetal distress. Ultrasonography can aid in the assessment of maternal abdominal injury or bleeding (Dittrich, 1996; Ma, Mateer, & DeBehnke, 1996). Although ultrasonography is a critical tool in detecting abruptio placenta, the diagnosis of abruptio placenta cannot be made based solely on ultrasound findings (Clark; 1999; Ma et al., 1996).

Routine laboratory testing for a pregnant trauma patient is the same as that for a nonpregnant patient. In addition, diagnostic testing should include a serum bicarbonate level, which is perhaps the most sensitive indicator of tissue hypoperfusion, even in the presence of normal maternal vital signs (Agnoli & Deutchman, 1993; Biester et al., 1997; Coleman et al., 1997; Dittrich, 1996). The normal bicarbonate level is a pregnant woman is 27 to 32 mm Hg, which is significantly lower than that of a nonpregnant woman (Esposito, 1994). Coagulation studies should be performed because the incidence of severe coagulopathy is higher with concealed, traumatic abruptio placenta than with atraumatic abruptio placenta (Cunningham et al., 1997).

A Kleihauer-Betke test is used to assess fetal well-being. The Kleihauer-Betke stain indicates the presence and volume of fetomaternal hemorrhage and should be considered for all pregnant trauma patients, especially those who are Rh negative (Dahmus & Sibai, 1993; Pimentel, 1991).

Radiographic testing should not be avoided in the pregnant patient. The most critical time for radiation exposure is 2 to 7 weeks of gestation (Neufeld, 1993). With proper shielding of the abdomen, the fetus is exposed to minimal radiation from the routine screening series after trauma (Coleman et al., 1997).

Although previously contraindicated in pregnant patients, peritoneal lavage can be performed safely using the supraumbilical technique (Oakley & Johnson, 1991; Rozycki, 1993; Rowe et al., 1996). Peritoneal lavage is helpful in diagnosing intraperitoneal bleeding, which may be obscured by the gravid uterus.

MANAGEMENT

Stabilization

Restoration of maternal circulation and thus fetal circulation is the goal of effective management. It is difficult to establish clear management protocols because maternal symptomology is a poor predictor of fetal outcome (Connolly, Katz, Bash, McMahon, & Hansen, 1997). During maternal resuscitation, adequate oxygenation, fluid replacement, and left lateral positioning should be implemented. It is also important to remember that any medication given to the mother may affect the fetus (Smart, 1994).

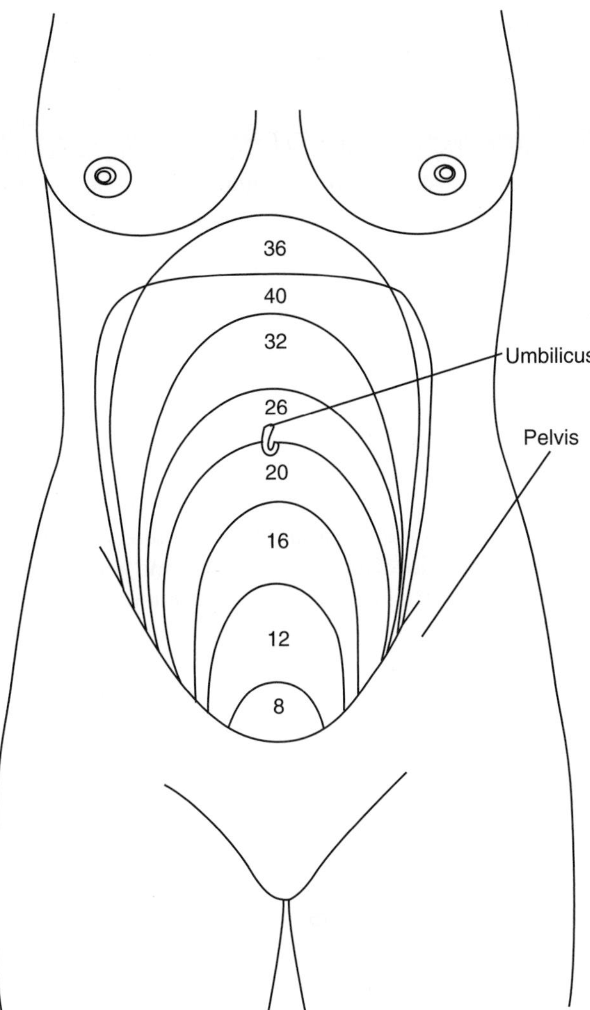

FIGURE 21-1 Uterine size at different weeks of gestation. (From Neufeld, J. D. G. [1993]. Trauma in pregnancy, what if ...? *Emergency Medicine Clinics of North America, 11*[1], 215.)

Respiratory support of the pregnant patient is critical because of her decreased pulmonary reserve and the fetal intolerance of hypoxia (Pimentel, 1991). High-flow 100% oxygen should be administered to pregnant women as soon as possible to meet increased maternal needs and maintain a well-oxygenated fetus (Esposito, 1994; Harrahill, 1997).

The pregnant woman should be positioned in the left lateral decubitus position as soon as possible to prevent compression of the aorta and the IVC (Cunningham et al., 1997; Smart, 1994; Troiano, 1991). If the patient requires a backboard, manual deflection of the uterus to the side or a roll placed under the board at a 15-degree angle can relieve pressure from the IVC and minimize the effects of compression.

Aggressive fluid resuscitation is critical to stabilize maternal blood pressure and improve uteroplacental circulation. Two large-bore catheters should be inserted for rapid fluid administration. Placement of intravenous lines in the lower extremities should be avoided because of the possibility of IVC syndrome and the tendency for fluid and/or blood to pool in the pelvic veins (Coleman et al., 1997). When possible, the use of vasopressors should be avoided to minimize uteroplacental vasoconstriction and fetal hypoxia (Coleman et al., 1997; Gregoire, 1997).

Aggressive maternal resuscitation and prolonged vascular collapse may prevent delivery of a viable fetus (Henderson & Mallon, 1998; Neufeld, 1993). If there is no response to maternal resuscitation within 4 to 5 minutes, a thoracotomy and perimortem cesarean section should be performed in an attempt to save both the mother and the fetus (Pearlman et al., 1990a; Pimentel, 1991). Increased venous return from decompression of the IVC, as well as return flow of blood previously pooled in the uterus and pelvic vessels, contributes to maternal resuscitation (Henderson & Mallon, 1998).

Surveillance

Continuous monitoring of fetal heart rate and for uterine contractions is the most effective method of fetal assessment after maternal trauma. Most authors agree that 4 hours of continuous monitoring after the trauma is sufficient if no other signs and/or symptoms of fetal distress develop (Clark, 1999; Connolly et al., 1997; Dahmus & Sibai, 1993; Gabbe et al., 1996; Pearlman & Tintinalli, 1991; Pearlman et al., 1990a). Towery et al. (1993) documented that all complications after blunt trauma developed within 6 hours of injury. Fetal monitoring may benefit the mother because the fetus is more sensitive to maternal hemodynamic changes and can be used to guide interventions to restore normal parameters (Cunningham et al., 1997; Neufeld, 1993). If signs of fetal distress or maternal vaginal bleeding develop, a minimum of 24 hours of fetal monitoring is recommended (Clark, 1999; Smart, 1994). Once discharged home, the mother should be instructed to report to her physician any decrease in fetal movement, vaginal bleeding, contractions, or uterine pain (Neufeld, 1993). The pregnancy is rarely affected in most women who do not suffer immediate adverse outcomes (Connolly et al., 1997; Goodwin & Breen, 1990; Pearlman et al., 1990a).

Delivery of the Infant

The obstetrician and neonatal team should be called to the emergency department before the arrival of the trauma victim. If the mother is hemodynamically unstable or if there is evidence of severe fetal distress, an emergency cesarean section should be performed (Coleman et al., 1997). A multidisciplinary approach should be taken to optimize maternal and fetal outcomes.

A perimortem cesarean should be performed if maternal resuscitation is unsuccessful within 4 to 5 minutes (Pearlman et al., 1990a; Pimentel, 1991; Rozycki, 1993). Survival of the infant after perimortem cesarean section is inversely proportional to the time interval between the onset of maternal cardiac arrest and delivery of the infant (Lanoix, Akkapeddi, & Goldfeder, 1995).

NEONATAL RESUSCITATION AND STABILIZATION

If the delivery begins before arrival of the neonatal team, the trauma team should prepare the equipment necessary for resuscitation and stabilization of the infant. The first few moments of the infant's life are critical. Making the transition from intrauterine to extrauterine life is difficult for many infants, especially those already compromised from maternal trauma. It is the responsibility of the team to facilitate this transition using the principles of neonatal resuscitation as established by the American Heart Association and American Academy of Pediatrics (2000).

EQUIPMENT

A radiant warmer with stethoscope and cardiorespiratory monitor should be set up in the emergency department, with equipment for suctioning, intubating, and establishing venous access in an infant. Staff should be familiar with the equipment and adequately trained to use it. Emergency medications and volume expanders should be available. A person trained in neonatal resuscitation and stabilization should be present at each delivery. Box 21-2 gives a complete list of equipment required for newborn resuscitation.

STEPS

Initial steps in neonatal resuscitation include thermal management, positioning, suctioning, and tactile stimulation. All neonates have difficulty maintaining their body temperature. Heat loss is minimized by placing the infant on a preheated warmer and quickly drying the infant. Hypothermia delays recovery from acidosis, and these critical steps require only a few seconds. The infant should be positioned supine with the neck in a neutral position. The mouth should be suctioned first, then the nose. If meconium-stained fluid is present, the infant should be intubated with a meconium aspirator and suctioned to prevent aspiration of meconium into the lungs.

Drying and suctioning generally provide enough tactile stimulation to induce effective respirations in most newborns. However, compromised infants will require further evaluation and resuscitation. During initial stabilization, evaluation begins with assessment of respiratory effort, heart rate, and color. The Apgar scoring system (Table 21-2) provides a method of documenting status, but it should not be used to determine the need for further intervention.

Most infants in distress are hypoxic and require 100% oxygen administration. If respiratory effort is minimal, positive-pressure ventilation using a face mask or endotracheal tube should be initiated. After adequate ventilation is established, heart rate should be evaluated. Chest compressions should be initiated if the heart rate is less than 60

BOX 21-2 Neonatal Resuscitation Supplies and Equipment

Suction Equipment

Bulb syringe
Mechanical suction and tubing
Suction catheters, 5 or 6 Fr, 8 Fr, and 10 or 12 Fr
8-Fr feeding tube and 20-ml syringe
Meconium aspiration device

Bag-and-Mask Equipment

Neonatal resuscitation bag with a pressure-release valve or pressure manometer (the bag must be capable of delivering 90% to 100% oxygen)
Face masks, newborn and premature sizes (masks with cushioned rim preferred)
Oxygen with flowmeter (flow rate upto 10 L/min) and tubing (including portable oxygen cylinders)

Intubation Equipment

Laryngoscope with straight blades, no. 0 (preterm) and no. 1 (term)
Extra bulbs and batteries for laryngoscope
Tracheal tubes, 2.5, 3.0, 3.5, and 4.0 mm ID
Stylet (optional)
Scissors
Tape or securing device for tracheal tube
Alcohol sponges
CO_2 detector (optional)
Laryngeal mask airway (optional)

Medications

Epinephrine 1:10,000 (0.1 mg/ml)—3- or 10-ml ampules
Isotonic crystalloid (normal saline or Ringer's lactate) for volume expansion—100 or 250 ml
Sodium bicarbonate 4.2% (5 mEq/10 ml)—10-ml ampules
Naloxone hydrochloride 0.4 mg/ml—1-ml ampules; or 1.0 mg/ml—2-ml ampules
Normal saline, 30 ml
Dextrose 10%, 250 ml
Normal saline "fish" or "bullet" (optional)
Feeding tube, 5 Fr (optional)
Umbilical vessel catheterization supplies
- Sterile gloves
- Scalpel or scissors
- Povidone-iodine solution
- Umbilical tape
- Umbilical catheters, 3.5 and 5 Fr
- Three-way stopcock

Syringes, 1, 2, 5, 10, 20, and 50 ml
Needles, 25, 21, and 18 gauge or puncture device for needleless system

Miscellaneous

Gloves and appropriate personal protection
Radiant warmer or other heat source
Firm, padded resuscitation surface
Clock (timer optional)
Warmed linens
Stethoscope
Tape, ½ or ¾ inch
Cardiac monitor and electrodes and/or pulse oximeter with probe (optional for delivery room)
Oropharyngeal airways

From American Heart Association and American Academy of Pediatrics. (2000). *Textbook of neonatal resuscitation.* Elk Grove, IL: Author.
ID, Internal diameter.

TABLE 21-2 **Apgar Scoring System**

Sign	0	1	2
Heart rate (beats/min)	Absent	<100	>100
Respiratory effort	Absent	Slow, irregular	Good, crying
Muscle tone	Flaccid	Some flexion of extremities	Active motion
Reflex irritability	No response	Grimace	Vigorous cry
Color	Blue, pale	Body pink, extremities blue	Completely pink

From Cunningham, F. G., MacDonald, P. C., Gant, N. F., Leveno, K. J., Gilstrap, L. C., Hankins, G. D. V., & Clark, S. I. (1997). *Williams obstetrics* (20th ed.). Stamford, CT: Appleton & Lange.

beats/min. If prolonged positive-pressure ventilation is required or if bag-mask ventilation is ineffective, an endotracheal tube should be inserted.

Sustained bradycardia is usually a sign of profound hypoxia. Medications should be administered if the heart rate remains less than 60 beats/min despite adequate ventilation and chest compressions. Volume expanders are necessary in infants with hypovolemia, and the need for expanders should be anticipated in infants with a history of abruptio placenta. Intravascular access may be obtained easily via the umbilical vein for administration of volume, medications, and glucose. Epinephrine and naloxone hydrochloride can be given via the endotracheal tube when vascular access is not readily available.

It is important to remember that the key to successful neonatal resuscitation is a coordinated multidisciplinary approach. Anticipation and adequate preparation of personnel and equipment are critical to a successful outcome for both mother and infant.

PREVENTION STRATEGIES

Prevention strategies for pregnant patients are similar to those for nonpregnant patients. Because trauma is more likely to affect pregnancy now than ever before, it is important to incorporate trauma prevention strategies into routine prenatal care. Pregnant women should be taught to recognize changes in their bodies that may contribute to trauma. They should be taught preventive measures, especially women in colder climates where falls on slippery surfaces are more likely to occur.

Most authors agree that the use of three-point restraints decreases fetal and maternal injuries caused by motor vehicle accidents. Use of the lap belt alone does not prevent forward movement of the mother. One study indicated an 8% fetal death rate with a three-point restraint versus a 50% death rate with the lap belt only (Stafford et al., 1988). Pearlman, Klinich, Schneider, Rupp, Moss, & Ashton-Miller (2000) reported adverse fetal outcome in 27% of women properly restrained with a three-point restraint compared with 62% of improperly restrained women. Current recommendations are that the three-point restraint should be worn with the lap belt below the distended abdomen and the shoulder sash across the chest above the abdomen.

The role of domestic violence in trauma in pregnancy is of paramount concern. Prevention must be aimed at early detection and intervention. Because most women will receive prenatal care at some time during their pregnancy, it is an ideal setting for screening and education (Greenblatt, Dannenberg, & Johnson, 1997).

BIBLIOGRAPHY

Agnoli, F. R., & Deutchman, M. E. (1993). Trauma in pregnancy. *Journal of Family Practice, 37*(6), 588-592.

Akhtar, M. A., Mulawkar, P. M., & Kulkarni, H. R. (1994). Burns in pregnancy: Effect on maternal and fetal outcomes. *Burns, 20*(4), 351-355.

Ali, J., Yeo, A., Gana, T. J., & McLellan, B. A. (1997). Predictors of fetal mortality in pregnant trauma patients. *Journal of Trauma: Injury, Infection, and Critical Care, 42*(5), 782-785.

American Heart Association and American Academy of Pediatrics. (2000). *Textbook of neonatal resuscitation.* Elk Grove, IL: Author.

Anquist, K. W., Parnes, S., Cargill, Y., & Tawagi, G. (1994). An unexpected fetal outcome following a severe maternal motor vehicle accident. *Obstetrics and Gynecology, 84*, 656-659.

Awwad, J. T., Azar, G. B., Seoud, M. A., Mroueh, A. M., & Karam, K. S. (1994). High-velocity penetrating wounds of the gravid uterus: Review of 16 years of civil war. *Obstetrics and Gynecology, 83*(2), 259-264.

Baethmann, M., Kahn, T., Lenard, H-G., & Voit, T. (1996). Fetal CNS damage after exposure to maternal trauma during pregnancy. *Acta Paediatrics, 85*, 1331-1338.

Biester, E. M., Tomich, P. G., Esposito, T. J., & Weber, L. (1997). Trauma in pregnancy: Normal revised trauma score in relation to other markers of maternofetal status—A preliminary study. *American Journal of Obstetrics and Gynecology, 176*(6), 1206-1210.

Clark, S. L. (1999). Placenta previa and abruptio placentae. In R. K. Creasy & R. Resnik (Eds.), *Maternal-fetal medicine* (4th ed., pp. 621-628). Philadelphia: WB Saunders.

Coleman, M. T., Trianfo, V. A., & Rund, D. A. (1997). Nonobstetric emergencies in pregnancy: Trauma and surgical conditions. *American Journal of Obstetrics and Gynecology, 177*(3), 497-502.

Connolly, A., Katz, V. L., Bash, K. L., McMahon, M. J., & Hansen, W. F. (1997). Trauma and pregnancy. *American Journal of Perinatology, 14*(6), 331-336.

Cunningham, F. G., MacDonald, P. C., Gant, N. F., Leveno, K. J., Gilstrap, L. C., Hankins, G. D. V., & Clark, S. I. (1997). *Williams obstetrics* (20th ed., pp. 749, 1070-1074). Stamford, CT: Appleton & Lange.

Dahmus, M. A., & Sibai, B. M. (1993). Blunt abdominal trauma: Are there any predictive factors for abruptio placentae or maternal-fetal distress? *American Journal of Obstetrics and Gynecology, 169*(4), 1054-1059.

Dittrich, K. C. (1996). Rupture of the gravid uterus secondary to motor vehicle trauma. *Journal of Emergency Medicine, 14*(2), 177-180.

Eaton, D. G. M., Ahmed, Y., & Dubowitz, L. M. S. (1991). Maternal trauma and cerebral lesions in preterm infants: Case reports. *British Journal of Obstetrics and Gynaecology, 98*, 1292-1294.

Einarson, A., Bailey, B., Inocencion, G., Ormond, K., & Koren, G. (1997). Accidental electric shock in pregnancy: A prospective cohort study. *American Journal of Obstetrics and Gynecology, 176*(3), 678-681.

Emergency Nurses Association. (1995). *Trauma in pregnancy. Trauma nursing core course* (pp. 285–304). Park Ridge, IL: Author.

Esposito, T. J. (1994). Trauma during pregnancy. *Emergency Medicine Clinics of North America, 12*(1), 167-198.

Esposito, T. J., Gens, D. R., Smith, L. G., Scorpio, R., & Buchman, T. (1991). Trauma during pregnancy: A review of 79 cases. *Archives of Surgery, 126*, 1073-1078.

Evrard, J. R., Sturner, W. Q., & Murray, E. J. (1989). Fetal skull fracture from an automobile accident. *American Journal of Forensic Medicine and Pathology, 10*(3), 232-234.

Fatovich, D. M. (1993). Electric shock in pregnancy. *Journal of Emergency Medicine, 11*, 175-177.

Gabbe, S. G., Niebyl, J. R., & Simpson, J. L. (1996). *Obstetrics: Normal and problem pregnancies* (pp. 505-510, 632-633). New York: Churchill Livingstone.

Gilles, M. T., Blair, E., Watson, L., Badawi, N., Alessandri, L., Dawes, V., Plant, A. J., & Stanley, F. J. (1996). Trauma in pregnancy and cerebral palsy: Is there a link? *Medical Journal of Australia, 164*(8), 500-501.

Goodwin, T. M., & Breen, M. T. (1990). Pregnancy outcome and feto-maternal hemorrhage after noncatastrophic trauma. *American Journal of Obstetrics and Gynecology, 162*(3), 665-671.

Greenblatt, J. F., Dannenberg, A. L., & Johnson, C. J. (1997). Incidence of hospitalized injuries among pregnant women in Maryland, 1979-1990. *American Journal of Preventive Medicine, 13*(5), 374-379.

Gregoire, A. S. (1997). When the trauma patient is pregnant. *RN, 60*, 44-49.

Grubb, D. K. (1992). Nonsurgical management of penetrating uterine trauma in pregnancy: A case report. *American Journal of Obstetrics and Gynecology, 166*(2), 583-584.

Harrahill, M. (1997). Maternal trauma care: A brief review. *Journal of Emergency Nursing, 23*(6), 649-650.

Hartl, R., & Ko, K. (1996). In utero skull fracture: Case report. *Journal of Trauma: Injury, Infection, and Critical Care, 41*(3), 549-552.

Harvey, M. G., & Troiano, N. H. (1992). Trauma during pregnancy. *NAACOG's Clinical Issues in Perinatal and Women's Health Nursing, 3*(3), 521-529.

Henderson, S. O., & Mallon, W. K. (1998). Trauma in pregnancy. *Emergency Medicine Clinics of North America, 16*(1), 209-228.

Jaffe, R., & Fejgin, M. (1997). Accidental electric shock in pregnancy's: A prospective cohort study [Letter to the editor]. *American Journal of Obstetrics and Gynecology, 177*(4), 983-984.

Jordan, B. D. (1994). Maternal head trauma during pregnancy. In O. Devinsky, E. Feldmann, & B. Hainline (Eds.), *Neurological complications of pregnancy* (pp. 131-138). New York: Raven Press.

Lanoix, R., Akkapeddi, V., & Goldfeder, B. (1995). Perimortem cesarean section: Case reports and recommendations. *Academic Emergency Medicine, 2*(12), 1063-1067.

Lifschultz, B. D., & Donoghue, E. R. (1991). Fetal death following maternal trauma: Two case reports and a survey of the literature. *Journal of Forensic Sciences, 36*(6), 1740-1744.

Lipitz, S., Achiron, R., Horoshovski, D., Rotstein, Z., Sherman, D., & Schiff, E. (1997). Fetomaternal haemorrhage discovered after trauma and treated by fetal intravascular transfusion. *European Journal of Obstetrics, Gynecology, and Reproductive Biology, 71*, 21-22.

Ma, O. J., Mateer, J. R., & DeBehnke, D. J. (1996). Use of ultrasonography for the evaluation of pregnant trauma patients. *Journal of Trauma: Injury, Infection, and Critical Care, 40*(4), 665-668.

Matthews, G., & Hammersley, B. (1997). A case of maternal pelvic trauma following a road traffic accident, associated with fetal intracranial haemorrhage. *Journal of Accident and Emergency Medicine, 14*, 115-117.

Neufeld, J. D. G. (1993). Trauma in pregnancy, what if ...? *Emergency Medicine Clinics of North America, 11*(1), 207-224.

Oakley, L. E., & Johnson, J. D. (1991). Traumatic injury during pregnancy. *Critical Care Nurse, 11*(6), 64-73.

O'Shaughnessy, M. J. (1997). Conservative obstetric management of a gunshot wound to the second-trimester gravid uterus. *Journal of Reproductive Medicine, 42*(9), 606-608.

Pearlman, M. D., Klinich, K. D., Schneider, L. W., Rupp, J., Moss, S., & Ashton-Miller, J. (2000). A comprehensive program to improve safety for pregnant women and fetuses in motor vehicle crashes: A preliminary report. *American Journal of Obstetrics and Gynecology, 182*(6), 1554-1564.

Pearlman, M. D., & Tintinalli, J. E. (1991). Evaluation and treatment of the gravida and fetus following trauma during pregnancy. *Obstetrics and Gynecology Clinics of North America, 18*(2), 371-380.

Pearlman, M. D., Tintinalli, J. E., & Lorenz, R. P. (1990a). A prospective controlled study of outcome after trauma during pregnancy. *American Journal of Obstetrics and Gynecology, 162*(6), 1502-1510.

Pearlman, M. D., Tintinalli, J. E., & Lorenz, R. P. (1990b). Blunt trauma during pregnancy. *New England Journal of Medicine, 323*(23), 1609-1613.

Pimentel, L. (1991). Mother and child: Trauma in pregnancy. *Emergency Medicine Clinics of North America, 9*(3), 549-563.

Polko, L. E., & McMahon, M. J. (1997). Burns in pregnancy. *Obstetrical and Gynecological Survey, 53*(1), 50-56.

Poole, G. V., Martin, J. N., Perry, K. G., Griswold, J. A., Lambert, C. J., & Rhodes, R. S. (1996). Trauma in pregnancy: The role of interpersonal violence. *American Journal of Obstetrics and Gynecology, 174*(6), 1873-1878.

Prasanna, M., & Singh, K. (1996). Early burn wound excision in major burns with pregnancy: A preliminary report. *Burns, 22*(3), 234-237.

Ribe, J. K., Teggatz, J. R., & Harvey, C. M. (1993). Blows to the maternal abdomen causing fetal demise: Report of three cases and a review of the literature. *Journal of Forensic Sciences, 38*(5), 1092-1096.

Rowe, T. F., Lafayette, S., & Cox, S. (1996). An unusual fetal complication of traumatic uterine rupture. *Journal of Emergency Medicine, 14*(2), 173-176.

Rozycki, G. (1993). Trauma during pregnancy: Predicting pregnancy outcome. *Archives of Gynecology and Obstetrics, 253*(Suppl.), 15-20.

Scorpio, R. J., Esposito, T. J., Smith, L. G., & Gens, D. R. (1992). Blunt trauma during pregnancy; Factors affecting fetal outcome. *Journal of Trauma, 32*, 213.

Smart, P. (1994). Care of the injured pregnant patient. *Orthopaedic Nursing, 13*(6), 43-49.

Stafford, P. A., Biddinger, P. W., & Zumwalt, R. E. (1988). Lethal intrauterine fetal trauma. *American Journal of Obstetrics and Gynecology, 159*(2), 485-489.

Steer, R. G. (1992). Delayed fetal death following electrical injury in the first trimester. *Australia and New Zealand Journal of Obstetrics and Gynaecology, 32*(4), 377-378.

Towery, R., English, T. P., & Wisner, D. (1993). Evaluation of pregnant women after blunt injury. *Journal of Trauma, 35*(5), 731-736.

Troiano, N. H. (1991). Trauma during pregnancy. In C. Harvey (Ed.), *Critical care obstetrical nursing* (pp. 147-159). Rockville, MD: Aspen.

Ullmann, Y., Blumenfeld, Z., Hakim, M., Mahoul, I., Sujov, P., & Peled, I. J. (1997). Urgent delivery, the treatment of choice in term pregnant women with extended burn injury. *Burns, 23*(2), 157-159.

Unsur, V., Oztopcu, C., Atalay, C., Alpay, E., & Turhanoglu, B. (1996). A retrospective study of 11 pregnant women with thermal injuries. *European Journal of Obstetrics, Gynecology, and Reproductive Biology, 64*, 55-58.

Vaizey, C. J., Jacobson, M. J., & Cross, F. W. (1994). Trauma in pregnancy. *British Journal of Surgery, 81*, 1406-1415.

Viljoen, D. L. (1995). Porencephaly and transverse limb defects following severe maternal trauma in early pregnancy. *Clinical Dysmorphology, 4*, 75-78.

Weiss, H. B. (1999). Pregnancy-associated injury hospitalizations in Pennsylvania, 1995. *Annals of Emergency Medicine, 34*(5), 626-636.

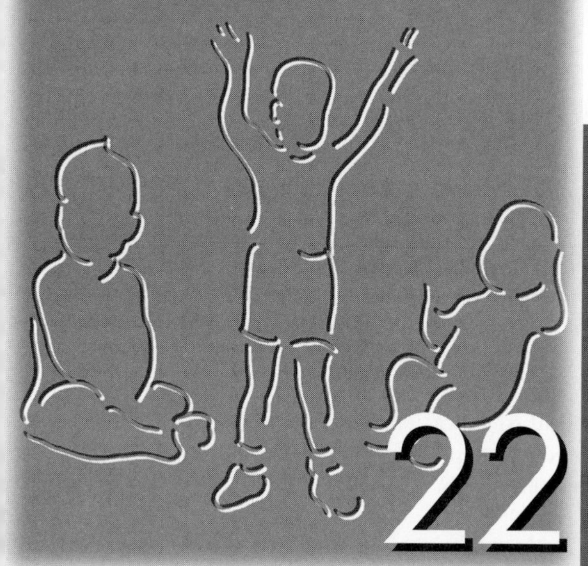

22 Sequelae of Pediatric Trauma: Multiple Organ Dysfunction Syndrome

Tara Trimarchi • Judy Trivits Verger

Approximately 50% of deaths in children between 1 and 19 years of age are attributed to traumatic injury. Head injury and intractable hemorrhage are common causes of death within 48 hours of traumatic injury. However, as early trauma care has improved in quality, survival of children beyond the time of initial injury is increasing. Along with the increase in survival comes an increase in the incidence of the sequelae of traumatic injury. Multiple organ dysfunction syndrome (MODS) is a potential sequela of traumatic injury. During the Vietnam conflict, respiratory dysfunction in soldiers who survived combat injuries was reported. In the early 1970s, multiple organ system failure in individuals who survived severe hemorrhage was first described. Since then, much effort has focused on elucidating the causes of the multiple organ system dysfunction that follows traumatic injury. An understanding of the multisystem effects of trauma is important for planning and providing comprehensive nursing care to the pediatric trauma patient (Bone, 1996; Division of Injury Control, 1990; Moloney-Harmon & Adams, 2001; Simms, 1999; Tobin & Wetzel, 1996).

Occasionally, organ systems fail because they are directly injured during a traumatic event. However, the failure of multiple organ systems in the child who experiences trauma is typically precipitated by the onset of shock and a systemic inflammatory response. Injured children may develop shock secondary to any physiologic derangement that disrupts the delivery and utilization of oxygen and metabolic substrates by cells. Cells of organs that are deprived of oxygen and metabolic substrates lose their ability to generate energy, perform metabolic processes, and synthesize proteins and other essential biomolecules. Cells deprived of oxygen during states of low perfusion generate toxic oxygen free radicals that are activated and released during reperfusion and cause further damage to multiple organ systems (Border, 1995; Kirton, Windsor, Wedderburn, Hudson-Civetta, Shartz, & Mataragas, 1998; McMahon, 1995; Nast-Kolb, Waydhas, Gippner-Steppert, Schneider, Trupka, & Ruchholtz, 1997; Sauaia, Moore, Moore, & Lezotte, 1996; Tobin & Wetzel, 1996).

Direct injury to cells and/or cellular deprivation of oxygen and substrates incites an inflammatory response. Inflammation starts locally, for example, at the site of the injury or an area of low perfusion, and then progresses to a systemic response. The systemic inflammatory response leads to circulatory failure and vascular occlusion, which add to inadequate organ perfusion. Diffuse damage to the endothelium of blood vessels induced by hypoperfusion and inflammation causes many of the physiologic derangements that contribute to injury of the cells of multiple organ systems. Mediators of the systemic inflammatory response cause direct damage to cells of organs and disrupt cellular processes. As function fails at a cellular level, abnormalities in overall organ system function ensue (Border, 1995; McMahon, 1995; Nast-Kolb et al., 1997; Sauaia et al., 1996; Tobin & Wetzel, 1996) (Figure 22-1).

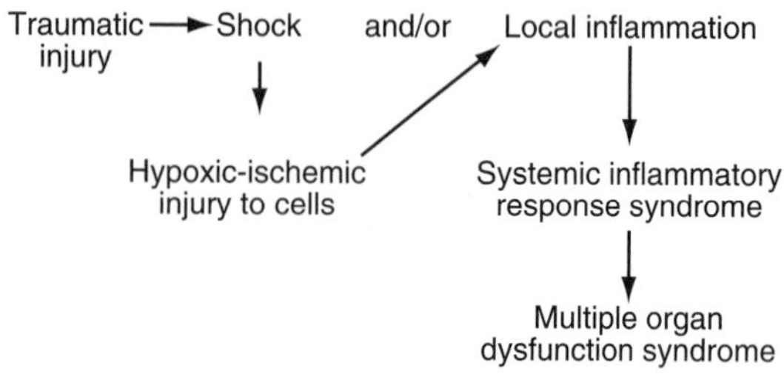

FIGURE 22-1 Progression of traumatic injury to multiple organ dysfunction syndrome.

SHOCK

DEFINITION

Shock is a state of disrupted circulatory function with a resulting decrease in tissue perfusion and inadequate oxygen and substrate delivery to cells. Shock results when the metabolic demands of cells exceed the amount of oxygen and substrates delivered to cells by the circulatory system. Hypotension is often considered a hallmark feature of shock. However, children can be in a state of shock with a normal or even an elevated blood pressure. Although not a defining characteristic of shock, hypotension contributes greatly to inadequacies in meeting the metabolic needs of cells (Curley, 2001; Morgan & O'Neill, 1998; Tobin & Wetzel, 1996).

CLASSIFICATIONS

Shock usually results from the loss of circulating blood volume, the inability of the heart to pump blood, and/or the loss of vascular tone. Shock is often categorized according to cause. Tobin and Wetzell (1996) classify shock as hypovolemic, distributive, septic, and cardiogenic (Table 22-1). Hypovolemic shock resulting from hemorrhage is commonly encountered in the traumatically injured child. Hypovolemic shock resulting from hemorrhage is second only to brain injury as the cause of mortality in children who experience traumatic injury (Morgan & O'Neill, 1998). Injured children may also experience cardiogenic shock from myocardial contusion, distributive shock from loss of vascular tone from a spinal cord injury, or septic shock induced by infection. In the physically traumatized child, a state of inadequate oxygen delivery may be the result of hypoxemia caused by a lung injury such as a pulmonary contusion, neurogenic pulmonary edema in the case of head trauma, or lipid embolism of the pulmonary vasculature after a bone fracture. In some cases, such as carbon monoxide poisoning, shock may result from the inability of hemoglobin to deliver oxygen to cells. Damaged or abnormal cells that are unable to extract or use oxygen, a condition called *dysoxia,* may lead to shock. Furthermore, the injured child may simultaneously experience more than one form of shock (Curley, 2001; Tobin & Wetzel, 1996; Tuit, 1997).

TABLE 22-1 **Classification of Shock**

Type of Shock	Characteristics of the Shock State
Hypovolemic	• Decreased intravascular volume • External or internal fluid loss
Distributive	• Abnormal vascular tone • Maldistribution of vascular tone
Cardiogenic	• Myocardial dysfunction • Decreased cardiac output
Septic	• Associated with infection • Related to the systemic inflammatory response triggered by infection • Characteristic of hypovolemic, distributive, and cardiogenic shock

STAGES

There are three phases of shock: compensated, uncompensated, and irreversible. *Compensated shock* occurs in the early phase of disrupted of circulatory function. In early shock, compensatory mechanisms maintain circulation and organ perfusion is not compromised. Compensatory mechanisms maintain circulation by stimulating water retention and promoting vasoconstriction to selectively shunt available blood volume to vital organs. There are several compensatory mechanisms that play a role. Baroreceptors are located in the carotid sinus, aortic arch, right and left atria, junction of the superior vena cava and inferior vena cava, and pulmonary veins. There is communication between the baroreceptors and the sympathetic and parasympathetic nervous systems. Activation of the parasympathetic nervous system decreases blood pressure by causing decreases in heart rate and stroke volume of the heart. Activation of the sympathetic nervous system increases blood pressure by increasing heart rate and stroke volume of the heart and by promoting vasoconstriction.

Baroreceptors fire impulses when stretched by high blood pressure and cease to fire when blood pressure is low. An increase in impulses from baroreceptors stimulates parasympathetic activity. However, when blood pressure is low, as in a state of shock, a decrease in baroreceptor impulses triggers sympathetic activity, thus causing an increase in blood pressure.

Renal hypoperfusion stimulates the secretion of renin from the juxtaglomerular apparatus of the kidneys. Renin converts angiotensinogen from the liver to angiotensin I. Angiotensin I is then converted to angiotensin II by the angiotensin-converting enzyme in endothelium (primarily in the lungs). Angiotensin II is a potent vasoconstrictor.

Angiotensin II stimulates aldosterone release from the adrenal gland. Aldosterone acts on the kidneys to promote sodium reabsorption. Water is reabsorbed along with sodium, and intravascular volume is increased.

Angiotensin II stimulates antidiuretic hormone (AHD), or vasopressin, from the hypothalamus. ADH promotes water reabsorption by the kidneys, and intravascular volume is increased (Figures 22-2 and 22-3).

Uncompensated shock occurs as the compensatory mechanisms that maintain circulation deteriorate and perfusion of organs fail. In uncompensated shock, cells of organ systems are injured, manifestations of organ system dysfunction ensue, and supportive therapies are required to prevent

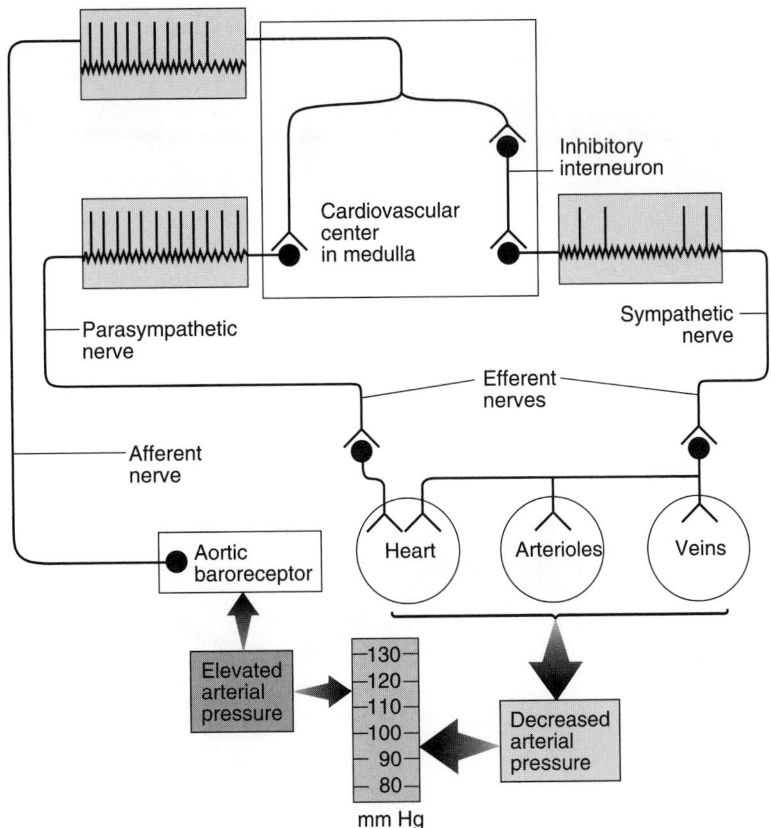

FIGURE 22-2 Compensatory mechanisms in shock: baroreceptors and neural reflexes. (From Rhoades, R., & Pflanzer, R. [Eds.]. [1996]. *Human physiology* [6th ed.]. Reprinted with permission of Wadsworth, a division of Thomson Learning: www.thomsonrights.com. Fax 800-730-2215.)

permanent damage to organs. *Irreversible shock* develops when there is a prolonged state of disrupted circulatory function with a resulting decrease in tissue perfusion and inadequate oxygen and substrate delivery to cells. Despite supportive therapies, in irreversible shock, cells die and permanent cessation of organ function results (Curley, 2001; McMahon, 1995; Tobin & Wetzel, 1996; Tuit, 1997).

SYSTEMIC INFLAMMATORY RESPONSE SYNDROME

HYPERIMMUNE RESPONSE

An immune response occurs when cells are damaged by direct mechanical injury during the traumatic event or as a result of uncompensated shock. Injured cells activate leukocytes. Leukocytes trigger the release of the mediators of inflammation, such as cytokines, eicosanoids, and the complement system. The coagulation cascade is also stimulated. The immune response and inflammation initially are triggered as local mechanisms of defense against further cellular injury. An antiinflammatory response is stimulated simultaneous with the onset of the immune response. A detrimental systemic inflammatory response develops as a consequence of the persistent hyperactivation of the immune system and the inability of antiinflammatory mechanisms to counteract the mediators of inflammation (Bone, 1996; Border, 1995; Davies & Hagen, 1997; Moore, Sauaia, Moore, Haenel, Burch, & Lezotte, 1996; Neidhardt, Keel, Steckholzer, Safret, Ungethuem, & Trentz, 1997; Simms, 1999). These mediators and their major effects are listed in Table 22-2.

OXYGEN FREE RADICAL PRODUCTION AND ISCHEMIA-REPERFUSION INJURY

In states of inadequate perfusion and oxygen delivery, cells produce oxygen free radicals. When perfusion is restored, the oxygen free radicals are activated and then released into the circulation (Figure 22-4). Oxygen free radicals cause further cellular damage and heighten the inflammatory response. Injury related to oxygen free radical release after a state of inadequate perfusion is known as *ischemia-reperfusion injury* (Border, 1995; Flowers & Zimmerman, 1998; Kirton & Civetta, 1999; McMahon, 1995; Tobin & Wetzel, 1996).

ENDOTHELIOPATHY

The endothelial cells of capillary networks are a part of all organ systems and are implicated as precipitating and moderating the inflammatory response. Endothelial cells are damaged during states of low perfusion, from exposure to oxygen free radicals during reperfusion, and from exposure to inflammatory mediators. Derangement of endothelial cell function is referred to as *endotheliopathy*. Endotheliopathy is a final common pathway of MODS (Border, 1995; Tobin & Wetzel, 1996) (Figure 22-5).

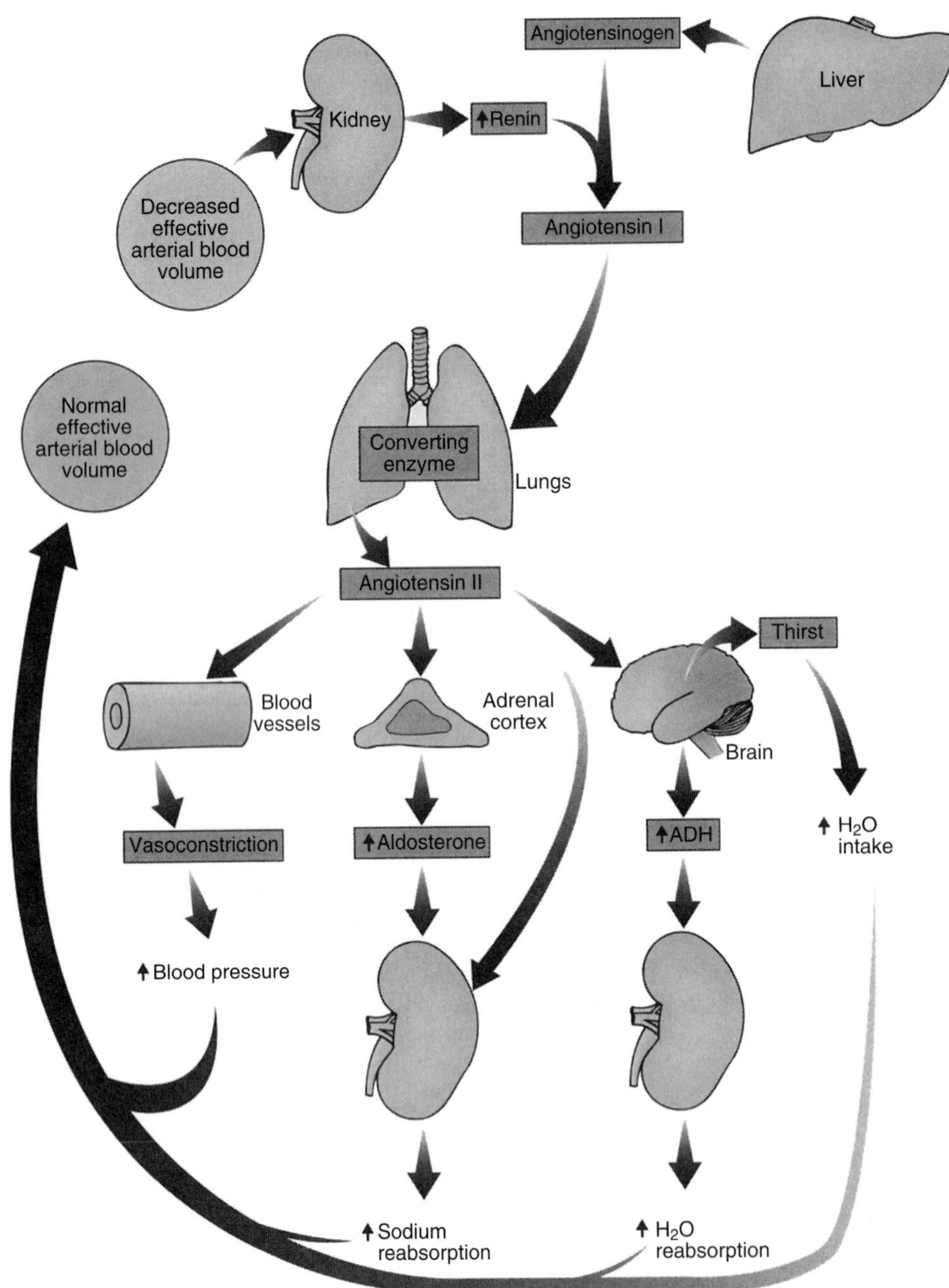

FIGURE 22-3 Compensatory mechanisms in shock: humoral responses: renin-angiotensin, aldosterone, and antidiuretic hormone. (From Rhoades, R., & Pflanzer, R. [Eds.]. [1996]. *Human physiology* [6th ed.]. Reprinted with permission of Wadsworth, a division of Thomson Learning: www.thomsonrights.com. Fax 800-730-2215.)

Defining Characteristics

Many insults trigger the clinical condition of heightened systemic inflammation. Because bacteremia is a well-known stimulus for a systemic inflammatory response, definitions for distinguishing sepsis and septic shock from other insults that cause a systemic inflammatory response were developed in 1992 by the American College of Chest Physicians and the Society of Critical Care Medicine (Table 22-3). One study has shown that early multiple organ system failure in traumatized individuals is associated with severe systemic inflammation (Smail, Messiah, Edouard, Descorps-Declere, Duranteau, & Vigue, 1995). In this study hypovolemic shock and the need for massive volume resuscitation, but not infection, were considered the cause of the inflammatory response and ultimately organ system failure in trauma patients. The diagnosis of systemic inflammatory response syndrome (SIRS) is usually designated to cases of systemic inflammation of noninfectious origin (American College of Chest Physicians and the Society of Critical Care Medicine, 1992; Moore et al., 1996; Nathens & Marshall, 1996; Neidhardt et al., 1997; Parker, 1998). Figure 22-6 shows the relationship among infection, sepsis, and SIRS.

TABLE 22-2 Mediators of Inflammation and Major Effects

Cytokines (polypeptides activated by white blood cells)
- Tumor necrosis factor
- Interleukins
- Interferons
  - Many direct effects on endothelium
  - Amplify, orchestrate, and suppress the inflammatory response

Complement Proteins
- Amplification of the inflammatory response/leukocyte activation
- Histamine release from mast cells
- Breaks down cell membranes
- Enhances platelet aggregation

Eicosanoids (generated from the breakdown of the phospholipid membrane of cells)
- Prostaglandins
  - Vasodilation
- Prostacyclin
  - Vasodilation
  - Inhibits platelet aggregation
- Leukotrienes
  - Leukocyte activation
  - Vasoconstriction, particularly pulmonary vasculature
- Thromboxane
  - Vasoconstriction
  - Enhances platelet aggregation

Platelet-activating factor (PAF)
- Platelet aggregation
- Vasoconstriction, including increased pulmonary vascular resistance
- Amplification of inflammatory response/leukocyte activation
- Cell membrane breakdown and synthesis of eicosanoids

Histamine and bradykinins (from stimulation of mast cells)
- Peripheral vasodilation
- Pulmonary vasoconstriction
- Increased capillary membrane permeability

Cell adhesion proteins
- P-selectin
- L-selectin
  - Encourage adhesion of white blood cells to endothelium

Data from Sclag, G., & Redl, H. (1996). Mediators of inflammation. *World Journal of Surgery, 20*(4), 406-410; and Tobin, J., & Wetzel, R. (1996). Shock and multi-organ system failure. In M. Rogers (Ed.), *Textbook of pediatric critical care* (3rd ed., pp. 568-576). Baltimore: Williams & Wilkins.

Although the findings of Smail et al. (1995) suggest that early SIRS is not related to infection, later sepsis is a cause of systemic inflammation and MODS in individuals who experience trauma. The systemic inflammatory response elicited by the initial injury may alter the function and deplete mediators of the immune system and induce a state of immunosuppression. The resulting state of immunosuppression then predisposes the injured individual to infection. Sepsis after trauma is closely linked to the development of MODS. Moore et al. (1996) report a bimodal presentation of systemic inflammation and MODS after trauma. The authors demonstrate that late-onset MODS is more common and more often associated with infection than is early-onset MODS (Bone, 1996; Moore et al., 1996; Neidhardt et al., 1997; Simms, 1999; Wichmann, Ayala, & Chaudry, 1998). Figure 22-7 shows the progression of SIRS to immunosuppression.

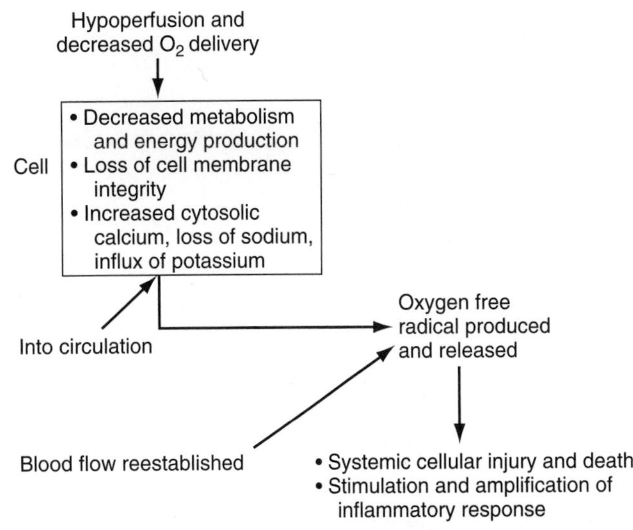

FIGURE 22-4 Hypoxic-ischemic injury and oxygen free radical production.

MANIFESTATIONS

The clinical findings associated with SIRS are the result of the activation of the immune system and the resulting increase in membrane permeability of cells, changes in vascular tone, myocardial depression, consumptive coagulopathy, and hypermetabolic state associated with the response. Mediators of the immune response cause direct damage to multiple types of cells, precipitate organ system dysfunction, and create or contribute to a preexisting state of circulatory failure.

CHANGES IN CELL MEMBRANES AND CAPILLARY LEAK

Loss of endothelial cell integrity results from the direct effects of multiple mediators of inflammation. Loss of cell membrane integrity creates fluxes in the movement of electrolytes and fluid into cells and contributes to cellular injury and death. Disruption of cellular membranes also changes the permeability of tissue barriers. As mediators of inflammation are released into the circulation, the endothelium of blood vessels is affected. The increased permeability of capillaries leads to loss of fluid from the intravascular space with resulting hypovolemia. Leukotrienes, histamine, and complement are examples of inflammatory mediators that increase capillary membrane permeability (McMahon, 1995).

LOSS OF VASOMOTOR TONE

Multiple stimuli of endothelial cells during an inflammatory response, as well as the direct effects of certain biomolecules and toxins, generate the production of nitric oxide (NO). Spack, Hvens, and Griffith (1997) report that high serum

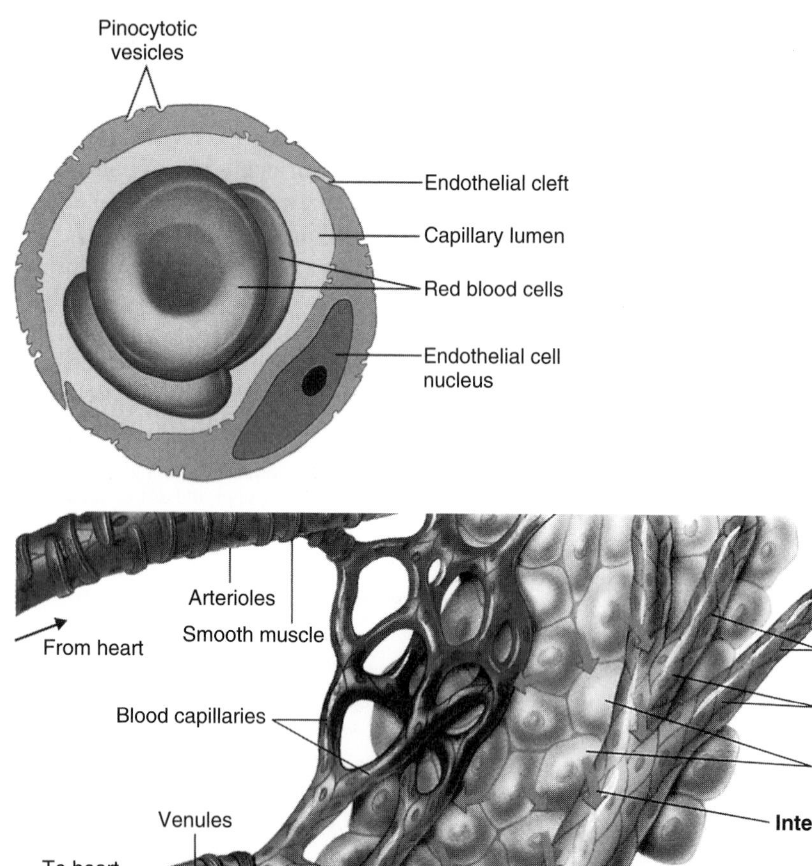

FIGURE 22-5 Endothelium and vascular bed. (From Rhoades, R., & Pflanzer, R. [Eds.]. [1996]. *Human physiology* [6th ed.]. Reprinted with permission of Wadsworth, a division of Thomson Learning: www.thomsonrights.com. Fax 800-730-2215.)

concentrations of nitrite/nitrate levels are strongly correlated with the clinical diagnosis of SIRS in children. NO produced by affected vascular endothelium acts on the adjacent smooth muscles of blood vessels to cause vasodilation. Hypotension from low peripheral vascular resistance results from vasodilation. Many exotoxins and endotoxins released by bacteria are known to induce the production of NO and cause the low peripheral resistance often encountered in children with sepsis and septic shock. Duke, Butt, and South (1997) report that in children with sepsis, elevated NO metabolite levels are associated with an increased incidence of organ system failures. Other inflammatory mediators, such as histamine and prostacyclin, also act as vasodilators (Bengur & Meliones, 1998; McMahon, 1995; Tobin & Wetzel, 1996; Wong, Carcillo, Burckhart, & Kaplan, 1996). The process of NO production is outlined in Figure 22-8.

Myocardial Depression

Early SIRS presents as high-output circulatory failure. Compensatory increases in heart rate and stroke volume occur in response to the decreased peripheral vascular resistance and hypotension induced by SIRS. However, as SIRS progresses, myocardial depressants are released, which can result in decreased contractile force of the heart and diminish cardiac output. NO, tumor necrosis factor-α interleukin-1, and interleukin-6 are known myocardial depressant factors produced by the systemic inflammatory response (Bengur & Meliones, 1998; McMahon, 1995; Tobin & Wetzel, 1996).

Microvasculature Constriction, Thrombosis, and Consumptive Coagulopathy

SIRS results in vasoconstriction of microvasculature. Inflammatory mediators such as thromboxane and leukotrienes cause vasoconstriction. Disseminated intravascular coagulation (DIC) may develop. Gando, Kameue, Nanzaki, and Nakanishi (1996) report an 83% incidence of DIC in adults with SIRS and a high correlation between severity of DIC in patients with SIRS and mortality. DIC is activated when tissue factor is released from damaged vascular endothelium. Tissue factor initiates the extrinsic coagulation pathway and the production of thrombin (Figure 22-9). Thrombin formation results in vascular occlusion and ischemia to dependent tissue. Feedback mechanisms take over and the breakdown of formed clots takes place after initiation of coagulation. However, a decrease in endogenously produced anticoagulants, such as antithrombin III, occurs and further promotes thrombosis. In addition, platelet aggregation stimulated by the inflammatory mediator platelet-activating factor fosters clot formation and vascular occlusion. Ischemia resulting from vasoconstriction, thrombosis, and platelet aggregation leads directly to organ damage and MODS (Gando et al., 1996; Gando, Kameue, Nanzaki, Hayakawa, & Nakanishi, 1997; Penner, 1998).

TABLE 22-3 Definition of Systemic Inflammatory Response Syndrome (SIRS) and Septic States

Standard Adult Criteria

Diagnosis	Definition	Criteria
SIRS	Systemic inflammatory response to various severe clinical insults	Two or more of the following: Temperature >38° C or <36° C Heart rate >90 beats/min Respiratory rate >20 breaths/min or PaCO_2 <32 mm Hg WBC count >12,000 cells/mm^3, 4000 cells/mm^3, or >10% bands
Sepsis	Systemic response to infection	Two or more of the following: Temperature >38° C or <36° C Heart rate >90 beats/min Respiratory rate >20 breaths/min or PaCO_2 <32 mm Hg WBC count >12,000 cells/mm^3, 4000 cells/mm^3, or >10% bands
Septic shock	Sepsis with hypotension, despite adequate fluid resuscitation, persistent perfusion abnormalities (lactic acidosis, oliguria, acute alteration in mental status)	Systolic BP <90 mm Hg or a reduction of >40 mm Hg from baseline

Values for Children

Age	Heart Rate (beats/min)	Respiratory Rate (breaths/min)	Systolic BP (mm Hg)
1-12 mo	>170	>40	<70
1-5 yr	>150	>30	<80
5-10 yr	>130	>25	<80
>10 yr	>120	>20	<90

Definitions from American College of Chest Physicians and the Critical Care Medicine Consensus Conference. (1992). American College of Chest Physicians/Society of Critical Care Medicine consensus conference: Definitions for sepsis and organ failure and guidelines for the use of innovative therapies in sepsis. *Critical Care Medicine, 20,* 864-875. Modified from Parker, M. (1998). Pathophysiology of cardiovascular dysfunction in septic shock. *New Horizons, 6*(2), 130-138.
WBC, White blood cell.

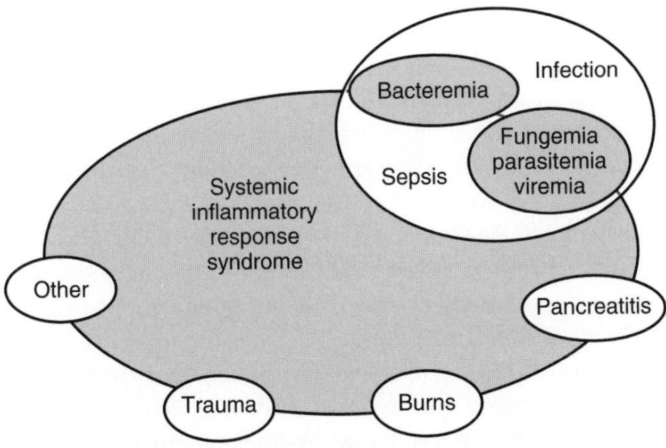

FIGURE 22-6 Relationship among infection, sepsis, and systemic inflammatory response syndrome. (Redrawn from Nathens, A. B., & Marshall, J. C. [1996]. Sepsis, SIRS and MODS: What's in a name? *World Journal of Surgery, 20*[4], 388. Originally appeared in American College of Chest Physicians and the Society of Critical Care Medicine. [1992]. Consensus conference: Definitions for sepsis and organ failure and guidelines for the use of innovative therapies in sepsis. *Critical Care Medicine, 20,* 864-875.)

In SIRS, after clotting factors and platelets have been consumed by the stimulation of coagulation cascades and platelet aggregation, a state of hypocoagulation results. The effect of hypocoagulation is impaired hemostasis. Hemorrhage from impaired hemostasis may precipitate or worsen hypovolemic shock (Gando et al., 1997; Penner, 1998).

Hypermetabolic State

Shock and the systemic inflammatory response induce a state of hypermetabolism, as shown in Table 22-4. Hypermetabolic cells have excessive requirements for oxygen and important metabolic substrates such as phosphates and essential amino acids. Increased metabolic requirements of cells, coupled with the state of low delivery, result in significant cellular energy debt during episodes of shock and systemic inflammation. Energy debt contributes to cell dysfunction, cell death, and a heightened immune response (Border, 1995; Lennie, 1997; McMahon, 1995; Tobin & Wetzel, 1996).

MULTIPLE ORGAN DYSFUNCTION SYNDROME

Stages

MODS is the failure of two or more organ systems in association with shock and a systemic inflammatory response. Four stages of MODS exist. The first stage is the time of the initiating event, such as traumatic injury, and typically includes a period of shock. Removal of the insult and

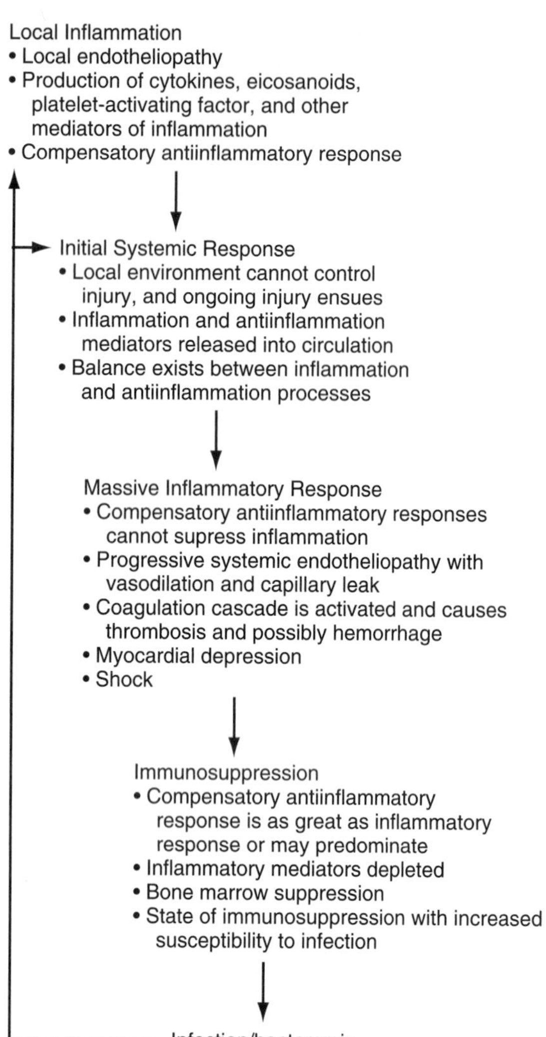

FIGURE 22-7 Progression of the systemic inflammatory response syndrome. (From Bone, R. [1996]. Immunologic dissonance: A continuing evolution in our understanding of systemic inflammatory response syndrome [SIRS] and the multiple organ dysfunction syndrome [MODS]. *Annals of Internal Medicine, 125*[8], 680-687.)

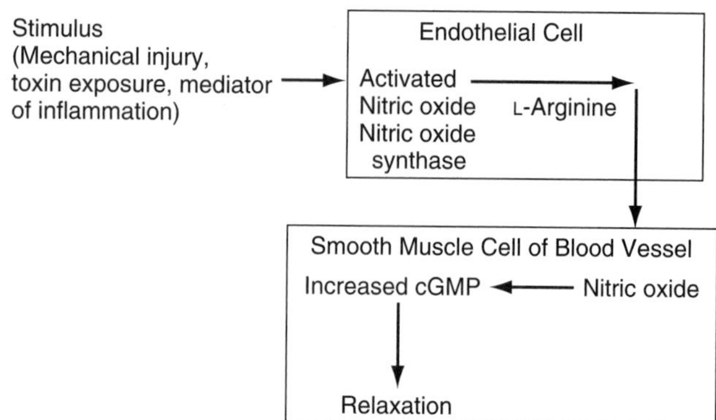

Nitric oxide (NO) is produced when the enzyme nitric oxide synthase (NOS) in an endothelial cell is stimulated. NOS converts the L-arginine (an amino acid) to NO. NO then diffuses out of the endothelial cell and acts on adjacent smooth muscle cells. In the smooth muscle cell, NO triggers an increase in cyclic guanylate monophosphate (cGMP). The increased levels of cGMP promote smooth muscle relaxation, and the blood vessel dilates.

FIGURE 22-8 Nitric oxide production in the systemic inflammatory response syndrome.

attempts at resuscitation of circulatory function takes place during the second stage. The third stage includes the development of systemic inflammation hypermetabolism and often a persistent shock state. The onset of abnormalities in organ system function begins in this third stage. Finally, in the fourth stage of MODS, organ systems fail secondary to prolonged inadequate delivery of oxygen and metabolic substrates and the effects of inflammation (Duke et al., 1997; McMahon, 1995).

Pattern and Progression

MODS typically begins with circulatory collapse that creates the state of shock and triggers SIRS. Dysfunction of the respiratory system usually occurs soon after the onset of circulatory failure, particularly as SIRS progresses. The lungs are particularly susceptible to injury from inflammation. The onset of hypoxemia from early respiratory failure worsens shock and SIRS by contributing to a decrease in oxygen available to already poorly perfused cells. Along with, or after, respiratory dysfunction, abnormalities of the gastrointestinal (GI) tract and hepatic dysfunction soon occur. The GI tract and liver are prone to relatively early dysfunction during states of hypoperfusion because compensatory mechanisms shunt circulation away from the splanchnic vascular beds to preferentially allow for cardiac, respiratory, and cerebral perfusion. As GI perfusion decreases, breakdown of the gut and translocation of bacteria into the bloodstream takes place. Bacteremia serves to further heighten the inflammatory response and maintain a state of shock. Decreased blood flow to the kidneys follows soon after a decrease in splanchnic blood flow and results in renal insufficiency. Myocardial depression and hematologic dysfunction occur at various times throughout the illness and are associated with acute SIRS. Decreased cardiac output and hemorrhage induced by coagulopathy further worsen circulatory failure. A depressed level of consciousness may accompany acute shock and SIRS, but significant neurologic dysfunction tends to develop later and is ominous. When shock and SIRS are prolonged, organ system dysfunction evolves into organ system failure (Bone, 1996; Deitch, 1990; McMahon, 1995; Regel, Grotz, Weltner, Sturm, & Tscherne, 1996; Swank & Deitch, 1996; Tobin & Wetzel, 1996). The definitions of organ system failure are provided in Table 22-5.

Specific Organ System Dysfunction

Cardiac

Cardiac depression from the release of myocardial depressant factors induced by SIRS was previously discussed. In addition to myocardial depression from the direct effects of inflammatory mediators, the excessive workload of the heart during compensation for shock increases myocardial oxygen demand. As shock persists, the increased oxygen demand of

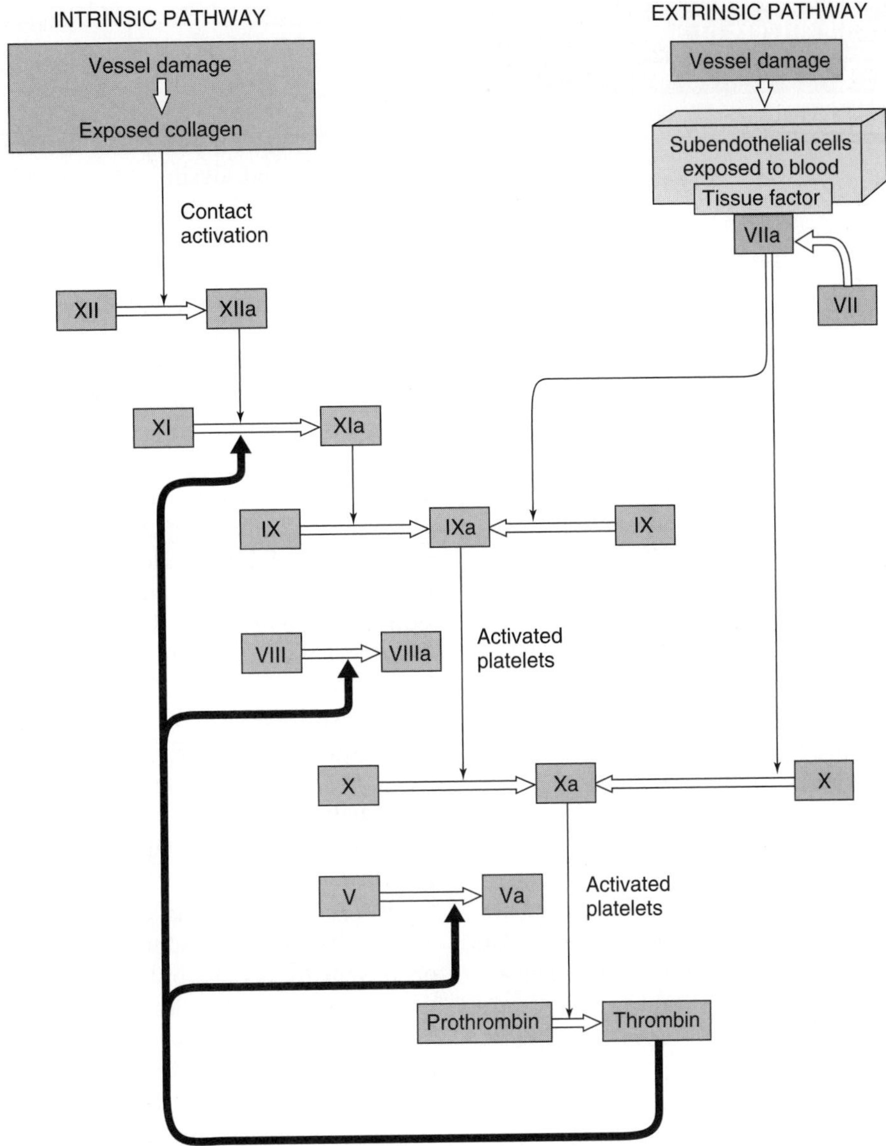

FIGURE 22-9 Coagulation cascade. (Redrawn from Vander, A., Sherman, J., & Luciano, D. [Eds.]. [1994]. *Human physiology: The mechanisms of body function* [6th ed., p. 745]. New York: McGraw-Hill.)

the heart is not met and myocardial ischemia occurs. Myocardial ischemia further contributes to low cardiac output and may precipitate arrhythmias. Changes in cell membranes as a result of inflammation may promote the development of pericardial effusions and contribute to heart failure by creating tamponade (Chang, 1999; Parker, 1998).

RESPIRATORY

Acute respiratory distress syndrome (ARDS) often occurs after shock secondary to traumatic injury. ARDS is considered an essential contributor to the progression of SIRS to MODS. Regel et al. (1996) report that respiratory failure is the most commonly encountered dysfunction in patients with MODS after trauma and that patients with ARDS have the highest mortality. The incidence of death in children with ARDS is estimated to be as high as 50% (Davis, Furman, & Costario, 1993; Fackler, Arnold, Nichols, & Rogers, 1996; Regel et al., 1996; Simms, 1999; Timmons, Havens, & Fackler, 1995; Verbrugge, Sorm, & Lachmann, 1997).

Lung injury is caused by the systemic inflammatory response. In ARDS, platelet and leukocyte aggregation and vasoconstriction lead to lung perfusion abnormalities and pulmonary hypertension. Interestingly, although increased NO production and vasodilation manifests systemically during an inflammatory response, injury to the pulmonary system results in low NO production and vasoconstriction, which contributes to ventilation/perfusion mismatch. Concurrently, increased capillary membrane permeability of the pulmonary vascular bed results in pulmonary edema. Pulmonary edema compromises oxygen diffusion into the blood and decreases lung compliance. Changes in cell membranes caused by mediators of systemic inflammation may also promote the development of pericardial effusions and contribute to respiratory failure. In addition, surfactant

TABLE 22-4 Metabolic Effects of Systemic Inflammatory Response Syndrome

Cytokines released during the inflammatory response that affect metabolism
Interleukin-1 (IL-1)
Interleukin-6 (IL-6)
Tumor necrosis factor (TNF)

Metabolic Response	Effects
Stimulation of adrenocorticotropic hormone with subsequent cortical release from the adrenal cortex and catecholamine (epinephrine) release from the adrenal medulla	Insulin suppression/ glucagon release • Increased metabolic rate • Hyperglycemia • Mobilization of fatty acids • Negative nitrogen balance
Release of amino acids from skeletal muscle	Provides essential amino acids for wound healing Creates net loss of body protein with muscle wasting

From Lennie, T. A. (1997). The metabolic response to injury: Current perspectives and nursing implications. *Dimensions of Critical Care Nursing, 16*(2), 79-87.

deficiency and the production of abnormal surfactant are induced by lung injury and result in atelectasis and decreased lung compliance. Ultimately, ARDS results in severe hypoxemia. Hypercarbia is problematic in individuals with ARDS. The criteria used for diagnosis of ARDS are presented in Box 22-1.

RENAL

Hypoperfusion of the kidneys results in acute tubular necrosis. Impaired renal tubular function results in electrolyte imbalance. Because hyperkalemia can precipitate cardiac arrest, it is the most serious electrolyte abnormality associated with renal dysfunction. Renal dysfunction also causes hypocalcemia. Hypocalcemia contributes to low cardiac output states by decreasing the strength of myocardial contraction. In addition, excessive bicarbonate loss as a result of renal tubular damage causes acidosis. Acidosis depresses myocardial function (Curley, 2001; Hand, Harmon, & McManus, 1996; Morgan-Madder & Milberger, 1996; Vincent, 1996).

Although the electrolyte imbalances and acidosis associated with renal diseases contribute to circulatory collapse, decreased kidney perfusion results in diminished glomerular filtration rate, water retention, and systemic vasoconstriction. Initially in shock states, there is a need for compensatory fluid retention and peripheral vasoconstriction to maintain blood volume and a normal blood pressure. After restoration of circulatory function, however, fluid retention and vasoconstriction may persist and cause intravascular volume overload and hypertension (Curley, 2001; Hand et al., 1996; Morgan-Madder & Milberger, 1996; Vincent, 1996).

HEPATIC

Hypoxic-ischemic injury to the liver results in hepatocyte dysfunction and death. Without adequate hepatocyte function, protein synthesis is impaired. Hypoalbuminemia and lack of coagulation factor production result from impaired protein synthesis. Low albumin decreases the oncotic pressure of the blood and promotes fluid shifts from the vascular space to the interstitial space. Hypoalbuminemia in conjunction with capillary leak from the breakdown of vascular endothelium caused by systemic inflammation leads to extensive intravascular fluid depletion and hypovolemia. Decreased production of clotting factors worsens coagulopathy and increases the potential for hemorrhage. At the same time, the inability of the damaged liver to clear toxins results in an increase of circulating vasoactive molecules, which causes hypotension. The inability of the damaged liver to clear toxins may cause encephalopathy and cerebral edema. In addition, the failing liver may be unable to orchestrate carbohydrate metabolism, and hypoglycemia can occur (Furuta, Rogers, & Leichtner, 1996; Martin, 1992).

GASTROINTESTINAL

Dysfunction of the GI system typically is not used as a defining characteristic of MODS. However, the problems that result from GI injury can contribute greatly to shock, systemic inflammatory responses, and dysfunction of other organ systems. Because of the importance of GI damage in the overall process, it is described here.

Damage to the GI tract from inadequate perfusion and inflammation results in loss of mucosal integrity. Without an intact mucosal layer, acidic gastric cause gastritis with erosions, or *stress ulcers*. Bleeding from stress ulcers, particularly in conjunction with a state of hypocoagulability such as that in DIC, may contribute to hypovolemia and shock.

As previously mentioned, ischemia to the bowel causes breakdown in barrier tissues, translocation of bacteria into the bloodstream, and potential sepsis. Swank and Deitch (1996) reviewed the phenomena and reported that in up to 30% of the cases of bacteremia in seriously ill patients with MODS, no source of infection is identified. Swank and Deitch and other investigators propose that bacteremia in these cases results from bacterial translocation from the gut (Furuta et al., 1996; Stechmiller, Treloar, & Allen, 1997; Swank & Deitch, 1996).

Trauma can also induce pancreatitis. Berney, Belli, Bugmann, Beghetti, Morel, and LeCoultre (1996) report that approximately 30% of the cases of pancreatitis treated in a pediatric intensive care unit were induced by abdominal trauma and an additional 33% of cases were precipitated by hypovolemic shock from multiple causes. Also in that study, low Glasgow Coma Scale scores demonstrated good specificity in correlating with pancreatitis. Enzymes released from

TABLE 22-5 Definitions of Organ System Failure

Body System	Definition
Cardiac	Presence of one or more of the following: MAP: Neonate-3 mo: <30 mm Hg 3 mo-1 yr: <35 mm Hg 1-6 yr: <40 mm Hg >6 yr: <50 mm Hg Arterial blood pH <7.25 and Pao_2 <45 mm Hg
Respiratory	Presence of one or more of the following: $Paco_2$ >50 mm Hg with serum pH <7.25 $A\text{-}aDo_2$ >350 mm Hg Oxygenation index >30
Renal	Requirement for renal replacement therapy Presence of one or more of the following: Urine output <0.5 ml/kg/hr for 4 consecutive hr or <300 ml/m^2/24 hr Serum creatinine: 1 day-1 month: >0.15 mmol/L 1 mo-1 yr: >0.04 mmol/L 1-4 yr: >0.05 mmol/L 5-10 yr: >0.06 mmol/L 10 yr: >0.1 mmol/L
Hepatic	Presence of three or more of the following: Prolonged PT (in absence of warfarin anticoagulation) AST >100 U/L Serum albumin: <12 mo: <23 g/L ≥12 mo: <30 g/L Conjugated bilirubin >10 mmol/L
Hematologic	Presence of two or more of the following: WBC count <1000 cells/mm^3 Platelets <20,000/mm^3 Prolonged PT (in absence of warfarin anticoagulation) D-Dimers >0.25/presence of fibrin split productions Prolonged PTT (in the absence of heparin anticoagulation)
Neurologic	Glasgow Coma Scale score <6 in the absence of sedation

Modified from Duke, T., Butt, W., & South, M. (1997). Predictors of mortality and multiple organ failure in children with sepsis. *Intensive Care Medicine, 23,* 690.

AST, Aspartate aminotransferase; *MAP,* mean arterial pressure; *PT,* prothrombin time; *PTT,* partial thromboplastin time; *WBC,* white blood cell.

BOX 22-1 Criteria for Diagnosis of Acute Respiratory Distress Syndrome (ARDS)

Murray's Criteria

Acute respiratory insufficiency requiring mechanical ventilation
Pao_2/Fio_2 ≤250 mm Hg with PEEP ≥5 cm H_2O
Bilateral pulmonary infiltrates on chest radiograph
Pulmonary capillary wedge pressure ≤18 mm Hg
ARDS is diagnosed when respiratory failure occurs without preexisting left-sided heart failure (pulmonary capillary wedge pressure ≤18 mm Hg)

Modified from Bernard, G., Artigas, A., & Brigham, K. (1994). The American European Consensus Conference on ARDS. *American Journal of Respiratory and Critical Care Medicine, 149,* 818.
PEEP, Positive end-expiratory pressure.

the damaged pancreas amplify the systemic inflammatory response. Pancreatitis alone is a known cause of SIRS (Berney et al., 1996; Furuta et al., 1996).

Neurologic

Inadequate oxygen delivery to the brain results in hypoxic-ischemic encephalopathy (HIE). Ischemia of the brain results in neuronal membrane breakdown. Loss of membrane integrity precipitates the flux of electrolytes, such as calcium, and fluid into neurons and results in the death of neurons. Local mediators of inflammation and the activation of excitatory amino acids during brain injury contribute to the process of neuronal injury and death. Neurons swell as they are damaged, and cerebral edema ensues. Cerebral edema causes an elevation in intracranial pressure and further disruption of blood flow to the brain. Neurologic injury with elevated intracranial pressure may worsen circulatory failure via blood pressure and heart rate instability from brainstem compression. In addition, pituitary-hypothalamic axis dysfunction may cause diabetes insipidus (DI). Free water loss from DI may cause or worsen preexisting hypovolemia. In 1996, Lee, Hunang, Shen, Kao, Ho, and Shyur reviewed the literature and reported cases of DI associated with HIE. It was found that hemorrhagic shock was a major cause of HIE-induced DI and that approximately 99% of children with DI secondary to HIE died (Haun, Kirsch, & Dean, 1996; Lee et al., 1996).

Hematologic

The development of DIC and thrombocytopenia associated with shock and SIRS was previously described. Disorders of coagulation and platelets initially result in thrombosis and contribute to tissue ischemia. Microvascular occlusion is a final common pathway of MODS. As coagulation factors and platelets are consumed during the state of hypercoagulation and platelet aggregation, a state of hypocoagulability then results. Hypocoagulation may cause hemorrhage and add to preexisting hypovolemia.

Bone marrow suppression may also result during episodes of shock and SIRS. The cause of bone marrow suppression in the case of MODS is not fully understood. Bone marrow suppression contributes to an immunocompromised state and anemia and, thus increases the risk of sepsis and decreases the oxygen-carrying capacity of the blood (Bone, 1996; Gando et al., 1997; Penner, 1998).

ASSESSMENT AND MANAGEMENT OF SHOCK, SIRS, AND MODS

Initial Resuscitation and Stabilization

Prevention is the best treatment for MODS. Successful initial resuscitation and stabilization of the trauma patient are imperative to the prevention of the systemic inflammatory response and the failure of multiple organ systems. Prolonged hypovolemic shock, the need for massive volume resuscitation, and persistent signs of decreased organ perfusion, such as acidosis, are directly linked to the development of MODS and to mortality (Kirton et al., 1998; Orliaguet et al., 1998; Sauaia et al., 1996; Smail et al., 1995).

Early surgical intervention is often warranted for the trauma patient. In a hallmark study in 1985, Johnson, Cadambi, and Seibert (1985) demonstrated decreased length of time on mechanical ventilation and decreased incidence of ARDS in patients who underwent early fixation of pelvic and long-bone fractures. Stopping blood loss through surgical intervention and facilitating mobilization are likely reasons for improved outcomes with early surgical intervention (Baue, Durham, & Mazuski, 1996; Johnson, Cadambi, & Seibert, 1985; Kirton et al., 1998; Smail et al., 1995).

Prevention and Treatment of Infection and Provision of Nutrition

After the phase of initial resuscitation and stabilization, assessment and management strategies to prevent MODS revolve around the maintenance of circulatory function and adequate oxygen delivery to cells. However, prevention of infection and provision of nutrition are also important components of the care plan for the child at risk for MODS. As with any seriously ill or postsurgical patient, early identification of the signs of infection, prompt initiation of antimicrobial treatment, and wound debridement and drainage (when necessary) are imperative (Box 22-2). Preventing infection through close attention to aseptic technique when providing care is as important as treating existing infections. Decontamination of the GI tract to reduce the likelihood of bacterial translocation from the gut has been proposed as a measure preventive against bacteremia. However, the findings of studies investigating the usefulness of GI decontamination are inconclusive (Baue et al., 1996; Gullo & Berlot, 1996; Vincent, 1996).

Providing adequate nutrition promotes wound healing and complements strategies to prevent and treat infection. Providing adequate nutrition is necessary to meet the needs of cells in the hypermetabolic state induced by SIRS. Parenteral nutrition is necessary in the child who is unable to eat. Enteral nutrition, however, should be initiated whenever safe and possible. Enteral nutrition has been demonstrated to protect against the breakdown of the GI tract and may help prevent bacterial translocation. Diets rich in glutamine are believed to promote generation of the epithelial lining of the gut and growth of intestinal villi. Specialized diets that contain nutrients believed to enhance immune system function are often recommended for trauma patients experiencing SIRS who are at risk for infection (Box 22-3). Antioxidants such as glutathione, vitamin E, and β-carotene are recommended to counteract the deleterious effects of oxygen free radicals. Nutrients such as glutamine, arginine, vitamin C, and omega-3 fatty acids are recommended for their immune system–enhancing properties. Adult formulas containing antioxidants and immune system–enhancing nutrients are available, but such pediatric formulations are limited (Bengmark & Gianotti, 1996; Gullo & Berlot, 1996; Sax, 1993; Stechmiller et al., 1997).

BOX 22-2 Signs of Infection in Children

- Changes in body temperature
  - Fever or hypothermia
- Changes in white blood cells
  - Leukocytosis or leukopenia
- Hypotension (usually late in cases of sepsis and septic shock)
- Changes in respiratory pattern and heart rate
  - Bradypnea, apnea, or tachypnea
  - Bradycardia or tachycardia
- Generalized malaise/lethargy or irritability
- Purulent or malodorous drainage from wounds
- Erythema of wound
- Ecchymosis or petechiae of the skin
- Hypoglycemia (infants)
- Gastrointestinal upset

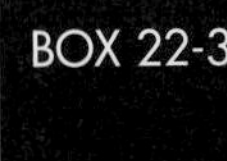

BOX 22-3 Dietary Nutrients Recommended for Patients With Actual or Potential Systemic Inflammatory Response Syndrome and Multiple Organ Dysfunction Syndrome

Glutamine
- Promotes integrity of the lining of the gastrointestinal tract
- Enhances immune system function

Glutathione, vitamin E, and β-carotene
- Antioxidants/protect cells against damage from oxygen free radicals

Arginine, vitamin C, and omega-3 fatty acids
- Enhance immune system function

Data from Bengmark, S., & Gianotti, L. (1996). Nutritional support to prevent and treat multiple organ failure. *World Journal of Surgery, 20*(4), 474-481.

Modulation of the Systemic Inflammatory Response

At present, there are no established pharmacologic therapies that successfully control or stop the systemic inflammatory response. However, the ability to modulate the inflammatory response is a potential strategy to prevent MODS. Potential therapies for modulating the systemic inflammatory response are presented in Table 22-6.

Maintaining Oxygen Delivery: Cardiovascular and Respiratory Dysfunction

Components of Oxygen Delivery

Inadequate oxygen delivery to cells because of poor perfusion or hypoxemia is the main cause of cellular injury, SIRS, and MODS. Maximization of oxygen delivery to cells is the most important component of caring for the traumatically injured child. Oxygen delivery (DO_2) is dependent on

TABLE 22-6 Potential Therapies for Modulation of the Systemic Inflammatory Response

Therapy	Rationale
Monoclonal antibodies to inflammatory mediators such as tumor necrosis factor, interleukin-1, and complement proteins	Destruction of inflammatory mediators by antibodies decreases initiation and amplification of the inflammatory response, severity of cell membrane damage, changes in vascular tone, and hypermetabolism
Monoclonal antibodies to endotoxin and exotoxin	Prevent the inflammatory response produced by the endotoxins and exotoxins released by bacteria in sepsis and septic shock and prevent vasodilation secondary to activation of nitric oxide
Complement 1 inhibitor	Prevents cell membrane damage, histamine release, platelet aggregation, and amplification of the inflammatory response
Prostaglandin inhibitor	Prevents changes in vasomotor tone associated with prostagandins
Arachidonic acid inhibitor	Prevents production of eicosanoids
Neutrophil inhibitors	Prevent white blood cell function, which activates and amplifies inflammation and contributes to cell damage and vascular obstruction
Antioxidants	Prevent cellular damage from oxygen free radicals
Free radical scavengers	Prevent cellular damage from oxygen free radicals
Antithrombin III, protein C, and plasminogen activator	Replenish levels of anticoagulant factors to prevent or lessen severity of disseminated intravascular coagulation
Antihistamines	Prevent histamine release and associated capillary leak and hypotension
Calcium channel blockers	Prevent calcium influx into damaged cells, which contributes to cell dysfunction and death and may prevent vascular constriction
Receptor antagonists to inflammatory mediators, such as tumor necrosis factor, interleukin-1, platelet-activating factor, thromboxane, and bradykinin	Blocking the actions of mediators decreases initiation and amplification of the inflammatory response, severity of cell membrane damage, changes in vascular tone, thrombosis, andhypermetabolism
Catecholamines	Reduce levels of tumor necrosis factor and interleukins and may activate antiinflammatory cytokines
Glucocorticoids	Alter cytokine function

Modified from Curley, M. A., & Moloney-Harmon, P. A. (Eds.). (1996). *Critical care nursing of infants and children* (p. 942) Philadelphia: WB Saunders. Additional data from Guirao, X. & Lowry, S. E. (1996). Biologic control of injury and inflammation: Much more than too little or too late. *World Journal of Surgery, 20*(4), 437-446.

cardiac index, which is a measurement of cardiac output based on body surface area. Cardiac output and cardiac index are functions of blood volume, heart rate, myocardial contractile force, and resistance of the blood vessels (Bloedel-Smith, Ley, Curley, Elixson, & Dodds, 1996; Chang, 1999; Cornwell, Kennedy, & Rodriquez, 1996; Yu, 1999).

Oxygen delivery is also dependent on the content of oxygen in the arterial blood (Cao_2). Arterial blood oxygen content consists of both the partial pressure of oxygen dissolved in the blood (Pao_2) and the amount of hemoglobin saturated with oxygen (Sao_2). Only oxygen bound to hemoglobin is available to cells (Bloedel-Smith et al., 1996; Chang, 1999; Peruzzi & Martin, 1995; Yu, 1999).

The amount of oxygen delivered to cells of the body is reduced when there is a decrease in cardiac index related to myocardial failure, hypovolemia, or vasodilation with decreased venous return to the heart. Decreased oxygen content of arterial blood (hypoxemia) and decreased hemoglobin (anemia) also reduce the amount of oxygen delivered to cells. Monitoring for myocardial depression, hypovolemia, decreased peripheral vascular resistance, hypoxemia, and anemia is the key to identifying states of inadequate oxygen delivery (Bloedel-Smith et al., 1996; Chang, 1999; Peruzzi & Martin, 1995; Yu, 1999).

Evaluation of Oxygen Delivery and Consumption

Oxygen consumption by cells (Vo_2) is reflected by the arteriovenous oxygen difference (a-vDo_2). The a-vDo_2 is the difference between the content of oxygen in the arterial blood (Cao_2) and the content of oxygen in venous blood (Cvo_2) as it returns to the heart after perfusing the cells of the body. A large a-vDo_2 indicates that cells are extracting a great deal of the oxygen delivered to them. Cells may be extracting a great deal of oxygen from the arterial blood because their demand for oxygen is extremely high and perfusion is marginal or low. A normal a-vDo_2 indicates adequate oxygen delivery to the cells. A small a-vDo_2 may be the result of the lack of extraction of oxygen by cells because of severely compromised delivery from inadequate perfusion or, less frequently, because critically injured and dead cells can no longer extract oxygen (Bloedel-Smith et al., 1996; Chang, 1999; Yu, 1999).

Similarly, evaluation of the hemoglobin oxygen saturation of venous blood (Svo_2) returning to the heart can be used to assess the adequacy of oxygen delivery. A normal Svo_2 indicates adequate oxygen delivery to the cells. A high Svo_2 may be the result of the lack of extraction of oxygen by cells because of severely compromised delivery from inadequate perfusion or, less frequently, because critically injured and dead cells can no longer extract oxygen (Chang, 1999; Craig, Smith, & Fineman, 2001; Sanders, 1997; Yu, 1999). Normal oxygenation profile values are presented in Table 22-7.

Serum lactate levels can be used to assess the adequacy of oxygen delivery to cells. When cells are deprived of oxygen, they use alternative pathways for energy production that result in the formation of lactate. The use of alternative pathways for energy production because of oxygen debt is called *anaerobic metabolism.* Under normal conditions cells produce energy from oxidative phosphorylation using glycolysis, the citric acid cycle, and the electron transport chain. Thiry-six high-energy adenosine triphosphate (ATP) molecules are produced. Oxidative phosphorylation cannot take place in low-oxygen states. In the absence of oxygen, pyruvate formed from glycolysis is converted to lactate in an alterative pathway that produces only 2 ATP. Lactate accumulation causes acidosis (Figure 22-10). A normal serum lactate level is less than 2 mmol/L. An increase in serum lactate level creates a metabolic acidosis. Multiple studies demonstrate a correlation among lactate levels, metabolic acidosis, and states of low oxygen delivery (Chang, 1999).

The arterial base deficit is an indicator of the severity of metabolic acidosis. A low serum pH and a base deficit, in conjunction with a normal arterial carbon dioxide level, are indicative of metabolic acidosis. Like lactate level, base deficit can be used to follow the trend of the severity of a shock state. Davis, Kaups, and Parks (1998) report that base deficit is a more sensitive indicator than serum pH in the evaluation of acidosis after traumatic injury (Chang, 1999; Davis et al., 1998).

TABLE 22-7 **Normal Oxygenation Profile Values**

Parameter	Calculation	Norms
Cao_2	$Cao_2 = (Hgb \times 1.34 \times Sao_2) + (Pao_2 \times 0.003)$	20 ml/dl
Cvo_2	$C\bar{v}o_2 = (Hgb \times 1.34 \times S\bar{v}o_2) + (P\bar{v}o_2 \times 0.003)$	15 ml/dl
a-vDo_2	$Cao_2 - C\bar{v}o_2$	3.5-5 ml/dl
$\dot{D}o_2$	$\dot{D}o_2 = Cao_2 \times CI \times 10$	620 ± 50 ml/min/M^2
$\dot{V}o_2$	$\dot{V}o_2 = (Cao_2 - C\bar{v}o_2) \times CI \times 10$	120-200 ml/min/M^2
O_2ER	$(Cao_2 - C\bar{v}o_2)/Cao_2 \times 100$	25% ± 2%
$S\bar{v}o_2$		75% (60%-80%)

From Curley, M. A. Q., & Moloney-Harmon, P. A. (2001). *Critical care nursing of infants and children.* Philadelphia: WB Saunders.
Cao_2, Arterial oxygen content; *Hgb*, hemoglobin; *Sao_2*, arterial oxygen saturation; *CI*, cardiac index; *$\dot{D}o_2$*, oxygen delivery; *Pao_2*, arterial partial pressure of oxygen; *$C\bar{v}o_2$*, venous oxygen content; *$S\bar{v}o_2$*, venous oxygen saturation; *$P\bar{v}o_2$*, venous partial pressure of oxygen; *a-$\bar{v}$ Do_2*, arteriovenous oxygen difference; *$\dot{V}o_2$*, oxygen consumption; *O_2ER*, oxygen extraction ratio.

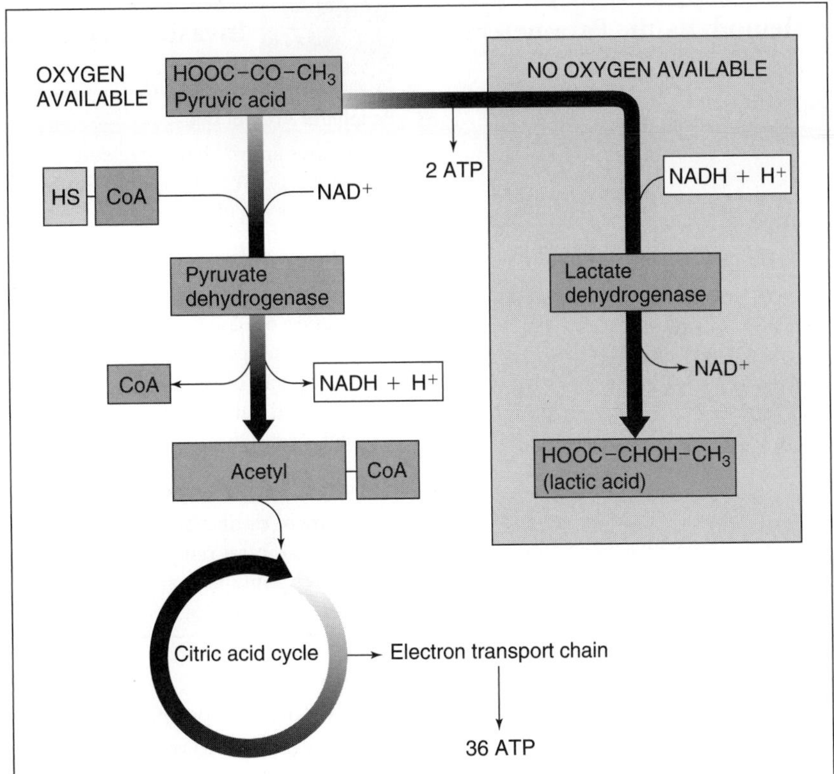

FIGURE 22-10 Lactate production in anaerobic metabolism. (From Rhoades, R., & Pflanzer, R. [Eds.]. [1996]. *Human physiology* [6th ed.]. Reprinted with permission of Wadsworth, a division of Thomson Learning: www.thomsonrights.com. Fax 800-730-2215.)

The pH of GI mucosa can be used to follow the trend of severity of shock. Early in states of hypoperfusion, the GI tract develops local ischemia and acidosis. Probes placed into the GI tract can continuously measure changes in the pH of GI mucosa. Measurement of the pH of GI mucosa is called *tonometry.* Multiple studies have demonstrated a correlation between low GI mucosa pH on tonometry and decreased oxygen delivery. Low GI mucosa pH has been reported to be prognostic of increased mortality in critically ill children (Casado-Flores, Mora, Perez-Corral, Martinez-Azagra, Garcia-Teresa, and Ruiz-Lopex; Chang, 1999; Davis et al., 1998; Ferguson, 1996).

Methods of Assessing and Supporting Cardiovascular and Respiratory Function

Assessment of the Cardiovascular System. Examination of the quality of pulses and the temperature, color, and capillary refill time of the extremities assess cardiovascular status. Weak pulses and cool, pale extremities with delayed capillary refill time are evidence of poor perfusion. In states of excessive vasodilation, however, extremities may be warm and pulses may be bounding. This phenomenon is commonly called *warm shock.* Tachycardia, hypotension, decreased urine output, and decreased level of consciousness are other signs of cardiovascular failure.

Measurement of cardiac function is performed noninvasively by echocardiography. Echocardiography provides estimations of ejection fraction or shortening fraction of the heart, valve quality, and direction of blood flow. Echocardiography can assist in the diagnosis of a pericardial effusion (Chang, 1999; Jalonen, 1997; Parker, 1998).

Measurement of cardiovascular function is performed invasively through the placement a pulmonary artery catheter. Pulmonary artery catheters provide measurements of cardiac output, cardiac index, central venous pressure, peripheral vascular resistance, and pulmonary vascular resistance (Box 22-4). Oxygen availability and consumption can be calculated based on data from pulmonary artery catheters. Pulmonary artery catheters, however, are rarely used in pediatric critical care. The risks of vascular injury, such as lethal perforation of the pulmonary artery, outweigh the benefit of their use in most cases (Pulmonary Artery Catheter Consensus Conference: Consensus Statement, 1997; Thompson, 1997). Useful surrogates for the data obtained from pulmonary artery catheters include calculation of a-vDO_2 from blood samples taken from a peripheral arterial catheter and a simple, central venous catheter. A peripheral arterial catheter provides continuous monitoring of blood pressure, and a central venous catheter provides continuous monitoring central venous pressure. In addition, a central venous catheter provides access to blood samples for SvO_2 measurement (Chang, 1999; Jalonen, 1997; Parker, 1998; Sanders, 1997). Box 22-5 lists the functions of the three types of catheters.

BOX 22-4 Derived Hemodynamic Parameters

Cardiac Index (CI)

Normal = 2.5 to 5 L/min/m^2
CI = Cardiac output/body surface area

Stroke Index (SI)

Normal = 30 to 60 ml/beat/m^2
SI = Cardiac index/heart rate

Stroke Work Index (SWI)

LVSWI Normal = 56 ± 6 g-m/m^2
LVSWI = (MAP – PAWP) × SI × 0.0136
RVSWI Normal = 6 ± 0.9 g-m/m^2
RVSW = (PAM – CVP) × SI × 0.0136
Where
LV = left ventricular
RV = right ventricular
CVP = central venous pressure
MAP = mean arterial pressure
PAM = pulmonary artery mean (pressure)
PAWP = pulmonary artery wedge pressure
SI = stroke index
0.0136 = conversion factor for pressure to work (measured in grams)

Systemic Vascular Resistance Index (SVRI)*
SVRI = MAP – CVP/CI × 80

Normal = 800-1600 dynes/sec/cm^{-5} or 10-15 Woods units/m^2 infants;
15-20 Woods units/m^2 1-2 yr;
15-30 Woods units/m^2 child/adolescent
Where
MAP = mean arterial pressure
CVP = central venous pressure
CI = cardiac index

Pulmonary Vascular Resistance Index
(PVRI) PVRI = PAM – PAWP(or LAP)/CI × 80

Normal = 80-240 dynes/sec/cm^{-5} or 1-3 Woods units/m^2 >8 wk old;
8-10 Woods units/m^2 <8 wk old
Where
PAM = pulmonary artery mean (pressure)
PAWP = pulmonary artery wedge pressure
CI = cardiac index
LAP = left atrial pressure

From Curley M. A. Q., & Moloney-Harmon, P. A. (2001). *Critical care nursing of infants and children.* Philadelphia: WB Saunders.
*Vascular resistance can be expressed as dynes/sec/cm^{-5} or Woods units. Dynes/sec/cm^{-5} are primarily used in the ICU and Woods units in the cardiac catheterization laboratory. Dynes/sec/cm^{-5} can be converted to Woods units by dividing by 80.

BOX 22-5 Invasive Hemodynamic Monitoring Techniques

Peripheral Arterial Line

- Measures arterial blood pressure
- Used to assess cardiac output, intravascular volume status, and peripheral vascular resistance

Central Venous Line

- Measurement of venous oxygen saturation Svo_2 (oxygen saturation of blood returning to the heart)
- Used to assesses oxygen delivery and extraction
- Measurement of central venous pressure
- Used to estimate intravascular volume status and peripheral vascular resistance

Pulmonary Artery Catheter

- Measure of cardiac output and cardiac index
- Measures central venous pressure
- Measures pulmonary and peripheral vascular resistance
- Measures Svo_2 and calculates oxygen availability and consumption

Management of Cardiovascular Dysfunction. Support of cardiovascular function includes the administration of intravenous fluid and transfusion of blood products to maintain intravascular volume. Cardiovascular function is maintained through the administration of positive inotropic agents (increase myocardial contractile force), positive chronotropic agents (increase heart rate), and vasopressors (increase peripheral vascular resistance). Table 22-8 describes pharmacologic therapy used in shock. Correction of hypocalcemia, acidosis, and hypoglycemia will improve myocardial function. Arteriovenous extracorporeal membrane oxygenation (ECMO) can be applied in exceptional cases of refractory heart failure. During arteriovenous ECMO, circulation and oxygenation of the blood are entirely supported by a circuit that is outside of the body (Chang, 1999; Parker, 1998).

Assessment of the Respiratory System. The child in respiratory failure will exhibit tachypnea and, depending on the cause of respiratory failure, may have adventitious breath sounds such as crackles or decreased breath sounds on physical examination. Evaluation of blood gases provides information regarding the ability of the lungs to perform oxygenation and ventilation. In most cases of respiratory failure, there are both abnormalities of oxygenation and ventilation. Decreased oxygenation secondary to respiratory failure contributes greatly to inadequate oxygen delivery to cells.

Respiratory variables measured in mechanically ventilated children include mean airway pressure as an indication of lung compliance and the degree of positive end-expiratory pressure (PEEP) required for increased functional residual capacity. Mean arterial pressure and PEEP requirements are used to determine the severity of respiratory insufficiency. The amount of supplemental oxygen needed to maintain the Pao_2 is used to gauge respiratory function (see Box 22-1 for diagnostic criteria for ARDS) (Davis et al., 1993; Fackler et al., 1996; Johannigman, Campbell, Branson, & Hurst, 1999; Regel et al., 1996; Simms, 1999; Timmons et al., 1995; Verbrugge et al., 1997).

Management of Respiratory Dysfunction. Supplemental oxygen administration and mechanical venti-

TABLE 22-8 **Pharmacologic Therapy Used in Shock**

Drug	Site of Action	Dosage (μg/kg/min)	Primary Effect*	Secondary Effect
Dopamine	Dopaminergic Dopaminergic and β_1 α	2-5 2-10 10-20	Increase renal perfusion Inotropy Chronotropy Increase renal perfusion Vasoconstriction	Arrhythmias
Norepinephrine	$\alpha > \beta$	2-10	Vasoconstriction Inotropy	$>MVO_2$ Arrhythmias <Renal BF
Epinephrine	α and β	0.05-1.5	Vasoconstriction Inotropy Chronotropy	$>MVO_2$ Arrhythmias <Renal BF
Dobutamine	β_1	5-20	Inotropy	Tachycardia Arrhythmias Vasodilation Hypotension
Sodium nitroprusside	NA	0.5-10 (light sensitive)	Vasodilation (balanced)	<PVR $>\dot{V}/\dot{Q}$ mismatch Cyanide toxicity
Nitroglycerin	NA	0.2-20	Vasodilation (venous)	<PVR >ICP
Amrinone	NA	5-10 (load with up to 3 mg/kg over 20 min)	Inotropy Vasodilation	Arrhythmias <PVR Thrombocytopenia
Milrinone	NA	0.75-1.0 (load with 75 μg/kg over 20 min)	Inotropy Vasodilation Improves diastolic function	Arrhythmias <PVR

From Curley M. A. Q., & Moloney-Harmon, P. A. (2001). *Critical care nursing of infants and children.* Philadelphia: WB Saunders.
BF, Blood flow; *ICP,* intracranial pressure; *MVO_2,* myocardial oxygen consumption; *NA,* no specific receptor; *PVR,* pulmonary vascular resistance; $\dot{V}/\dot{Q}$, ventilation/perfusion.
*Difficult to predict the dose-response effect. Management requires individual titration at the bedside.

lation are the major forms of support for the child with respiratory failure. As previously described, respiratory failure caused by ARDS is common in patients who have experienced shock and SIRS secondary to trauma. Management of ARDS includes both conventional mechanical ventilation and nonconventional support, such as inverse inspiration/exhalation ratio, high PEEP, permissive hypercapnia, and oscillation or high-frequency ventilation. ARDS can be treated with inhalation of NO to promote vasodilation of the pulmonary vasculature for improved ventilation/perfusion matching. In addition, exogenous surfactant instillation can be used to treat abnormalities in surfactant production associated with ARDS. ECMO can be applied in exceptional cases of refractory respiratory failure. During ECMO, oxygenation of the blood is performed by a circuit external to the body (Davis et al., 1993; Fackler et al., 1996; Marini, 1998; Regel et al., 1996; Simms, 1999; Timmons et al., 1995; Verbrugge et al., 1997). Table 22-9 summarizes therapies used to treat respiratory failure and ARDS.

Organ System–Specific Care

Detailed discussions of specific organ system dysfunction and failure are beyond the scope of this text. Textbooks of critical care nursing and medicine provide extensive information regarding the management of different forms of organ system failure. The following provides an overview of the findings of physical examination, important studies, and the most essential components of treating various organ system problems. Emphasis is placed on describing key signs of dysfunction and the most important aspects of supportive care. The cardiovascular and respiratory systems were presented in the discussion of oxygen delivery.

Renal Dysfunction

Renal insufficiency presents with a decrease in urine output (less than 0.5 ml/kg/hr). Progressive renal insufficiency can result in cessation of urine production or oliguria. Monitoring urine output for a trend suggestive of decreasing urine production is essential in the care of the child with potential or actual shock and SIRS. Urine output is a sensitive indicator of cardiac output. Indwelling bladder drainage catheters are usually placed in severely injured children to accurately monitor urine production (Morgan-Madder & Milberger, 1996).

Increases in blood urea nitrogen (BUN) and serum creatinine suggest renal insufficiency. An elevated BUN with a normal or only slightly elevated creatinine is suggestive of

TABLE 22-9 Treatment of Respiratory Failure/Acute Respiratory Distress Syndrome

Therapy	Rationale
Conventional mechanical ventilation	• Takes over work of breathing • Supports oxygenation and ventilation • Supplies supplemental oxygen • May need to use high mean airway pressure which can result in barotrauma/volutrauma to the lungs
High positive end-expiratory pressure	• Increased functional residual capacity • Prevents atelectasis/improves airway compliance • Improves oxygenation
Inverse inhalation-to-exhalation ratio	• Improves oxygenation and recruitment of alveoli
Oscillation and high-frequency ventilation	• Takes over work of breathing • Supports oxygenation and ventilation • Theoretically allows for lower mean airway pressures and decreased barotrauma/volutrauma to lungs
Nitric oxide	• Dilates pulmonary vasculature to promote matching of ventilation and perfusion • Improved oxygenation and ventilation
Surfactant instillation	• Replaces deficient and dysfunctional surfactant • Prevents atelectasis/improves airway compliance
Permissive hypercarbia	• Allowing for elevated carbon dioxide levels uses ventilator settings that reduce the risk of barotrauma/volutrauma to the lungs
Extracorporeal membrane oxygenation	• Takes over oxygenation • Some techniques can also remove carbon dioxide • Prevents barotrauma/volutrauma to lungs • Can also support circulation • Multiple associated risks include stroke, infection, and hemorrhage

hypovolemia. Increased urine specific gravity (greater than 1.020) is also an indicator of hypovolemia. Children with severe renal failure may exhibit signs of volume overload and may have hypertension. Increased bodily edema can be suggestive of severe renal failure. Management of renal failure often requires the application of continuous venovenous hemofiltration (CVVH) or continuous arteriovenous hemofiltration (CAVH). In the child with an unstable circulatory status, CVVH or CAVH is preferred over conventional hemodialysis because these techniques allow slow and controlled removal of fluid and electrolytes (Curley, 2001; Hand et al., 1996; Morgan-Madder & Milberger, 1996; Vincent, 1996).

Serum electrolytes must be monitored closely in children with potential or actual renal insufficiency. Hyperkalemia and hypocalcemia are important electrolyte abnormalities associated with renal insufficiency. Hyperkalemia may precipitate cardiac arrest. Performance of an electrocardiogram to evaluate for peaked T waves, which indicate the effects of hyperkalemia on the heart, is an important surveillance step in the care of the child with renal insufficiency. Hyperkalemia can be treated with sodium polystyrene sulfonate and/or insulin and glucose infusions. Hypocalcemia may cause seizures and myocardial depression and can be treated with intravenous calcium supplementation (Curley, 2001; Hand et al., 1996; Morgan-Madder & Milberger, 1996; Vincent, 1996).

Renal insufficiency may disrupt acid-base balance. A serum pH of less than 7.2 indicates significant acidosis. Acidosis decreases myocardial contractility. Acidosis secondary to renal insufficiency is treated with bicarbonate replacement (Curley, 2001; Hand et al., 1996; Morgan-Madder & Milberger, 1996).

Hepatic Dysfunction

An elevation in serum liver enzymes, particularly transaminases (aspartate aminotransferase and alanine aminotransferase), which represent hepatocyte function, indicates hepatic disease. Hepatic dysfunction results in decreased protein synthesis. Replacement of important proteins is essential to the care of the child with hepatic dysfunction. Children with hepatic dysfunction require the administration of albumin to maintain serum oncotic pressure and fresh frozen plasma or cryoprecipitate to replace clotting factors. Albumin levels, prothrombin time (PT), and partial thromboplastin time (PTT) need to be followed. Monitoring for hypotension and increased bodily edema, such as ascites, is important for the identification of fluid losses. Assessing for ecchymosis, petechiae, or excessive bleeding from sites of vascular catheters aids in the identification of coagulopathy (Furuta et al., 1996; Martin, 1992).

Hepatic failure can lead to encephalopathy. Hyperammonemia secondary to liver failure is a known cause of encephalopathy. Ammonia levels should be followed, but ammonia level is not directly related to the severity of encephalopathy. Other, unidentified toxins associated with liver failure also cause hepatic encephalopathy. Serial neurologic examinations must be used in the care of the child with

BOX 22-6 Signs of Elevated Intracranial Pressure

- Decreased level of consciousness
- Decreased pupil reactivity to light
- Impaired lateral and upward gaze
- Bradycardia
- Hypertension
- Changes in respiratory pattern

(Bradycardia, Hypertension, Changes in respiratory pattern: Cushing's triad)

liver failure to identify encephalopathy and signs of intracranial hypertension associated with cerebral edema (Box 22-6). Occasionally, severe hepatic failure with significant coagulopathy and encephalopathy is treated with plasmapheresis (Furuta et al., 1996; Martin, 1992).

Hepatic failure results in disrupted carbohydrate metabolism. Lack of gluconeogenesis may result in hypoglycemia. Because infants have decreased glycogen stores, they are particularly prone to hypoglycemia. Serum glucose should be monitored closely in the child with hepatic dysfunction (Martin, 1992).

Gastrointestinal Dysfunction and Pancreatitis

Preservation of GI integrity through the delivery of enteral nutrition was discussed previously. Prevention of gastritis and stress ulcers associated with shock and SIRS is accomplished with the administration of antacids. Histamine-2 (H_2) blockers such as ranitidine are commonly used antacids. There is evidence suggesting that alkalinizing gastric contents allows for overgrowth of bacteria and may increase the risk of aspiration pneumonia. Results of investigations of the incidence of aspiration pneumonia secondary to the use of antacids are conflicting. At present, many clinicians believe the risk of developing a stress ulcer outweighs the risk of aspiration pneumonia. However, the gastric coating agent sucralfate can be used instead of an antacid in older children (Furuta et al., 1996; Stechmiller et al., 1997; Vincent, 1997).

Assessment of the GI tract includes serial examinations of the abdomen and testing of stool, vomitus, and nasogastric tube drainage for blood. Treatment of identified GI bleeding includes the administration of antacids or sucralfate, placement of a nasogastric tube, and lavage. In severe cases of GI bleeding, endoscopy is performed to isolate and cauterize the site of blood loss. Hemoglobin level should be monitored closely in the child with actual or potential GI bleeding (Furuta et al., 1996).

Pancreatitis is an additional problem of the GI system that can occur in the trauma patient. Signs of pancreatitis include epigastric pain and vomiting. An ileus may also be present. Serum levels of the pancreatic enzymes amylase and lipase are elevated in cases of pancreatitis. In addition, pancreatitis may cause hypocalcemia and hypoglycemia. Holding enteral fluid, nutrition, and medications (when possible) is the treatment for pancreatitis (Furuta et al., 1996).

Neurologic Dysfunction

It is important to perform serial neurologic examinations on the child who is at risk for or is experiencing shock and SIRS. Decreased level of consciousness indicates poor cerebral perfusion related to circulatory failure. The child with preexisting head injury may already be receiving therapies to reduce intracranial pressure. Signs of elevated intracranial pressure are presented in Box 22-6. Elevated intracranial pressure is typically managed with elevation of the head, support of blood pressure, normocarbia, and in severe cases, hyperosmolar fluid and/or diuretic administration. The child who develops HIE because of poor cerebral perfusion may receive these therapies. The development of HIE in the patient with shock and SIRS after trauma is ominous. Children in whom DI develops are treated with fluid replacement and vasopressin (Haun et al., 1996; Lee et al., 1996).

Hematologic Dysfunction/Disseminated Intravascular Coagulation

The management of DIC is variable. Heparin is often used to enhance the effects of antithrombin III (AT-III) and inactivate thrombin. Inactivation of thrombin prevents vascular occlusion and further cellular injury and limits further consumption of coagulation factors. However, if thrombin formation accelerates because of persistent SIRS, AT-III is depleted and heparin is no longer therapeutic. The administration of exogenous AT-III is a potential treatment for DIC and is currently under investigation (Penner, 1998).

Protein factors that promote coagulation are eventually depleted in DIC, and then a state of hypocoagulation exists. As clotting factors are depleted, replacement with fresh frozen plasma is necessary to promote hemostasis. Fibrinogen, the precursor to thrombin, is also depleted. Cryoprecipitate can be administered to replenish serum fibrinogen levels. In addition, platelet aggregation is heightened during DIC and may ultimately lead to platelet consumption and thrombocytopenia. Transfusions of platelets are used to correct thrombocytopenia (Penner, 1998).

The child with potential or actual DIC must be monitored closely for signs of coagulopathy, such as ecchymosis and petechiae of the skin and excessive bleeding from intravascular catheter sites. Hemoglobin levels should be followed closely to identify anemia from blood loss. Platelet count, PT, PTT, and fibrinogen levels and the presence of fibrin split products and elevated D-dimer (generated by clot degeneration) are followed closely to track the progression of DIC. In fulminant DIC, platelet count is low, PT and PTT are prolonged, fibrinogen level is low, fibrin split products are present, and D-dimer level is elevated (Penner, 1998).

SUMMARY

Caring for children in whom MODS develops after traumatic injury requires knowledge of complex pathophysiology, astute assessment skills, and expert collaborative management. MODS is precipitated in the pediatric trauma victim by shock and the development of a systemic inflammatory response.

Care is directed at preventing the sequelae of the inflammatory response, which result in disruption of cellular processes. Nursing's important contribution to care will enhance the child's potential for a good outcome.

BIBLIOGRAPHY

American College of Chest Physicians and the Society of Critical Care Medicine. (1992). American College of Chest Physicians/Society of Critical Care Medicine consensus conference: Definitions for sepsis and organ failure and guidelines for the use of innovative therapies in sepsis. *Critical Care Medicine, 20,* 864-875.

Baue, A. E., Durham, R. M., & Mazuski, J. E. (1996). Clinical trials of new and novel therapeutic agents. *World Journal of Surgery, 20*(4), 493-498.

Bengmark, S., & Gianotti, L. (1996). Nutritional support to prevent and treat multiple organ failure. *World Journal of Surgery, 20*(4), 474-481.

Bengur, A. R., & Meliones, J. N. (1998). Cardiogenic shock. *New Horizons, 6*(2), 139-150.

Berney, T., Belli, D., Bugmann, P., Beghetti, M., Morel, P., & LeCoultre, C. (1996). Influence of severe underlying pathology and hypovolemic shock on the development of acute pancreatitis in children. *Journal of Pediatric Surgery, 31*(9), 1256-1261.

Bone, R. (1996). Immunologic dissonance: A continuing evolution in our understanding of systemic inflammatory response syndrome (SIRS) and the multiple organ dysfunction syndrome (MODS). *Annals of Internal Medicine, 125*(8), 680-687.

Border, J. (1995). Death from severe trauma; open fractures to multiple organ dysfunction syndrome. *Journal of Trauma: Injury, Infections and Critical Care, 39*(1), 12-22.

Casado-Flores, J., Mora, E., Perez-Corral, R., Martinez-Azagra, A., Garcia-Teresa, M., & Ruiz-Lopex, M. (1998). Prognostic value of gastric intramucosal pH in critically ill children. *Critical Care Medicine, 26*(6), 1123-1127.

Chang, M. (1999). Monitoring of the critically injured patient. *New Horizons, 7*(1), 35-45.

Cornwell, E. E., Kennedy, F., & Rodriquez, J. (1996). The critical care of severely injured patients: Assessing and improving oxygen delivery. *Surgical Clinics of North America, 76*(4), 959-969.

Craig, J., Smith, J. B., & Fineman, L. D. (2001). Tissue perfusion. In M. A. Q. Curley & P. A. Moloney-Harmon (Eds.), *Critical care nursing of infants and children* (2nd ed., pp. 131-232). Philadelphia: WB Saunders.

Curley, M. (2001). Shock. In M. A. Curley, J. B. Smith, & P. A. Moloney-Harmon (Eds.), *Critical care nursing of infants and children* (pp. 921-946). Philadelphia: WB Saunders.

Davies, M., & Hagen, P. (1997). Systemic inflammatory response syndrome. *British Journal of Surgery, 84*(7), 920-935.

Davis, S. L., Furman, D. P., & Costario, A. J. (1993). Adult respiratory distress syndrome in children: Associated disease, clinical course and predictors of death. *Journal of Pediatrics, 123,* 35-45.

Davis, J., Kaups, K., & Parks, S. (1998). Base deficit is superior to pH in evaluating clearance of acidosis after traumatic shock. *Journal of Trauma: Injury, Infections and Critical Care, 44*(1), 114-118.

Deitch, E. (1990). Multiple organ failure: Summary and overview. In E. Deitch (Ed.), *Multiple organ failure* (pp. 285-299). New York: Thieme Medical Publishers.

Division of Injury Control, Center for Environmental Health and Injury Control, Centers for Disease Control. (1990). Childhood injuries in the United States. *American Journal of Diseases of Children, 144,* 627-646.

Duke, T., Butt, W., & South, M. (1997). Predictors of mortality and multiple organ failure in children with sepsis. *Intensive Care Medicine, 23,* 684-692.

Fackler, J., Arnold, J., Nichols, D., & Rogers, M. (1996). In M. Rodgers (Ed.), *Textbook of pediatric intensive care* (3rd ed., pp. 197-234). Baltimore: Williams & Wilkins.

Ferguson, A. (1996). Gastric tonometry: Evaluating tissue oxygenation. *Critical Care Nurse, 16*(6), 48-55.

Flowers, F., & Zimmerman, J. (1998) Reactive oxygen species in the cellular pathophysiology of shock. *New Horizons, 6*(2), 170-180.

Furuta, G., Rogers, E., & Leichtner, A. (1996). Gastrointestinal and hepatic failure in the pediatric intensive care unit. In M. Rogers (Ed.), *Textbook of pediatric intensive care* (3rd ed., pp. 1163-1192). Baltimore: Williams & Wilkins.

Gando, S., Kameue, T., Nanzaki, S., Hayakawa, T., & Nakanishi, Y. (1997). Participation of tissue factor and thrombin in posttraumatic systemic inflammatory syndrome. *Critical Care Medicine, 25*(11), 1820-1826.

Gando, S., Kameue, T., Nanzaki, S., & Nakanishi, Y. (1996). Disseminated intravascular coagulation is a frequent complication of systemic inflammatory response syndrome. *Thrombosis and Haemostasis, 75*(2), 224-228.

Guirao, X., & Lowry, S. F. (1996). Biologic control of injury and inflammation: Much more than too little or too late. *World Journal of Surgery, 20*(4), 437-446.

Gullo, A., & Berlot, M. D. (1996). Ingredients of organ system dysfunction or failure. *World Journal of Surgery, 20*(4), 430-436.

Hand, M., Harmon, W., & McManus, M. (1996) Renal disorders in pediatric intensive care. In M. Rogers (Ed.), *Textbook of pediatric intensive care* (3rd ed., pp. 1217-1246). Baltimore: Williams & Wilkins.

Harris, B., & Gelfand, J. (1995). The immune response to trauma. *Seminars in Pediatric Surgery, 4*(2), 77-82.

Haun, S., Kirsch, J., & Dean, J. M. (1996). Theories of brain resuscitation. In M. Rogers (Ed.), *Textbook of pediatric intensive care* (3rd ed., pp. 699-734). Baltimore: Williams & Wilkins.

Jalonen, J. (1997). Invasive hemodynamic monitoring: Concepts and practical approaches. *Annals of Medicine, 29*(4), 313-318.

Johannigman, J., Campbell, R., Branson, R., & Hurst, J. (1999) Ventilatory support of the critically injured patient. *New Horizons, 7*(1), 116-129.

Johnson, K. D., Cadambi, A., & Seibert, B. (1985). Incidence of adult respiratory distress syndrome in patients with multiple skeletal injuries: Effect of early operative stabilization. *Journal of Trauma, 25,* 375.

Kirton, O., & Civetta, J. (1999) Ischemia-reperfusion injury in the critically ill: A progenitor of multiple organ failure. *New Horizons, 7*(1), 87-95.

Kirton, O., Windsor, J., Wedderburn, R., Hudson-Civetta, J., Shartz, D., & Mataragas, N. (1998). Failure of splanchnic resuscitation in the acutely injured trauma patient correlates with multiple organ system failure and length of stay in the ICU. *Chest, 113*(4), 1064-1069.

Lee, Y., Hunang, F., Shen, E., Kao, H., Ho, M., & Shyur, S. (1996). Neurogenic diabetes insipidus in children with hypoxic encephalopathy: Six new cases and a review of the literature. *European Journal of Pediatrics, 155*(3), 245-248.

Lennie, T. (1997). The metabolic response to injury: Current perspectives and nursing implications. *Dimensions of Critical Care Nursing, 16*(2), 78-87.

Marini, J. J. (1998). A lung-protective approach to ventilating ARDS. *Respiratory Care Clinics of North America, 4*(4), 633-663.

Martin, S. A. (1992). The ABCs of pediatric LFTs. *Pediatric Nursing, 18*(5), 445-449.

McMahon, K. (1995). Multiple organ failure: The final complication of critical illness. *Critical Care Nurse, 15*(6), 20-30.

Moloney-Harmon, P., & Adams, P. (2001). Trauma. In M. A. Curley, P. A. Moloney-Harmon (Eds.), *Critical care nursing of infants and children* (pp. 947-980). Philadelphia: WB Saunders.

Moore, F., Sauaia, A., Moore, E., Haenel, J., Burch, J., & Lezotte, D. (1996). Postinjury multiple organ failure: A bimodal phenomenon. *Journal of Trauma: Injury, Infections and Critical Care, 40*(4), 510-512.

Morgan, W., & O'Neill, J. (1998). Hemorrhagic and obstructive shock in pediatric patients. *New Horizons, 6*(2), 150-154.

Morgan-Madder, S., & Milberger, P. M. (1996). Renal critical care problems. In M. A. Curley, J. B. Smith, & P. A. Moloney-Harmon (Eds.), *Critical care nursing of infants and children* (pp. 695-723). Philadelphia: WB Saunders.

Nathens, A. B., & Marshall, J. C. (1996). Sepsis, SIRS and MODS: What's in a name? *World Journal of Surgery, 20*(4), 386-391.

Nast-Kolb, D., Waydhas, C., Gippner-Steppert, C., Schneider, I., Trupka, A., & Ruchholtz, S. (1997). Indicators of posttraumatic inflammatory response correlate with organ failure in patients with multiple injuries. *Journal of Trauma, 42*(3), 446-454.

Neidhardt, R., Keel, M., Steckholzer, U., Safret, A., Ungethuem, U., & Trentz, O. (1997). Relationship of interleukin-10 plasma levels to severity of injury and clinical outcome in injured patients. *Journal of Trauma: Injury, Infections and Critical Care, 42*(5), 863-871.

Orliaguet, G. A., Meyer, P. G., Blanot, S., Jarreau, M., Charron, B., Buisson, C., & Carli, P. A. (1998). Predictive factors of outcome in severely traumatized children. *Anesthesia and Analgesia, 87*(3), 537-542.

Parker, M. (1998). Pathophysiology of cardiovascular dysfunction in septic shock. *New Horizons, 6*(2), 130-138.

Penner, J. (1998). Disseminated intravascular coagulation in patients with multiple organ failure of non-specific origin. *Seminars in Thrombosis and Hemostasis, 24*(1), 45-52.

Peruzzi, W. T., & Martin, M. (1995). Oxygen transport. *Respiratory Care Clinics of North America, 1*(1), 23-34.

Pulmonary Artery Catheter consensus conference: Consensus statement. (1997). *Critical Care Medicine, 25*(60), 910.

Regel, G., Grotz, M., Weltner, T., Sturm, J. A., & Tscherne, H. (1996). Pattern of organ system failure following severe trauma. *World Journal of Surgery, 20*(4), 422-429.

Sanders, C. L. (1997). Making clinical decisions using Svo_2 in PICU patients. *Dimensions in Critical Care Nursing, 16*(5), 257-264.

Sauaia, A., Moore, F. A., Moore, E. E., & Lezotte, D. C. (1996). Early risk factors for postinjury multiple organ failure. *World Journal of Surgery, 20*(4), 392-400.

Sax, H. C. (1993). Can early enteral feeding reduce postoperative sepsis and multiple organ failure? A review of recent studies. *Journal of Critical Care Nutrition, 1*, 5-14.

Schlag, G., & Redl, H. (1996). Mediators of injury and inflammation. *World Journal of Surgery, 20*(4), 406-410.

Simms, H. H. (1999). Mechanisms of immune suppression in critically ill patients. *New Horizons, 7*(1), 147-157.

Smail, N., Messiah, A., Edouard, A., Descorps-Declere, A., Duranteau, J., & Vigue, B. (1995). Role of systemic inflammatory response syndrome and infection in the occurrence of early multiple organ dysfunction syndrome following severe trauma. *Intensive Care Medicine, 21*(10), 813-816.

Spack, L., Hvens, P., & Griffith, O. (1997). Measurements of total plasma nitrite and nitrate in pediatric patients with the systemic inflammatory response syndrome. *Critical Care Medicine, 25*(6), 1071-1078.

Stechmiller, J. K., Treloar, D., & Allen, N. (1997). Gut dysfunction in ill patients: A review of the literature. *American Journal of Critical Care, 6*(3), 204-209.

Swank, G. M., & Deitch, E. A. (1996). Role of gut in multiple organ failure: Bacterial translocation and permeability changes. *World Journal of Surgery, 20*(4), 411-417.

Thompson, M. (1997). Pulmonary artery catheterization in children. *New Horizons, 5*(3), 244-250.

Timmons, O. D., Havens, P. L., & Fackler, J. C. (1995). Predicting death in patients with acute respiratory failure. *Chest, 108*, 789.

Tobin, J., & Wetzel, R. (1996). Shock and multi-organ system failure. In M. Rogers (Ed.), *Textbook of pediatric intensive care* (3rd ed., pp. 555-606). Baltimore: Williams & Wilkins.

Tuit, P. K. (1997). Recognition and management of shock in the pediatric patient. *Critical Care Nursing Quarterly, 20*(1), 52-61.

Ushay, H., & Notterman, D. (1997). Pharmacology of pediatric resuscitation. *Pediatric Clinics of North America, 44*(1), 207-233.

Verbrugge, S., Sorm, V., & Lachmann, B. (1997). Mechanisms of acute respiratory distress syndrome: Role of surfactant changes and mechanical ventilation. *Journal of Physiology and Pharmacology, 48*(4), 537-557.

Vincent, J. (1996). Prevention and therapy of multiple organ failure. *World Journal of Surgery, 20*(4), 465-470.

Wichmann, M. W., Ayala, A., & Chaudry, I. H. (1998). Severe depression of host immune functions following closed-bone fracture, soft tissue trauma and hemorrhagic shock. *Critical Care Medicine, 26*(8), 1372-1379.

Wong, H. R., Carcillo, J. A., Burckhart, G., & Kaplan, S. S. (1996). Nitric oxide production in critically ill patients. *Archives of Diseases in Childhood, 74*(6), 482-489.

Yu, M. (1999). Oxygen transport optimization. *New Horizons, 7*(1), 46-53.

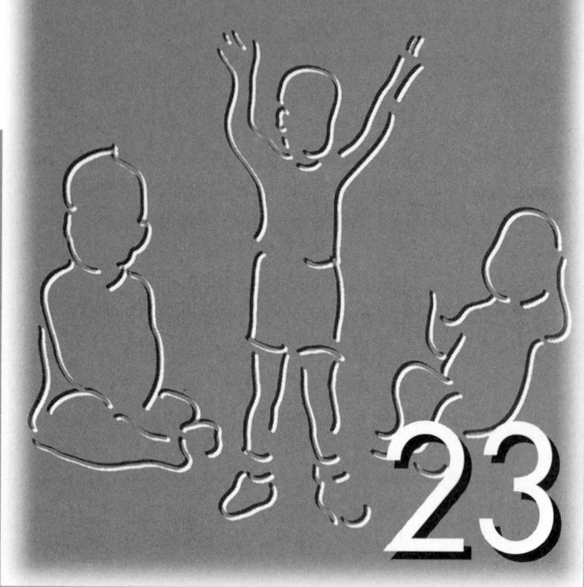

23 Psychosocial Aspects of Pediatric Trauma

Linda A. Lewandowski • Emily Frosch

Walking across the road to get the mail, Sara is hit by a speeding truck and thrown into the air as her mother and young brother watch in horror...

At a large family gathering for his mother's birthday party, 6-year-old Kevin trips over the cord of the coffee pot and scalding coffee splashes over his back, arm, and leg...

Sitting on the front porch, Devon's grandmother hears a gunshot and sees her young grandson, who was playing next to her, fall over, shot in the abdomen...

Playing in the park, little Felicia toddles over to a nearby dog and reaches for his ball; the dog growls and then attacks, sinking his teeth into her neck...

A drunk driver slams into a car carrying four teenagers to their junior prom; all are seriously injured, one is killed...

And in these moments, the world is changed forever for these children and their families and sometimes for the communities in which they live.

Nothing bad is supposed to happen to children, but sometimes bad things do happen. When the "something bad" includes a significant injury of a child, the psychological impact is often far reaching and may last long after the physical injuries have healed.

The injury of a child is a multifaceted phenomenon (Figure 23-1). The trauma associated with pediatric injury is not all physical. Psychological trauma may occur to the injured child; the child's parents, siblings, other family members, friends, or school community; the family's religious community; and the wider community, as well as to the emergency and hospital personnel who treat the child. For many the psychological effects will be acute, that is, short-term symptoms that go away in time. For others the psychological implications will be long lasting and may even become pathologic, interfering with normal functioning and development. This chapter focuses on the psychological and psychosocial implications for the injured child, family, caregivers, and community of unintentional injury and injury resulting from community violence.

RISK FACTORS FOR INJURY

Several years ago, trauma specialists advocated for changing the term *accidental injury* to *unintentional injury.* The rationale was that "accidental" implied a randomness to injury and an inability to do anything about it. To the contrary, it is known that a number of factors and characteristics place some children at greater risk for injury and that many of these factors can be identified and addressed. Numerous epidemiologic studies demonstrate that environmental determinants and psychosocial characteristics of both the child and caregiver are related to pediatric injury.

One child characteristic that increases the risk of injuries resulting from child-initiated activities (e.g., bicycling, swimming, playing) is gender. Boys are more likely than girls to be injured in these types of situations, and this gender differential increases with age (Baker, O'Neill, Ginsburg, & Li, 1992; Irwin, Cataldo, Matheny, & Peterson, 1992). In injury situations in which the child has no influence over the situation, such as motor vehicle accidents (MVAs), the male/female injury ratio is similar (Baker et al., 1992). Other child characteristics that place children at risk for injury include hyperactivity, impulsivity, lower attentiveness and adaptability, negative mood, higher aggressiveness, higher risk-taking behaviors, arrhythmic sleep habits, and previous psychological or emotional problems (Bussing, Menvielle, & Zima, 1996; Christoffel, Donovan, Schofer, Wills, & Lavigne, 1996; Irwin et al., 1992; Schwebel & Plumert, 1999; Wilson, Baker, Teret,

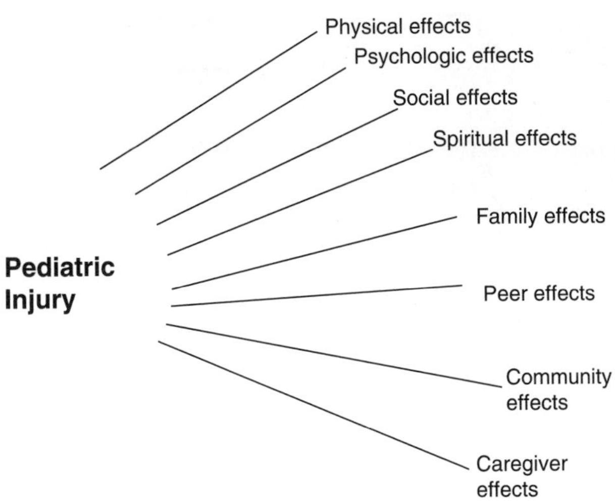

FIGURE 23-1 Effects of pediatric injury.

Shock, & Garbarino, 1991). Some developmental factors associated with pediatric injury include nonrecognition of hazards, unchecked curiosity, incomplete development of motor skills, and need for supervision (Baker et al., 1992). A number of studies have shown that a previous injury experience is a risk factor for subsequent injuries (Bijur, Golding, & Haslum, 1988; Jaquess & Finney, 1994; Kendrick, 1993). A recent study of 41,242 unintentionally injured children 0 to 15 years old who were enrolled in Medicaid found that there was a period of increased risk for unintentional injury that lasted at least 90 days after the index injury and affected not only the child who was injured but also his or her siblings (Johnston, Grossman, Connell, & Koepsell, 2000). The authors note that this effect on siblings suggests risk factors in the social or physical environment may affect all children in the family. They also note that some high-risk families may experience transient high-risk periods for childhood injury rather than existing at a permanently elevated risk. Counseling families about taking special care to prevent the possibility of another injury to a child in their family during the several months after a child's injury may be warranted.

Family-related factors that place children at higher risk for injury include low family cohesion and support, high stress, high disorganization, high conflict, less active engagement between parents and children, and parental mental illness or emotional instability (Christoffel et al., 1996; Irwin et al., 1992; Wilson et al., 1991). Children who live in low-income areas are at greater risk of being injured and dying from their injuries, as are children who live in rural areas (Baker et al., 1992; Crawley, 1996; Irwin et al., 1992; Laflamme & Diderichsen, 2000; Wilson et al., 1991). Unintentional gun-related injuries are most likely to occur when a gun is available in the home and children are left unsupervised at home (Christoffel, 1992; Crawley, 1996). Some headway has been made in decreasing some environmental hazards with mandatory car seat, seat belt, and bicycle helmet legislation. However, risk of injury increases markedly when parents or children do not follow through on the use of these safety devices.

Children's Responses to Traumatic Events

Pediatric Injury as a Traumatic Event

To develop a posttraumatic response, one must have been exposed to a traumatic event. The characteristics of a traumatic event include actual or threatened death or injury to self or another person; intense stimuli (e.g., large amounts of blood, sirens, screaming); high uncertainty and unpredictability; and a response that involves intense fear, helplessness, and/or horror (American Psychiatric Association [APA], 1994). Clearly, these characteristics are encompassed in the experience of pediatric injury. The sudden, unexpected physical assault, the frenzied pace of rescue, the actual injury and pain, the invasiveness of treatment, the overriding unpredictability and uncertainty, the presence of strangers, the strange environments (e.g., inside the ambulance, the emergency department trauma bay), the loss of control, the periods of separation from parents or significant caretakers, and the social drama all contribute to the trauma of the experience of unintentional or violent injury (Horowitz, Wilner, & Kultreider, 1980; Lewandowski & Baranoski, 1994). For injured children the "trauma" may last past the injury event itself well into the treatment period, particularly when significant pain or separation is involved.

Traumatic injury and treatment are often viewed as a "one-time" acute stressor. The reality for many families, however, is that they are dealing with multiple stressors at the same time, some of which may be intense chronic stressors (e.g., divorce and ongoing discord, poverty, exposure to community violence). The possible different reactions and needs related to a one-time acute traumatic event versus an acute traumatic event that takes place in the context of cumulative stressors is an area that needs exploration. It is important for the clinician to take into account the context of the injury event and to recognize the psychological trauma potential of the pediatric injury experience.

Possible responses of children to stressful, traumatic situations include cognitive, emotional, physiologic, and behavioral responses (Box 23-1). Family members, friends, witnesses to the injury event, emergency personnel, and hospital staff may experience similar symptoms. Many affected individuals experience some posttraumatic symptoms as described later; others will develop the full posttraumatic stress disorder (PTSD).

Posttraumatic Stress Symptoms and Disorder

PTSD has become an increasingly recognized phenomenon in adults. Although it was first associated with war experiences, it is now clear that various types of stressors may lead to this type of reaction (Figley, 1983; Fletcher, 1996). However, the recognition that children experience posttraumatic stress reactions to stressful, traumatic events is a relatively recent one (APA, 1987; Yule & Williams, 1990). Even well into the 1980s it was believed that children were not much affected by traumatic events and then not for very long (Fletcher, 1996; Garmezy & Rutter, 1985; Rigamer, 1986). Now it is known that depending on the number, nature, and

BOX 23-1 Possible Responses of Children to Acute Trauma

Cognitive

Confusion
Time distortions
Hyperalertness
Disbelief, denial
Difficulty concentrating
Difficulty problem solving
Modified sense of reality
Memories of incorrect perceptions
Persistent thoughts of the trauma
Belief/fear that another traumatic event will occur
Thought suppression
Memory problems
Misidentification of involved persons and/or hallucinations of "at fault" persons
Belief in omens and prediction
Pessimism about the future
Fear of sleeping alone
Recurrent nightmares
Fear of death; dreams of own death
Increased sensitivity to further stresses
Fear of reexperiencing traumatic anxiety
Trauma-specific and mundane fears

Emotional

Anxiety
Fear
Irritability
Decreased frustration tolerance
Guilt, shame, blaming
Anger
Depression
Grief
Fear of separation from parents or primary caretakers
Embarrassment
Avoidance, psychological numbing
Worry about physical health
Constricted affect, emotional withdrawal

Physiologic

Tendency to startle easily
Increased nervous tension
Somatic symptoms
Repetitions of psychophysiologic disturbances that began with traumatic event

Behavioral

Regressive behaviors, e.g., clinging, enuresis, thumb sucking
Fatigue
Slowness
Withdrawal into uncustomary behavior patterns
Behavioral reenactments
Posttraumatic play
Hyperactivity
Difficulty falling asleep
Nighttime awakenings
Night terrors
Inhibited, avoidant, or phobic behaviors
Conduct disturbances
Lowered school performance

From Lewandowski, L. A., & Baranoski, M. V. (1994). Psychological aspects of acute trauma: Intervening with children and families in the inpatient setting. *Child and Adolescent Clinics of North America, 3*, 513-529.

pattern of traumatic events, 27% to 100% of children develop PTSD, especially those exposed to events that are sudden, unexpected, life threatening, and violent in nature (McNally, 1993). In a meta-analysis of 2697 children from 34 samples, Fletcher (1996) reports that an average of 36% of children exposed to traumatic events were diagnosed with PTSD compared with 24% of adults based on 3495 adults from five samples (den Velde et al., 1993; Kilpatrick & Resnick, 1993; Smith & North, 1993). More children and adults develop posttraumatic symptoms than those who meet the criteria for the actual disorder (Fletcher, 1996). PTSD cannot be diagnosed until 1 month after the traumatic event (APA, 1994). If posttraumatic symptoms interfere with functioning in the first month after injury, the diagnosis of "acute stress disorder" is given (APA, 1994; Daviss, Mooney, Racusin, Ford, Fleischer, & McHugo, 2000; Robert, Meyer, Villarreal, Blakeney, Desai, & Herndon, 1999).

Although a considerable amount of literature is evolving regarding the prevalence of PTSD in children who witness violence (Cooley-Quille, Turner, & Beidel, 1995; Garbarino, 1995; Horowitz, Weine, & Jekel, 1995; Nader, Pynoos, Fairbanks, & Frederick, 1990; Osofsky, 1995; Richters, 1993), children who are injured through violence and their families have not been studied systematically in terms of posttraumatic response. There have been reports of PTSD in adults after unintentional injuries such as MVAs (Blanchard, Hickling, Taylor, Loos, & Gerardi, 1994; Blanchard, Hickling, Vollmer, Loos, Buckley, & Jaccard, 1995; Burstein, 1989; Mayou, Bryant, & Duthrie, 1993). Similar findings in injured children are only beginning to be reported (Aaron, Zaglul, & Emery, 1999; Daviss et al., 2000; deVries, Kassam-Adams, Cnaan, Sherman-Slate, Gallagher, & Winston, 1999; Jones & Peterson, 1993; Lewandowski, Berent, Frosch, & Weissberg, in press; Mirza, Bhadrinath, Goodyer, & Gilmour, 1998). A significant amount of literature on children after head injury and their families (Levi, Drotar, Yeates, & Taylor, 1999; Max et al., 1998; Rivara et al., 1993, 1994) confirms the presence of PTSD in children after injuries.

A traumatic event that affects a child can lead to traumatic responses in other family members (Kelly, 1990). Parent and family factors (such as functioning style) can determine the development of PTSD in the child (Fletcher, 1996; McFarlane, 1987; Schwarz & Perry, 1994). Children's PTSD and other behavioral symptoms after a traumatic event have been found to be correlated with parents' PTSD symptoms (Green et al., 1991). Thus intervening with parents to decrease their trauma response is an indirect way of benefitting the child.

TABLE 23-1 **Factors Affecting Children's Responses to Acute Trauma**

Factors	Implications
Developmental stage of the child	Cognitive and emotional development affect the child's perceptions, understanding, and coping ability.
Cause of the trauma	Child's interpretation of cause of trauma (e.g., self, other, nature, unknown) influences meaning of and coping with event; violent acts further undermine trust in others and view of world as safe and controllable.
Reactions of parents/significant others	For young children, emotional empathy anxiety transmission, and social referencing are key in determining child's reaction; for older children, a supportive stance vs. guilt-inducing, blaming, angry stance is important.
Child's perception/understanding/ appraisal of the trauma	Have implications for shaping child's self and world view. Adult objective view may be of little or no relevance to child's view of the trauma.
Pain/anxiety/sleep deprivation	Influence child's ability to process, understand, and cope. May lower frustration tolerance sap energy, and deprive child of psychological focus for working through.
Available situational support	Supportive adults, peers, and environment mitigate stresses of traumatic situations.
Number and type of other stressess recently experienced	Psychological risk for child may be higher if family has experienced recent stressors or many daily hassles.
Acute or chronic nature of the injury	Children with long-term or chronic losses, disfigurements, or disabilities face additional body image, self-concept, and functional issues.
Injury or death of family member due to same traumatic event	Grief, guilt, blame, and worry about others increase child's psychological burden. Added family disruption may decrease support available to the child.
Community/societal response	Public attention and response (support, outrage) may influence impact of trauma on the child and family.
Preexisting psychological problems	May influence vulnerability and response of child and family.

From Lewandowski, L. A., & Baranoski, M. V. (1994). Psychological aspects of acute trauma: Intervening with children and families in the inpatient setting. *Child and Adolescent Clinics of North America, 3,* 513-529.

Both adults and children respond to traumatic events with three types of symptoms: reexperiencing, avoidance of stimuli associated with the trauma, and increased arousal (APA, 1994). Reexperiencing phenomena demonstrate that elements of the traumatic experience remain active in the individual's mental life. They include intrusive thoughts, images, and perceptions; behavioral reenactments; distressing dreams; and physiological reactivity to cues that remind the individual of the trauma (Pynoos & Nader, 1993). Avoidance of associated stimuli and a psychological numbing both indicate efforts to restrict or regulate emotions or behavior in an attempt to control recurrent impressions and the associated affect (Pynoos & Nader, 1993). Examples of these symptoms include avoidance of thoughts, feelings, places, and people associated with the trauma; memory disturbances; decreased interest or participation in usual activities; feelings of detachment or estrangement from others; a restricted range of affect; and a sense of a foreshortened future (APA, 1994). Hyperarousal symptoms, consistent with increased sympathetic nervous system activity, are thought to be less common in children than in adults (McNally, 1993; Putnam, 1996). They include hypervigilance, exaggerated startle response, difficulty concentrating, irritability or outbursts of anger, and difficulty falling or staying asleep (APA, 1994).

Several studies have found a "hidden morbidity" in pediatric trauma (Harris, Schwaitzberg, Seman, & Herrmann, 1989) that manifests even years after the injury event. The morbidity consists of not only physical disability but also changes in cognition, personality, behavior, and family functioning (Emanuelson, vonWendt, Beckung, & Hagberg, 1998; Hu, Wesson, Kenney, Chipman, & Spence, 1993; Wesson, Scorpio, Spence, Filler, Armstrong, & Pearl, 1989; Wesson et al., 1992).

Factors Affecting Children's Responses: Risk and Protective Factors

As noted earlier, not all children and family members develop significant negative symptoms after a pediatric injury. A number of factors have been identified as affecting children's responses to trauma. Some of these factors are summarized in Table 23-1. Considerable attention in recent years has been given not only to children who show major upset after traumatic events but also to children who experience some sort of trauma and adversity but who are able to integrate the difficult experience into their lives without experiencing significant symptoms and disruption in functioning (Rutter, 1987). Studies of the children who "do well" have led to the concept of *resiliency.* These studies have identified various factors, termed *risk factors,* that appear to make children and families more vulnerable to negative reactions after stressful or traumatic events. *Protective factors* work just the opposite. They appear to act as buffers or protectors for the child or family member, thus decreasing the long-term negative impact of the event. A number of risk and protective factors have been identified in studies of injured children and their families and in studies of children and families coping with other types of traumatic events.

Risk Factors

It has been noted that posttraumatic psychological distress influences most aspects of everyday life and may have a significant negative effect on everyday functioning (Norman, 1989; Richmond, 1997). Perceived life threat, intrusive horrific memories, and early avoidance of traumatic reminders have been identified as predictors of PTSD in children (Mayou et al., 1993). Poverty, poor preinjury family functioning, family conflict and disorganization, preexisting mental health problems in the child or parent, and the presence of traumatic brain injury have been identified as other possible risk factors (Garmezy & Rutter, 1985; Rutter 1987; Stancin, Taylor, Thompson, Wade, Drotar, & Yeates, 1998). Individuals who dissociate during the traumatic experience have been found to be at higher risk for the later development of PTSD (Putnam, 1997; Shalev, Peri, Canetti, & Schreiber, 1996). Injury severity has not consistently been identified as a predictor of subsequent dysfunction (deVries et al., 1999; Malt et al., 1993), although several studies of children with head injuries have identified injury severity as a risk factor. Extent of injury, fear of death, preexisting depression, and active litigation regarding the crash predicted PTSD in adults after an MVA (Blanchard & Hickling, 1997). Prior psychopathology, high levels of parental distress, parental PTSD, greater thought suppression, prior sexual abuse, older child age, and female gender have been found to be predictors of PTSD in children after MVAs (deVries et al., 1999; Mirza et al., 1998) and other types of pediatric injury (Aaron et al., 1999; Daviss et al., 2000).

Protective Factors

Family cohesion, absence of marital discord, presence of a supportive adult, consistent social support, religious participation, and higher intelligence have been repeatedly demonstrated to mitigate the impact of negative life events and to serve as significant protective factors (Garmezy, 1985, 1987; Garmezy & Rutter, 1985; Rutter, 1987; Tennant, 1988). Immediate intervention may reduce the negative impact of traumatic events (Galante & Foa, 1986; Gislason & Call, 1982; Pynoos & Nader, 1993; Terr 1989).

Special Injury Situations

Motor Vehicle Accidents

MVA is the most common cause of unintentional injury in children (deVries et al., 1999). However, despite the frequency of these events, there have been few empirical data about the mental health sequelae of MVA until recently. More attention has been focused on adults injured in MVA. These studies found that up to 40% of adults injured in MVAs develop PTSD after the event. The adults may show other psychiatric symptoms, including depression and travel avoidance/distress (Blanchard et al., 1994, 1995; Burstein, 1989; Mayou et al., 1993; Taylor & Koch, 1995). Initial studies have found the prevalence of PTSD in children after traffic injuries to be about 25% to 28% at 6 weeks after injury and 17% to 25% at 6 to 12 months after injury (deVries et al., 1999; Mirza et al., 1998). Individuals who experience dissociative symptoms, such as depersonalization, derealization, or time distortion, are at greater risk of developing acute or chronic PTSD than individuals who do not dissociate after this type of traumatic event (Ursano et al., 1999). Clinical reports of children's responses to MVAs have noted nightmares, avoidance of the locale or setting in which the MVA occurred, and altered play patterns with repetitive reenactment of the event (Jaworski, 1992; Jones & Peterson, 1993).

Traumatic Brain Injury

Children and adolescents who sustain head injuries have been the most studied population in terms of the long-term effect of pediatric injury on the child and the family. Numerous studies indicate that most often, after the initial medical stabilization and treatment, individual and family psychosocial functioning and adjustment problems overshadow the recovery from the actual physical injury (Guerriere & McKeever, 1997; Jacobson et al., 1986; Wade, Drotar, Taylor, & Stancin, 1995; Wade, Taylor, Drotar, Stancin, & Yeates, 1998). The most crucial disabling component in a sample of adolescents with severe traumatic brain injury was poor social integration (Emanuelson et al., 1998). In one study, families of children with traumatic brain injuries expressed greater concern about the functioning of the injured child and their interactions with persons outside of the immediate family than families of children who sustained only orthopedic injuries (Stancin et al., 1998). In another study, parents of children ages 6 to 12 years with severe traumatic brain injury reported higher levels of posttraumatic symptoms in their children at 12 months than the parents of children with moderate traumatic brain injury or orthopedic injuries (Levi et al., 1999). Traumatic brain injury in a child and the resultant deficits, changes in personality and functioning, and increased care demands all take a toll on the child, the primary caregivers, and the rest of the family (Kreutzer, Gervaio, & Camplair, 1994; Livingston & Brooks, 1988; Testani-Dufour, Chappel-Aiken, & Gueldner, 1992).

Burns

Long-term pain and painful treatments, significant scarring, and multiple surgeries are some factors that are unique to the burn injury experience. Some studies have found the potential for dysfunction in families of pediatric patients with burns (Kendall-Grove, Ehde, Patterson, & Johnson, 1998). Other studies have stressed the resiliency and potential for positive outcome for burned children and their families (Blakeney, Meyer, Robert, Desai, Wolf, & Herndon, 1998; Tarnowski, Rasnake, Linscheid, & Mulick, 1989). The potential for positive psychosocial adjustment can be enhanced by working with the family to promote cohesion, decrease conflict, enhance stability, and promote the expectation of positive achievement (LeDoux, Meyer, Blakeney, & Herndon, 1998).

Injuries Resulting From Interpersonal or Community Violence

Violence is now recognized as a major public health epidemic in the United States (Satcher, 1995, 2001). The American

Academy of Pediatrics Task Force on Adolescent Assault Victim Needs (Christoffel et al., 1997) notes that youths who are injured through violence most often are treated like children injured through unintentional injury, without an understanding that violent injury is a special circumstance. Although there are many similarities between these types of injuries, such as the sudden, unexpected nature of the injury event; emergency treatment; and high emotions, there are also major differences. With injuries resulting from violence, there is the element of malevolence, that is, someone intended to harm someone, even if the child or adolescent was not the intended victim. It may be that the perceptions, needs, and responses of families of children injured through violence differ in some respects from those of families of children injured by other, nonviolent means in which there was not an actual intent to do harm (Lewandowski et al., in press), but these differences need further investigation. It is clear that exposure to violence and chronic danger has pervasive effects on cognitive, emotional, and behavioral functioning and affects the day-to-day and the long-term functioning for children, families, and communities (Hutson, Anglin, Mallon, & Pratts, 1994; Osofsky, 1995; Ozmar, 1994; Schuman, Silbernagel, Chesney, & Villarreal, 1996). Hamrin (1998) interviewed hospitalized gunshot patients ages 11 to 15 years and found a 56% rate of acute stress disorder. However, to date, little effort has been made by most health care facilities to address the developmental and psychological sequelae of children and families exposed to violence, especially with injuries resulting from violence, although evidence suggests that intervention is crucial to preventing PTSD and repeated violence exposure (Bell, Jenkins, Kpo, & Rhodes, 1994; Hamrin, 1998; Kharasch, Yuknek, Vinci, Herbert, & Zuckerman, 1997; Pynoos & Nader, 1988; Sanders-Phillips, 1997; Satcher, 2001).

Street gangs have existed in the United States for more than 100 years. They are active in 94% of U.S. cities with populations of over 100,000, in many smaller cities and towns, and even in rural areas (Hutson, Anglin, & Spears, 1995). In the 1970s, firearms started to become the weapons of choice. Drive-by shootings have become more common as gang members seek to create fear, terror, and intimidation among rival gang members, with the secondary intent being to kill. Sometimes people other than the intended victims get in the way. The number of gang members and innocent bystanders who are seriously injured or killed each year has increased. In 1991 more children in the city of Los Angeles died as a result of violent street gang activity than from child abuse (Hutson et al., 1995). Prevention of injuries resulting from this type of violence is challenging; however, some optimism has been expressed (Hutson, Anglin, & Mallon, 1992).

INTERVENING WITH CHILDREN AND THEIR FAMILIES

Interventions after pediatric injury and trauma must be family-centered and developmentally appropriate. The specialized expertise of all members of the multidisciplinary team is important to the optimal recovery of the child and family (Mangini, Confessore, Girard, & Spadola, 1995). Specific considerations and suggestions for caring for seriously injured children at each developmental stage have been detailed previously (Denholm, 1995; Lanning, 1985; Lewandowski, 1992b; Reynolds & Ramenofsky, 1988; Wong, 1982).

In the immediate postinjury period the child may be dazed, disoriented, and in "shock." Adults recognize with relief that help has arrived when ambulance and rescue personnel come to the scene. Young children, however, may not have the same reaction. Personnel at the scene or in the emergency department may need to help the stressed and perhaps traumatized child realize that the initial traumatic event is over and that people are seeking to help the child, not do more harm (Lewandowski & Baranoski, 1994). For example, a child with significant burns may need reassurance that he or she is no longer on fire. A child injured by gunfire may need to know that the perpetrator has been arrested and the gun danger is past.

Children should be given initial, brief, developmentally appropriate explanations of what happened to them, who the helpers are, what is being done, where they are being taken, and where their parents or significant others are. For example, one may say to a young child, "Hi, Michael, my name is Pat. Your arm is hurt, and we are going to put you on special bed in the ambulance and take you to the hospital. Your mom is going to come with us, and we are going to take good care of you." Children or adolescents who experienced loss of consciousness may need brief explanations of where they are and why they are in the hospital. If the child is conscious and there is time, brief explanations should be given about each procedure that is to be done and why. Staff should be aware of the hyperstartle response and high arousal after traumatic events and avoid surprises and sudden, unexpected entries and movements.

Injured children's questions should be answered reassuringly but honestly. During the initial treatment, it may not be necessary or advisable to tell children bad news about the death or serious injury of a family member or friend involved in the same incident. The child may have witnessed the injury and treatment of others, however, and direct questions should not be ignored. Giving children false information or lying to them has many later negative repercussions, including erosion of the child's ability to trust adults and reinforcement of the child's posttraumatic view of the world as unsafe and unpredictable (Lewandowski & Baranoski, 1994). It is important not to get out of phase with the child by not giving enough information or providing too much information too fast (Ravenscroft, 1982). The clinician must take cues from the child about what the child is ready to hear and what the child may already know but feels is not acceptable to talk about. Avoiding direct discussion when a child is ready for it may reinforce the child's belief that the situation is too overwhelming to talk about, even for adults. Because of anxiety, medications, possible head trauma, and the new and strange environment and language, children may need repeated explanations of why they are in the hospital, what happened, what is being done, and why. When a death has occurred, children need particular support, reassurance (e.g., who will take care of them, how they will be kept safe), and understanding (Mangini et al., 1995).

Talking About What Happened: Debriefing

After an injury event, children should be allowed and facilitated in expressing their feelings, thoughts, and perceptions of their injury experience and the events in the aftermath. This can be done directly, indirectly, or symbolically through verbal expression, reenactment of the events through play, drawing of pictures, or use of other means of expression. Children should be facilitated but not forced to talk about their experiences as a means of communicating, "working through," and ultimately integrating the experience. Various approaches to facilitating this process have been described (Lewandowski & Baranoski, 1994; Pynoos & Eth, 1986). Children often describe their injury experience and its aftermath in detailed, graphic ways that may be difficult for adults to hear. However, this expression and "debriefing" are important tasks for the child, and adults must find ways to cope with their own feelings so that they can be appropriately supportive to the child engaged in this process. Listening to children's descriptions allows parents and staff to identify and correct any inaccuracies or misconceptions that may be causing the child distress. Normalizing the child's feelings, concerns, and questions will help allay some older children's fears of being "weird" or different. Comments such as, "A lot of kids who get hurt like you did talk about feeling that way," or prefacing information with phrases such as, "Many kids your age wonder about . . . maybe you have been wondering that, too," may help children deal with their feelings and be more receptive to accepting new information.

Some children will experience avoidance and will not wish to engage in discussion of the event. They may become distressed when the event is mentioned. Other children need to talk about the experience repeatedly in an attempt to gain mastery over what happened. Most children will eventually talk about their experience in their own time (which may not be until they are back in the "safe" and familiar surrounding of their own home). Parents may need anticipatory guidance to expect this sometime after discharge. Children who never wish to talk about the event and who show other avoidance and posttraumatic symptoms may need professional intervention to help them deal with the trauma.

Sometimes well-meaning family members or staff seek to "protect" the child by cutting off this needed verbal expression. When this occurs, the nurse might assist the individuals in understanding the child's need for "telling his or her story." Adults, siblings, friends, and others involved in the injury event and the aftermath may have this pressing need to talk about what happened and process their feelings. Often, after being given an opportunity to talk about what happened, individuals will thank the nurse or make comments about "feeling better now." The literature on critical incident stress debriefing (Mitchell & Everly, 1996; Ragaisis, 1994) and emotional processing (Rachman, 1980) supports the view that postevent processing can be helpful in preventing or minimizing later posttraumatic symptoms. Pennebaker (1990) and Pennebaker and Susman (1988) report the numerous benefits, including physical health benefits, of disclosure of traumatic experiences and the negative physical and psychological effects of "holding them in."

After the child is stabilized, every effort should be made to prepare the child for treatments, examinations, x-ray films, or scans. Various cognitive and behavioral techniques such as distraction (e.g., use of a kaleidoscope), controlled breathing by helping the child blow bubbles or into a party blower, and guided imagery have been shown to decrease children's distress during venipunctures and other painful procedures (Vessey & Carlson, 1996; Vessey, Carlson, & McGill, 1994). These techniques can easily be put to use in the emergency department and on the hospital units. Some children may feel guilty or responsible for their injury (even when they had no control over the event) and thus may believe that treatments are punishments for their "bad" behavior in becoming hurt. They may need reassurance that the injury was not their fault (or if their behavior caused it that they did not mean for the injury to happen) and that they are not being punished. It may be confusing for young children to differentiate the "good" hurt of treatments from the "bad" hurt of the injury event. Ongoing emotional support is vital (Zink, 1996).

When discharge is being planned, a number of issues must be taken into account. Some children have fears about going back to the setting where they were injured or about going back "out into the world" at all if they perceive it to be unsafe. Open discussion of their fears and concerns, as well as a focus on coping skills or changes in behavior that will help keep them safe, may be helpful (e.g., always wear a helmet, only cross streets with an adult, duck down on the car floor if you hear gunfire). What to tell their friends and going back to school are other areas of concern to older children. Having children role-play talking with their friends and planning what information they wish to share can help smooth the transition back home and into regular activities. In some situations in which significant injuries occurred (e.g., traumatic amputations or extensive scarring), the nurse can plan with the child, family, and school personnel how to give appropriate information to school staff and other students and how to facilitate the injured child's transition back to normal activities. Families need to be educated about "normal" expected responses that the child and family might experience (see Box 23-1), when to become concerned (significant symptoms lasting more than a few weeks and interfering with functioning), and where and how to get help if they need it. Ensuring effective pain control after discharge is crucial for child and family well-being (Chan, Russell, & Robak, 1998).

FAMILY TRAUMA

A child's trauma is a family's trauma (Braulin, Rook, & Sills, 1982; Ravenscroft, 1982). Who constitutes "family" for the injured child may include one, two, or four parents (as in the case of remarried couples); extended family members who are primary caretakers; or foster parents. Other family members may be siblings, extended family members, close friends, or community support people such as clergy or day-care or school personnel. It is important to identify and accept the family's own definition of "family" and to refrain from judgments about the family's structure and unnecessary restrictiveness. The composition of a family is not the key factor in determining the family's ability to support and nurture the injured child and each other through the difficult injury situation.

A family-centered care model is needed in cases of pediatric injury because the effects of the injury situation and its aftermath clearly reverberate through the family, and how the family copes will have a direct effect on the child. The injured child may not be the only casualty. The traumatic event may have other direct effects on the family. Other family members may have been injured or killed; the family's home and all of their possessions may have been destroyed by a fire, a tornado, or other natural disaster; or the family car may have been "totaled" in the crash. Family conflict may be heightened because of the stress of the child's injury and treatment demands, or dysfunctional coping patterns such as substance abuse may add to the family's stress (Frosch, 1996; Frosch & Lewandowski, 1998). Feelings of guilt, blame, and anger and different styles of coping may interfere with optimal family functioning (Lewandowski et al., in press). Uncertainty, fear for the child's survival and long-term functioning, and competing demands of the injured and well children may add to the family's stress. Although all hospitalizations of children are stressful for families, sudden, unplanned, emergency hospitalizations have the added dimension of taking the family by surprise and allowing no time for advance preparation (Eberly, Miles, Carter, Hennessey, & Riddle, 1985; Epperson, 1977; Roskies, Bedard, Gauvreau-Guilbault, & Lafortune, 1975). The family's ethnic, cultural, and/or religious beliefs may be of extreme importance to the family in this type of traumatic situation. Family members' abilities to be supportive, available, and effective in caring for the injured child and each other may be affected by all of these factors, as well as family communication and functioning styles before the traumatic event. It is critical to assess the context in which the injury event and treatment occur and to identify the family's strengths, vulnerabilities, and risk and protective factors to provide support and assistance to the family during this difficult time. Assessing families for characteristics of functional and dysfunctional coping (Table 23-2) will give the clinician further direction to the targeting of interventions.

PARENTAL PRESENCE AND PARTICIPATION IN CARE

Parental presence and support over time have repeatedly been shown to be pivotal factors that determine a child's ability to cope effectively with stressful experiences (Freud & Burlingham, 1944; Visintainer & Wolfer, 1975). Still, parents are often not given the option to be present. They may be asked to leave while the child receives emergency treatment and later during hospitalization when other treatments, especially painful procedures, are carried out on the child. In 1994 the Emergency Department Nurses Association first issued a position statement supporting family presence during the treatment of a loved one (Emergency Nurses Association, 1998; Figure 23-2). The issue of family presence during emergency department treatment has received attention on national radio (Suarez, 1999) and television (Dateline NBC, 1999), in the media, and on the Internet (MSNBC, 1999). Parental presence during pediatric procedures and resuscitations remains an area of controversy in pediatric practice today.

It is important that parents and children be kept together or reunited if they have been separated during transport as soon as possible after the child arrives at the emergency department. The parents' presence and participation in the child's care should be supported and facilitated throughout the injured child's treatment, as desired by the family. There is strong support in the child development literature for the child's need for parental presence and support (Ainsworth, Blehar, Waters, & Wall, 1978; Bowlby, 1980). During times of

TABLE 23-2 Family Coping

Functional Family Coping	Dysfunctional Family Coping
1. Clear acceptance of the the stressor	1. Denial or misperception of the stressor
2. Family-centered locus of the problem	2. Individual-centered locus of the problem
3. Solution-oriented problem solving	3. Blame-oriented problem solving
4. High tolerance for each other	4. Low tolerance for each other
5. Clear and direct expressions of commitment and affections	5. Indirect or missing expressions of commitment and affections
6. Open and effective communication	6. Closed and ineffective communication
7. High family cohesion	7. Low or poor family cohesion
8. Flexible family roles	8. Rigid family roles
9. Efficient resource utilization	9. Inefficient resource utilization
10. Absence of violence	10. Use of violence
11. Infrequency of substance use	11. Frequent use of substances

From Figley, C. R. (1983). Catastrophes: An overview of family reaction. In C. R. Figley & H. I. McCubbin (Eds.), *Stress and the family: Volume 2. Coping with catastrophe* (p. 3020). New York: Brunner/Mazel.

EMERGENCY NURSES ASSOCIATION
POSITION STATEMENT

FAMILY PRESENCE AT THE BEDSIDE DURING
INVASIVE PROCEDURES AND RESUSCITATION

STATEMENT OF PROBLEM

In most instances, the family is the patient's primary support system. Family members are frequently not given the opportunity to remain with the patient during invasive procedures, including resuscitation efforts.

This separation during treatment occurs for a variety of reasons. Health care personnel often feel concerned performing these procedures in the presence of non-medically oriented individuals. Additionally, family members are perceived to be overwhelmed or intimidated in these situations.

Family-centered care recognizes the role of the family in the health and well being of the patient. It is characterized by collaboration among the patient, family, and health care professionals and recognizes that the family is a constant in the patient's life (Eckle, 2001; Eckle & MacLean, 2001). In most instances, families are the patient's primary support system.

In 1993, the Emergency Nurses Association adopted a resolution to support the option of family presence during invasive procedures (IP) and resuscitation (CPR) (ENA, 1993). However, written policies allowing the option of family presence during IP and CPR are infrequent in emergency departments (MacLean et al., 2001). In a recent study of 456 emergency nurses and 473 critical care nurses (MacLean et al., 2001), only 9% of the emergency nurses indicated that their emergency department had written policies allowing the option of family presence during CPR and IP. A greater percentage reported that the emergency department had no written policy but allowed the option during CPR (68%) and IP (80%). Emergency nurses reported that only 1% of their emergency departments had written policies prohibiting family presence during IP and CPR, however, the option of family presence was prohibited for IP (20%) and CPR (32%) in the absence of a written policy. Written policies and practices allowing the option of family presence during IP and CPR continue to be underutilized in U.S. emergency departments.

Several investigators documented the benefits of family presence during IP and CPR which includes knowing that everything possible was being done for their loved one; reducing anxiety and fear; feeling of being supportive and helpful to the patient and the staff; sharing critical information about the patient and the patient's condition; maintaining the patient-family relationship; closure on a life shared together; and facilitating the grieving process in the emergency department and later at home (Bauchner, Waring, & Vinci, 1991; Meyers et al., 2000; MacLean et al., 2001; Robinson, MacKenzie-Ross, & Campbell-Hawson, 1998; Sacchetti et al., 1996; Timmermans, 1997). Patients indicated that having family present provided comfort, helped with coping and pain control, maintained the family bond, and reminded health providers that the patient was a person with a family who deserved dignity, and respect (Eichhorn et al., 2001; Robinson et al., 1998). In addition, the American Heart Association's Guidelines 2000 recommended that providers offer families the option to remain with their loved one during resuscitation (AHA, 2000).

Although many patients, family members, and health care providers support the option of family presence, family members frequently are not given the option to remain with the patient during invasive procedures and resuscitation efforts. This separation during treatment occurs for a variety of reasons. Health professionals express concern that the event may be too traumatic for the family; clinical care might be impeded; family members might become too emotional or out of control; staff may experience increased stress with family present; ED rooms are too crowded; staff are focused on the patient and may not be available to assist family members; there is a shortage of nurses; and the risk of increased liability might increase (Belanger & Reed, 1997; Eichhorn, Meyers, & Guzzetta, 1995; Eichhorn, Meyers, Mitchell, & Guzzetta, 1996; Eichhorn et. al, 2001; MacLean et al., 2001; Meyers et al., 2000; Redley & Hood, 1996; Rosenczweig, 1998; Sacchetti et al., 1996; Timmermans, 1997; Van der Woning, 1997). Yet, families reported that they would be present again if a similar event occurred (Belanger & Reed, 1997; Powers & Rubenstein, 1999; Meyers et al., 2000). In addition, investigators reported that there were no adverse psychological effects among family members and the operations of the emergency care providers was not disrupted when the option of family presence was used (Belanger & Reed, 1997; Meyers et al., 2000; Robinson et al., 1998; Sacchetti et al., 1996).

ASSOCIATION POSITION

ENA supports the option of family presence during invasive procedures and /or resuscitation efforts.

ENA supports further research related to the presence of family members during invasive procedures and/or resuscitation efforts and the impact it has upon family members, patients, and health care personnel.

ENA supports the development and dissemination of educational resources for emergency department health care personnel concerning the issues, policies, practices, and programs supporting the option of related to family presence.

ENA supports the development and dissemination of educational resources for the public concerning the option of family presence during invasive procedures and resuscitation.

The ENA supports collaboration with other specialty organizations (including, but not limited to nursing, social and family services, pastoral care, physicians, and pre-hospital care providers) to develop multidisciplinary guidelines related to family presence during invasive procedures and/or resuscitation.

ENA supports healthcare facilities having in place policies and procedures allowing the option of family presence during invasive procedures and resuscitation.

FIGURE 23-2 Position statement on family presence at bedside during resuscitation. (From Emergency Nurses Association. (2001). *Family presence at the bedside during invasive procedures and resuscitation. Emergency Nurses Association position statement.* Park Ridge, IL: Author.)

Continued

REFERENCES

American Heart Association in Collaboration with the International Liaison Committee on Resuscitation. Guidelines 2000 for cardiopulmonary resuscitation and emergency cardiovascular care. *Circulation, 102*(8 Suppl.), I-374.

Bauchner, H., Vinci, R., & Waring, C. (1989). Pediatric procedures: Do parents want to watch? *Pediatrics, 84,* 907-909.

Bauchner, H., Waring, C., & Vinci, R. (1991). Parental presence during procedures in an emergency room: Results from 50 observations. *Pediatrics, 87,* 544-548.

Belanger, M., & Reed, S. (1997). A rural community hospital's experience with family-witnessed resuscitation. *Journal of Emergency Nursing, 23*(3), 238-239.

Eckle, N. (Ed). (2001). *Presenting the option of family presence* (2nd ed.). Des Plaines, IL: Emergency Nurses Association.

Eckle, N., & MacLean, S. (2001). Assessment of family-centered care for pediatric patients in the emergency department. *Journal of Emergency Nursing, 27*(3), 238-245.

Eichhorn, D. J., Meyers, T. A., & Guzzetta, C. E. (1995). Family presence during resuscitation: It is time to open the door. *Capsules Comments Critical Care Nursing, 3,* 1-5.

Eichhorn, D. J., Meyers, T. A., Mitchell, T. G., & Guzzetta, C. E. (1996). Opening the doors: Family presence during resuscitation. *Journal of Cardiovascular Nursing, 10*(4), 59-70.

Eichhorn, D. J., Meyers, T. A., Guzzetta, C. E., Clark, A. P., Klein, J. D., Taliaferro, E., & Calvin, A. O. (2001). Family presence during invasive procedures and resuscitation: Hearing the voice of the patient. *American Journal of Nursing, 101*(5), 26-33.

Emergency Nurses Association. (1993). Family presence at the bedside during invasive procedures and/or resuscitation. *Resolution, 93,* 2.

Institute for Family Centered Care. (1998). Core principles of family-centered health care. *Advances in Family Centered-Care, 4,* 2-4.

MacLean, S., White, C., Guzzetta, C. E., Fontaine, D., Eichhorn, D. J., Meyers, T. A., & Desy, P. (2001). *Family presence practices of critical care and emergency nurses in the United States (raw data).* Des Plaines, IL: Emergency Nurses Association,

Meyers, T. A., Eichhorn, D. J., Guzzetta, C. E., Clark, A. P., Klein, J. D., Taliaferro, E., & Calvin, A. O. (2000). Family presence during invasive procedures and resuscitation: The experience of family members, nurses, and physicians. *American Journal of Nursing, 100*(2), 32-42.

Molter, N. (1979). Needs of relatives of critically ill patients: A descriptive study. *Heart and Lung, 8,* 332-339.

Powers, K. S., & Rubenstein, J. S. (1999). Family presence during invasive procedures in the pediatric intensive care unit. *Archives of Pediatric Adolescent Medicine, 153,* 955-958.

Redley, B., & Hood, K. (1996). Staff attitudes towards family presence during resuscitation. *Accident and Emergency Nursing, 4*(3), 145-151.

Robinson, S., MacKenzie-Ross, S., Campbell-Hawson, G., et al. (1998). Psychological effect of witnessed resuscitation on bereaved relatives. *Lancet, 352,* 614-617.

Rosenczweig, C. (1998). Should relatives witness resuscitation? *Canadian Medical Association Journal, 158*(5), 617-620.

Sacchetti, A., Lichenstein, R., Carraccio, C., et al. (1996). Family member presence during pediatric emergency department procedures. *Pediatric Emergency Care, 12*(4), 268-271.

Timmermans, S. (1997). High touch in high tech: The presence of relatives and friends during resuscitation efforts. *Scholarly Inquiry of Nursing Practice, 11*(2), 153-168.

Van der Woning, M. (1997). Should relatives be invited to witness a resuscitation attempt? *Accident and Emergency Nursing, 5*(4), 215-218.

FIGURE 23-2, *cont'd*

stress and/or pain, young children want their parents to be with them and protect them or, if that is not possible, then at least to comfort them and provide security (Baucher, Vinci, & Wading, 1989). Because regression often occurs during stressful times such as after an injury, even older children may have a strong need for the security of their parent or primary caretaker.

It is clear from numerous studies that parents wish to be involved with the care of their ill or injured child, with some individual variation in the actual care they wish to perform and extent to which they wish to or can be involved (Broome, Knafl, Pridham, & Feetham, 1998; Brown & Ritchie, 1990; Knafl, 1985; Knafl, Cavalleri, & Dixon, 1988; Romaniuk & Kritsjanson, 1995). Providing emotional support, performing basic care, entertaining the child, and participating in technical aspects of care all have been identified by parents of hospitalized children as activities they wish to perform (Hill, 1978; Knafl et al., 1988; Merrow & Johnson, 1968; Snowden & Gottlieb, 1989). Although nurses have been found to be in agreement with parents regarding the parents' participation in providing support, entertainment, and basic care activities, some have expressed less comfort with parents performing technical tasks (Brown & Ritchie, 1990).

Some clinicians believe that parental presence during procedures increases the anxiety of the child, the parents themselves, and the clinicians performing the procedure. However, converging research evidence does not support these concerns. Numerous studies have shown that most parents, when given the option, wish to be with their child during procedures and that, in most cases where parents have been prepared for their support role, parental presence is beneficial for the child and parent (decreased anxiety and increased satisfaction). The studies show that parental presence does not make the clinician more nervous or prolong the procedure (Baucher, Vinci, Bak, Pearson, & Corwin, 1996; Baucher, Vinci, & Wading, 1989; Baucher, Wading, & Vinci, 1991; Haimi-Cohen, Amir, Harel, Straussberg, & Varsano, 1996; Wolfram & Turner, 1996).

A study of parents who experienced the unexpected admission of their child to the intensive care unit reports that the highest rated stressors for the parents are being unable to protect the child from pain, not knowing how to best help the child during the crisis, being separated from the child for long periods, seeing the child acting or looking as if he or she were in pain, not being able to be with the crying child, and not being able to hold the child, as well as the inability of the child to talk or cry (Eberly et al., 1985). It is clear that being kept from their child's bedside is a major stressor for parents who experience a strong need to fulfill their parental supportive role. Although it is evident that parental presence during procedures may not be for everyone, the evidence is clear that most parents wish to stay with their children and that both children and parents tend to benefit from this practice. More research is needed with regard to parental presence during the various phases of pediatric injury transport and treatment.

PARENTAL ANXIETY

The issue of parental anxiety is an important one. Parental anxiety is a significant predictor of child anxiety and a possible problematic issue with parental presence when parental anxiety is very high (Bevan et al., 1990; Broome & Endsley, 1989; Cameron, Bond, & Pointer, 1996; Vessey, Bogetz, Caserza, Liu, & Cassidy, 1994). It is frightening and upsetting for children to see their parents exhibiting high anxiety and distress; still, children have a strong need for the presence, support, and reassurance of their parents during times of stress. Assisting parents or primary caretakers to work through and effectively cope with their own feelings is crucial to the well-being of the injured child and their noninjured siblings (Lewandowski & Baranoski, 1994). Some parents will choose not to be present, often because of their anxiety, and they should be supported in their decision. If a parent is so distressed that he or she is unable to function in a support role, another close family member, friend, or staff person may be a temporary substitute to provide support to the child while other staff members intervene with the distressed parent. Extended family members or friends can help parents who are in a state of shock and high anxiety to organize and carry out needed tasks (e.g., arranging for child care for noninjured children; notifying employers, the child's school, or the family's religious community about the incident; providing transportation). It may be helpful for the family to designate a "spokesperson" (Mangini et al., 1995) who serves a liaison between the parents and the rest of the family and friends in terms of relaying information, coordinating visitors, making phone calls, and sending emails. Another family member or friend might take over the coordination of child care arrangements or manage daily routines in the home. Pastoral care staff or the family's clergy may provide important support during the child's treatment, particularly during times of high anxiety, if the family wishes this type of assistance.

Providing adequate information paced in a manner that is sensitive to the family's readiness to receive it and helping the family formulate questions and concerns so that they can be addressed by the health care staff can play a large role in decreasing parental anxiety. Although it is important not to withhold vital information from the family, it is also important to read the family members' cues and not to overwhelm them with too much information at once (Mangini et al., 1995). It may be necessary to repeat important information more than once because stressed individuals often have trouble "taking in" and remembering new information. Ongoing assessment of the family's understanding of the child's condition, course of treatment, options being considered, and decisions that need to be made is necessary (Mangini et al., 1995). Ongoing support, education, and preparation may help decrease family members' anxiety so that they can be of better assistance to their child and experience less upset themselves (LaRosa-Nash & Murphy, 1997; LaRosa-Nash, Murphy, Wade, & Clasby, 1995).

Parents who are highly stressed and who are in a new, strange, and possibly threatening environment may need assistance in knowing how they can participate in their child's care and ways in which they can support their child. Melnyk (1995) provided mothers of 2- to 5-year-old children who had unplanned hospital admissions with audio taped information regarding possible behavioral responses of their children, suggestions regarding how the mothers could participate in their child's care and assist their child in coping with the experience, and details about the hospital's services and policies. Melnyk found that mothers who received this information had increased confidence and certainty regarding their role during the child's hospitalization, which resulted in increased participation in their child's care and decreased maternal anxiety.

During phases of high anxiety, distress, and uncertainty, family members may need to be reminded and encouraged to take care of themselves so that they can better attend to their child. It is important that family members eat, drink, rest, and take periodic breaks. Sleep deprivation, hypoglycemia, and dehydration can add to already stressed parents' difficulties in processing information and functioning in an optimal manner given the circumstances.

In rare instances some parents or other family members may become angry, belligerent, intrusive, and/or demanding. They may displace their anger at the situation onto the staff, criticizing staff behavior, demanding fast results or information that is not yet known, and inadvertently interfering with staff functioning (Ravenscroft, 1982). This behavior is usually defensive in nature, springing from the family member's own anxiety or guilt. It requires special staff intervention to help the family member better understand his or her own feelings and reactions and the impact of this type of behavior. Staff should help these individuals redirect the energy into more constructive ways of benefiting the child and family. In rare cases family members come to the emergency department, unit, or clinic obviously inebriated or "high." In most instances these individuals will not be of benefit to the injured child. If they are disruptive, they may be asked to leave or, if necessary, be escorted by security from the building.

Parents facing the death of their child may react in many different ways as they begin the grief process for their tragic loss. Parents may request to hold their child after the death and may request locks of hair, fingerprints, or pictures in an attempt to hold on to a precious memory of their lost child (Mangini et al., 1995). Some parents may become withdrawn and immobilized in their grief; others may become loudly expressive. Allowing parents and other family members time to grieve in private (as much as possible) and to take the time they need to say their good-byes is important in helping them move successfully through the grief process. Calling upon the services of pastoral care staff or other clergy as the family desires can be a vitally important resource for the family. In emergency situations, fulfilling the family's request for prayers or a religious service at the child's bedside can be accomplished by a member of the health care staff, depending on the staff member's own comfort level. Family members need to hear that their child and family will not be forgotten and that they may benefit from an "aftercare bereavement program" (Mangini et al., 1995). Oliver and Fallat (1995) report that risk factors for pathologic grieving in families include the lack of a support network beyond the extended family, an avoidant stance to grieving, and a view of God as distant and punitive.

Siblings of Injured Children

Siblings of injured children may also have experienced the injury event, may have witnessed their sibling being injured, or may have heard about what happened in graphic detail; therefore they may themselves be experiencing posttraumatic symptoms. Older siblings may have played important support roles for their younger sibling who was injured, such as running for help or holding the younger child until help arrived (Lewandowski et al., in press). Younger siblings may not really understand what has happened and may react more to the absence of their parent and injured, hospitalized sibling. Siblings of all ages may have intense feelings about the situation and may feel responsible in some way for what happened, even if they had no role in the injury. Using a family-centered approach to care means that the feelings, reactions, and well-being of the injured child's siblings must be taken into account in the plan of care (Craft, Wyatt, & Sandell, 1986; Murray, 2000). Although in the immediate acute period the family's attention may be focused on the injured child, an assessment of the siblings' needs and well-being should be conducted as soon as possible and appropriate suggestions or referrals made. Siblings have a strong need for ongoing, developmentally appropriate information and honest answers to their questions (Lewandowski, 1992a). They need to feel important and to be included. Sibling visitation may be considered, and some siblings may benefit from the opportunity to speak with a member of the injured child's treatment team directly to have their questions and concerns addressed (Lewandowski & Baranoski, 1994). Close or "best" friends of the injured child may experience posttraumatic symptoms, needs, and concerns similar to those of the siblings.

Impact of the Media

In some cases children or adolescents are injured in situations that spark community interest, and their treatment and hospital course become topics of community (and sometimes national) interest (Lewandowski & Baranoski, 1994). This community interest has both positive and negative aspects. On the positive side, intense media coverage may result in tangible shows of community support, such as cards, gifts, prayers, and donations to help cover medical bills. In some situations, other families in the community benefit by learning of possible dangers to their children that they can work to prevent. On the negative side, some families may experience the media interest as intrusive and disturbing at a critical time for their family.

Different families experience and react to media interest in different ways. Some prefer to avoid it and to maintain as much privacy as possible. Others view it as a positive support and willingly share personal information with the media. Some seem to get caught up with a sense of importance and notoriety. Some families may feel an obligation to agree to interviews, press conferences, or media coverage of their child's discharge, particularly if they have received much community support, even though they would prefer their privacy. Some families may be so overwhelmed with their own feelings and concerns that they are not able to think through the possible impact of media coverage on their child. Some children may benefit from the opportunity, such as an 11-year-old boy who used his television appearance in a positive manner to encourage other children to wear their bicycle helmets, something he had not been doing at the time of his injury. At other times children may need to be protected from media appearances. For example, a young child who has sustained a gunshot wound, is voicing concerns about leaving the hospital to go back out where it is "unsafe," and is showing posttraumatic symptoms of hypervigilance and arousal will likely be further upset by being met by a hospital lobby full of photographers and reporters as he or she is discharged (Lewandowski & Baranoski, 1994). Because nurses often have strong rapport with families and may be able to view the situation in a somewhat objective, holistic manner, the nurse can be of assistance to the family, unit and institutional staff, and hospital's public relations personnel (usually charged with liaisons with the media but not necessarily informed about clinical aspects or family preferences) in planning, "on the spot" or in advance, the best way to meet the needs of the family, the institution, and the media. The nurse can also provide some anticipatory guidance for the family about the time when the media spotlight fades, the community interest turns elsewhere, and the family is left to deal with the aftermath of the experience.

Community Trauma

In recent years the media have been replete with graphic and comprehensive coverage of high-profile traumatic events, such as school shootings, bombings, tornados, floods, and other types of disasters leading to pediatric injuries and deaths. Local media coverage often details more local "disasters," such as MVAs in which several teenagers are injured or killed, community shootings in which children are the innocent victims, and near-drownings at a community pool. These events can affect large numbers of people who directly experience or witness the event, who have family members or friends who were involved, or who just hear about what happened via the media. Often, a more comprehensive community response may be needed to allow affected community members a meaningful way to grieve, share feelings and support, and ultimately find meaning (if possible) and closure for the event. Memorial services, candlelight vigils, and crisis counseling services may help meet these needs. Giving out ongoing information that safeguards the affected family's privacy and confidentiality and meets the community's need to know what happened and is happening is a challenge, but it also is important in giving a sense of control to all parties and in bringing about a sense of order and closure. Many times, giving family, friends, and community members something meaningful to do will help decrease their sense of helplessness and powerlessness. For example, they can contribute to a fund to cover medical expenses, join the local MADD (Mothers Against Drunk Driving) chapter, help a family rebuild after a house fire, or place flowers or notes at a meaningful site. Nurse and other health care professionals can play a role in assisting a community coping with these types of high-profile injury events by becoming involved in or facilitating meaningful ways in which the community can share in and work through their own feelings regarding these traumatic events in a positive way.

It is important to remember the 1-year and perhaps annual anniversaries of the traumatic events because these are times when strong feelings are often rekindled. Oklahoma City has provided a positive model of community response to the yearly anniversary of a traumatic event by planning a meaningful memorial service each year. In the service, community members can come together, remember those who were injured or killed, and gain support from each other in dealing with difficult feelings and memories. Other significant events, such as birthdays and high school graduations, may engender strong feelings, particularly if one or more deaths resulted from the injury event. Anticipatory guidance for families and school officials regarding the responses that may occur and ways in which acknowledgments can be made can help mitigate some of the feelings of family, friends, and community members.

Caregiver Trauma

Children who are injured may provoke many reactions in the health care providers who care for them and their families, even if the interactions are brief (Tuckman, 1973). Table 23-3 list the signs and symptoms of distress and distress sig-

TABLE 23-3 Critical Incident Stress Information Sheets

You have experienced a traumatic event or a critical incident (any event that causes unusually strong emotional reactions that have the potential to interfere with the ability to function normally). Even though the event may be over, you may now be experiencing, or may experience later, some strong emotional or physical reactions. It is very common, in fact quite *normal,* for people to experience emotional aftershocks when they have passed through a horrible event.

Sometimes the emotional aftershocks (or stress reactions) appear immediately after the traumatic event. Sometimes they may appear a few hours or a few days later. And, in some cases, weeks or months may pass before the stress reactions appear.

The signs and symptoms of a stress reaction may last a few days, a few weeks, a few months, or longer, depending on the severity of the traumatic event. The understanding and the support of loved ones usually cause the stress reactions to pass more quickly. Occasionally, the traumatic event is so painful that professional assistance may be necessary. This does not imply craziness or weakness. It simply indicates that the particular event was just too powerful for the person to manage by himself or herself.

Here are some common signs and signals of a stress reaction:

Physical*	Cognitive	Emotional	Behavioral
Chills	Confusion	Fear	Withdrawal
Thirst	Nightmares	Guilt	Antisocial acts
Fatigue	Uncertainty	Grief	Inability to rest
Nausea	Hypervigilance	Panic	Intensified pacing
Fainting	Suspiciousness	Denial	Erratic movements
Twitches	Intrusive images	Anxiety	Change in social activity
Vomiting	Blaming someone	Agitation	Change in speech patterns
Dizziness	Poor problem solving	Irritability	Loss or increase in appetite
Weakness	Poor abstract thinking	Depression	Hyperalert to environment
Chest pain	Poor attention/decisions	Intense anger	Increased alcohol consumption
Headaches	Poor concentration/memory	Apprehension	Change in visual communications
Elevated BP	Disorientation of time/place or person	Emotional shock	etc.
Rapid heart rate	Difficulty identifying objects or people	Emotional outbursts	
Muscle tremors	Heightened or lowered awareness	Feeling overwhelmed	
Shock symptoms	Increased or decreased awareness of surroundings	Loss of emotional control	
Grinding of teeth	etc.	Inappropriate emotional response	
Visual difficulties		etc.	
Profuse sweating			
Difficulty breathing			
etc.			

**Any of these symptoms indicate the need for medical evaluation. When in doubt, contact a physician.*

From Mitchell, J. T., & Everly, G. S. (2001). *The basic critical incident stress management course: Basic group crisis intervention* (3rd ed.). Baltimore: International Critical Incident Stress Foundation, Inc.

nals that indicate immediate intervention is needed. It is important to recognize that self-care and recognizing and responding to the each other's needs help staff provide more effective care for children and families. Staff may become upset about the type or circumstances of the injury, angry about the role the child played in the event, angry at the child's caretakers who were not able to prevent the injury, angry at bystanders who did not help the child, or outraged at a perpetrator such as a gunman or a drunk driver. In addition to anger, staff may experience feelings of sadness, depression, grief, or blame. Emergency and hospital staff who work closely with traumatized children may themselves experience psychological trauma to varying extents, ranging from mild upset to symptoms of PTSD (Mitchell, 1986; Mitchell & Everly, 1996; Spitzer & Burke, 1993).

The care of an injured child may take place in the context of other job stressors, such as physical and mental overload, inadequate or low staffing, already existing concerns related to emotional and ethical patient care issues, different lifestyles and coping mechanisms of families, staff conflicts, and self-expectation of perfection in patient care (Back, 1992; Lawson, 1987; Schottenfeld & Cullen, 1985; Triolo, 1989). In most situations health care personnel are able to develop and use effective coping strategies that enable them to adequately cope with and manage their job-related stresses. However, an event is sometimes so traumatic or overwhelming that emergency responders and health care professionals experience significant stress reactions. It is increasingly clear that the job stresses associated with pediatric injuries and the context in which they are addressed must be monitored by staff members themselves, as well as by their managers. Appropriate intervention must take place on an ongoing basis to safeguard the health and well-being of the staff members, as well as to safeguard quality patient care.

Critical Incidents and Compassion Fatigue

A *critical incident* is any situation that generates an unusually strong emotional reaction with the potential to interfere with physical and psychological function and health (Mitchell, 1983). The significant stress that is associated with critical incidents, usually situations that are dramatic and emotionally overwhelming, may render professionals' usual coping mechanisms ineffective (Mitchell, 1983; Mitchell & Bray, 1990; Spitzer & Burke, 1993). These types of situations may occur in emotionally charged situations, such as the sudden death of a child and/or other family members, loss of life after extraordinary and prolonged professional interventions, situations in which multiple children are seriously injured or killed, serious injury or death resulting from human-to-human violence, actual or potential threats to professionals' well-being, or injury or death of colleagues or relatives of co-workers (Mitchell, 1986; Mitchell & Everly, 1996). These types of situations are viewed as critical incidents not only by emergency rescue personnel but also by hospital-based nurses (Burns & Harm, 1993).

Figley (1995) suggests that "there is a cost to caring," noting that professionals who are exposed to patients' stories of fear, pain, and suffering may themselves experience posttraumatic symptoms. He identifies two types of stress reactions resulting from situations involving critical incidents and contact with traumatized persons (Figley, 1991, 1995). *Compassion stress*, or *secondary traumatic stress reaction*, is described as the manageable tension or demand associated with feeling compassion or sympathy in difficult situations. *Compassion fatigue*, or *secondary posttraumatic stress disorder*, is characterized by feelings of helplessness, confusion, isolation, numbness or avoidance, and persistent arousal and requires intervention. Other symptoms associated with excessive acute or sustained stress include cognitive effects such as problems with decision making, memory, and attention span; emotional reactions such as increased anxiety, anger, irritability, guilt, fear, paranoia, and depression; and physical problems such as fatigue, dizziness, chest pain, headaches, hypertension, and even illnesses such as diabetes and cancer (Everly, 1990; Mitchell, 1986; Mitchell & Bray, 1990; Spitzer & Burke, 1993).

Intervening to Decrease Staff Trauma

There is extensive literature on stress management. Many articles, books, tapes, and websites are available to assist individuals in managing stress. Some "things to try" in managing critical incident stress are listed in Box 23-2. Staff meetings, groups, and psychiatric liaison services have long been identified as helpful in facilitating staff expression of feelings, mutual support, problem solving, and conflict resolution (Eisendrath & Dunkel, 1979; Kunkler & Whittick, 1991; Lewandowski, & Baranoski, 1994; Matheson, 1990).

One system that has been receiving increasing attention for its effectiveness in decreasing critical incident stress in emergency and hospital personnel is *critical incident stress management* (CISM) (Everly & Mitchell, 1997; Mitchell & Everly, 1997). CISM is a comprehensive, multicomponent crisis intervention system that covers the precrisis phase, acute crisis phase, and postcrisis intervention. It is composed of seven core components, which underscores the importance of using multiple interventions to achieve the goals of crisis stabilization and prevention of significant long-term posttraumatic stress reactions (Everly & Mitchell, 1997; Mitchell & Everly, 1997).

The first component entails *precrisis preparation*, including stress management education, anticipatory guidance, and crisis mitigation training for both individuals and organizations. The second component is *one-on-one crisis intervention* and counseling or provision of psychological support throughout the full range of the crisis spectrum. The third component, *family crisis intervention*, recognizes a dual purpose: to decrease secondary traumatization in the family members and to assist family members in supporting the member most involved in the incident and/or each other. Specialized training is necessary to carry out the fourth and fifth components, defusing and debriefing. *Defusings* are short, informal meetings held in the first few hours after a traumatic event that help immediately stabilize personnel involved in the critical incident so that they can either

BOX 23-2 Managing Critical Incident Stress

Things to Try

- WITHIN THE FIRST 24-48 HOURS, periods of appropriate physical exercise alternated with relaxation will alleviate some of the physical reactions.
- Structure your time; keep busy.
- You are normal and having normal reactions; do not label yourself crazy.
- Talk to people; talk is the most healing medicine.
- Be aware of *numbing* the pain with overuse of drugs or alcohol; you do not need to complicate this with a substance abuse problem.
- Reach out; people do care.
- Maintain as normal a schedule as possible.
- Spend time with others.
- Help your co-workers as much as possible by sharing feelings and checking out how they are doing.
- Give yourself permission to feel rotten and share your feelings with others.
- Keep a journal; write your way through those sleepless hours.
- Do things that feel good to you.
- Realize those around you are under stress.
- Do not make any big life changes.
- Do make as many daily decisions as possible that will give you a feeling of control over your life (e.g., if someone asks you what you want to eat, answer him or her even if you are not sure).
- Get plenty of rest.
- Do not try fighting reoccurring thoughts, dreams, or flashbacks—they are normal and will decrease over time and become less painful.
- Eat well-balanced and regular meals (even if you do not feel like it).

For Family Members and Friends

- Listen carefully.
- Spend time with the traumatized person.
- Offer your assistance and a listening ear if he or she has not asked for help.
- Reassure the person that he or she is safe.
- Help the person with everyday tasks such as cleaning, cooking, caring for the family, and minding children.
- Give the person some private time.
- Do not take his or her anger or other feelings personally.
- Do not tell the person that he or she is "lucky it wasn't worse"; a traumatized person is not consoled by those statements. Instead, tell the person that you are sorry such an event has occurred and you want to understand and assist him or her.

From Mitchell, J. T., & Everly, G. S. (2001). *The basic critical incident stress management course: Basic group crisis intervention* (3rd ed.). Baltimore: International Critical Incident Stress Foundation, Inc.

reenter the situation and carry on their jobs or return home after the reduction of potentially debilitating stress.

Critical incident stress debriefing (CISD) is the component that has received the most attention in the literature (Burns & Harm, 1993; Freehill, 1992; Jimmerson,1988; Pickett, Brennan, Greenberg, Licht, & Worrell, 1994; Rubin, 1990; Spitzer & Burke, 1993). CISD is not intended to stand alone as a sole intervention but is only as a component of the more comprehensive CISM system (Everly & Mitchell, 1997; Mitchell & Everly, 1997). CISD sessions are more formalized group crisis intervention meetings that are designed to include all staff members or emergency personnel who were involved in the critical incident in any capacity. The sessions occur 24 to 72 hours after a critical incident and often last about 3 hours. Debriefings are intended to accelerate the normal recovery of normal people who are suffering through normal but difficult and painful reactions to abnormal events (Mitchell, 1986; Mitchell & Bray, 1990). They are not intended to be psychotherapy or situational critique sessions. CISD sessions consist of progressive phases in a structured format conducted by personnel with specific training in the technique (to contact the International Critical Incident Stress Foundation for a schedule of training workshops held throughout the United States and internationally, see the website www.icisf.org). Debriefings are designed to decrease symptoms of those attending the sessions, assess the need for follow-up of individuals, and if possible, provide a sense of postcrisis closure (Mitchell, 1983; Mitchell & Bray, 1990). Debriefings can enhance group cohesiveness, team building, and interagency cooperation (Spitzer & Burke, 1993).

The sixth component of CISM is *follow-up and referral mechanisms* for further assessment and treatment, if necessary. Referrals can be made to employee assistance programs (Spitzer & Burke, 1993) or to other types of resources as appropriate. The seventh component of CISM relates to intervening in disasters or other large-scale incidents in which *demobilizations and staff advisement* become important. CISM is becoming a "standard of care" in addressing critical incident stress in many communities and organizations (Everly & Mitchell, 1997). However, whether CISM or another system of intervention is used, it is clear that the potential for staff trauma in situations of pediatric injury is real and is a possibility that can no longer be ignored. For the health and safety of staff and patients, critical incident stress must be recognized and addressed.

SUMMARY

The best pediatric psychological trauma intervention strategy is to prevent the injury from occurring in the first place. Because unintentional, preventable injury is the leading cause of death and disability among children in the United States (U.S. Department of Health and Human Services, 1999), primary, secondary, and tertiary prevention strategies are essential priorities for all pediatric caregivers, no matter what the setting in which they have contact with children and families. The frequency of occurrence and severity of injuries can be reduced by the consistent and appropriate use of safety precautions and safety equipment by informed children, families, and communities (Crawley, 1996). Although many parents are aware of the general risk of childhood injury, more time must be spent educating parents about specific injury risks at each developmental stage and effective countermeasures (Coffman, Martin, Prill, &

Langley, 1998; Hu, Wesson, Parkin, & Rootman, 1996). It will be time well spent. Many children and families can be saved the trauma, physical pain, mental anguish, and long-term disabilities and dysfunction associated with a sudden injury event that can change their lives and their world forever. For those families for whom prevention strategies come too late to prevent the trauma of an injury event, informed, family-centered, developmentally appropriate care can help reduce the psychological trauma and enhance long-term coping toward successful adaptation and functioning.

BIBLIOGRAPHY

Aaron, J., Zaglul, H., & Emery, R. E. (1999). Posttraumatic stress in children following acute physical injury. *Journal of Pediatric Psychology, 24,* 335-343.

Ainsworth, M. D. S., Blehar, M. C., Waters, E., & Wall, S. (1978). *Patterns of attachment.* Hillsdale, NJ: Erlbaum.

American Psychiatric Association. (1987). *Diagnostic and statistical manual of mental disorders* (3rd rev. ed.). Washington, DC: Author.

American Psychiatric Association. (1994). *Diagnostic and statistical manual of mental disorders* (4th ed.). Washington, DC: Author.

Back, K. J. (1992). Critical incident stress management for care providers in the pediatric emergency department. *Critical Care Nurse, 12,* 78-83.

Baker, S., O'Neill, B., Ginsburg, M., & Li, G. (1992). *The injury fact book* (2nd ed.). New York: Oxford University Press.

Baucher, H., Vinci, R., Bak, S., Pearson, C., & Corwin, M. J. (1996). Parents and procedures: A randomized controlled trial. *Pediatrics, 98,* 861-867.

Baucher, H., Vinci, R., & Wading, C. (1989). Pediatric procedures: Do parents want to watch? *Pediatrics, 84,* 907-909.

Baucher, H., Wading, C., & Vinci, R. (1991). Parental presence during procedures in an emergency room: Results from 50 observations. *Pediatrics, 87,* 544-548.

Bell, C. C., Jenkins, E. J., Kpo, W., & Rhodes, H. (1994). Response of emergency rooms to victims of interpersonal violence. *Hospital and Community Psychiatry, 45,* 142-146.

Bevan, J. C., Johnson, C., Haig, M. J., Tousignant, G., Lucy, S., Kimon, V., Assimes, I. K., & Carranza, R. (1990). Preoperative parental anxiety predicts behavioral and emotional responses to induction of anaesthesia in children. *Canadian Journal of Anesthesiology, 37,* 177-182.

Bijur, P. E., Golding, J., & Haslum, M. (1988). Persistence of occurrence of injury: Can injuries of preschool children predict injuries of school-age children? *Pediatrics, 82,* 707-712.

Blakeney, P., Meyer, W., Robert, R., Desai, M., Wolf, S., & Herndon, D. (1998). Long-term psychosocial adaptation of children who survive burns involving 80% or greater total body surface area. *Journal of Trauma, 44,* 625-634.

Blanchard, E. B., & Hickling, E. J. (1997). *After the crash: Assessment and treatment of motor vehicle accident survivors.* Washington, DC: American Psychological Association.

Blanchard, E. B., Hickling, E. J., Taylor, A. E., Loos, W. R., & Gerardi, R. J. (1994). Psychological morbidity associated with motor vehicle accidents. *Behavioral Research and Therapy, 32,* 283-290.

Blanchard, E. B., Hickling, E. J., Vollmer, A. J., Loos, W. R., Buckley, T. C., & Jaccard, J. (1995). Psychological morbidity associated with motor vehicle accidents. *Behavioral Research and Therapy, 33,* 369-377.

Bowlby, J. (1980). *Attachment and loss: Volume 3. Loss, sadness, and depression.* New York: Basic Books.

Braulin, J. L. D., Rook, J., & Sills, G. M. (1982). Families in crisis: The impact of trauma. *Critical Care Quarterly, 5,* 38-46.

Broome, M. E., & Endsley, R. C. (1989). Maternal presence, childrearing practices, and children's response to an injection. *Research in Nursing and Health, 12,* 229-235.

Broome, M. E., Knafl, K., Pridham, K., & Feetham, S. (Eds.). (1998). *Children and families in health and illness.* Thousand Oaks, CA: Sage Publications.

Brown, J., & Ritchie, J. (1990). Nurses' perceptions of parent-nurse roles in caring for hospitalized children. *Childrens Health Care, 19*(1), 28-36.

Burns, C., & Harm, N. J. (1993). Emergency nurses' perceptions of critical incidents and stress debriefing. *Journal of Emergency Nursing, 19,* 431-436.

Burstein, A. (1989). Posttraumatic stress disorder in victims of motor vehicle accidents. *Hospital and Community Psychiatry, 40,* 295-297.

Bussing, R., Menvielle, E., & Zima, B. (1996). Relationship between behavioral problems and unintentional injuries in US children. *Archives of Pediatric and Adolescent Medicine, 150,* 50-56.

Cameron, J. A., Bond, M. J., & Pointer, S. C. (1996). Reducing the anxiety of children undergoing surgery: Parental presence during anesthetic induction. *Journal of Pediatric Health, 32,* 51-56.

Chan, L., Russell, T. J., & Robak, N. (1998). Parental perception of the adequacy of pain control in their child after discharge from the emergency department. *Pediatric Emergency Care, 14,* 251-253.

Christoffel, L. (1992). Pediatric firearm injuries: Time to target a growing population. *Pediatric Annals, 21,* 430-436.

Christoffel, K. K., Barlow, B., Bell, C., Dowd, D., Godbold, L. T., Kitchen, A., Reynolds, M., & Staggers, B. C. (1997). AAP Task Force report: Adolescent assault victim needs: A review of issues and a model protocol. *Pediatrics, 98,* 991-1001.

Christoffel, K. K., Donovan, M., Schofer, J., Wills, K., & Lavigne, J. V. (1996). Psychosocial factors in childhood pedestrian injury: A matched case-control study. Kid's'n'Cars Team. *Pediatrics, 97,* 33-42.

Coffman, S., Martin, V., Prill, N., & Langley, B. (1998). Perceptions, safety behaviors, and learning needs of parents of children brought to an emergency department. *Journal of Emergency Nursing, 24,* 133-139.

Cooley-Quille, M. R., Turner, S. M., & Beidel, D. C. (1995). Emotional impact of children's exposure to community violence: A preliminary study. *Journal of the American Academy of Child and Adolescent Psychiatry, 34,* 1362-1368.

Craft, M. J., Wyatt, N., & Sandell, B. (1986). Behavior and feeling changes in siblings of hospitalized children. *Clinical Pediatrics, 24,* 374-377.

Crawley, T. (1996). Childhood injury: Significance and prevention strategies. *Journal of Pediatric Nursing, 11,* 225-232.

Dateline NBC. (1999, July 30). *Who should be allowed behind the ER's closed doors?* New York: National Broadcasting Corporation.

Daviss, W. B., Mooney, D., Racusin, R., Ford, J. D., Fleischer, A., & McHugo, G. J. (2000). Predicting posttraumatic stress after hospitalization fro pediatric injury. *Journal of the American Academy of Child and Adolescent Psychiatry, 39,* 76-83.

Denholm, C. J. (1995). Survival from a wild animal attack: A case study analysis of adolescent coping. *Maternal-Child Nursing Journal, 23,* 26-34.

deVries, A. P. J., Kassam-Adams, N., Cnaan, A., Sherman-Slate, E., Gallagher, P. R., & Winston, F. K. (1999). Looking beyond the physical injury: Posttraumatic stress disorder in children and parents after pediatric traffic injury. *Pediatrics, 104,* 1293-1299.

den Velde, W. O., Falger, P. R. J., Havens, J. E., de Groen, J. H. M., Lasschuit, L. J., Van Duijn, H., & Schouten, E. G. W. (1993). Posttraumatic stress disorder in Dutch resistance veterans from World War II. In J. P. Wilson & B. Raphael (Eds.), *International handbook of traumatic stress syndromes* (pp. 219-230). New York: Plenum Press.

Eberly, T. W., Miles, M. S., Carter, M. C., Hennessey, J., & Riddle, I. (1985). Parental stress after the unexpected admission of a child to the intensive care unit. *Critical Care Quarterly, 8,* 57-65.

Eisendrath, S. J., & Dunkel, J. (1979). Psychological issues in intensive care unit staff. *Heart & Lung, 7*, 756-760.

Emanuelson, I., vonWendt, L., Beckung, E., & Hagberg, I. (1998). Late outcome after severe traumatic brain injury in children and adolescents. *Pediatric Rehabilitation, 2*, 65-70.

Emergency Nurses Association. (1998). *Family presence at the bedside during invasive procedures and/or resuscitation. ENA position statement.* Available at: www.ena.org/services/posistate/data/fampre.

Epperson, M. M. (1977). Families in sudden crisis: Process and intervention in a critical care center. *Social Work in Health Care, 2*, 265-273.

Everly, G. S. (1990). *A clinical guide to the treatment of the human stress response.* New York: Plenum Press.

Everly, G. S., & Mitchell, J. T. (1997). *Critical incident stress management (CISM): A new era and standard of care in crisis intervention.* Ellicott City, MD: Chevron.

Figley, C. R. (1983). Catastrophes: An overview of family reaction. In C. R. Figley & H. I. McCubbin (Eds.), *Stress and the family: Volume 2. Coping with catastrophe* (p. 3020). New York: Brunner/Mazel.

Figley, C. R. (1991). Compassion stress: Toward its measurement and management. *Family Therapy News, 24*, 3, 16.

Figley, C. R. (1995). Compassion fatigue: Coping with secondary traumatic stress disorder in those who treat the traumatized. New York: Brunner/Mazel.

Fletcher, K. E. (1996). Childhood posttraumatic stress disorder. In E. J. Marsh & R. A. Barkley (Eds.), *Child psychopathology.* New York: The Guilford Press.

Freehill, K. M. (1992). Critical incident stress debriefing in health care. *Critical Care Clinics of North America, 8*, 491-500.

Freud, A., & Burlingham, D. (1944). *Infants without families.* New York: International Universities Press.

Frosch, E. (1996). Acute physical injury in children: Psychological consequences and treatment implications. *American Psychiatric Press Review of Psychiatry, 15*, 429-445.

Frosch, E., & Lewandowski, L. A. (1998). Psychological issues associated with acute physical injury: After the pediatric emergency department. *International Review of Psychiatry, 10*, 216-223.

Galante, R., & Foa, D. (1986). An epidemiological study of psychic trauma and treatment effectiveness for children after a natural disaster. *Journal of the American Academy of Child and Adolescent Psychiatry, 25*, 357-363.

Garbarino, J. (1995). The American war zone: What children can tell us about living with violence. *Developmental and Behavioral Pediatrics, 16*, 431-435.

Garmezy, N. (1985). Stress-resistant children: The search for protective factors. In J. Stevenson (Ed.), *Recent research in developmental psychopathology* (pp. 213-233). Oxford, UK: Pergamon Press.

Garmezy, N. (1987). Stress, competence, and development: Continuities in the study of schizophrenic adults, children vulnerable to psychopathology, and the search for stress-resistant children. *American Journal of Orthopsychiatry, 57*, 159-174.

Garmezy, N., & Rutter, M. (1985). Acute reactions to stress. In M. Rutter & L. Hersov (Eds.), *Child and adolescent psychiatry: Modern approaches* (2nd ed., pp. 152-176). Oxford, UK: Blackwell.

Gislason, I. L., & Call, J. (1982). Dog bite in infancy: Trauma and personality development. *Journal of the American Academy of Child Psychiatry, 22*, 203-207.

Green, B. L., Korol, M., Grace, M. C., Vary, M. G., Leonard, A. C., Gleser, G. C., & Smitson-Cohen, S. (1991). Children and disaster: Age, gender, and parental effects on PTSD symptoms. *Journal of the American Academy of Child and Adolescent Psychiatry, 30*, 945-951.

Guerriere, D., & McKeever, P. (1997). Mothering children who survive brain injuries: Playing the hand you're dealt. *Journal of the Society of Pediatric Nurses, 2*, 105-115.

Haimi-Cohen, Y., Amir, J., Harel, L., Straussberg, R., & Varsano, Y. (1996). Parental presence during lumbar puncture. *Clinical Pediatrics, 35*, 2-4.

Hamrin, V. (1998). Psychiatric interviews with pediatric gunshot patients. *Journal of Child and Adolescent Psychiatric Nursing, 11*, 61-68.

Harris, B. H., Schwaitzberg, S. D., Seman, T. M., & Herrmann, C. (1989). The hidden morbidity of pediatric trauma. *Journal of Pediatric Surgery, 24*, 103-106.

Hill, C. J. (1978). The mother on the pediatric ward: insider or outlawed? *Pediatric Nursing, 5*, 26-29.

Horowitz, K., Weine, S., & Jekel, J. (1995). PTSD symptoms in urban adolescent girls: Compounded community trauma. *Journal of the American Academy of Child and Adolescent Psychiatry, 34*, 1353-1361.

Horowitz, M. J., Wilner, M., & Kultreider, N. (1980). Signs and symptoms of post-traumatic stress disorder. *Archives of General Psychiatry, 37*, 85-92.

Hu, X., Wesson, D. E., Kenney, B. D., Chipman, M. L., & Spence, L. J. (1993). Risk factors for extended disruption of family function after severe injury to a child. *Canadian Medical Association Journal, 149*, 421-427.

Hu, X., Wesson, D, Parkin, P., & Rootman, I. (1996). Pediatric injuries: Parental knowledge, attitudes, and needs. *Canadian Journal of Public Health, 87*, 101-105.

Hutson, H. R., Anglin, C., & Spears, K. (1995). The perspectives of violent street gang injuries. *Neurosurgery Clinics of North America, 6*, 621-628.

Hutson, H. R., Anglin, D., & Mallon, W. (1992). Injuries and deaths from gang violence: They are preventable. *Annals of Emergency Medicine, 21*, 1234-1236.

Hutson, H. R., Anglin, D., Mallon, W., & Pratts, M. J. (1994). Caught in the crossfire of gang violence: Small children as innocent victims of drive-by shootings. *Journal of Emergency Medicine, 12*, 385-388.

Irwin, C. E., Jr., Cataldo, M. F., Matheny, A. P., Jr., & Peterson, L. (1992). Health consequences of behaviors: Injury as a model. *Pediatrics, 90*, 798-807.

Jacobson, M. S., Rubenstein, E. M., Bohannon, W. E., Sonheimer, D. L., Cicci, R., Toner, J., Gong, E., & Heald, F. P. (1986). Follow-up of adolescent trauma victims: A new model of care. *Pediatrics, 77*, 236-241.

Jaquess, D. L., & Finney, J. W. (1994). Previous injuries and behavior problems predict children's injuries. *Journal of Pediatric Psychology, 19*, 79-89.

Jaworski, S. (1992). Traffic accident injuries of children: The need for prospective studies of psychiatric sequelae. *Israeli Journal of Psychiatry and Related Science, 29*, 174-184.

Jimmerson, C. (1988). Critical incident stress debriefing. *Journal of Emergency Nursing, 14*, 43A-45A.

Johnston, B. D., Grossman, D. C., Connell, F. A., & Koepsell, T. D. (2000). High-risk periods for childhood injury among siblings. *Pediatrics, 105*, 562-568.

Jones, R. W., & Peterson, L. W. (1993). Post-traumatic stress disorder in a child following an automobile accident. *Journal of Family Practice, 36*, 222-225.

Kelly, S. (1990). Parental stress responses to sexual abuse and ritualistic abuse of children in daycare centers. *Nursing Research, 39*, 25-29.

Kendall-Grove, Ehde, D. M., Patterson, D. R., & Johnson, V. (1998). Rates of dysfunction in parents of pediatric patients with burns. *Journal of Burn Care Rehabilitation, 19*, 312-316.

Kendrick, D. (1993). Accidental injury attendances as predictors of future admission. *Journal of Public Health Medicine, 15*, 171-174.

Kharasch, J. S., Yuknek, J., Vinci, R. J., Herbert, B., & Zuckerman, B. (1997). Violence-related injuries in a pediatric emergency department. *Pediatric Emergency Care, 13*, 95-97.

Kilpatrick, D., & Resnick, H. (1993). PTSD associated with exposure to criminal victimization in clinical and community populations. In J. Davidson & E. Foa (Eds.), *Post-traumatic stress disorder in review: Recent research and future directions* (pp. 113-143). Washington, DC: American Psychiatric Press.

Knafl, K. A. (1985). How families manage a pediatric hospitalization. *Western Journal of Nursing Research, 7*, 151.

Knafl, K. A., Cavalleri, K. A., & Dixon, D. M. (1988). *Pediatric hospitalization: Family and nurse perspectives.* Glenview, IL: Scott, Foresman.

Kreutzer, J. S., Gervaio, A. H., & Camplair, P. S. (1994). Primary caregivers' psychological status and family functioning after traumatic brain injury. *Brain Injury, 8*, 197-210.

Kunkler, J., & Whittick, J. (1991). Stress management groups for nurses: Practical problems and possible solutions. *Journal of Advanced Nursing, 16*(2), 172-176.

Laflamme, L., & Diderichsen, F. (2000). Social differences in traffic injury risks in childhood and youth: A literature review and a research agenda. *Injury Prevention, 6*, 293-298.

Lanning, J. (1985). Pediatric trauma: Emotional aspects. *AORN Journal, 42*, 345-351.

LaRosa-Nash, P. A., & Murphy, J. M. (1997). An approach to pediatric perioperative care: Parent-present induction. *Nursing Clinics of North America, 32*, 183-199.

LaRosa-Nash, P. A., Murphy, J. M., & Wade, L. A., & Clasby, L. L. (1995). Implementing a parent-present induction program. *AORN Journal, 61*, 526-531.

Lawson, B. Z. (1987). Work-related post-traumatic stress reactions: The hidden dimension. *Health and Social Work, 12*, 250-258.

LeDoux, J., Meyer, W. J., Blakeney, P. E., & Herndon, D. N. (1998). Relationship between parental emotional states, family environment and the behavioral adjustment of pediatric burn survivors. *Burns, 24*, 425-432.

Levi, R. B., Drotar, D., Yeates, K. O., & Taylor, H. G. (1999). Posttraumatic stress symptoms in children following orthopedic or traumatic brain injury. *Journal of Clinical Child Psychology, 28*, 232-243.

Lewandowski, L. A. (1992a). Needs of children during the critical illness of a parent or sibling. *Critical Care Nursing Clinics of North America, 4*, 573-585.

Lewandowski, L. A. (1992b). Psychosocial aspects of pediatric critical care. In M. F. Hazinski (Ed.), *Pediatric critical care nursing.* St. Louis: Mosby.

Lewandowski, L. A., & Baranoski, M. V. (1994). Psychological aspects of acute trauma: Intervening with children and families in the inpatient setting. *Child and Adolescent Psychiatric Clinics of North America, 3*, 513-529.

Lewandowski, L. A., Berent, L. L., Frosch, E., & Weissberg, E. (in press). Unintentional or violent injury in children and adolescents: Family perceptions and experiences. *Journal of Advanced Nursing.*

Livingston, M. G., & Brooks, D. N. (1988). The burden on families of the brain injured: A review. *Journal of Head Trauma Rehabilitation, 3*, 6-15.

Malt, U. F., Karlehagen, S., Hoff, H., Herrstromer, U., Hildingson, K., Tibell, E., & Leymann, H. (1993). The effect of major railway accidents on the psychological health of train drivers—I. Acute psychological responses to accident. *Journal of Psychosomatic Research, 37*, 793-805.

Mangini, L., Confessore, M. T., Girard, P., & Spadola, T. (1995). Pediatric trauma support program: Supporting children and families in emotional crisis. *Critical Care Nurse Clinics of North America, 7*, 557-567.

Matheson, K. (1990). Stress and stress counseling. *Postgraduate Medical Journal, 66*, 738-742.

Max, J. E., Castillo, C. S., Robin, D. A., Lindgren, S. D., Smith, W. L., Sato, Y., & Arndt, S. (1998). Posttraumatic symptomatology after childhood traumatic brain injury. *Journal of Nervous and Mental Diseases, 186*, 589-596.

Mayou, R., Bryant, B., & Duthrie, R. (1993). Psychiatric consequences of road traffic accidents. *British Medical Journal, 307*, 647-651.

McFarlane, A. (1987). Family functioning and overprotection following a natural disaster: The longitudinal effects of post-traumatic morbidity. *Australia and New Zealand Journal of Psychiatry, 21*, 210-218.

McNally, R. (1993). Stressors that produce posttraumatic stress disorder in children. In J. Davidson & E. Foa (Eds.), *Posttraumatic stress disorder: DSM-IV and beyond* (pp. 57-74). Washington, DC: American Psychiatric Association Press.

Melnyk, B. M. (1995). Coping with unplanned childhood hospitalization: The mediating functions of parental beliefs. *Journal of Pediatric Psychology, 20*, 299-312.

Merrow, D. L., & Johnson, B. S. (1968). Perceptions of the mother's role with her hospitalized child. *Nursing Research, 17*, 155-156.

Mirza, K. A., Bhadrinath, B. R., Goodyer, I. M., & Gilmour, C. (1998). Post-traumatic stress disorder in children and adolescents following road traffic accidents. *British Journal of Psychiatry, 172*, 443-447.

Mitchell, J. T. (1983). When disaster strikes: The critical incident stress debriefing process. *Journal of Emergency Medical Services, 8*, 36-39.

Mitchell, J. T. (1986). Critical incident stress management. *Response!, September/October*, 24-25.

Mitchell, J. T., & Bray, G. (1990). *Emergency services stress: Guidelines for preserving the health and careers of emergency services personnel.* Englewood Cliffs, NJ: Prentice Hall.

Mitchell, J. T., & Everly, G. S. (1996). Critical incident stress debriefing: CISD: An operations manual for the prevention of traumatic stress among emergency service and disaster workers (2nd ed.). Ellicott City, MD: Chevron Publishing Corp.

Mitchell, J. T., & Everly, G. S. (1997). Scientific evidence for CISM. *Journal of Emergency Medical Services, 22*, 87-93.

MSNBC. (1999, July 39). *Open door policy: Who should be allowed behind the ER's closed doors?* Available at: www.msnbc.com/news/295067.

Murray, J. S. (2000). Understanding sibling adaptation to childhood cancer. *Issues in Comprehensive Pediatric Nursing, 23*, 39-47.

Nader, K. O., Pynoos, R. S., Fairbanks, L. A., & Frederick, C. (1990). Children's PTSD reactions one year after a sniper attack at their school. *American Journal of Psychiatry, 147*, 1526-1530.

Norman, E. M. (1989). Analysis of the concept of post-traumatic stress disorder. *Journal of Advanced Medical Surgical Nursing, 1*, 55-64.

Oliver, R. C., & Fallat, M. E. (1995). Traumatic childhood death: How well do parents cope? *Journal of Trauma, 39*, 303-308.

Osofsky, J. D. (1995). The effects of exposure to violence on young children. *American Psychologist, 50*, 782-788.

Ozmar, B. (1994). Encountering victims of interpersonal violence: Implications for critical care nursing. *Critical Care Nursing Clinics of North America, 6*, 515-523.

Pennebaker, J. W. (1990). *Opening up: The healing power of confiding in others.* New York: Avon Books.

Pennebaker, J. W., & Susman, J. R. (1988). Disclosure of traumas and psychosomatic processes. *Social Science & Medicine, 26*, 327-332.

Pickett, M., Brennan, A. M. W., Greenberg, H. S., Licht, L., & Worrell, J. D. (1994). Use of debriefing techniques to prevent compassion fatigue in research teams. *Nursing Research, 43*, 250-252.

Putnam, F. W. (1996). Posttraumatic stress disorder in children and adolescents. In M. Lewis (Ed.), *Child and adolescent psychiatry: A comprehensive textbook* (pp. 447-467). Baltimore: Williams & Wilkins.

Putnam, F. W. (1997). *Dissociation in children and adolescents: A developmental perspective.* New York: The Guilford Press.

Pynoos, R. S., & Eth, S. (1986). Witness to violence: the child interview. *Journal of the American Academy of Child and Adolescent Psychiatry, 25*, 306-319.

Pynoos, R. S., & Nader, K. (1993). Issues in the treatment of posttraumatic stress in children and adolescents. In J. P. Wilson & B. Raphael (Eds.), *International handbook of traumatic stress syndromes* (pp. 535-549). New York: Plenum Press.

Pynoos, R. S., & Nader, K. (1988). Psychological first aid and treatment approach to children exposed to community violence: Research implications. *Journal of Traumatic Stress, 1*, 445-473.

Rachman, S. (1980). Emotional processing. *Behavioral Research and Therapy, 18*, 51-60.

Ragaisis, K. M. (1994). Critical incident stress debriefing: A family nursing intervention. *Archives of Psychiatric Nursing, 8*, 38-43.

Ravenscroft, K. (1982). Psychiatric consultation to the child with acute physical trauma. *American Journal of Orthopsychiatry, 52*, 298-307.

Reynolds, E. A., & Ramenofsky, M. L. (1988). The emotional impact of trauma on toddlers. *MCN: The American Journal of Maternal Child Nursing, 13,* 106-109.

Richmond, T. S. (1997). An explanatory model of variables influencing postinjury disability. *Nursing Research, 46,* 262-269.

Richters, J. E. (1993). Community violence and children's development: Toward a research agenda for the 1990's. *Psychiatry, 56,* 3-6.

Rigamer, E. F. (1986). Psychological management of children in a national crisis. *Journal of the American Academy of Child Psychiatry, 25,* 364-369.

Rivara, J. B., Jaffe, K. M., Fay, G. C., Polissar, N. L., Martin, K. M., Shurtleff, H. A., & Liao, S. (1993). Family functioning and injury severity as predictors of child functioning one year following traumatic brain injury. *Archives of Physical Medicine and Rehabilitation, 74,* 1047-1055.

Rivara, J. B., Jaffe, K. M., Fay, G. C., Polissar, N. L., Fay, G. C., Martin, K. M., Shurtleff, H. A., & Liao, S. (1994). Family functioning and children's academic performance and behavior problems in the year following traumatic brain injury. *Archives of Physical Medicine and Rehabilitation, 75,* 369-379.

Robert, R., Meyer, W. J., Villarreal, C., Blakeney, P. E., Desai, M., & Herndon, D. (1999). An approach to the timely treatment of acute stress disorder. *Journal of Burn Care Rehabilitation, 20,* 250-258.

Romaniuk, D. K., & Kritsjanson, L. J. (1995). The parent nurse relationship from the perspective of parents of children with cancer. *Journal of Pediatric Oncology Nursing, 12*(2), 80-89.

Roskies, E., Bedard, P., Gauvreau-Guilbault, H., & Lafortune, D. (1975). Emergency hospitalization of young children: Some neglected psychological considerations. *Medical Care, 13,* 570-581.

Rubin, J. G. (1990). Critical incident stress debriefing: Helping the helpers. *Journal of Emergency Nursing, 16,* 255-258.

Rutter, M. (1987). Psychosocial resilience and protective mechanisms. *American Journal of Orthopsychiatry, 57,* 316-331.

Sanders-Phillips, K. (1997). Assault violence in the community: Psychological responses of adolescent victims and their parents. *Journal of Adolescent Health, 21,* 356-365.

Satcher, D. (1995). Violence as a public health issue. *Bulletin of the New York Academy of Medicine, 72,* 46-56.

Satcher, D. (2001). *Youth violence: A report of the Surgeon General.* Available at: www.surgeongeneral.gov/library/youthviolence.

Schottenfeld, R. S., & Cullen, M. R. (1985). Occupation-induced posttraumatic stress disorders. *American Journal of Psychiatry, 142,* 198-202.

Schuman, M., Silbernagel, K. H., Chesney, M. A., & Villarreal, S. (1996). Interventions among adolescents who were violently injured and those who attempted suicide. *Psychiatric Services, 47,* 755-757.

Schwarz, E. D., & Perry, B. D. (1994). The post-traumatic response in children and adolescents. *Psychiatric Clinics of North America, 17,* 311-326.

Schwebel, D. C., & Plumert, J. M. (1999). Longitudinal and concurrent relations among temperament, ability estimation, and injury proneness. *Child Development, 70,* 700-712.

Shalev, A. Y., Peri, T., Canetti, L., & Schreiber, S. (1996). Predictors of PTSD in injured trauma survivors: A prospective study. *American Journal of Psychiatry, 153,* 219-225.

Smith, E. M., & North, C. S. (1993). Posttraumatic stress disorder in natural disasters and technological accidents. In J. P. Wilson & B. Raphael (Eds.), *International handbook of traumatic stress syndromes* (pp. 405-419). New York: Plenum Press.

Snowden, A. W., & Gottlieb, L. N. (1989). The maternal role in the pediatric intensive care unit and hospital ward. *Maternal-Child Nursing Journal, 18,* 97-115.

Spitzer, W. J., & Burke, L. (1993). A critical-incident stress debriefing program for hospital-based health care personnel. *Health & Social Work, 18,* 149-156.

Stancin, T., Taylor, H. G., Thompson, G. H., Wade, S., Drotar, D., & Yeates, K. O. (1998). Acute psychosocial impact of pediatric orthopedic trauma with and without accompanying brain injuries. *Journal of Trauma, 45,* 1031-1038.

Suarez, R. (1999). *Talk of the nation: Should family members be allowed in the emergency department?* National Public Radio, March 1999.

Tarnowski, K. J., Rasnake, L. K., Linscheid, T. R., & Mulick, J. A. (1989). Behavioral adjustment of pediatric burn victims. *Journal of Pediatric Psychology, 14,* 607-615.

Taylor, S., & Koch, W. (1995). Anxiety disorders due to motor vehicle accidents: Nature and treatment. *Clinical Psychology Review, 15,* 721-738.

Tennant, C. (1988). Parental loss in childhood: Its effect in adult life. *Archives of General Psychiatry, 45,* 1045-1049.

Terr, L. C. (1989). Family anxiety after traumatic events. *Journal of Clinical Psychiatry, 50,* 15-19.

Testani-Dufour, L., Chappel-Aiken, L., & Gueldner, S. (1992). Traumatic brain injury: A family experience. *Journal of Neuroscience Nursing, 24,* 317-323.

Triolo, P. K. (1989). Occupational health hazards of hospital staff nurses. *Journal of the American Association of Occupational Health Nursing, 37,* 232-237.

Tuckman, A. J. (1973). Disaster and mental health intervention. *Community Mental Health Journal, 9,* 151-157.

Ursano, R. J., Fullerton, C. S., Epstein, R. S., Crowley, B., Vance, K., Kao, T. C., & Baum, A. (1999). Peritraumatic dissociation and post-traumatic stress disorder following motor vehicle accidents. *American Journal of Psychiatry, 156,* 1808-1810.

U.S. Department of Health and Human Services. (1999). *Healthy people 2010* (DHHS Publication No. (PHS)91-50212). Washington, DC: Author.

Vessey, J. A., Bogetz, M. S., Caserza, C. L., Liu, K. R., & Cassidy, M. D. (1994). Parental upset associated with participation in induction of anesthesia in children. *Canadian Journal of Anesthesiology, 41,* 276-280.

Vessey, J. A., & Carlson, K. L. (1996). Nonpharmacological intervention to use with children in pain. *Issues in Comprehensive Pediatric Nursing, 19,* 169-182.

Vessey, J. A., Carlson, K. L., & McGill, J. (1994). Use of distraction with children during an acute pain experience. *Nursing Research, 43,* 369-372.

Visintainer, M., & Wolfer, J. (1975). Psychological preparation for pediatric surgical patients: The effect on children's and parents' stress responses and adjustment. *Pediatrics, 56,* 187-197.

Wade, S., Drotar, D., Taylor, H. G., & Stancin, T. (1995). Assessing the effects of traumatic brain injury on family functioning: Conceptual and methodological issues. *Journal of Pediatric Psychology, 20,* 737-752.

Wade, S. L., Taylor, H. G., Drotar, D., Stancin, T., & Yeates, K. O. (1998). Family burden and adaptation during the initial year after traumatic brain injury in children. *Pediatrics, 102,* 110-116.

Wesson, D. E., Scorpio, R., Spence, L., Filler, R. M., Armstrong, P. F., & Pearl, R. H. (1989). Functional outcome in pediatric trauma. *Journal of Trauma, 29,* 589-592.

Wesson, D., Scorpio, R., Spence, L., Kenny, B., Chipman, M., Netley, C., & Hu, X. (1992). The physical, psychological, and socioemotional costs of pediatric trauma. *Journal of Trauma, 33,* 252-257.

Wilson, M., Baker, S., Teret, S., Shock, S., & Garbarino, J. (1991). *Saving children: A guide to injury prevention.* New York: Oxford University Press.

Wolfram, R. W., & Turner, E. D. (1996). Effects of parental presence during children's venipuncture. *Academic Emergency Medicine, 3,* 58-64.

Wong, D. L. (1982). Childhood trauma: Its developmental aspects and nursing interventions. *Critical Care Quarterly, 5,* 47-60.

Yule, W., & Williams, W. (1990). Post-traumatic stress reactions in children. *Journal of Traumatic Stress, 3,* 279-295.

Zink, K. A. (1996). Emotional support in pediatric trauma: Remembering children like Caleb. *Journal of Pediatric Nursing, 11,* 345-346.

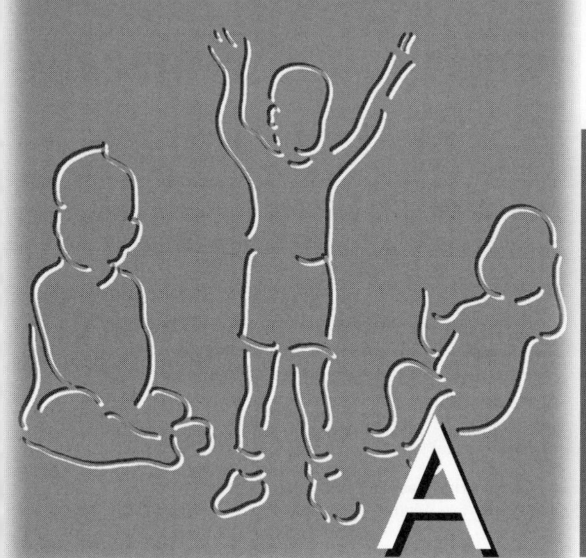

Interdisciplinary Admission Data Base

CHILDREN'S SEASHORE HOUSE

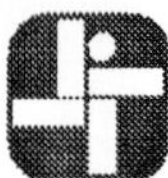

INTERDISCIPLINARY ADMISSION DATA BASE

Addressograph

PAGE 1

Name:________ Nickname:________ D.O.B:______ Age:______ Sex:___

Admission Date & Time:________ Admitted From:________ Admitted Via:________ ELOS: ______

Primary Care Physician:________ Telephone:________ Person Interviewed/Relationship to Patient:________ Whom to Notify in an Emergency/Phone#:________

ORIENTATION TO UNIT: T.V. ❒ Meal Schedule ❒
ID Band ❒ Call System ❒ Smoking ❒ Side Rails ❒ Leaving Unit ❒ Phone Use ❒ Visitation/Overnight ❒
Tour of Unit ❒ Kitchen ❒ CR Monitor ❒ Caring for Other Patients ❒ Electrical Equip ❒ Isolation ❒
Safety Crib ❒ Foot Wear ❒ Special Safety Needs/Describe________

Vital Signs: T________ HR________ RR ________

BP & location:________ ❒ RUE ❒ LUE ❒ RLE ❒ LLE Cuff size______

Ht/Length (cm):________ Wt (kg)______ Scale / Type ______ Head Circumference (cm)______

Admitting Diagnosis:________ Secondary Diagnosis:________

Caregiver's Expectations of Admission/Reason for Admission:________

Child's Expectations of Admission/Reason for Admission:________

Previous Hospitalizations (Date & Reason):________

MEDICATIONS:

	NAME	DOSE	ROUTE	FREQUENCY	TIMES TO BE GIVEN	LAST DOSE
1.						
2.						
3.						
4.						
5.						

Were you able to obtain prescriptions ? ❒ Yes ❒ No Why Not ? ________
Did you take your prescriptions as prescribed ? ❒ Yes ❒ No Why Not ? ________
Form of Medications Preferred: Pill ❒ Crushed ❒ Chewable ❒ Liquid ❒ Other________

HEALTH MANAGEMENT/HEALTH PERCEPTION:

Allergies: (Drug, Food, Latex)________

____

Recent Exposure to Communicable Disease (Type of Disease/Date):________

Immunization Status (up to date ?) ❒ Yes ❒ No ________

Initials ______ **Initials** ______ **Initials** ______ **Initials** ______
Date ______ **Date** ______ **Date** ______ **Date** ______

Courtesy Children's Seashore House of the Children's Hospital of Philadelphia, Philadelphia, PA.

CHILDREN'S SEASHORE HOUSE

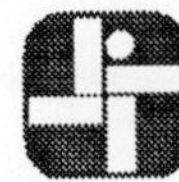

INTERDISCIPLINARY ADMISSION DATA BASE

Addressograph

PAGE 2

History of Hearing Problems: ☐ Yes ☐ No ______________________

History of Vision Problems: ☐ Yes ☐ No ______________________

Nose: Drainage: ☐ Yes ☐ No ______________________
Mouth: Mucous membranes: moist ☐ dry ☐ Lesions of mucosa:__________
Comments:______________________

RESPIRATORY:

Lung Sounds:
Productive Cough: Yes ☐ No ☐ Frequency of suctioning __________
Color:________ Amount:________ Consistency:__________
Tracheotomy: Yes ☐ No ☐
Type:____________ Size:__________
Capped: Yes ☐ No ☐ Time tolerates capping:__________
Passey Muir: Yes ☐ No ☐
Supplemental Oxygen:
Yes ☐ No ☐ Amount/Flow Rate:__________ Delivery Method:__________
Supplemental Humidification:
Yes ☐ No ☐ Constant/Intermittent:__________
Mechanical Ventilation:
Yes ☐ No ☐ Brand Type:__________ Settings:__________
Other:______________________

CARDIOVASCULAR:

Rhythm: Regular ☐ Irregular ☐
Peripheral Pulses (Keys: **S**-Strong, **W**-Weak, **A**-Absent): RUE________LUE________RLE________LLE________
Capillary Refill Time:__________

ABDOMEN:

Soft ☐ Firm ☐ Distended ☐ Tender ☐ Non-Tender ☐
Bowel Sounds: Normal ☐ Hyperactive ☐ Diminished ☐ Absent ☐
Bowel Elimination Pattern: Last Bowel Movement__________ Continent/Incontinent__________ Frequency________
Character__________ Frequency__________ Regular__________ Frequency________
Bowel Training Program: Yes ☐ No ☐ Adaptive Equipment:__________ Yes ☐ No ☐
Laxatives Needed: Yes ☐ No ☐ Type:______________________

Initials ______	**Initials** ______	**Initials** ______	**Initials** ______
Date ______	**Date** ______	**Date** ______	**Date** ______

CHILDREN'S SEASHORE HOUSE

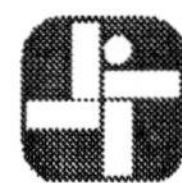

INTERDISCIPLINARY ADMISSION DATA BASE

Addressograph

PAGE 3

NUTRITION:

❒ Diet:__________

Likes/Dislikes:__________

❒ NG size _____ Placed_______ Formula / Feed Time__________

❒ GT size _____ Placed_______ Formula / Feed Time __________

❒ JT size _____ Placed_______ Formula / Feed Time __________

❒ TPN type of line__________ Placed_______

Additional Comments:__________

Dietary Restrictions (ethnic / cultural / religious): __________

CRITERIA FOR NUTRITION SCREENING

- ❒ Patient is < 1 year old
- ❒ Patient is tube fed or receiving Parental Nutrition
- ❒ Diagnosis of FTT, Malnutrition, Inborn Errors of Metabolism, Cerebral Palsy, Food Allergies/Sensitivities, Diabetes Mellitus, Burn
- ❒ Patient is ventilator dependent
- ❒ Patient is receiving a calorie, protein, fat or sodium controlled diet, or a renal, Ketogenic or o concentrated sweet diet
- ❒ Patient's Wt/Ht is < 5th percentile based on National Center of Health Statistics (NCHS) Standard Growth Charts
- ❒ Patient's Wt/Ht is > 95th percentile based on NCHS Standard Growth Charts

Note:
If patient meets any of above criteria, forward this page to Dietician for a complete nutrition assessment.

Initials _____	**Initials** _____	**Initials** _____	**Initials** _____
Date _____	**Date** _____	**Date** _____	**Date** _____

Courtesy Children's Seashore House of the Children's Hospital of Philadelphia, Philadelphia, PA.

CHILDREN'S SEASHORE HOUSE

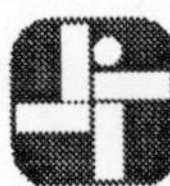

INTERDISCIPLINARY ADMISSION DATA BASE

Addressograph

PAGE 4

GENITOURINARY/URINARY SYSTEM:

Frequency/Recent Urinary Tract Infections: Yes ❒ No ❒

Characteristics of Urine:__________

Frequency: Regular ❒ Irregular ❒ Method__________

Continent/Incontinent: Frequency__________

Intermittent Catheterization Program: Yes ❒ No ❒ Adaptive equipment__________

Level of Assistance:__________ Catheter Type______ Frequency______

Technique: Clean______ Sterile______

Position used: Bed (head of bed elevated/Flat)______ Toilet:______ Chair (erect/reclined)______

Other:__________

NEUROLOGIC:

Level of Consciousness: Awake ❒ Alert ❒ Oriented x3 ❒ High-pitched Cry ❒ Comatose ❒

Rancho Level: __________

Eye Opening: Spontaneous ❒ To Voice ❒ To Pain ❒ None ❒

Verbal Response: Oriented ❒ Confused ❒ Inappropriate Words ❒ Incomprehensible ❒ None ❒ Appropriate ❒

Motor Response: Obeys Commands ❒ Localizes (pain) ❒ Withdraws (pain) ❒ Flexion (Pain) ❒ Extension (Pain) None ❒

Seizure History: Yes ❒ No ❒ *(if Yes please describe)*__________

HOME ENVIRONMENT ASSESSMENT:

Home Adaptive Equipment: Yes ❒ No ❒ (**O**-Owns, **B**-Borrows, **R**-Rents)

1.__________

2.__________

Home Telephone: Yes ❒ No ❒

Home Entrance: Steps Front ❒ Steps Back ❒ No. of Steps to 2nd Floor ____ Railing ____ What side____

Bedroom: What Floor ______

Bathrooms: Walk in Shower______ Tub Shower______ What Floor______

Transportation: **Primary Means of Transportation:** Car ❒ Cab ❒ Other ____

Car Seat: ❒ Has appropriate car seat ❒ Needs appropriate car seat ❒ N/A

Current Client's Driver's License: Yes ❒ No ❒

Comments:__________

SEXUALITY/REPRODUCTIVE PATTERN:

Sexualy Active: Yes ❒ No ❒ Not applicable ❒

History of Pregnancy/Fathering a Child:______ Sexually Transmitted Diseases______

Currently using birth control: Yes ❒ Method ______ No ❒ Not Applicable ❒

Last Menstrual Period:______ Change in flow: No ❒ Not Applicable ❒

Other Pertinent data:__________

Initials ______	**Initials** ______	**Initials** ______	**Initials** ______
Date ______	**Date** ______	**Date** ______	**Date** ______

CHILDREN'S SEASHORE HOUSE

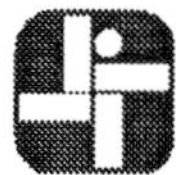

INTERDISCIPLINARY ADMISSION DATA BASE

Addressograph

PAGE 5

SKIN:

Color:	Pink ❒	Pale ❒	Flushed ❒	Cyanosis ❒	Acrocyanosis ❒	
Mucous Membranes:	Moist ❒	Dry ❒	Cracked ❒	Ulcers ❒		
Temperature:	Warm ❒	Cool ❒	Hot ❒	Diaphoretic ❒		
Assessment:	Edema ❒	Scaling/Dryness ❒	Bruises ❒	Rash ❒	Scar ❒	Birthmark ❒
	Lesions ❒	Breakdown ❒	Description ______			

Bathing Habits/Ointments: ______

Vascular Access/Site: ______

WOUNDS			
LOCATION	STAGE	MEASUREMENT	CHARACTER

MODIFIED BRADEN Q SCORE:

Initials ______	**Initials** ______	**Initials** ______	**Initials** ______
Date ______	**Date** ______	**Date** ______	**Date** ______

Courtesy Children's Seashore House of the Children's Hospital of Philadelphia, Philadelphia, PA.

CHILDREN'S SEASHORE HOUSE

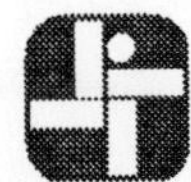

INTERDISCIPLINARY ADMISSION DATA BASE

Addressograph

PAGE 6

POSITIONING (describe posture and ability to tolerate these positions) ☐ NOT APPLICABLE

Supine____________________________

Side-lying____________________________

Prone____________________________

Wheelchair____________________________

Head control ☐GOOD ☐ POOR

FUNCTION: (✓ appropriate box)

	DEPENDENT	REQUIRES A (LEVEL)	SUPERVISION	INDEPENDENT	UNABLE TO ASSESS
Rolling in bed					
Come to sit in bed					
Sitting in bed (dangling)					
Standing					
Transfer To/From mat					
To/From bed					

AMBULATION: (✓ appropriate)

- ☐ unable to ambulate
- ☐ unable to ambulate but able to stand in the parallel bars for ________(time) with _________assistance.
- ☐ able to ambulate in parallel bars with _______assistance
- ☐ able to ambulate with _________________assistance for ________ feet (with/without) assistive device (specify type ____________________________)

GAIT QUALITY: (describe)

____

____

STAIRS:

Is able to ascend/descend_____________ stairs with ____________(level of assistance) and (right/left/no) railing.

ENDURANCE:

Patient is able to perform ______________ minutes of aerobic exercise with heart rate at ______________.

Type of Equipment:____________________________

Time for heart rate to return to baseline_________ SaO2 (resting)______% (exercise)______%

Respiratory Rate(resting) ________________ (exercise)________________

Further Testing Required________________ Not appropriate at this time________________

Initials _______ **Initials** _______ **Initials** _______ **Initials** _______

Date _______ **Date** _______ **Date** _______ **Date** _______

CHILDREN'S SEASHORE HOUSE

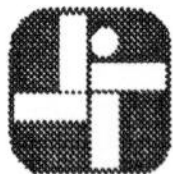

INTERDISCIPLINARY ADMISSION DATA BASE

Addressograph

PAGE 7

ORTHOSES/SPLINTS (✓ if appropriate and describe)

LEs

Has/Owns__________ Needs__________ Not Applicable__________

UEs

Has/Owns__________ Needs__________ Not applicable __________

MOTOR ASSESSMENT

Hand Dominance: R/L (circle)

LEFT					RIGHT			
ROM			STRENGTH (MMT)	MOTION	STRENGTH (MMT)	ROM		
Limited but not affecting function	Limited and affecting function	WNL				WNL	Limited and affecting function	Limited but not affecting function
				Shoulder Flexion				
				Extension				
				Abduction				
				Adduction				
				Ext Rot				
				Int Rot				
				Elbow flexion				
				Extension				
				Forearm Supination				
				Pronation				
				Wrist flexion				
				Extension				
				Finger flexion				
				Extension				
				Hip Flexion				
				Extension				
				Abduction				
				Adduction				
				Int Rot				
				Ext Rot				
				Knee flexion				
				Extension				
				Ankle dorsi				
				Plantar flexion				
				Eversion				
				Inversion				

Initials ______ **Initials** ______ **Initials** ______ **Initials** ______

Date ______ **Date** ______ **Date** ______ **Date** ______

TONE (✓ APPROPRIATE BLOCK)

Courtesy Children's Seashore House of the Children's Hospital of Philadelphia, Philadelphia, PA.

CHILDREN'S SEASHORE HOUSE

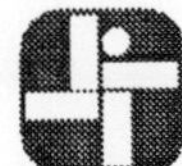

INTERDISCIPLINARY ADMISSION DATA BASE

Addressograph

PAGE 8

	FLACCID	NORMAL	SPASTIC
Right Upper Extremity			
Left Upper Extremity			
Right Lower Extremity			
Left Lower Extremity			

Describe:

ADL SKILLS

AREA EVALUATED	LEVEL OF ASSIST (INCLUDE TRANSFER)	ADAPTIVE EQUIPMENT		COMMENTS
		YES	NO	
EATING/SELF FEEDING				
GROOMING/HYGIENE				
BATHING				
UE DRESSING				
LE DRESSING				
TOILETING				

COGNITIVE/PERCEPTUAL:

	COMMENTS	IMPAIRED	WNL	ASSESSMENT REQUIRED
Direction Following				
Spatial Perceptual				
Visual Perceptual				
Visual Motor				
Praxis				
Attention				
Memory				

Initials _______ Initials _______ Initials _______ Initials _______

Date _______ Date _______ Date _______ Date _______

FINE MOTOR

CHILDREN'S SEASHORE HOUSE

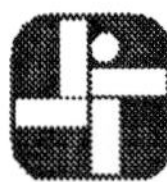

INTERDISCIPLINARY ADMISSION DATA BASE

Addressograph

PAGE 9

AREA EVALUATED	WNL	IMPAIRED BUT NOT LIMIT FUNCTION	IMPAIRED LIMITING FUNCTION	FURTHER TESTING NEEDED	FUNCTIONAL AREA
PROXIMAL STABILITY					
SHOULDER POSITION					
FOREARM POSITION					
WRIST MOBILTY					
MANIPULATIVE SKILL					
DEXTERITY					
GRASP PATTERNS					
BIMANUAL SKILLS					
EYE – HAND COORD.					

SENSORY STATUS: GLOBAL ASSESSMENT OF CHILD (UE/LE)

WNL	IMP	ASSMT REQ.		COMMENTS
			Sensory Modulation (Hyper/Hypo Sensitive)	
			Touch	
			Pain	
			Temperature	
			Auditory	
			Olfaction	
			Vision	
			Position Sense	
			Proprioception	
			Sensory Motor/Motor Planning	
			Stereognosis	

Initials _______ Initials _______ Initials _______ Initials _______

Date _______ Date _______ Date _______ Date _______

PRIMARY LANGUAGE: ☐ English ☐ Spanish ☐ Other ____________________

Courtesy Children's Seashore House of the Children's Hospital of Philadelphia, Philadelphia, PA.

CHILDREN'S SEASHORE HOUSE

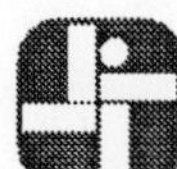

INTERDISCIPLINARY ADMISSION DATA BASE

Addressograph

PAGE 10

HISTORY OF DEVELOPMENTAL COMMUNICATION DELAYS: ❒ Yes ❒ No

DIAGNOSIS(ES): ______________________________

NEW COMMUNICATION DEFICITS: ❒YES ❒ NO

I. If "No" new deficits, then complete items a–>c. Only fill out the remainder of this form if appropriate. Write "N/A" in areas applicable.

II. If "Yes" new deficits with "Yes" for history of delays, then complete items a–>c , as well as remainder of this form.

III. If "Yes" new deficits, with "No" history of delays, then skip items a–>c and complete remainder of the form.

A. Child receives speech therapy in school ❒ Yes ❒ No
Intensity / Focus of therapy: ______________________________

B. During this admission, a full speech/language evaluation IS / IS NOT warranted (circle one)

C. During this admission, speech therapy IS / IS NOT warranted (circle one)
If therapy will be provided, check all those that apply:
❒ Group ❒ Individual ❒ focus of therapy to be in accordance with child's IEP
Comments: ______________________________

COGNITIVE/BEHAVIOR OBSERVATIONS:

❒ Agitation	❒ Flat Affect	❒ Pleasant	❒ Attention Problems/Distractibility
❒ Aggression	❒ Lethargy	❒ Cooperative	❒ Physical Restlessness
❒ Hostility	❒ Fatigue	❒ Interactive	❒ Short-Term Memory Problems
❒ Irritability	❒ Low Endurance	❒ Emotional Lability	❒ Concrete/Literal Thinking
❒ Impulsivity	❒ Perseveration	❒ Slow Processing	❒ Word Retrieval Problems
❒ Disinhibition	❒ Confabulation	❒ Response Delay	❒ Reduced Problem Solving
❒ Poor Judgment	❒ Confusion	❒ Reduced Initiation	❒ Reduced Critical Thinking
❒ Lack of Insight	❒ Disorientation	❒ Poor Safety Awareness	❒ Linguistic Disorganization

Comments: ______________________________

Initials _______	**Initials** _______	**Initials** _______	**Initials** _______
Date _______	**Date** _______	**Date** _______	**Date** _______

CHILDREN'S SEASHORE HOUSE

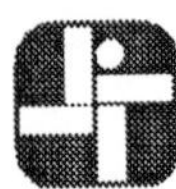

INTERDISCIPLINARY ADMISSION DATA BASE

Addressograph

PAGE 11

FEEDING SKILLS:

History of Feeding Difficulties: ______

CURRENT STATUS:

Oral Phase: ☐ WNL ☐ impaired for certain textures ☐ slow ☐ drools / unable to handle secretions

Pharyngeal Phase: ☐ WNL ☐ delayed trigger of swallow

Laryngeal Phase: ☐ WNL ☐ wet breath sounds ☐ cough / choke ☐ clinical signs of aspiration

RECOMMENDATIONS AT THIS TIME:

Diet: ☐ Regular ☐ Chopped ☐ Pureed ☐ Thick liquids (consistency: ______) ☐ Thin Liquids ☐ NPO

Positioning: ☐ N/A ☐ in wheelchair only ☐ in highchair ☐ other ☐ modifications ______

Pacing: ☐ N/A ☐ alternate solids & liquids ☐ multiple swallows needed ☐ wait____ seconds between bites /sips

Special Equipment: ☐ N/A ☐ ______

Level of Assistance: ☐ Independent ☐ Supervision ☐ Hand over Hand ☐ Fed by Caregiver ☐ Fed by Therapist Only

Further Assessment: ☐ Modified Barium Swallow Study ☐ Blue Dye Test ☐ Feeding Team Consult

Comments: ______

ORAL MOTOR SKILLS: ☐ Normal ☐ Impaired ☐ Functional

Comments: ______

SPEECH: ☐ Normal ☐ Nonverbal ☐ Impaired ☐ Functional for Communication

Area(s) Impaired: ☐ Articulation ☐ Voice ☐ Fluency ☐ Resonance (hypo / hyper-nasal)

Overall Intelligibility: ☐ Excellent ☐ Good ☐ Fair ☐ Poor

Comments: ______

LANGUAGE: ☐ Normal ☐ Impaired ☐ Functional for basic needs / wants

Area(s) Impaired: ☐ Receptive Language (Auditory & Reading Comprehension)

Comments: ______

☐ Expressive Language (Verbal, Written, Gestural Communication)

Comments: ______

☐ Cognitive / Communication (i.e. Pragmatics, Abstract Language)

Comments: ______

Primary means of communication: ☐ Verbal ☐ Nonverbal ☐ No communicative intent observed

Augmentative/alternative needs: ☐ Yes ☐ No ☐ Type: ______

Comments: ______

Initials ______ **Initials** ______ **Initials** ______ **Initials** ______

Date ______ **Date** ______ **Date** ______ **Date** ______

Courtesy Children's Seashore House of the Children's Hospital of Philadelphia, Philadelphia, PA.

CHILDREN'S SEASHORE HOUSE

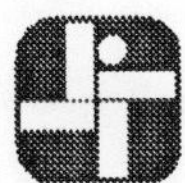

INTERDISCIPLINARY ADMISSION DATA BASE

Addressograph

PAGE 12

EVALUATION RESULTS:

Children's Orientation & Amnesia Test ❒ Pass ❒ Fail ❒ N/A

Language Testing	STANDARD SCORE	AGE EQUIVALENT

Comments:____

AUDIOLOGY EVALUATION: ❒ Warranted ❒ Not Warranted ❒ Complete

Comments:____

Initials _______ **Initials** _______ **Initials** _______ **Initials** _______

Date _______ **Date** _______ **Date** _______ **Date** _______

CHILDREN'S SEASHORE HOUSE

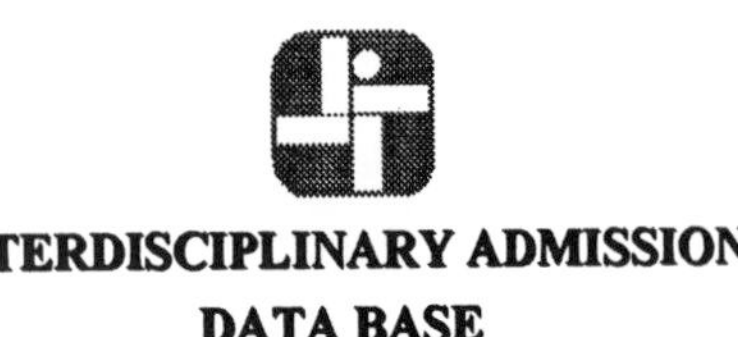

INTERDISCIPLINARY ADMISSION DATA BASE

Addressograph

PAGE 13

Legal Guardian:_______________ Relationship:_______________

Address:_______________

Phone:_______________

Physical Caregiver:_______________

Address:_______________

Phone:_______________

Discharge Disposition:_______________

Patients' Religion:_______________ Patient's Social Security Number:_____-_____-_____

Mother:_______________ DOB:_______ Marital Status:_______________

Education:_______________ Social Security Number:_______________

Address:_______________ County:_______________

Religion:_______ Home #:_______ Work #:_______ Occupation:_______

Father:_______________ DOB:_______ Marital Status:_______________

Education:_______________ Social Security Number:_______________

Address:_______________ County:_______________

Religion:_______ Home #:_______ Work #:_______ Occupation:_______

HOUSEHOLD MEMBERS	RELATIONSHIP	DOB/AGE	PHONE/OCCUPATION
OTHER PERSONS INVOLVED			

Advanced Directives ❒ **Yes** ❒ **No** ❒ **N/A**

Additional Information: _______________

____

Initials _______ **Initials** _______ **Initials** _______ **Initials** _______

Date _______ **Date** _______ **Date** _______ **Date** _______

Courtesy Children's Seashore House of the Children's Hospital of Philadelphia, Philadelphia, PA.

CHILDREN'S SEASHORE HOUSE

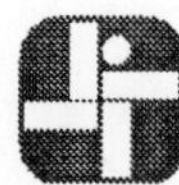

INTERDISCIPLINARY ADMISSION DATA BASE

Addressograph

PAGE 14

COMMUNITY RESOURCES	Y	N	N/A	SERVICE/AGENCY	CONTACT PERSON #
Financial Resources					
Outpatient Services					
Support Services					
Educational Services					
DHS/C&Y					
Recreational Services					
Counseling / Therapy Services					
Other					

CULTURAL / ETHNIC / RELIGIOUS PRACTICES THAT NEED TO BE CONSIDERED IN PLAN OF CARE ☐ YES ☐ NO

DESCRIBE: ______

Current Stresses/Problems Identified

______

Summary/Impression/Plan

______

Initials ______ Initials ______ Initials ______ Initials ______

Date ______ Date ______ Date ______ Date ______

CHILDREN'S SEASHORE HOUSE

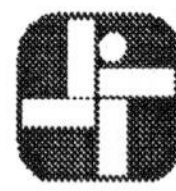

INTERDISCIPLINARY ADMISSION DATA BASE

Addressograph

PAGE 15

EDUCATIONAL HISTORY: (Information provided by school).

School Name: ______________________

Address: ______________________

Phone: ______________________ Fax: ______________________

Teacher: ______________________ School Nurse/Phone: ______________________

Guidance Counselor /Phone: ______________________ Principal/Phone: ______________________

Accessible Building: ❐ Yes ❐ No Explain: ______________________

Nursing Availability: ❐ Full-Time ❐ Part-Time

CURRENT EDUCATIONAL STATUS: (✓ all that apply).

❐ Daycare ❐ Preschool ❐ Kindergarten ❐ Elementary (Grade __)

❐ Middle School (Grade ___) ❐ Junior High (Grade __) ❐ High School (Grade _____)

❐ Other*

*Please Explain: ______________________

Current School Placement: ❐ Regular Ed. ❐ Special Ed.* ❐ Gifted

Indicate: ❐ Classroom ❐ Homebound* ❐ Intermittent Homebound*

*Please Explain: ______________________

Attendance:

❐ No Attendance Problems

❐ Recent problems related to illness/treatment. Explain: ______________________

❐ Problems not related to illness/treatment. Explain: ______________________

Additional Information:

IEP ❐ Yes ❐ No

Therapies provided under IEP (include duration & frequency) ______________________

____

504 Plan ❐ Yes ❐ No

Accommodations / Provisions under 504: ______________________

____

Has classification of health impairment / chronically ill ❐ Yes ❐ No ❐ NA

Concerns expressed by the school: ______________________

____

____

Initials _______ **Initials** _______ **Initials** _______ **Initials** _______

Date _______ **Date** _______ **Date** _______ **Date** _______

Courtesy Children's Seashore House of the Children's Hospital of Philadelphia, Philadelphia, PA.

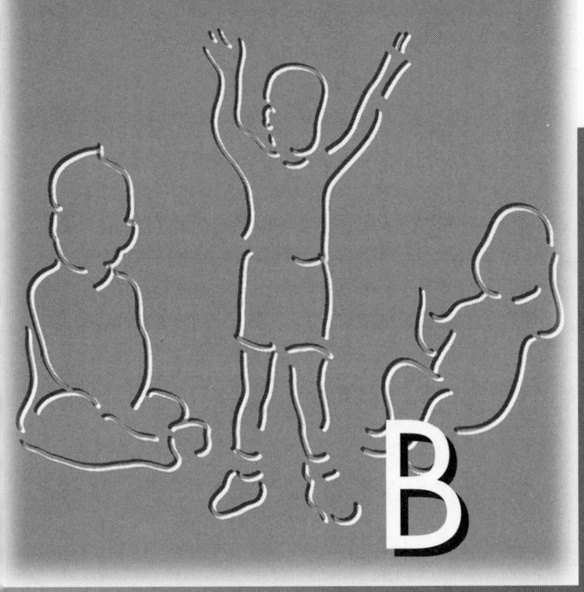

B Resources for Health Care Providers and Families

PROFESSIONAL ORGANIZATIONS

American Academy of Pediatrics
141 Northwest Point Boulevard
Elk Grove Village, IL 60007
Phone: 847-434-4000
Fax: 847-434-8000
Website: www.aap.org

National Association of Pediatric Nurse Practitioners (NAP-NAP)
1101 Kings Highway North
Suite 206
Cherry Hill, NJ 08034-1912
Phone: 856-557-1773; 877-662-7627 (toll-free)
Fax: 856-667-7187
Website: www.napnap.org

National Association of School Nurses (Eastern Office)
P.O. Box 1300
Scarborough, ME 04070
Phone: 207-883-2177; 877-623-6476 (toll-free)
Fax: 207-883-2683
Website: www.nasn.org

National Association of School Nurses (Western Office)
1416 Park Street, Suite A
Castle Rock, CO 80104
Phone: 303-663-2329; 866-627-6767 (toll-free)
Fax: 303-663-0403
Website: www.nasn.org

Society of Pediatric Nurses
7794 Grow Drive
Pensacola, FL 32514-7072
Phone: 850-494-9467; 800-723-2902 (toll-free)
Fax: 850-484-8762
Website: www.pedsnurses.org

GENERAL PEDIATRIC RESOURCES

National Center for Education in Maternal and Child Health
2000 15th Street, N, Suite 701
Arlington, VA 22201-2617
Phone: 703-524-7802
Fax: 703-524-9335
Website: www.ncemch.org

National Center for Health Statistics
Centers for Disease Control and Prevention
Website: www.cdc.gov/nchs

National Health Information Center
Department of Health and Human Services
Website: www.health.gov/nhic

Office of Disease Prevention and Health Promotion Objectives
Department of Health and Human Services
Website: www.health.gov/healthypeople

ABUSE, PHYSICAL OR SEXUAL

See also *Domestic Violence*
National Committee to Prevent Child Abuse (NCPCA)
332 South Michigan Avenue, Suite 1600
Chicago, IL 60604
Phone: 312-663-3520
Fax: 312-939-8962
Website: www.childabuse.org

Parents Anonymous
675 West Foothill Boulevard, Suite 220
Claremont, CA 91711
Phone: 909-621-6184
Website: www.parentsanonymous.org

AIDS/HIV

The Names Project Foundation
310 Townsend Street, Suite 310
San Francisco, CA 94107
Phone: 415-882-5500
Fax: 415-882-6200
Website: www.aidsquilt.org

ATTENTION DEFICIT-HYPERACTIVITY DISORDER

Children and Adults with Attention Deficit Disorders (CHADD)
8181 Professional Place, Suite 201
Landover, MD 20785
Phone: 301-306-7070; 800-233-4050 (toll-free)
Fax: 301-306-7090
Website: www.chadd.org

National Attention Deficit Disorder Association (NADDA)
1788 Second Street, Suite 200
Highland Park, IL 60085
Phone: 847-432-ADDA
Fax: 847-432-5874
Website: www.add.org

AUTISM

Autism Society of America
7910 Woodmont Avenue, Suite 300
Bethesda, MD 20814-3067
Phone: 301-657-0881; 800-3 AUTISM (toll-free)
Fax: 301-657-0869
Website: www.autism-society.org

Center for the Study of Autism
P.O. Box 4538
Salem, OR 97302
Website: www.autism.org

National Institute of Mental Health
6001 Executive Boulevard
Room 8184, MSC 9663
Bethesda, MD 20892-9663
Phone: 301-443-4513
Fax: 301-443-4279
Website: www.nimh.nih.gov

BLINDNESS, VISUAL IMPAIRMENT

American Council of the Blind
1155 15th Street, NW, Suite 1004
Washington, DC 20005
Phone: 202-457-5081; 800-424-8666 (toll-free)
Fax: 202-467-5085
Website: www.acb.org

American Foundation for the Blind
11 Penn Plaza, Suite 300
New York, NY 10001
Phone: 212-502-7600; 800-AFB-LINE (toll-free)
Fax 212-502-7777
Website: www.afb.org

The Blind Children's Center
4120 Marathon Street
Los Angeles, CA 90029-3584
Phone: 323-664-2153; 800-222-3566 (U.S. t.o. toll-free); 800-222-3567 (California toll-free)
Fax: 323-665-3828
Website: www.blindcntr.org

Helen Keller National Center for Deaf-Blind Youth and Adults
111 Middle Neck Road
Sands Point, NY 11050
Phone: 516-944-8900 (voice, TTY); 516-944-8637 (TTY)
Fax: 516-944-7302
Website: www.helenkeller.org

National Association for Parents of the Visually Handicapped
P.O. Box 317
Watertown, MA 02471
Phone: 617-972-7441; 800-562-6265 (toll-free)
Fax: 617-972-7444
Website: www.napvi.org

BURNS

American Burn Association
625 North Michigan Avenue, Suite 1530
Chicago, IL 60611
Phone: 312-642-9260
Fax: 312-642-9130
Website: www.ameriburn.org

Camp I-Thonka-Chi
Parkland Health and Hospital System
Physical Medicine and Rehabilitation Department
5201 Harry Hines Boulevard
Dallas, TX 75235-7757
Phone: 214-590-8139

International Shrine Headquarters
2900 Rocky Point Drive
Tampa, FL 33607-1460
Phone: 813-281-0300; 800-237-5055 (U.S. toll-free); 800-361-7256 (Canada toll-free)
Website: www.shriners.com

CANCER

American Cancer Society
1599 Clifton Road, NE
Atlanta, GA 30329
Phone: 800-ACS-2345 (toll-free)
Website: www.cancer.org

Association of Pediatric Oncology Nurses
4700 West Lake Avenue
Glenview, IL 60025-1485
Phone: 847-375-4724
Fax: 847-375-6324
Website: www.apon.org

Candlelighters Childhood Cancer Foundation
3910 Warner Street
Kensington, MD 20895
Phone: 301-962-3520; 800-366-2223 (toll-free)
Fax: 301-962-3521
Website: www.candlelighters.org

The Center for Attitudinal Healing
33 Buchanan Drive
Sausalito, CA 94965
Phone: 415-331-6161
Fax: 415-331-4545
Website: www.healingcenter.org

Corporate Angel Network
Westchester County Airport
1 Loop Road
West Plains, NY 10604
Phone: 914-328-1313
Website: www.corpangelnetwork.org

Leukemia & Lymphoma Society
1311 Mamaroneck Avenue
White Plains, NY 10605
Phone: 914-949-5213; 800-955-4572 (toll-free)
Fax: 914-949-6691
Website: www.leukemia.org

Make-A-Wish Foundation of America
3550 North Central Avenue, Suite 300
Phoenix, AZ 85012
Phone: 602-279-9474; 800-722-WISH (toll-free)
Fax: 602-279-0855
Website: www.wish.org

National Childhood Cancer Foundation
440 East Huntington Drive
P.O. Box 60012
Arcadia, CA 91066-6012
Phone: 626-447-1674; 1-800-458-NCCF (toll-free)
Fax: 626-447-6359
Website: www.nccf.org

Ronald McDonald House Charities
1 Kroc Drive
Oak Brook, IL 60523
630-623-7048
Website: www.rmhc.com
Provides housing near treatment centers for children with life-threatening diseases and their families

Sunshine Kids Foundation
2814 Virginia
Houston, TX 77098
Phone: 713-524-1264; 800-594-5756 (toll-free)
Fax: 713-524-7165
Website: www.sunshinekids.org

CARDIOVASCULAR DISORDERS

American Heart Association
7272 Greenville Avenue
Dallas, TX 75231
Phone: 214-373-6300; 800-AHA-USA1 (toll-free)
Website: www.americanheart.org

March of Dimes Birth Defects Foundation
1275 Mamaroneck Avenue
White Plains, NY 10605
Phone: 914-428-7100; 1-888-MODIMES (toll-free)
Website: www.modimes.org

COMMUNICATION WITH CHILDREN

Child Life Council, Inc.
11820 Parklawn Drive, Suite 202
Rockville, MD 20852-2529
Phone: 301-881-7090
Fax: 301-881-7092
Website: www.childlife.org

Family Voices
National Office
3411 Candelaria NE, Suite M
Albuquerque, NM 87107
Phone: 505-872-4774; 888-835-5669 (toll-free)
Fax: 505-872-4780
Website: www.familyvoices.org

Institute for Family-Centered Care
7900 Wisconsin Avenue, Suite 405
Bethesda, MD 20814
Phone: 301-652-0281
Fax: 301-652-0186
Website: www.familycenteredcare.org

National Association for the Education of Young Children
1509 16th Street, NW
Washington, DC 20036-1426
Phone: 202-232-8777; 800-424-2460 (toll-free)
Website: www.naeyc.org

Zero to Three
National Center for Infants, Toddlers, and Families
2000 M Street, NW, Suite 200
Washington, DC 20036
Phone: 202-638-1144
Fax: 202-638-0851
Website: www.zerotothree.org

DEAFNESS, HEARING IMPAIRMENT

Alexander Graham Bell Association for the Deaf and Hard of Hearing
3417 Volta Place, NW
Washington, DC 20007-2778
Phone: 202-337-5220 (voice and TTY)
Fax: 202-337-8314
Website: www.agbell.org

American Society for Deaf Children (ASDC)
ASDC Headquarters
P.O. Box 3355
Gettysburg, PA 17325
Phone: 717-334-7922 (voice and TTY)
Fax: 717-334-8808
Website: www.deafchildren.org

Helen Keller National Center for Deaf-Blind Youth and Adults
111 Middle Neck Road
Sands Point, NY 11050
Phone: 516-944-8900 (voice, TTY); 516-944-8637 (TTY)
Fax: 516-944-7302
Website: www.helenkeller.org

National Information Center on Deafness
Gallaudet University
800 Florida Avenue, NE
Washington, DC 20002-3695
Phone: 202-651-5050 (voice and TTY)
Fax: 202-651-5054
Website: www.gallaudet.edu

DENTAL CARE

American Dental Association
211 East Chicago Avenue
Chicago, IL 60611
Phone: 312-440-2500
Fax: 312-440-2800
Website: www.ada.org

American Society of Dentistry for Children
211 East Chicago Avenue, Suite 710
Chicago, IL 60611
Phone: 312-943-1244
Fax: 312-943-5341
Website: www.asdckids.org

National Foundation of Dentistry for the Handicapped
1800 15th Street, Unit 100
Denver, CO 80202
Phone: 303-534-5360
Fax: 534-5290
Website: www.nfdh.org

DEVELOPMENTAL MATERIALS

Denver Developmental Materials, Inc.
P.O. Box 37107
Denver, CO 80237
Phone: 303-355-4729; 800-419-4729 (toll free)

DIABETES

American Association of Diabetes Educators
100 West Monroe Street, Suite 400
Chicago, IL 60603-1901
Phone: 312-424-2426; 800-338-DMED (toll-free)
Fax: 312-424-2427
Website: www.aadenet.org

American Diabetes Association
1701 North Beauregard
Alexandria, VA 22311
Phone: 703-549-1500; 800-DIABETES (toll-free)
Website: www.diabetes.org

Human Biological Database Interchange
1880 John F. Kennedy Boulevard
Sixth Floor
Philadelphia, PA 19103
Phone: 800-345-4234 (toll-free)
Fax: 215-557-7154
Website: www.hbdi.org

International Diabetes Center
3800 Park Nicollet Boulevard
Minneapolis, MN 55416
Phone: 952-993-3393; 888-825-6315 (toll-free)
Fax: 952-993-1302
Website: www.idcdiabetes.org

Juvenile Diabetes Research Foundation International
120 Wall Street
New York, NY 10005
Phone: 212-785-9500; 800-533-CURE (toll-free)
Fax: 212-785-9595
Website: www.jdrf.org

National Institute of Diabetes, Digestive, and Kidney Diseases
31 Center Drive
Building 31, Room 9A04
Bethesda, MD 20892-2560
Phone: 301-496-3583
Website: www.niddk.nih.gov

DOMESTIC VIOLENCE

See also *Abuse*
American Bar Association Commission on Domestic Violence
740 15th Street, NW
Ninth Floor
Washington, DC 20005-1002
Website: www.abanet.org/domviol

Center for the Prevention of Sexual and Domestic Violence (CPSDV)
2400 45th Street, No. 10
Seattle, WA 98103
Phone: 206-634-1903
Fax: 206-634-0115
Website: www.cpsdv.org

Domestic Violence Awareness Handbook
Website: www.usda.gov/da/shmd/aware.htm

Domestic Violence Handbook
Website: www.domesticviolence.org

National Domestic Violence Hotline
P.O. Box 161810
Austin, TX 78716
Phone: 800-799-SAFE (toll-free); 800-787-3224 (TTY)
Website: www.ndvh.org

GASTROINTESTINAL ALTERATIONS

American Celiac Society/Dietary Support Coalition
59 Crystal Avenue
West Orange, NJ 07052
Phone: 973-325-8837
Email: bentleac@umdnj.edu

Cleft Palate Foundation (CPF)
104 South Estes Drive, Suite 204
Chapel Hill, NC 27514
Phone: 919-933-9044
Fax: 919-933-9604
Website: www.cleftline.org

American Pseudo-obstruction and Hirschsprung Disease Society (APHS)
158 Pleasant Street
North Andover, MA 01845-2797
Phone: 978-685-4477
Fax: 978-685-4488
Email: aphs@tiac.net

Celiac-Sprue Association USA
(CSA/USA On-Line)
P.O. Box 31700
Omaha, NE 68131-0700
Phone: 402-558-0600
Fax: 402-558-1347
Website: www.csaceliacs.org

Crohn's and Colitis Foundation of America
386 Park Avenue South
17th Floor
New York, NY 10016
Phone: 212-685-3440; 800-932-2423 (toll-free)
Fax: 212-779-4098
Website: www.ccfa.org

Gluten Intolerance Group of North America (GIG)
15110 10th Avenue, SW, Suite A
Seattle, WA 98166-1820
Phone: 206-246-6652
Fax: 206-246-6531
Email: info@gluten.net

March of Dimes Birth Defects Foundation
1275 Mamaroneck Avenue
White Plains, NY 10605
Phone: 914-428-7100; 1-888-MODIMES (toll-free)
Website: www.modimes.org

National Institute of Diabetes, Digestive, and Kidney Diseases
31 Center Drive
Building 31, Room 9A04
Bethesda, MD 20892-2560
Phone: 301-496-3583
Website: www.niddk.nih.gov

Pull-Thru Network
316 Thomas Street
Bessemer, AL 35020
Phone: 205-428-5953
Website: www.pullthrough.org

GENITOURINARY ALTERATIONS

American Association of Kidney Patients (AAKP)
100 South Ashley Drive, Suite 280
Tampa, FL 33602
Phone: 813-223-7099; 800-749-2257 (toll-free)
Fax: 813-223-0001
Website: www.aakp.org

American Foundation for Urologic Disease
1128 North Charles Street
Baltimore, MD 21201
Phone: 410-468-1800; 800-242-2383 (toll-free)
Website: www.afud.org

American Kidney Fund, Inc.
6110 Executive Boulevard, Suite 1010
Rockville, MD 20852
Phone: 301-881-3052; 800-638-8299 (toll-free)
Website: www.akfinc.org

National Kidney Foundation
30 East 33rd Street
New York, NY 10016
Phone: 212-889-2210; 800-622-9010 (toll-free)
Fax: 212-689-9261
Website: www.kidney.org

National Institute of Diabetes, Digestive, and Kidney Diseases
31 Center Drive
Building 31, Room 9A04
Bethesda, MD 20892-2560
Phone: 301-496-3583
Website: www.niddk.nih.gov

HEMATOLOGIC ALTERATIONS

Aplastic Anemia Foundation of America
P.O. Box 613
Annapolis, MD 21404-0613
Phone: 410-867-0242; 800-747-2820 (toll-free)
Fax: 410-867-0240
Website: www.aplastic.org

Cooley's Anemia Foundation (CAF)
129-09 26th Avenue, No. 203
Flushing, NY 11354
Phone: 718-321-CURE; 800-522-7222 (toll-free)
Fax: 718-321-3340
Website: www.thalassemia. org

The ITP Society*
333 East 38th Street, Room 830
New York, NY 10016
Website: www.ultranet.com/~itpsoc

National Hemophilia Foundation
HANDI
116 West 32nd Street
Eleventh Floor
New York, NY 10001
Phone: 212-328-3700; 800-42-HANDI (toll-free)
Fax: 212-328-3777
Website: www.hemophilia.org

Sickle Cell Disease Association of America (SCAA)
200 Corporate Pointe
Suite 495
Culver City, CA 90230-8727
Phone: 310-216-6363; 800-421-8453 (toll-free)
Fax: 310-215-3722
Website: www.sicklecelldisease.org

LATEX ALLERGY

Latex Allergy Information Services (LAIS)
176 Roosevelt Avenue
Torrington, CT 06790
Phone: 860-482-6869
Fax: 860-482-7640
Email: 76500.1452@compuserve or debid@ix.netcom.com

MENTAL RETARDATION

American Association of Mental Retardation
444 North Capitol Street, NW, Suite 846
Washington, DC 20001-1512
Phone: 202-387-1968; 800-424-3688 (toll-free)
Fax: 202-387-2193
Website: www.aamr.org

The ARC* of the United States
1010 Wayne Avenue, Suite 650
Silver Spring, MD 20910
Phone: 301-565-3842
Fax: 301-565-3843
Website: www.thearc.org

*ITP is Thrombocytopenia Purpura, a division of the Children's Blood Foundation
*Formerly Association of Retarded Citizens

National Down Syndrome Society
666 Broadway
Eighth Floor
New York, NY 10012-2317
Phone: 212-460-9330; 800-221-4602 (toll-free)
Fax: 212-979-2873
Website: www.ndss.org

National Fragile-X Foundation
P.O. Box 190488
San Francisco, CA 94119-0488
Phone: 510-763-6030
Fax: 510-763-6223
Website: www.FragileX.org

MUSCULOSKELETAL ALTERATIONS

Arthritis Foundation
P.O. Box 7669
Atlanta, GA 30357-0669
Phone: 800-283-7800 (toll-free)
Website: www.arthritis.org

Arthritis Society (Canada)
393 University Avenue, Suite 1700
Toronto, Ontario M5G 1E6
Canada
Phone: 416-979-7228
Fax: 416-979-8366
Website: www.arthritis.ca

Muscular Dystrophy Association of America, Inc.
3300 East Sunrise Drive
Tucson, AZ 85718
Phone: 800-572-1717 (toll-free)
Website: www.mdausa.org

Muscular Dystrophy Association of Canada
2345 Yonge Street, Suite 900
Toronto, Ontario M4P 2E5
Canada
Phone: 416-488-0030; 800-567-2873 (toll-free)
Fax: 416-488-7523
Website: www.mdac.ca

National Scoliosis Foundation, Inc.
5 Cabot Place
Stoughton, MA 02072
Phone: 781-341-6333; 800-673-6922 (toll-free)
Fax: 781-341-8333
Website: www.scoliosis-assoc.org

Scoliosis Association, Inc.
P.O. Box 811705
Boca Raton, FL 33481-1705
Phone: 800-800-0669 (toll-free)
Website: www.scoliosis-assoc.org

Osteogenesis Imperfecta Foundation, Inc.
804 West Diamond Avenue, Suite 210
Gaithersburg, MD 20878
Phone: 301-947-0083; 800-981-2663 (toll-free)
Fax: 301-947-0456
Website: www.oif.org

NEUROLOGIC ALTERATIONS

Epilepsy Foundation
4351 Garden City Drive
Landover, MD 20785-7223
Phone: 301-459-3700; 800-EFA-1000 (toll-free)
Fax: 301-577-4941
Website: www.efa.org

Hydrocephalus Association
870 Market Street, Suite 705
San Francisco, CA 94102
Phone: 415-732-7040
Fax: 415-732-7044
Website: www.hydroassoc.org

Hydrocephalus Foundation, Inc. (HYFI)
910 Rear Broadway
Saugus, MA 01906
Phone: 781-942-1161
Website: www.hydrocephalus.org

Spina Bifida Association
4590 MacArthur Boulevard, NW, Suite 250
Washington, DC 20007-4226
Phone: 202-944-3285; 800-621-3141 (toll-free)
Fax: 202-944-3295
Website: www.sbaa.org

United Cerebral Palsy
1660 L Street, NW, Suite 700
Washington, DC 20036
Phone: 202-776-0406; 800-872-5827 (toll-free)
Fax: 202-776-0414
Website: www.ucp.org

NUTRITION

American Dietetic Association
216 West Jackson Boulevard, Suite 800
Chicago, IL 60606-6995
Phone: 312-899-0040; 800-877-1600 (toll-free)
Fax: 312-899-1979
Website: www.eatright.org

Food Research and Action Center
1875 Connecticut Avenue, NW, Suite 540
Washington, DC 20009
Phone: 202-986-2200
Fax: 202-986-2525
Website: www.frac.org

National Dairy Council
O'Hare International Center
10255 West Higgins Road, Suite 900
Rosemont, IL 60018
Phone: 847-803-2000; 800-426-8271 (toll-free)
Website: www.nationaldaircouncil.org

PAIN IN CHILDREN

American Pain Society
4700 W. Lake Avenue
Glenview, IL 60025
Phone: 847-375-4715
Fax: 877-734-8758
Website: www.ampainsoc.org

Association for the Care of Children's Health
19 Mantua Road
Mount Royal, NJ 08061
Phone: 609-224-1742
Fax: 609-423-3420
Website: www.acch.org

Center for Research Dissemination and Liaison
AHRQ Publications Clearinghouse
P.O. Box 8547
Silver Spring, MD 20907
Phone: 301-594-1364; 800-358-9295 (toll-free); 888-586-6340 (TDD)
Website: www.ahrq.gov

Pain and Palliative Care Resource Center
City of Hope National Medical Center
Department of Nursing Research and Education
1500 East Duarte Road
Duarte, CA 91010
Phone: 626-359-8111
Website: http://prc.coh.org

International Association for the Study of Pain
IASP Secretariat
909 NE 43rd Street, Room 306
Seattle, WA 98105-6020
Phone: 206-547-6409
Fax: 206-547-1703
Website: www.iasp-pain.org

Pediatric Pain Awareness Initiative (PPAI)
Phone: 888-569-5555 (toll-free)
Pediatric-Pain Mailing List*
Email: MAILSERV@ac.dal.ca

Books and Newsletters

Pain in Infants, Children, and Adolescents: An Overview (2nd ed., 2002)
N. L. Schechter & C. B. Berde (Eds.)
Lippincott Williams & Wilkins

Pain in Neonates (2nd ed., 2000)
K. J. S. Anand, B. J. Stevens, & P. J. McGrath
Elsevier Science Publications

Pediatric Pain Letter: Abstracts and Commentaries on Pain in Infants, Children, and Adolescents
P. J. McGrath & G. A. Finley (Eds.)
Psychology Department
Dalhousie University
Halifax, Nova Scotia B3H 4J1
Canada
Phone: 902-494-3417
Fax: 902-494-6585

Assessment Tools

Poker Chip Pain Assessment Tool
Nancy Hester, PhD, RN, FAAN
Campus Box C288-10
University of Colorado Health Sciences Center
4200 East 9th Avenue
Denver, CO 80262
Phone: 303-372-0000
Email: nancy.hester@uchsc.edu

Adolescent Pain Assessment Tool
Marilyn Savedra, RN, DNSc, FAAN
University of California, San Francisco
School of Nursing
Box 0606, N 411Y
San Francisco, CA 94143
Phone: 415-476-1435
Fax: 415-476-9707
Website: http://nurseweb.ucsf.edu

RESPIRATORY ALTERATIONS

American Academy of Allergy, Asthma, and Immunology
611 East Wells Street
Milwaukee, WI 53202
Phone: 414-272-6071; 800-822-2762 (toll-free)
Fax: 414-272-6070
Website: www.aaaai.org

*First line of the message should read as follows: subscribe PEDIATRIC-PAIN

American Allergy Association
1259 El Camino, No. 254
Menlo Park, CA 94025
Phone: 650-855-8036

American Lung Association
1740 Broadway
New York, NY 10019
Phone: 212-315-8700; 800-LUNG-USA (toll-free)
Website: www.lungusa.org

American SIDS Institute
2480 Windy Hill Road, Suite 380
Marietta, GA 30067
Phone: 770-612-1030; 800-612-1030 (toll-free)
Website: www.sids.org

Asthma and Allergy Foundation of America
1233 20th Street, NW, Suite 402
Washington, DC 20036
Phone: 202-466-7643; 800-7-ASTHMA (toll-free)
Fax: 202-466-8940
Website: www.aafa.org

National Jewish Medical Research Center
1400 Jackson Street
Denver, CO 80206
Phone: 303-388-4461; 800-222-LUNG (toll-free)
Website: www.njc.org

National Allergy and Asthma Network
Mothers of Asthmatics
2751 Prosperity Avenue, Suite 150
Fairfax, VA 22031
Phone: 703-641-9595; 800-878-4403 (toll-free)
Fax: 703-573-7794
Website: www.aanma.org

National Asthma Education and Prevention Program
National Heart, Lung, and Blood Institute Information Center (NHLBI)
National Institutes of Health
P.O. Box 30105
Bethesda, MD 20824-0105
Phone: 301-592-8573
Fax: 301-592-8563
Website: www.nhlbi.nih.gov/about/naepp

National Sudden Infant Death Syndrome Resource Center
Health Resources and Services Administration
Tycon Courthouse
2070 Chain Bridge Road, Suite 450
Vienna, VA 22182
Phone: 703-821-8955
Fax: 703-821-2098
Website: www.sidscenter.org

SAFETY

American Academy of Pediatrics
The Injury Prevention Program (TIPP)
141 Northwest Point Boulevard
Elk Grove Village, IL 60007
Phone: 847-434-4000
Fax: 847-434-8000
Website: www.aap.org

American Spinal Injury Association (ASIA)
2020 Peachtree Road, NW
Atlanta, GA 30309-1402
Phone: 404-355-9772
Fax: 404-355-1826
Website: www.asia-spinalinjury.org

American Trauma Society
8903 Presidential Parkway, Suite 512
Upper Malboro, MD 20772
Phone: 301-420-4189; 800-556-7890 (toll-free)
Website: www.amtrauma.org

U.S. Consumer Product Safety Commission
Washington, DC 20207
Phone: 301-504-0990; 800-638-CPSC (toll-free); 800-638-8270 (TTY)
Website: www.cpsc.gov

Harborview Injury Prevention and Research Center
Box 359960
325 Ninth Avenue
Seattle, WA 98104-2499
Phone: 206-521-1520
Fax: 206-521-1562
Website: http://depts.washington.edu/hiprc

National Head Injury Foundation
1776 Massachusetts Avenue, NW, Suite 100
Washington, DC 20036
Phone: 202-296-6443; 800-444-6443 (toll-free)

National Head and Spinal Cord Injury Prevention Program
American Association of Neurological Surgeons and Congress of Neurosurgical Surgeons
5550 Meadowbrook Drive
Rolling Meadows, IL 60088
Phone: 847-378-0500; 888-566-AANS (toll-free)
Fax: 847-378-0600
Website: www.aans.org

National Highway Traffic Safety Administration
400 7th Street, SW
Washington, DC 20590
Website: www.nhtsa.dot.gov/nhtsa

National Rifle Association of America
Education and Training Department
11250 Waples Mill Road
Fairfax, VA 22030
Phone: 800-672-3888 (toll-free)
Website: www.nrahq.org

National Safe Kids Campaign
1301 Pennsylvania Avenue, NW, Suite 1000
Washington, DC 20004-1707
Phone: 202-662-0600; 202-393-2072
Website: www.safekids.org

Self-Care Children (Books)

Latchkey Kids: Unlocking Doors for Children and Their Families (1998)
S. Lamorey & B. E. Robinson
Sage Publications

Self-Care for Children
Mississippi Cooperative Extension Service
Website: www.nncc.org/choose.quality.care/selfcare.html

TERMINAL ILLNESS SUPPORT, GRIEF, AND BEREAVEMENT

Association for Death Education and Counseling
342 North Main Street
West Hartford, CT 06117-2507
Phone: 860-586-7503
Fax: 860-586-7550
Website: www.adec.org

The Center for Attitudinal Healing
33 Buchanan Drive
Sausalito, CA 94965
Phone: 415-331-6161
Fax: 415-331-4545
Website: www.healingcenter.org

Children's Hospice International
901 North Pitt Street, Suite 230
Alexandria, VA 22314
Phone: 703-684-0330; 800-242-4453 (toll-free)
Fax: 703-684-0226
Website: www.chionline.org

Compassionate Friends
P.O. Box 3696
Oak Brook, IL 60522-3696
Phone: 630-990-0010
Fax: 630-990-0246
Website: www.compassionatefriends.org

Dougy Center for Grieving Children and Families
P.O. Box 86852
3909 SE 52nd Avenue
Portland, OR 97286
Phone: 503-775-5683
Fax: 503-777-3097
Website: www.dougy.org

Hospicelink
Hospice Education Institute
190 Westbrook Road
Essex, CT 06426-1510
Phone: 860-767-1620; 800-331-1620 (toll-free)
Fax: 860-767-2746
Website: www.hospiceworld.org

Make-A-Wish Foundation of America
3550 North Central Avenue, Suite 300
Phoenix, AZ 85012
Phone: 602-279-9474; 800-722-WISH (toll-free)
Fax: 602-279-0855
Website: www.wish.org

Ronald McDonald House Charities
1 Kroc Drive
Oak Brook, IL 60523
Phone: 630-623-7048
Website: www.rmhc.com

Starlight Foundation
International Headquarters
5900 Wilshire Boulevard, Suite 2530
Los Angeles, CA 90036
Phone: 323-634-0080; 800-274-STAR (toll-free)
Fax: 323-634-0090
Website: www.starlight.org

The Warm Place
1510 Cooper Street
Fort Worth, TX 76104
Phone: 817-870-2272
Website: www.thewarmplace.org

Periodicals and Online Services

Bereavement: A Magazine of Hope and Healing
Bereavement Publishing, Inc.
5125 North Union Boulevard, Suite 4
Colorado Springs, CO 80918
Phone: 719-266-0006; 888-60-4HOPE (toll-free)
Website: www.bereavementmag.com

Fernside Online
Fernside: A Center for Grieving Children
2303 Indian Mound Avenue
Cincinnati, OH 45212
Phone: 513-841-1012
Fax: 513-841-1546
Website: www.fernside.org

The Forum Newsletter
Association for Death Education and Counseling
342 North Main Street
West Hartford, CT 06117-2507
Phone: 860-586-7503
Fax: 860-586-7550
Website: www.adec.org

Professional Journals

Death Studies
Robert A. Neimeyer, Editor-in-Chief
Taylor & Francis Books
325 Chestnut Street, Suite 800
Philadelphia, PA 19106
Phone: 800-354-1420 (toll-free)
Fax: 215-625-8914
Website: www.taylorandfrancis.com

INDEX

Page numbers followed by f indicate figures; t, tables; b, boxes.